Diffuse Lung Disease

Robert P. Baughman
Roland M. du Bois
Editors

Diffuse Lung Disease

A Practical Approach

Second Edition

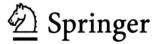

Editors
Robert P. Baughman, MD
Department of Internal Medicine
University of Cincinnati
College of Medicine
Cincinnati, OH, USA
bob.baughman@uc.edu

Roland M. du Bois, MD
Emeritus Professor of
Respiratory Medicine
Imperial College
London, UK
ron@du-bois.co.uk

ISBN 978-1-4419-9770-8   e-ISBN 978-1-4419-9771-5
DOI 10.1007/978-1-4419-9771-5
Springer New York Dordrecht Heidelberg London

Library of Congress Control Number: 2011939745

Printed on acid-free paper

Springer is part of Springer Science+Business Media (www.springer.com)

Preface

Introduction

Interstitial lung diseases, taken together, comprise a significant component of any respiratory medicine clinician's practice. This has been a rapidly changing field, with the emergence of new diagnostic techniques and therapies. In 2004, we edited the first edition of "Diffuse Lung Disease: a practical approach." In this second edition, we are not only updating what was presented in the first edition, but also providing information about many exciting new advances that have been made in many of this complex group of diseases over the last 7 years. The overall goal of this book remains the same – to provide the reader with clear and specific recommendations regarding the management of all forms of interstitial lung disease. These recommendations are provided by a group of physicians who are all experts in the areas on which they are contributing.

The book is divided into two major sections. The first section deals with general aspects of diagnosis and management of interstitial lung disease, including: the clinician's approach to patient evaluation (Myers and Raghu); the radiologist's approach to thoracic imaging with a major focus on the role of the high-resolution CT scan (Lynch); the added value of bronchoalveolar lavage (Drent and Linssen); a review of the histopathology of the various interstitial lung diseases (Colby and Leslie); a detailed review of the physiological changes produced by the various interstitial lung diseases including guidelines on what to monitor over time (Wells, Ward, and Cramer); the approach to classification and evaluation assimilating all aspects of clinical, radiographic and histopathologic information into a multidisciplinary process (Collard and King); a summary of the various treatments used for interstitial lung diseases, including suggested dosage, monitoring, and toxicity (Baughman, Costabel, and Lower); and the impact of pulmonary hypertension on interstitial lung diseases (Shlobin and Nathan).

The second section of the book deals with specific interstitial lung diseases: sarcoidosis, including extrapulmonary disease (Culver and Judson); the diagnosis, management, and outcome of idiopathic pulmonary fibrosis in which disease the most major advances have occurred over the last decade (Lynch and Belperio); the complexities of the diagnosis and management of nonspecific interstitial pneumonia including the similarities with but the quite different outcome from idiopathic pulmonary fibrosis (Flaherty and Martinez);

emerging understanding of collagen vascular-associated interstitial lung diseases, including the "grey" areas of subclinical disease (Fischer and du Bois); hypersensitivity pneumonitis (Selman, Mejia, Ortega, and Navarro); the impact of cigarette smoke on, and its interrelationship with interstitial lung disease (Solomon and Brown); the childhood interstitial lung diseases, in many of which the specific gene abnormality has been identified about which guidance is given regarding how and when further evaluation, including genetic testing, is appropriate (Young); an approach to the diagnosis and management of several of the rarer causes of interstitial lung disease including pulmonary alveolar proteinosis and lymphangioleiomyomatosis (Huie, Olson, Schwarz, and Frankel) an overview of occupational, environmental, and pharmaceutical causes of interstitial lung diseases (Pirozynski and Borg); the various forms of bronchiolitis, some of which are coexistent with interstitial lung disease (Cottin and Cordier); and the pulmonary vasculitides, focusing on the anti-neutrophil cytoplasmic antibody (ANCA)-associated conditions (Specks and Keogh).

All contributors were asked to provide clinician-focused practical guidance and all have keep to this goal admirably. As editors, we wish to thank them all for their hard work in the production of this practical guide to the management of interstitial lung disease. We also wish to thank Connie Walsh of Springer Science and Business Media for her help and patience in preparing this edition. Without her continuing and always friendly persistence, this volume would never have been completed!

Cincinnati, OH   Robert P. Baughman
London, UK   Roland M. du Bois

Contents

Contributors

Robert P. Baughman, MD
Department of Internal Medicine, University of Cincinnati
College of Medicine, Cincinnati, OH, USA

John A. Belperio, MD
Division of Pulmonary and Critical Care Medicine, David Geffen School
of Medicine at UCLA, Los Angeles, CA, USA

Roland M. du Bois, MA, MD, FRCP
National Heart & Lung Institute, Imperial College, London, UK

John Joseph Borg, PhD
Post-Licensing Directorate, Medicines Authority, Rue D'Argens Gzira
GZR 1368 MALTA

Kevin K. Brown, MD
Department of Medicine, National Jewish Health, University of Colorado,
Denver, CO, USA

Thomas V. Colby, MD
Mayo Clinic Scottsdale, Scottsdale, AZ, USA

Harold R. Collard, MD
Department of Medicine, University of California San Francisco,
San Francisco, CA, USA

Jean-François Cordier, MD
Department of Respiratory Medicine, Claude Bernard University,
Reference Center for Rare Pulmonary Diseases, Lyon, France

Department of Respiratory Medicine, Louis Pradel University Hospital,
Lyon, France

Ulrich Costabel, MD
Department of Pneumology/Allergy, Ruhrlandklinik, University Hospital,
Essen, Germany

Vincent Cottin, MD, PhD
Reference Center for Rare Pulmonary Diseases, Department of Respiratory
Medicine, Claude Bernard Lyon I University, Lyon, France

Department of Respiratory Medicine, Louis Pradel University Hospital,
Lyon, France

Derek Cramer
Lung Function Department, Royal Brompton Hospital, London, UK

Daniel A. Culver, DO
Respiratory Institute, Cleveland Clinic, Cleveland, OH, USA

Marjolein Drent, MD, PhD
Respiratory Medicine, ild care consultancy, Maastricht University Medical
Centre (MUMC+), Maastricht, The Netherlands

Aryeh Fischer, MD
Department of Medicine, National Jewish Health, Denver, CO, USA

Kevin R. Flaherty, MD, MS
Pulmonary/Critical Care Medicine, University of Michigan, Ann Arbor,
MI, USA

Stephen K. Frankel, MD
Health Sciences Center, Division of Pulmonary Sciences and Critical
Care Medicine, University of Colorado at Denver, Aurora, CO, USA

Tristan J. Huie, MD
Department of Medicine, National Jewish Health, Denver, CO, USA

Marc A. Judson, MD
Division of Pulmonary and Critical Care, Department of Medicine,
Medical University of South Carolina, Charleston, SC, USA

Karina A. Keogh, MB, BCh
Division of Pulmonary and Critical Care Medicine, Mayo Clinic,
Rochester, MN, USA

Talmadge E. King Jr., MD
Department of Medicine, University of California San Francisco,
San Francisco, CA, USA

Kevin O. Leslie, MD
Department of Pathology, Division of Anatomic Pathology,
Mayo Clinic College of Medicine, MN, USA

Laboratory Medicine and Pathology, Mayo Clinic Arizona,
Scottsdale, AZ, USA

Catharina F.M. Linssen, MD, PhD
Department of Medical Microbiology, Maastricht University
Medical Centre (MUMC+), Maastricht, The Netherlands

Elyse E. Lower, MD
Barnett Cancer Center, University of Cincinnati, Cincinnati, OH, USA

David A. Lynch, MD
Department of Radiology, National Jewish Health, Denver, CO, USA

Joseph P. Lynch III, MD
Division of Pulmonary and Critical Care Medicine, David Geffen School
of Medicine at UCLA, Los Angeles, CA, USA

Fernando J. Martinez, MD, MS
Pulmonary/Critical Care Medicine, University of Michigan, Ann Arbor,
MI, USA

Mayra Mejía, MD
Instituto Nacional de Enfermedades Respiratorias "Ismael Cosio Villegas",
Mexico D.F., Mexico

Keith C. Meyer, MD, MS
Department of Medicine, Section of Allergy,
Pulmonary and Critical Care Medicine, University of Wisconsin
School of Medicine and Public Health, Madison, WI, USA

Steven D. Nathan, MD, FCCP
Advanced Lung Disease and Transplant Program, Inova Fairfax Hospital,
Falls Church, VA, USA

Carmen Navarro, MD
Instituto Nacional de Enfermedades Respiratorias "Ismael Cosio Villegas",
Mexico D.F., Mexico

Amy L. Olson, MD, MSPH
Department of Medicine, National Jewish Health, Denver, CO, USA

Héctor Ortega, MD
Medicine Development Center, Glaxosmithkline, Research Triangle Park,
NC, USA

Michal Pirozynski, MD, PhD
Department of Anesthesiology and Critical Care Medicine CMKP,
Warszawa, Poland

Ganesh Raghu, MD, FCCP, FACP
Department of Medicine & Lab Medicine (Adjunct),
Division of Pulmonary & Critical Care Medicine, Interstitial Lung
Disease, Sarcoid and Pulmonary Fibrosis Program, Lung Transplant
Program, University of Washington, Seattle, WA, USA

Marvin I. Schwarz, MD
Division of Pulmonary Sciences and Critical Care Medicine,
University of Colorado at Denver, Aurora, CO, USA

Moisés Selman, MD
Instituto Nacional de Enfermedades Respiratorias "Ismael Cosio Villegas",
Mexico D.F., Mexico

Oksana A. Shlobin, MD, FCCP
Advanced Lung Disease and Transplant Program, Inova Fairfax Hospital,
Falls Church, VA, USA

Joshua J. Solomon, MD
Department of Medicine, National Jewish Health, University of Colorado,
Denver, CO, USA

Ulrich Specks, MD
Division of Pulmonary and Critical Care Medicine, Mayo Clinic, Rochester,
MN, USA

Simon Ward, BSc
Lung Function Department, Royal Brompton Hospital, London, UK

Athol U. Wells, MD
Interstitial Lung Disease Unit, Royal Brompton Hospital, London, UK

Lisa R. Young, MD
Division of Allergy, Immunology, and Pulmonary Medicine,
Department of Pediatrics, Vanderbilt University School of Medicine,
Nashville, TN, USA

Division of Allergy, Pulmonary, and Critical Care Medicine,
Department of Medicine, Vanderbilt University School of Medicine,
Nashville, TN, USA

Section I

General Considerations

Patient Evaluation

Keith C. Meyer and Ganesh Raghu

Abstract

The clinical evaluation of a patient with suspected interstitial lung disease (ILD) plays a key role in successfully making a confident clinical diagnosis. A secure diagnosis may be made with minimal radiologic imaging in some instances, but clinicians often need to obtain high-resolution computed tomography of the thorax (HRCT), lung specimens obtained via bronchoscopy, and, if needed, surgical lung biopsy and other appropriate testing. A well-performed patient interview and physical examination can provide key information that can assist in making a confident diagnosis when combined with appropriate laboratory testing, imaging, and/or specimens from invasive procedures. This chapter will outline an approach to the clinical evaluation of patients who undergo evaluation for possible ILD.

Keywords

Interstitial lung disease • Idiopathic interstitial pneumonia • Idiopathic pulmonary fibrosis • HRCT • Bronchoalveolar lavage • Lung biopsy

Introduction

The importance of the initial clinical evaluation of the patient with suspected interstitial lung disease (ILD) cannot be overemphasized. Elicitation of a thorough history provides key information that will help the clinician narrow the differential diagnoses as well as provide a sense of time of onset and tempo of disease progression. Additionally, the physical examination may detect both pulmonary and extrapulmonary findings that suggest or support specific diagnoses. When combined with key elements of subsequent evaluation that include measurements of lung function, appropriate blood tests, thoracic imaging, and invasive procedures (if required),

K.C. Meyer (✉)
Department of Medicine, Section of Allergy, Pulmonary and Critical Care Medicine, University of Wisconsin School of Medicine and Public Health, Madison, WI, USA
e-mail: kcm@medicine.wisc.edu

G. Raghu
Department of Medicine & Lab Medicine (Adjunct), Division of Pulmonary & Critical Care Medicine, Interstitial Lung Disease, Sarcoid and Pulmonary Fibrosis Program, Lung Transplant Program, University of Washington, Seattle, WA, USA

R.P. Baughman and R.M. du Bois (eds.), *Diffuse Lung Disease: A Practical Approach*,
DOI 10.1007/978-1-4419-9771-5_1, © Springer Science+Business Media, LLC 2012

a confident diagnosis of the specific form of ILD will be reached in most situations.

This chapter will review and examine salient aspects of the initial clinical evaluation and how findings in the history and physical examination can be used to narrow down the differential diagnosis or, on occasion, virtually make the diagnosis. All patients will require additional evaluation (if such has not been obtained prior to the initial visit) such as thoracic imaging and pulmonary function testing (PFT), but a thorough history combined with imaging studies may provide a confident diagnosis and obviate the need to proceed to invasive procedures such as bronchoscopy and/or surgical lung biopsy (SLB). Additionally, in the patient at high risk for complications with invasive studies or for those who do not wish to have such studies performed, aspects of the clinical presentation plus noninvasive studies (thoracic imaging, PFT) can provide a reasonably confident diagnosis or at least substantially reduce the number of possibilities.

Key Elements of the Clinical History

Respiratory Symptoms

The interval from the onset of symptoms can vary from weeks to years, and the rate of progression can vary considerably from patient to patient even with the same disease. Dyspnea is the most common symptom of ILD, and cough is a common complaint. Chest pain and wheezing are uncommon but may be present. Pleuritic chest pain may reflect pleuritis or spontaneous pneumothorax, and wheezing may be caused by bronchiolitis, hypersensitivity pneumonitis (HP), or eosinophilic pneumonia (EP) (Table 1.1). Sarcoidosis is occasionally associated with substernal or pleuritic chest pain, and collagen-vascular diseases (CVDs) can involve the pleura and cause pleurisy and/or pleural effusions. Spontaneous pneumothorax can occur with lymphangioleiomyomatosis (LAM), pulmonary Langerhans cell histiocytosis (LCH), or neurofibromatosis/tuberous sclerosis.

Hemoptysis is uncommon but would suggest the presence of an alveolar hemorrhage syndrome, vasculitis, and/or superimposed complications such as pulmonary embolism or lung neoplasm.

Acute vs. Chronic Onset

Most forms of ILD have a subacute or chronic course and presentation. However, some may develop quite rapidly over the course of a few days to weeks. These include acute interstitial pneumonia, acute EP, acute HP, drug reactions, and organizing pneumonia. Additionally, acute exacerbations of idiopathic pulmonary fibrosis (IPF) can occur in patients with early, previously unrecognized disease. Various infections, such as endemic fungal infections, community-acquired viral infection, or bacterial infections, can develop and progress over a few days and masquerade as noninfectious ILD.

The Occupational and Environmental Exposure History

Exposures in the workplace and in other settings may be the cause of ILD, and a careful and comprehensive exposure history must always be obtained including remote and sometimes transient exposures. Questionnaires provided to the patient in conjunction with a clinic visit can prove particularly helpful, and a comprehensive questionnaire is available via the American College of Chest Physicians website (www.chestnet.org) under the Interstitial and Diffuse Lung Disease NetWork webpage. Exposure to dusts, gases, and fumes can cause lung injury and lead to acute and subacute pneumonitis and pulmonary fibrosis. Exposures to potential fibrogenic factors in the domestic environment must be included in the elicitation of a thorough and detailed history (e.g., exposures to birds, poultry, hot tubs, visible molds, water leaks/damp conditions, etc.). Identification of an antigen exposure can be particularly helpful in diagnosing HP.

Table 1.1 Clues from the initial evaluation that suggest specific types of ILD

History elicited	Frequently associated ILD or its complications
Rapid onset and worsening	AIP
	Infection
	Acute HP, acute EP
	Drug reaction
	COP
	CVD (e.g., acute lupus pneumonitis)
	DAH (e.g., GPS)
Smoking	RB-ILD, DIP
	PLCH
Occupation: Pipefitter, foundry worker, coal miner	Pneumoconiosis
Pneumotoxic drug exposure	Drug-induced ILD
Hemoptysis	DAH, pulmonary capillaritis, pulmonary veno-occlusive disease, LAM
	Superimposed complications (e.g., pulmonary emboli, lung neoplasm)
Pleurisy	CVD (SLE, RA)
Wheezing	HP, EP
Eye symptoms	CVD, sarcoidosis, WG
Impaired vision combined with albinism and Puerto Rican heritage	HPS
Rash	Sarcoidosis, CVD
Exposure to organic antigens at home or at work (e.g., birds, grain dust, humidifiers, visible molds, hot tubs, etc.)	HP
	Occupational ILD
Abnormal GER/D, dysphagia	CVD (especially scleroderma)
	IPF
Sicca symptoms	Sjögren's disease
Raynaud's phenomenon	CVD
Arthralgias, arthritis	CVD, sarcoidosis
Myalgias, muscle weakness	DM-PM
Morning stiffness	RA, CVD
Age >70 years	IPF > other ILD if HRCT suspicious for IIP

AIP acute interstitial pneumonia, *COP* cryptogenic organizing pneumonia, *CVD* collagen-vascular disease, *DAH* diffuse alveolar hemorrhage, *DM-PM* dermatopolymyositis, *EP* eosinophilic pneumonia, *GER/D* gastroesophageal reflux disease, *GPS* Goodpasture's syndrome, *HP* hypersensitivity pneumonitis, *HPS* Hermansky–Pudlak syndrome, *IIP* idiopathic interstitial pneumonia, *IPF* idiopathic pulmonary fibrosis, *LAM* lymphangioleiomyomatosis, *PLCH* pulmonary Langerhans cell histiocytosis, *SLE* systemic lupus erythematosus, *RA* rheumatoid arthritis, *WG* Wegener granulomatosis

Smoking

The development of ILD in the setting of tobacco smoking suggests a number of specific entities that consist of respiratory bronchiolitis with interstitial lung disease (RB-ILD), desquamative interstitial pneumonia (DIP), and PLCH. Additionally, tobacco smoking is a risk factor for the development of IPF as well as rheumatoid arthritis (RA) and RA-associated ILD. Smoking crack cocaine can also lead to acute and subacute diffuse lung infiltrates.

Smokers who have emphysema may go on to develop superimposed ILD (IPF, Langerhans cell histiocytosis (LCH)). These individuals may have preserved lung volumes, although diffusing capacity for carbon monoxide, corrected for peripheral blood hemoglobin concentration

(DLCOc) can be very depressed. Patients with combined emphysema and IPF can have severely impaired lung function that progresses rapidly.

Demographic, Family, and Racial Factors

Epidemiologic studies have indicated that the incidence and prevalence of specific forms of ILD display some significant biases. Advanced age is associated with a much higher incidence and prevalence of IPF and it is unusual for idiopathic UIP/IPF to occur in individuals less than 50 years of age. One recent study has demonstrated that for individuals greater than 70 years of age with a high-resolution computed tomography (HRCT) that is consistent with idiopathic interstitial pneumonia (IIP), the diagnosis is almost exclusively IPF at SLB. A potential explanation for the greatly increased incidence and prevalence of IPF in the elderly is the finding that aging and pulmonary fibrosis are associated with telomere shortening due to hTERT gene dysfunction, and hTERT mutations have been identified in families with familial pulmonary fibrosis (FPF). Sarcoidosis tends to occur in young to middle age adults but occurs rarely in children and less often in the elderly. Additionally, sarcoidosis incidence and prevalence is significantly higher in individuals of northern European heritage (e.g., Scandinavian, German, Irish) and individuals of African descent who reside in the USA or United Kingdom. Hermansky–Pudlak syndrome (HPS), which is highly associated with pulmonary fibrosis in affected individuals, occurs virtually exclusively in individuals of Puerto Rican heritage.

Some forms of ILD can display an increased incidence in families and are undoubtedly due to inherited genetic factors that can sometimes be identified. These include FPF, familial sarcoidosis, and HPS. Some specific genes have been found in families with FPF (surfactant protein C, surfactant protein A-2, telomerase, and ELMOD-2), but the influence of other genes and environmental factors undoubtedly account for variable penetrance and development of disease. Individuals with multiple family members with pulmonary fibrosis should be encouraged to contact a center that is performing

research on genetic determinants that are linked to FPF to facilitate the identification of genetic abnormalities that can cause IPF.

Extrapulmonary Symptoms

The interview should seek to elicit extrapulmonary symptoms (see Table 1.1) that, if present, may provide clues to the diagnosis. Skin lesions, photosensitivity, and rash (with or without joint symptoms) should raise suspicion of CVD or sarcoidosis. Vision problems may be a consequence of eye involvement in sarcoidosis, Wegener's granulomatosis, (WG) Sjögren's syndrome (SS), or HPS, and the presenting symptom of dry eyes and mouth suggests the presence of SS. Arthralgias and/or myalgias may reflect the presence of a form of CVD. Severe gastroesophageal reflux (GER) is often present in patients with scleroderma, and abnormal GER is highly prevalent in IPF and in CVD. Symptoms consistent with Raynaud's phenomenon suggest the presence of CVD, and muscle aches and proximal muscle weakness suggest the presence of polymyositis. General constitutional symptoms such as night sweats and weight loss raise the possibility of systemic sarcoidosis (especially if generalized lymphadenopathy is present) and of chronic EP in women.

Drug and Radiation Exposures

A large number of prescribed drugs can cause pneumonitis that can progress to pulmonary fibrosis and, in some cases, progressive loss of lung function and death. Radiotherapy, typically performed for treatment of malignancy but also given for treatment of lymphoma or as conditioning for bone marrow or stem cell transplants, can also cause pneumonitis and pulmonary fibrosis. Some commonly used medications that are particularly notorious for causing pulmonary toxicity include bleomycin, methotrexate, amiodarone, and nitrofurantoin. The list of drugs associated with acute and chronic lung inflammation that can progress to irreversible fibrosis is increasing. The website www.pneumotox.com is an invaluable source that can provide key information concerning specific drugs and their potential to cause adverse pulmonary reactions as well as the specific type of reaction that they may cause.

The Physical Examination

Pulmonary Findings

The auscultatable sound that is most widely associated with ILD is that of crackles (also known as rales) that are best heard at the lung bases (Table 1.2). However, although crackles tend to be heard with certain forms of ILD that are characterized by extensive fibrosis, the physical examination of the chest can be entirely normal in several forms of ILD, such as sarcoidosis with parenchymal involvement or silicosis. Velcro crackles, which sound like strips of Velcro being pulled apart, are characteristically present when auscultating the lungs of patients with IPF,

Table 1.2 Clues from the physical examination and their disease associations

Organ system	Finding	Associated ILD or its complications
Lung	Velcro crackles	IPF, asbestosis >> other
	Squeaks	HP, bronchiolitis
	Pleural rub	RA, SLE
Skin	Erythema nodosum	Sarcoidosis, CVD, Behçet's disease
	Maculopapular rash	CVD, drugs, sarcoidosis, amyloid
	Heliotrope rash	DM-PM
	Gottron's papules	DM-PM
	Café-au-lait spots	Neurofibromatosis
	Albinism	HPS
	Telangiectasia	Scleroderma
	Calcinosis	Scleroderma, DM-PM
	Subcutaneous nodules	RA, neurofibromatosis, vasculitis
	Cutaneous vasculitis	WG, RA, MPA, SLE, drug reaction
	Mechanic's hands	DM-PM
	Tight skin/ulcerations over digits	Scleroderma
Eyes	Uveitis	Sarcoidosis, Behçet's disease, AS
	Scleritis	SLE, scleroderma, sarcoidosis, WG
	Keratoconjunctivitis sicca	Sjögren's disease, CVD
	Lacrimal gland enlargement	Sarcoidosis
	Horizontal nystagmus	HPS
Salivary glands	Enlarged	Sjögren's disease, sarcoidosis
Lymphatic	Lymphadenopathy	Sarcoidosis, lymphangitic CA, lymphoma
Reticuloendothelial	Hepatosplenomegaly	Sarcoidosis, LIP, CVD, LCH, amyloid, lymphoma
Musculoskeletal	Muscle weakness, myositis	CVD (especially DM-PM), sarcoidosis
	Synovitis, arthritis	CVD, sarcoidosis
Nervous system	Neurologic dysfunction	Sarcoidosis, lymphangitic CA, NF, TS, CVD, WG, MPA
Cardiovascular	Systemic hypertension	CVD, GPS, WG, MPA, NF
	Prominent P2	Suggests secondary PH (IPF, CVD, end-stage sarcoidosis)
	Pericardial rub	Sarcoidosis, SLE
Extremities	Digital clubbing	IPF, asbestosis > chronic HP, DIP > other fibrotic ILD
	Raynaud's phenomenon	CVD

AS ankylosing spondylitis, *CA* cancer, *CVD* collagen-vascular disease, *DAH* diffuse alveolar hemorrhage, *DIP* desquamative interstitial pneumonia, *DM-PM* dermatopolymyositis, *GPS* Goodpasture's syndrome, *HP* hypersensitivity pneumonitis, *HPS* Hermansky–Pudlak syndrome, *IPF* idiopathic pulmonary fibrosis, *LAM* lymphangioleiomyomatosis, *LCH* Langerhans cell histiocytosis, *LIP* lymphoid interstitial pneumonia, *MPA* microscopic polyangiitis, *NF* neurofibromatosis, *P2* auscultated pulmonic valve closure sound, *PH* pulmonary hypertension, *RA* rheumatoid arthritis, *SLE* systemic lupus erythematosus, *TS* tuberous sclerosis, *WG* Wegener granulomatosis particularly when more advanced disease that shows honeycomb change on HRCT is present. Velcro crackles at the lung bases are also characteristically present in asbestosis. Other forms of ILD, such as nonspecific interstitial pneumonia (NSIP) or CVD-associated ILD tend to be characterized by less prominent and finer crackles or may not display any crackles at all. Idiopathic bronchiectasis is often most prominent at the lung bases and characterized by crackles with deep inspiration–expiration, but these crackles are typically coarse and not Velcro like in nature.

Other sounds that may be heard on chest auscultation are wheezes or squeaks. These sounds are relatively uncommon, but may be heard with bronchiolitis, acute EP, or HP. Squeaks are often heard with fibrotic HP. Wheezing may also be present with bulky parenchymal sarcoidosis that impinges upon and constricts airways. If a rub is heard or if dullness to percussion is noted at the lung base, these findings may denote pleural involvement often associated with CVD.

Extrapulmonary Signs

The physical examination provides an opportunity to detect a variety of abnormalities that can provide extremely useful clues to the diagnosis (see Table 1.2). Saddle nose deformity, when present, raises the possibility of Wegener's granulomatosis. The presence of certain skin lesions can strongly support specific diagnoses. Erythema nodosum can be seen with sarcoidosis, and the finding of mechanic's hands (dry, cracking skin on the palmar surface of the digits) strongly supports a diagnosis of dermatopolymyositis (DM-PM). Some degree of finger swelling due to edema may herald the onset of systemic sclerosis (SSc) and be followed later by skin thickening and sclerodactyly. Other clues to the diagnosis of SSc or the CREST (calcinosis, Raynaud's phenomenon, esophageal dysmotility, sclerodactyly, and telangiectasias) syndrome include subcutaneous calcinosis (usually seen over the palmer aspects of the fingertips and over bony prominences), or telangiectasiae that usually occur on the palms, face,

lips, and mucus membranes. A violaceous rash over sun-exposed areas and bony prominences or the eyelids (heliotrope) strongly suggest DM-PM, as do Gottron's papules on the hands, which are erythematous, scaly eruptions that tend to appear over the metacarpal–phalangeal and interphalangeal joints. A malar or discoid rash, photosensitivity, mucosal ulcerations, and/or alopecia strongly point to a diagnosis of systemic lupus erythematosus (SLE). A thorough exam can also detect synovitis, nodules, tendon friction rubs, and/or muscle weakness, and the detection of dilated, tortuous capillary loops on nailfold capillary microscopy suggests the presence of SSc, PM-DM, or mixed connective tissue disease (MCTD). The presence of joint deformities of RA raises the probability of the ILD being secondary to RA, and the presence of a pericardial rub suggests the presence of pericarditis, which can be a manifestation of sarcoidosis or SLE. The presence of a loud P2 indicates the presence of pulmonary hypertension, which is often a manifestation of several ILD. Secondary pulmonary hypertension can occur at the onset or during the course of the ILD, although it is more likely to be present in advanced stages of the disease.

Thoracic Imaging

Most patients will already have had routine chest radiographs (CXRs) performed at the time of referral, and patterns on the CXR can be suggestive of specific entities (Table 1.3). Previous thoracic imaging studies should be obtained if available and reviewed to determine if changes have been present previously, which would suggest that the disease is chronic. Other previously obtained studies may also provide limited views of portions of the lungs (e.g., spine films, abdominal films) and show pulmonary changes that were present at the time these studies were obtained (but not necessarily mentioned in the imaging interpretations). Although the CXR almost always shows interstitial changes when ILD is present, it may rarely appear normal when lung involvement is mild. This situation can be

Table 1.3 Thoracic imaging patterns

Imaging modality	Pattern	Consistent ILD diagnoses, mimics of ILD, and/or complications of ILD
Routine CXR	Hilar lymphadenopathy	Sarcoidosis, silicosis, CBD, infection, malignancy
	Septal thickening	CHF, malignancy, infection, PVOD
	Lower lung zone predominance	IPF, asbestosis, DIP, CVD, NSIP
	Mid/upper lung zone predominance	Sarcoidosis, silicosis, acute HP, LCH, CBD, AS, chronic EP
	Peripheral lung zone predominance	COP, chronic EP, IPF
	Honeycomb change	IPF, asbestosis, chronic HP, sarcoidosis, fibrotic NSIP, CVD
	Small nodules	Sarcoidosis, HP, infection
	Cavitating nodules	WG, mycobacterial infection, CA
	Migratory or fluctuating opacities	HP, COP, DIP
	Pneumothorax	LCH, LAM, neurofibromatosis, TS
	Pleural involvement	Asbestosis, CVD, acute HP, malignancy, sarcoidosis, radiation fibrosis
	Kerley B line prominence	Lymphangitic carcinomatosis, CHF
HRCT	Nodules	Sarcoidosis HP, CBD, pneumoconiosis, RA, malignancy
	Septal thickening	Edema, malignancy, infection, drug toxicity, PVOD
	Cyst formation	LAM, LCH, LIP, DIP, SS
	Reticular lines	IPF, asbestosis, chronic EP, chronic HP, CVD, NSIP
	Traction bronchiectasis	IPF, other end-stage fibrosis
	Honeycomb change	IPF, chronic EP and HP, asbestosis, sarcoidosis
	Ground-glass opacity	AIP, acute EP, PAP, chronic EP, COP, lymphoma, sarcoidosis, NSIP, infection, hemorrhage

AIP acute interstitial pneumonia, *AS* ankylosing spondylitis, *CA* cancer, *CBD* chronic beryllium disease, *CHF* congestive heart failure, *CVD* collagen-vascular disease, *COP* cryptogenic organizing pneumonia, *DAH* diffuse alveolar hemorrhage, *DM-PM* dermatopolymyositis, *DIP* desquamative interstitial pneumonia, *EP* eosinophilic pneumonia, *HP* hypersensitivity pneumonitis, *HPS* Hermansky–Pudlak syndrome, *IPF* idiopathic pulmonary fibrosis, *LAM* lymphangioleiomyomatosis, *LCH* Langerhans cell histiocytosis, *LIP* lymphoid interstitial pneumonia, *NF* neurofibromatosis, *NSIP* nonspecific interstitial pneumonia, *PAP* pulmonary alveolar proteinosis, *P2* auscultated pulmonic valve closure sound, *PH* pulmonary hypertension, *PVOD* pulmonary veno-occlusive disease, *RA* rheumatoid arthritis, *SLE* systemic lupus erythematosus, *SS* Sjögren's syndrome, *TS* tuberous sclerosis, *WG* Wegener granulomatosis

encountered with HP, sarcoidosis, cellular NSIP, bronchiolitis, RB-ILD, or CVD.

The HRCT images, discussed in depth in Chap. 2, represent a key diagnostic tool, and the HRCT should be a standard test for evaluating a patient with possible ILD. Specific HRCT patterns in the appropriate clinical setting can be virtually diagnostic of specific ILD diagnoses or at least narrow the differential diagnosis considerably (see Table 1.3). A complete lack of pulmonary parenchymal changes in the HRCT images excludes IPF and the pattern compatible with usual interstitial pneumonia (UIP) due to other causes but does not exclude microscopic involvement of the lung parenchyma with mild changes of certain forms of ILD, such as granulomatous disease.

Laboratory Testing

Peripheral Blood and Urine

Basic blood and urine testing should be performed on all patients, and specific abnormalities may provide clues or strongly support specific diagnoses. Leukocytosis, cytopenia, or eosinophilia, and a very high erythrocyte sedimentation rate (ESR) or C-reactive protein (CRP) are suggestive of intense inflammation that can be seen in CVD or vasculitis. Blood chemistries should include electrolytes, calcium, and measures of liver and renal function. Antinuclear antibody (ANA), anticitrullinated peptide antibodies (anti-CCP, specific for RA) and rheumatoid factor (RF) titers should also be obtained. A urinalysis may detect evidence of renal inflammation and suggest the presence of CVD or a pulmonary-renal syndrome.

Additional Tests

Additional testing may provide key diagnostic information. A positive antineutrophil cytoplasmic antibody (C-ANCA; antiproteinase-3) is strongly suggestive of WG, and a positive perinuclear ANCA (P-ANCA; antimyeloperoxidase) is supportive

of vasculitis, pulmonary capillaritis such as microscopic polyangiitis (MPA) or Wegener's granulomatosis (WG). Various other antibodies (Table 1.4) may provide important diagnostic information, such as antiglomerular basement membrane (Goodpasture's syndrome (GPS)) and a beryllium lymphocyte proliferation test is specific for detecting beryllium sensitization that is required to diagnose chronic beryllium disease, but such testing should only be obtained when aspects of the history, exam, laboratory, and imaging studies suggest the possibility of these or other uncommon disorders as a diagnosis. Random panels for hypersensitivity are generally not helpful, although responses to specific antigens that correlate with a specific exposure can support a diagnosis of HP. However, a positive response only indicates sensitization following exposure, and a negative result does not rule out a diagnosis of HP. Angiotensin converting enzyme (ACE)

Table 1.4 Clues for specific diagnoses from blood and urine testing

Laboratory test	Abnormal result	Suggested disorder
CBC	Microcytic anemia	Occult pulmonary hemorrhage
	Normocytic anemia	CVD, chronic disease
	Leukocytosis	Infection, hematologic malignancy
	Eosinophilia	Eosinophilic pneumonia, drug toxicity
	Thrombocytopenia	CVD, sarcoidosis
Calcium	Hypercalcemia	Sarcoidosis
Creatinine	↑	CVD, pulmonary-renal syndrome, sarcoidosis; amyloidosis
Liver function	↑ GGT, ALT, AST	Sarcoidosis, amyloidosis, CVD (polymyositis)
Urine	Abnormal sediment with RBC casts and/or dysmorphic RBCs	Vasculitis (CVD, WG, GPS, MPA)
Muscle enzymes	↑ Increased CK, aldolase	PM, DM-PM
Angiotensin Converting Enzyme (ACE)	↑	Sarcoidosis (nonspecific; can be increased in other ILD)
Lymphocyte proliferation	Stimulated by beryllium	CBD
Serum antibodies	↓ Quantitative immunoglobulins	Immunodeficiency (CVID)
	↑ ANA, RF, anti-CCP	CVD, RA
	↑ C-ANCA	WG
	↑ P-ANCA	CVD, vasculitis
	↑ anti-GBM	GPS
	Positive specific precipitin	Supportive of HP
	↑ anti-Jo-1 or other antisynthetase autoantibodies	PM, DM-PM
	↑ SS-A, SS-B	Sjögren's syndrome

CBD chronic beryllium disease, *CVD* collagen-vascular disease, *COP* cryptogenic organizing pneumonia, *CVID* common variable immunodeficiency, *DAH* diffuse alveolar hemorrhage, *DM-PM* dermatopolymyositis, *DIP* desquamative interstitial pneumonia, *GPS* Goodpasture's syndrome, *HP* hypersensitivity pneumonitis, *MPA* microscopic polyangiitis, *PM* polymyositis, *RA* rheumatoid arthritis, *WG* Wegener granulomatosis levels are frequently elevated in sarcoidosis and have been used as a biomarker of sarcoidosis in the past. However, more recent analyses show that the use of the ACE level as a biomarker of the presence and activity of sarcoidosis has serious limitations. ACE levels can be elevated in a number of other pulmonary disorders, and ACE levels are frequently normal when sarcoidosis is present. Because of the nonspecificity and lack of sensitivity of serum ACE, there is no role for obtaining ACE as a routine lab test to evaluate ILD.

Pulmonary Function

Pulmonary function tests (PFTs), which are discussed extensively in Chap. 5, can provide useful information but are not diagnostic in and of themselves. Patients should receive basic testing with spirometry, determination of lung volumes, and measurement of DLCOc. However, PFTs provide a means of quantitatively assessing respiratory symptoms and are useful to monitor patients for disease progression and responses to therapeutic interventions. PFT can be within the normal range with early or mild disease. With more advanced disease, particularly when irreversible fibrosis is present, a restrictive ventilatory impairment pattern is present. Some disorders may display coexistent obstruction, as can be seen with certain disorders such as RB-ILD, sarcoidosis, LAM, HP, or PLCH. Alternatively, ILD associated with asthma (chronic EP, Churg–Strauss syndrome) may also display a mixed obstructive–restrictive pattern. Respiratory muscle weakness may also display a restrictive pattern, and measurement of maximal pressures and maximal voluntary (minute) ventilation (MVV) can be useful to detect significant respiratory muscle weakness. DLCOc typically declines in concert with other measures of lung function (forced vital capacity, total lung capacity), and the DLCO value typically increases considerably when adjusted for alveolar volume (DL/VA). Disproportionately low DLCOc may indicate the presence of significant pulmonary vascular disease (secondary pulmonary hypertension, pulmonary veno-occlusive disease, vasculitis, thromboembolic disease) but may occur with pulmonary alveolar proteinosis (PAP), LAM, or PLCH.

Oxyhemoglobin saturation can be readily measured via pulse oximetry (SpO2) at rest and during ambulation (6-min walk test, shuttle test) to detect exertional oxyhemoglobin desaturation when SpO2 is normal at rest. Both the severity of the decline in SpO2 and total walk distance on a standardized 6-min walk test (6-MWT) may be useful to monitor and assess the need for supplemental oxygen. Because of technical factors in measuring the pulse signals that determine SpO2 levels in patients with heavy and current cigarette smoking, the presence of carboxyhemoglobin (which cannot be differentiated from oxyhemoglobin via pulse oximetry) may yield falsely high values for SpO2. Additionally, patients with Raynaud's phenomenon or poor peripheral circulation may have unreliable values for SpO2 with exertion. An arterial blood gas (ABG) analysis will allow accurate measurement of SpO2 via direct measurement and provide a measure of partial pressures of O_2 and CO_2 as well as indicating acid–base status. Patients with mild disease may have a normal 6-MWT and resting ABG, and the only manifestation of their disease may be a widening of the A-a gradient during formal cardiopulmonary exercise testing. Lastly, some patients can have normal resting SpO2 in the wakeful state but may have significant nocturnal desaturation, which can be due to the presence of obstructive sleep apnea or altered gas exchange during sleep without the presence of sleep apnea. An overnight desaturation study with continuous pulse oximetry can be performed in the outpatient setting to detect nocturnal desaturation, and the presence of significant nocturnal desaturation may explain, in part, the presence of fatigue in the wakeful state that can be present in some patients with ILD.

Invasive Procedures

If the initial evaluation with the elicitation of a detailed and thorough medical and family history, a careful and thorough physical examination, laboratory testing, and thoracic imaging do not yield a confident diagnosis, invasive testing will be required to secure an accurate and confident diagnosis. Bronchoscopy is quite safe (if a stringent and adequate safety protocol is in place) and provides the opportunity to perform bronchoalveolar lavage (BAL) and endoscopic lung biopsies (endobronchial and/or transbronchial) in inpatient or outpatient settings. Additionally, needle biopsies can be performed, with or without ultrasound guidance, to sample enlarged lymph nodes for the possible diagnosis of sarcoidosis, malignancy, or infection.

BAL, which is discussed in Chap. 3, can be easily and safely performed in the right middle lobe or lingula when diffuse disease is present (although other lung regions such as the basilar segment of the lower lobes can also be safely lavaged), and the cell differential count may provide key findings (e.g., prominent eosinophilia or lymphocytosis) that points to a considerably narrowed differential diagnosis as discussed in Chap. 3. Additionally, BAL fluid and sediment can be analyzed for infection (bacteria, mycobacteria, fungi, virus) or malignant cells, and the gross appearance and nature of the retrieved BAL fluid at the time of bronchoscopy may indicate specific diagnostic entities (e.g., diffuse alveolar hemorrhage (DAH), PAP).

Transbronchial biopsies should be performed in areas away from honeycomb change, ideally in areas of ground-glass opacification, and the HRCT can be used to guide the choice of biopsy sites. Multiple biopsies (e.g., 3–6) with an adequately sized forceps (e.g., 2-mm alligator forceps) can provide good tissue sampling, and endobronchial biopsies of abnormal areas (e.g., endobronchial nodules or ulcerated mucosa) may yield diagnostic tissue sampling.

SLB is more invasive and entails some risk of morbidity and mortality and is discussed in Chap. 4. However, SLB is relatively safe and may be required if clinical findings, thoracic imaging, laboratory testing, and bronchoscopy do not provide a confident diagnosis. Video-assisted thoracoscopic surgery (VATS) has become a preferred approach and is associated with less morbidity and mortality than open lung biopsy. The VATS procedure appears to be safer, but series with both approaches have been reported from different centers that, on average, have a 30-day mortality that is less than 5%. When SLB is performed, areas with honeycomb change (advanced fibrosis) should be avoided, and two or more geographically distinct sites (e.g., upper lobe and lower lobe) should be sampled due to heterogeneous lung involvement in IPF with NSIP and UIP often coexisting in different areas of the same lung.

Other Testing

Additional testing may also provide key information that leads to an accurate diagnosis. The finding of bone lesions via imaging studies suggests LCH, sarcoidosis, lymphangitic cancer, or lymphoid interstitial pneumonia (LIP) as potential diagnoses, and the detection of diabetes insipidus suggests LCH or sarcoidosis. If glomerulonephritis is diagnosed via kidney biopsy, WG, CVD, GPS, MPA, or sarcoidosis are potential causes. Additionally, amyloid, drug toxicity, SLE, or sarcoidosis can all cause nephritic syndrome. The detection of a renal mass raises the possibility of LAM or tuberous sclerosis (TS). Finally, pericarditis can be associated with CVD and sarcoidosis. When PH (discussed in Chap. 8), which can be the cause of unexplained or disproportionate lowering of DLCOc, is suspected as a manifestation of ILD, echocardiography and especially right heart catheterization are indicated to detect and quantify the severity of PH.

Putting It All Together

Key components of the sequential evaluation of patients with suspected ILD are given in Table 1.5. A comprehensive interview plus a thorough and thoughtful physical examination provide both inclusionary and exclusionary data that can be invaluable in providing a secure and accurate diagnosis as the patient evaluation proceeds. When combined with appropriate laboratory analyses (including peripheral blood testing and PFTs) and thoracic imaging, especially HRCT, a reasonably confident diagnosis may be attainable in many instances without resorting to invasive studies (Fig. 1.1).

Table 1.5 Key elements of the patient evaluation

Patient interview with elicitation of the clinical history
How long have symptoms been present?
Are symptoms progressively worsening (if yes, how rapidly)?
Are significant exposures a factor?
Occupational
Environmental (domestic, work related, hobbies)
Drugs (prescribed and illicit)
Tobacco
Are extrapulmonary symptoms present (rash, arthralgias, GER, other)?
Examination
Are pulmonary signs present?
Evidence of dyspnea (increased respiratory rate, increased work of breathing)
Abnormal auscultation (crackles, wheezes, other)
Evidence of pulmonary hypertension
Are extrapulmonary signs present?
Eye signs
Skin changes
Digital clubbing
Synovitis
Cardiac manifestations
Laboratory testing
Routine tests abnormal?
Are special tests indicated?
Pulmonary function testing
Are test results normal?
What is the pattern and severity of abnormal test values?
Invasive testing
Bronchoscopy
Is it indicated and likely to aid diagnosis?
Should BAL be performed?
Should transbronchial biopsy (or needle or endobronchial biopsy) be performed?
What areas should be targeted (HRCT as guide)?
Surgical lung biopsy
Is it necessary for accurate/confident diagnosis?
Can it be performed safely?

Some presentations may be particularly challenging to the clinician. As mentioned earlier, patients with non-ILD lung disease may develop superimposed ILD. As an example, the presence of airflow obstruction and hyperinflation due to emphysema combined with the opposing restrictive physiology caused by the onset of a coexistent ILD may obscure the diagnosis and cause some confusion when PFTs and/or thoracic imaging produce atypical findings. An example of this type of situation is the patient with emphysema who develops coexistent IPF. These individuals tend to have more severe and more rapidly progressive disease that is often accompanied by relatively severe PH. Another situation that may be encountered is the patient who is quite breathless with poor exercise tolerance but relatively mild ILD as reflected by parenchymal imaging and PFTs. These individuals may have secondary PH or significant cardiac dysfunction due to coronary artery disease (CAD), and close attention to PH and/or CAD is essential in diagnosis as well as in formulating treatment plans. Lastly, some patients who present acutely and have no previous history of ILD may have a process that is superimposed on preexistent but clinically occult ILD. As an example, a patient with subclinical (clinically occult and previously undiagnosed) IPF may experience an acute exacerbation of IPF (AEIPF) with diffuse alveolar damage superimposed on chronic changes of UIP. Similarly, histopathologic changes of organizing pneumonia may occur in a patient with preexistent, clinically occult UIP and constitute the event that causes the appearance of prominent respiratory symptoms that lead to a clinical evaluation.

If the evaluation remains indeterminate without invasive testing, bronchoscopy with BAL and/or endoscopic biopsies may yield a confident diagnosis (Fig. 1.2). The pulmonologist should ensure that an adequate number of transbronchial biopsy specimens are retrieved, and an adequately sized forceps should be used when sampling distal lung parenchyma. Additionally, if likely to provide diagnostic specimens, needle biopsy of pathologic lymph nodes and/or endobronchial biopsies should be performed. If the diagnosis is still indeterminate after bronchoscopy has been performed, SLB should be considered and performed if safety issues do not contraindicate this procedure.

Histopathology slides from the endoscopic biopsies or SLB specimens should be examined and interpreted by pathologists with expertise in diffuse parenchymal lung diseases. Once these specimens have been obtained and examined, the ultimate diagnosis may be substantially influenced

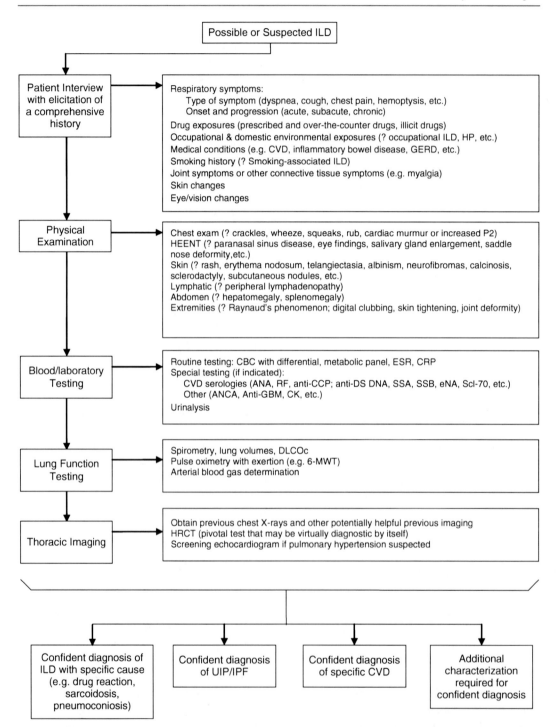

Fig. 1.1 Noninvasive evaluation of patients with suspected ILD. *ANA* antinuclear antibody, *CBC* complete lood count, *CCP* citrullinated peptides, *CK* creatine kinase, *CRP* C-reactive protein, *CVD* collagen-vascular disease, *GBM* glomerular basement membrane, *GERD* gastroesophageal reflux disease, *ESR* erythrocyte sedimentation rate, *ILD* interstitial lung disease, *P2* pulmonic valve closure sound, *RF* rheumatoid factor, *UIP* usual interstitial pneumonia

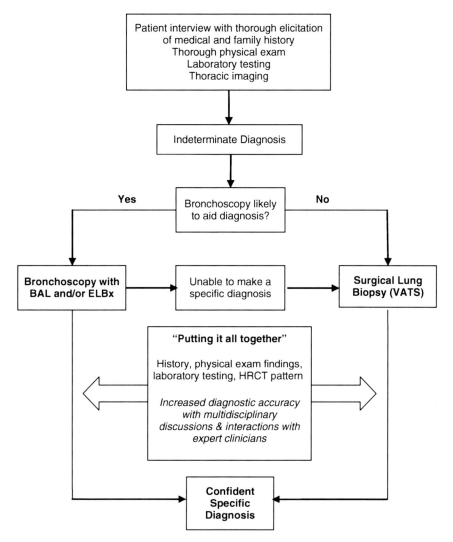

Fig. 1.2 Invasive testing for patients with suspected ILD. *BAL* bronchoalveolar lavage, *ELBx* endoscopic lung biopsy, *HRCT* high-resolution computed tomographic scan, *VATS* video-assisted thoracoscopic surgery

by the clinical data obtained from the interview, physical examination, laboratory testing, and thoracic imaging. Communication and discussion among the pulmonologist, radiologist, and pathologist will enhance the likelihood that a consensus diagnosis that is accurate and confident can be reached. Occasionally, the diagnosis may remain indeterminate even when a SLB has been obtained. In these instances, reviewing all the clinical findings, imaging results, and invasive testing in a multidisciplinary fashion will provide the best opportunity to reach a reasonably confident diagnosis. The accuracy of the diagnosis of IIPs and other forms of ILD is significantly increased when multidisciplinary interactions with experienced experts in ILD are incorporated into the diagnostic process.

Further Reading

ATS/ERS. International multidisciplinary consensus classification of the idiopathic interstitial pneumonias. Am J Respir and Crit Care Med. 2002;165:277–304.

Schwarz MI, King Jr TE, Raghu G. Approach to the evaluation and diagnosis of interstitial lung disease.

In: Schwarz MI, King Jr TE, editors. Interstitial lung disease. 4th ed. Hamilton: BC Decker; 2003. p. 1–30.

Raghu G, Brown KK. Interstitial lung disease: clinical evaluation and keys to an accurate diagnosis. Clin Chest Med. 2004;25:409–19.

Meyer KC. The role of bronchoalveolar lavage in interstitial lung disease. Clin Chest Med. 2004;25: 637–49.

Strange C, Highland KB. Interstitial lung disease in the patient who has connective tissue disease. Clin Chest Med. 2004;25:549–59.

Neralla S, Meyer KC. The keys to the diagnosis of interstitial lung disease. J Respir Dis. 2005;26:372–8 (part 1), 443–8 (part 2), 466–78 (part 3).

Judson MA. The diagnosis of sarcoidosis. Clin Chest Med. 2008;29:415–27.

Polomis D, Runo J, Meyer KC. Pulmonary hypertension in interstitial lung disease. Curr Opin Pulm Med. 2008;14:462–9.

Flaherty KR, King Jr TE, Raghu G, et al. Idiopathic interstitial pneumonia: what is the effect of a multidisciplinary approach to diagnosis? Am J Respir Crit Care Med. 2004;170:904–10.

Radiologic Evaluation

David A. Lynch

Abstract

High resolution CT is useful for early detection and characterization of diffuse lung diseases. Optimal CT evaluation requires careful attention to technique. Radiologic diagnosis is based on the use of standard descriptive terms and the distribution of abnormality in the craniocaudal and axial planes. Confident CT diagnoses of several diffuse diseases, including usual interstitial pneumonia, sarcoidosis, hypersensitivity pneumonitis, smoking-related lung injury, Langerhans histiocytosis, lymphangioleiomyomatosis, based on typical CT findings and made in the appropriate clinical context, are usually correct. However, certain other radiologic findings, particularly ground-glass abnormality, consolidation and reticular abnormality, are relatively nonspecific and will usually require further diagnostic evaluation.

Keywords

High resolution CT • Diagnosis • Usual interstitial pneumonia • Sarcoidosis • Hypersensitivity pneumonitis

Introduction

The purposes of this chapter are to explain optimal CT technique to evaluate diffuse lung disease, to describe and illustrate the common radiologic signs of diffuse lung disease, and to show how imaging can help elucidate some common clinical problems.

D.A. Lynch (✉)
Department of Radiology, National Jewish Health, Denver, CO, USA
e-mail: lynchd@njhealth.org

CT Techniques

The technique of high resolution CT (HRCT) requires thin (1–1.5 mm) sections and a special reconstruction algorithm to maximize detail in the lung parenchyma [1] (Fig. 2.1). HRCT images may be reconstructed from a volumetric dataset or may be acquired using noncontiguous images at 1–2 cm intervals. If volumetric acquisition is performed, coronal and sagittal reconstructions may be obtained, and may be very helpful in understanding distribution of disease.

Careful attention to technique is required to ensure high quality images. In particular,

R.P. Baughman and R.M. du Bois (eds.), *Diffuse Lung Disease: A Practical Approach*,
DOI 10.1007/978-1-4419-9771-5_2, © Springer Science+Business Media, LLC 2012

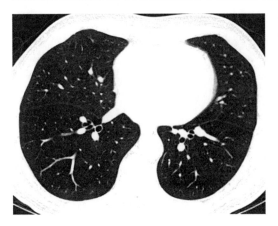

Fig. 2.1 Normal high resolution CT

technologists must work with the patient to ensure the absence of respiratory motion, which is the commonest cause of suboptimal images. Because atelectasis in the dependent lung can obscure detail, prone HRCT imaging is frequently performed to evaluate the posterior lung, where the early changes of asbestosis, collagen vascular-related lung disease, and idiopathic interstitial pneumonias may be first seen. Expiratory CT is often pivotal in identifying gas trapping in obstructive lung disease and hypersensitivity pneumonitis and sarcoidosis.

Radiologic Signs of Diffuse Lung Disease

Specificity of radiologic descriptors enhances the ability of radiologists to communicate their findings and generate appropriate differential diagnoses. The Fleischner Society has published a helpful glossary of descriptors used in thoracic imaging, which serves as standardized terminology [2]. Nonspecific terms such as alveolitis are best avoided. Table 2.1 illustrates the differential diagnosis of common patterns in diffuse lung disease.

Consolidation/Ground-Glass Attenuation

The term parenchymal opacification [3, 4] is applied to any homogeneous increase in lung density on chest radiographs or chest CT. When

this parenchymal opacification is dense enough to obscure the vessels and other parenchymal structures, it is called *consolidation* (Fig. 2.2). Since consolidation is usually due to a pathologic process filling the alveoli its differential diagnosis is broad, but may be narrowed when seen in relatively healthy outpatients, as given in Table 2.1.

Ground-glass attenuation is defined as an increase in lung density not sufficient to obscure vessels (see Fig. 2.2). Ground-glass attenuation is commonly, though not always, associated with reversible or potentially reversible lung disease. Because ground-glass attenuation may be due to any infiltrative process involving alveoli or alveolar septa, the differential diagnosis is broad. The differential presented in Table 2.1 may be applied to relatively healthy outpatients.

Nodules

Nodules seen on HRCT can be classified according to their size (micronodules or larger nodules), density (ground glass, soft tissue, or calcific densities), definition (well defined or poorly defined), and distribution. Micronodules measure less than 3 mm in diameter [5]. Gruden et al. [6] classified nodules on the basis of their location (random, perilymphatic, centrilobular, or airways associated). Perilymphatic micronodules are seen in subpleural and septal locations, most commonly in subjects with sarcoidosis (Fig. 2.3) or lymphangitic carcinoma, but may also be seen in pneumoconiosis. Scattered subpleural micronodules may be seen in normal subjects. Centrilobular nodules (see Table 2.2) are recognized by their characteristic location (Fig. 2.4), approximately 1–2 mm from each other, and separated by about the same distance from pleura and vessels. They are often of ground-glass attenuation. Small airways-associated nodules are identified when the tree-in-bud pattern is present (nodules closely related to small branching structures) (Fig. 2.5). These nodules are usually centrilobular.

Nodules of ground-glass density are typically seen in hypersensitivity pneumonitis (see Fig. 2.4), but may also be seen in respiratory bronchiolitis. Soft tissue density nodules are seen in patients with granulomatous lung diseases, malignancy,

Table 2.1 Differential diagnosis of infiltrative lung disease based on CT pattern

CT findings	Differential diagnosis
Consolidation[a]	Chronic infection (mycobacterial, fungal)
	Organizing pneumonia
	Sarcoidosis (pseudoalveolar)
	Bronchioloalveolar carcinoma
	Lymphoma
	Eosinophilic pneumonia
	Vasculitis
	Chronic aspiration (esp. lipid)
Ground-glass attenuation[a]	Hypersensitivity pneumonitis
	Nonspecific interstitial pneumonia
	Desquamative interstitial pneumonitis/respiratory bronchiolitis interstitial lung disease
	Hemorrhage
	Eosinophilic pneumonia
	Drug toxicity
Nodules	Malignancy
	Silicosis
	Coal workers' pneumoconiosis
	Granulomatous infection
	Sarcoidosis
	Berylliosis
	Langerhans cell histiocytosis
	Centrilobular nodules (see Table 2.3)
Fibrotic disease (reticular pattern, traction bronchiectasis, architectural distortion)	Usual interstitial pneumonia
	Nonspecific interstitial pneumonia
	Asbestosis
	Collagen vascular disease
	Sarcoidosis
	Chronic hypersensitivity pneumonitis
Honeycombing	Usual interstitial pneumonia
	Sarcoidosis
Cysts	Lymphangioleiomyomatosis
	Langerhans cell histiocytosis
	Lymphoid interstitial pneumonia
	Desquamative interstitial pneumonia
Crazy paving pattern[a]	Pulmonary alveolar proteinosis
	Lipoid pneumonia
	Bronchioloalveolar carcinoma
Decreased lung attenuation/mosaic attenuation	Hypersensitivity pneumonitis
	Obliterative bronchiolitis
	Thromboembolic disease
	Panlobular emphysema

Adapted from Lynch DA. Imaging of diffuse parenchymal lung diseases. In: Schwarz M, King T, editors. Interstitial lung disease. 5th ed. McGraw Hill; 2011. p. 105–49.

[a] The differential diagnosis provided here for consolidation, ground-glass attenuation, and crazy paving pattern is for relatively healthy patients presenting for routine high resolution CT evaluation. In acutely ill patients, the differential diagnosis of these findings is broader

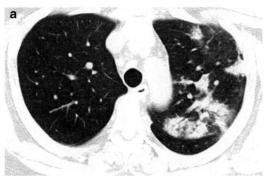
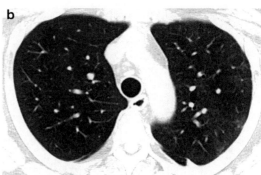

Fig. 2.2 Consolidation and ground-glass attenuation in a patient with cryptogenic organizing pneumonia. (**a**) Axial CT shows patchy consolidation and some ground-glass attenuation in the left upper lobe. (**b**) CT obtained 3 months later, after steroid treatment, shows resolution of the consolidation, but residual ground-glass attenuation

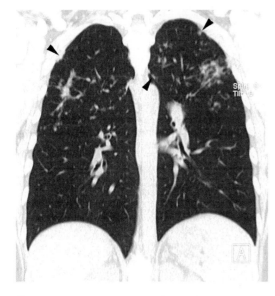

Fig. 2.3 Perilymphatic nodules in a patient with sarcoidosis. Coronal CT reconstruction shows bilateral upper lung predominant nodules, predominantly clustered along bronchovascular bundles and in the subpleural region (arrowheads)

or pneumoconiosis. Calcific nodules are seen in prior granulomatous infection or in pulmonary alveolar microlithiasis.

Lines

A variety of linear densities may be seen on HRCT. Thickened interlobular septa (Fig. 2.6) are identified because they are perpendicular to

Table 2.2 Lobular anatomy in differential diagnosis of infiltrative lung diseases on HRCT

Centrilobular nodules: soft tissue attenuation	Pneumoconiosis
	Langerhans cell histiocytosis
Centrilobular nodules: ground-glass attenuation	Respiratory bronchiolitis
	Hypersensitivity pneumonitis
Centrilobular nodules with tree-in-bud pattern	Infection
	Aspiration
	Diffuse panbronchiolitis
	Noninfectious bronchiolitis
Septal thickening	Left heart failure
	Lymphangitic carcinoma
	Acute eosinophilic pneumonia
	Drug hypersensitivity
	Sarcoidosis

Adapted from Lynch DA. Imaging of diffuse parenchymal lung diseases. In: Schwarz M, King T, editors. Interstitial lung disease. 5th ed. McGraw Hill; 2011. p. 105–49

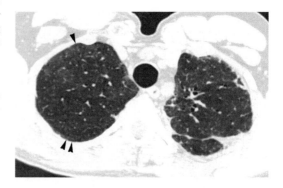

Fig. 2.4 Centrilobular ground-glass nodules in an individual with hypersensitivity pneumonitis. There are numerous poorly defined centrilobular nodules, most of which are of ground-glass attenuation (i.e., lower in attenuation than the vessels)

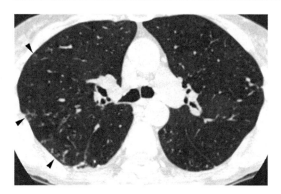

Fig. 2.5 Tree-in-bud pattern in a patient with nontuberculous mycobacterial infection. Axial CT shows multifocal tree-in-bud pattern in the right lung (arrowheads). There are some centrilobular nodules in the left lung

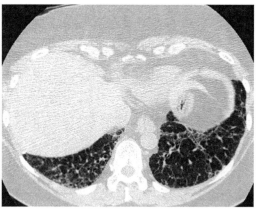

Fig. 2.7 Reticular pattern in a patient with usual interstitial pneumonia (UIP). Traction bronchiectasis is seen in the right lower lobe. Honeycombing is not present

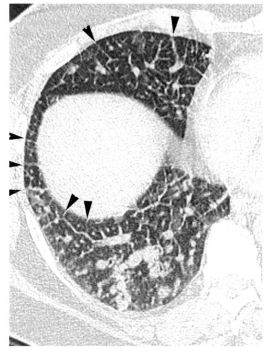

Fig. 2.6 Interlobular septal thickening in a patient with lymphangitic carcinoma from lung cancer. CT through the right lower lung shows smooth and nodular thickening of numerous interlobular septa, recognized as lines perpendicular to the pleura forming polygonal structures. The bronchovascular bundles are thickened. There is no traction bronchiectasis or architectural distortion to suggest fibrosis

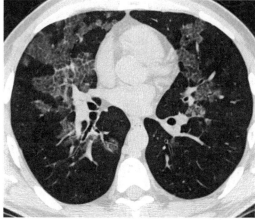

Fig. 2.8 Crazy paving pattern in a patient with pulmonary alveolar proteinosis. CT through the mid-lungs shows geographic areas of reticular abnormality, formed by thickened interlobular septa and interlobular lines, superimposed on a background of ground-glass attenuation. Traction bronchiectasis and architectural distortion are notably absent. The distribution is predominantly peribronchovascular

the pleura [7] or by the fact that they form polygonal structures [8]. Reticular lines are probably the commonest type of linear abnormality (Fig. 2.7). These lines are less than 5 mm long, forming a fine lace-like network which usually does not conform to lobular anatomy. They are seen in all types of fibrotic lung conditions, particularly idiopathic pulmonary fibrosis [9], collagen vascular disease, and asbestosis. They are usually associated with other evidence of lung fibrosis such as architectural distortion or traction bronchiectasis. Reticular lines are also a prominent CT feature in patients with the crazy paving pattern (Fig. 2.8)

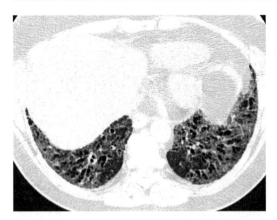

Fig. 2.9 Traction bronchiectasis in a patient with NSIP. CT shows marked ground-glass attenuation. The associated marked dilation of numerous bronchi indicates that this abnormality is due to fibrosis rather than an inflammatory process

(discussed below), but architectural distortion and traction bronchiectasis are absent.

Traction Bronchiectasis/ Bronchiolectasis

Traction bronchiectasis and bronchiolectasis (Fig. 2.9) refers to dilatation and distortion of the bronchi and bronchioles in areas of fibrosis, presumed to be due to the forces of increased elastic recoil acting on these structures [10]. It is usually associated with a reticular pattern or with ground-glass attenuation, and is reliable evidence of lung fibrosis [11].

Honeycombing

Honeycombing is defined as a subpleural cluster or row of cysts (Fig. 2.10). Honeycomb cysts are usually very small (less than 5 mm in diameter). This CT finding correlates with histologic honeycombing and is found in end-stage lung of any cause [12]. Larger honeycomb cysts may sometimes be found in patients with sarcoidosis.

Cysts

The cysts of interstitial lung disease are air-containing lucencies with a well-defined, complete wall (Fig. 2.11). They are usually round, but may

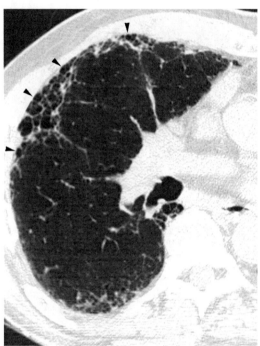

Fig. 2.10 Honeycombing in a patient with idiopathic pulmonary fibrosis (UIP). Axial CT through the right mid-lung shows clustered subpleural honeycomb cysts (arrowheads)

sometimes be irregular in shape, particularly in Langerhans histiocytosis. They must be distinguished from the "moth-eaten" lucencies of centrilobular emphysema, which are usually irregular in outline and do not have a definable wall (Fig. 2.12). Cysts may be distinguished from bronchiectatic bronchi by the fact that bronchi are usually accompanied by a smaller pulmonary artery, and can usually be traced back to the hilum on serial CT sections.

Crazy Paving Pattern

The crazy paving pattern is a distinctive pattern characterized by thickened interlobular and intralobular lines forming a geographic network superimposed on a background of ground-glass attenuation (see Fig. 2.8) [13]. In the correct clinical context, this pattern is strongly of pulmonary alveolar proteinosis. Lipoid pneumonia, and, rarely, bronchioloalveolar carcinoma may cause an identical appearance. The pattern can also be

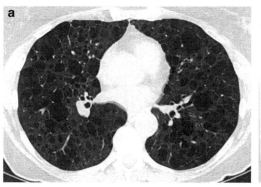
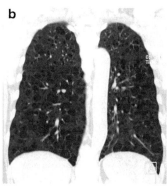

Fig. 2.11 Pulmonary cysts in a patient with lymphangioleiomyomatosis. (**a**) Axial CT through the mid-lungs shows numerous randomly distributed discrete cysts of varying sizes. Each cyst has a thin, well-defined wall. (**b**) Coronal image shows that distribution in the craniocaudal plane is diffuse

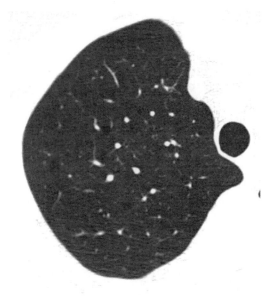

Fig. 2.12 Centrilobular emphysema. CT through the right upper lung shows well-defined lucencies without a discrete wall

seen in patients with other lung diseases including resolving pneumonia, ARDS, and mucinous bronchioloalveolar carcinoma, but in those conditions it is usually associated with other types of CT abnormality [14–16].

Decreased Lung Attenuation/Mosaic Pattern

The attenuation (density) of a given area of lung depends on the amount of parenchymal tissue, air, and blood in that area. Therefore, decreased attenuation of the lung may be due to lung destruction (in panlobular emphysema), to decreased blood flow (in vascular disease such as pulmonary thromboembolism), or to decreased ventilation with air trapping and reflex pulmonary oligemia (in small airways diseases with constrictive bronchiolitis) (Fig. 2.13). Panlobular emphysema differs from vascular lung disease and small airway disease in that it usually causes a diffuse decrease in lung attenuation (increased blackness), while thromboembolic disease and obliterative bronchiolitis are commonly (though not always) more patchy in distribution. Vascular disease can often be distinguished from airways disease by comparing inspiratory and expiratory scans. In airways disease, one will expect to see air trapping on the expiratory scans, resulting in an increase in the number of areas of decreased attenuation. In patients with occlusive vascular disease, the areas of decreased attenuation should not increase on expiration [17].

Patients with thromboembolic disease and obliterative bronchiolitis commonly present with a *mosaic pattern*, with lobules of normal attenuation adjacent to lobules or subsegments of decreased attenuation (see Fig. 2.13). A similar mosaic pattern may be caused by parenchymal disease which causes lobular areas of ground-glass attenuation (particularly hypersensitivity pneumonitis) (Fig. 2.14). With the mosaic pattern, it can be difficult to decide whether the abnormal areas are those of decreased attenuation or those of increased attenuation. This distinction can be made by observing the pulmonary

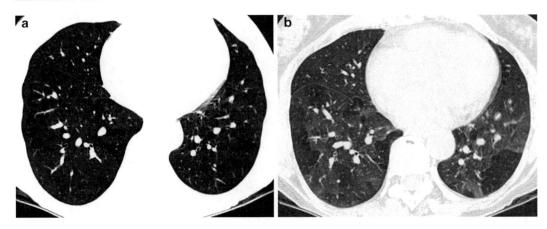

Fig. 2.13 Mosaic attenuation in a patient with bronchiolitis obliterans related to rheumatoid arthritis. (**a**) Inspiratory CT shows patchy geographic decrease in lung attenuation. Pulmonary vessels are decreased in size in the more lucent parts of lung. (**b**) Expiratory CT confirms that the areas of decreased attenuation on inspiratory images show gas trapping on expiration

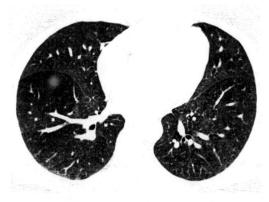

Fig. 2.14 Mosaic pattern in hypersensitivity pneumonitis. CT through the lower lungs shows diffuse ground-glass abnormality. However, there is focal decreased attenuation in the anterior right lower lobe

vessels, which will be reduced in size in areas affected by vascular occlusive disease or obliterative bronchiolitis, but will be normal in size in patients with parenchymal infiltrative lung diseases [17]. One can then use expiratory images to distinguish between airway obstruction and thromboembolic disease [18]. Of course, physiologic evaluation will also help to distinguish between vascular disease, airways obstruction, and parenchymal infiltration.

Distribution of Lung Diseases

Evaluation of disease distribution in the craniocaudal and axial planes is remarkably valuable for differential diagnosis of diffuse lung disease (Table 2.3). In the craniocaudal plane, distribution of disease may be characterized as upper lung predominant (Fig. 2.15), lower lung predominant (Fig. 2.16), or (uncommonly) mid-lung predominant. In the axial plane, disease distribution may be characterized as predominantly subpleural or perilymphatic. Perilymphatic abnormalities are usually predominantly distributed along the bronchovascular bundle (where most of the lymphatics of the lung reside), often associated with subpleural nodules and interlobular septal thickening (see Figs. 2.3 and 2.15).

Assessment of the secondary pulmonary lobule may also be valuable in some diffuse diseases (see Table 2.2) [19, 20]. The secondary pulmonary lobule is a basic anatomic and physiologic unit of mammalian lung [21]. In humans, it is an irregularly polyhedral structure composed of several acini, each supplied by a terminal bronchiole. In the center of the secondary pulmonary lobule are the distal bronchus and its terminal bronchioles with the associated distal pulmonary

Table 2.3 Differential diagnosis of infiltrative lung diseases by distribution within the lung

Peripheral distribution	UIP
	OP
	Asbestosis
	Collagen vascular disease
	Eosinophilic pneumonia
Perilymphatic distribution	Sarcoidosis
	Lymphangitic carcinoma
	Lymphoproliferative disorders
	Organizing pneumonia
Upper lobe predominance	Sarcoidosis
	Coal workers' pneumoconiosis
	Silicosis
	Eosinophilic pneumonia
	Langerhans cell histiocytosis
	Hypersensitivity pneumonitis
Lower lobe predominance	UIP
	NSIP
	OP
	Asbestosis
	Collagen vascular disease

UIP usual interstitial pneumonia, *OP* organizing pneumonia, *NSIP* nonspecific interstitial pneumonia
Adapted from Lynch DA. Imaging of diffuse parenchymal lung diseases. In: Schwarz M, King T, editors. Interstitial lung disease. 5th ed. McGraw Hill; 2011. p. 105–49

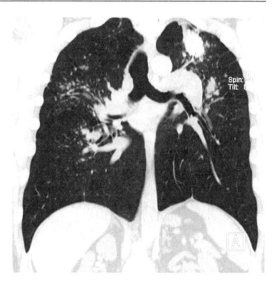

Fig. 2.15 Upper lung predominant nodules and conglomerate masses in a patient with silicosis. Coronal CT image shows the typical perilymphatic distribution, with predominance of the nodules along bronchovascular bundles, interlobular septa and pleura

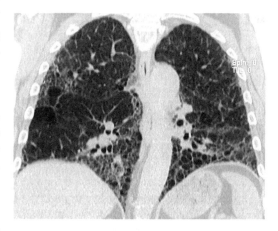

Fig. 2.16 Lower lung predominant reticular abnormality and honeycombing in a patient with idiopathic pulmonary fibrosis

artery branches. These structures are often called centrilobular or core structures and may be visible on HRCT as a dot or branching structure 1 to 3 mm deep to the pleural surface. In patients with inflammation or plugging of small airways, the normally invisible centrilobular structures become visible as nodules or short branching structures. The centrilobular nodules may either be of soft tissue attenuation or of ground-glass attenuation. When these branching structures terminate in a nodule, the "*tree-in-bud*" sign is present (see Fig. 2.5). The tree-in-bud sign is usually due either to infection or aspiration [22]. Nodules that are centrilobular without a "tree-in-bud" appearance are usually due to some form of inhalational disease (see Fig. 2.4).

The secondary lobules are separated from each other by interlobular septa, which contain branches of the pulmonary veins and lymphatics. On normal HRCT [21], the interlobular septa may be visible in the normal anterior lung as scattered, thin nontapering lines, 1–2 cm long, perpendicular to the pleura and often contacting the pleural surface. Thickening of interlobular septa is usually due to edema or infiltration of the lymphatic structures, and is often associated with thickening of the other lymphatic pathways (subpleural and peribronchovascular) (see Fig. 2.6).

Specific Imaging Issues in Evaluation of Diffuse Lung Disease

Detection of Early Interstitial Lung Disease

The chest radiograph is relatively insensitive for detection of diffuse lung disease. Although it is commonly stated that the chest radiograph is normal in 10–15% of patients with diffuse lung disease, the true sensitivity of the chest radiograph depends on the severity and type of disease present in the population being studied. CT has been shown to be more sensitive than the chest radiograph in many diseases including asbestosis [23], silicosis [24], sarcoidosis [25], scleroderma [26, 27], and hypersensitivity pneumonitis [28, 29]. In asbestosis, HRCT may detect abnormality before resting pulmonary function tests become abnormal [23, 30]. It is also clear that the HRCT scan may be normal despite the presence of biopsy-proven interstitial disease. In a population-based study of subjects with hypersensitivity pneumonitis who had normal resting pulmonary function the sensitivity of HRCT was 38% [31]. Similarly, in a paper by Gamsu and colleagues, CT scanning was normal or near normal in 5 of 25 patients with histologic asbestosis. These studies emphasize the fact that there is a phase in the evolution of any lung disease when the degree of parenchymal infiltration is too slight or too focal to cause a recognizable increase in lung attenuation on CT. Therefore, although CT is substantially more sensitive than the chest radiograph for ILD, normal findings on HRCT cannot be used to exclude ILD. In future, it is possible that computer-based characterization systems might help to detect lung disease in patients with visually normal CT.

Characterization of Interstitial Lung Disease

Several large retrospective studies have compared the diagnostic accuracy of chest CT and chest radiography for diagnosis of specific lung diseases. Mathieson et al. [32] examined the chest radiographs and CT scans of 118 patients with diffuse infiltrative lung diseases. For usual interstitial pneumonitis, the first choice diagnosis was correct in 75% of the cases on chest radiograph and 89% of the cases on CT. For silicosis, the corresponding figures were 63 and 93%, and sarcoidosis, 61 and 77%. For lymphangitic carcinomatosis, the first choice diagnosis was correct in 56% of cases on the chest radiograph and 85% on CT. In addition, interobserver variation appeared to be less for CT scanning than for chest radiographs. Overall, a correct first choice diagnosis was made with 57% of radiographs and 76% of CT scans.

One of the defects of these earlier studies was that they may have included patients with well-established disease. In a more recent study of 85 patients who were scanned prior to surgical lung biopsy, the accuracy of a confident first choice diagnosis of disease was 90%, but such a confident diagnosis was made in only about 25% of cases [33]. This relatively low level of diagnostic confidence was most likely due to selection bias (patients in whom confident CT diagnoses can be made are unlikely to undergo biopsy). However, it is also possible that confident diagnoses are more difficult to make in those with earlier disease.

A prospective, multicenter study of the accuracy of diagnosis of usual interstitial pneumonia (UIP) found that a confident CT diagnosis of UIP, based on typical features, was correct in 96% of cases [34], consistent with the results of several other studies indicating that the correctness of a confident first choice diagnosis of UIP, made by an experienced radiologist, is greater than 90% [33, 35, 36]. Univariate and multivariate analysis showed that radiologic features were the primary discriminants between UIP and other causes of diffuse lung disease [37]. However, it should be noted that in this study, a confident CT diagnosis

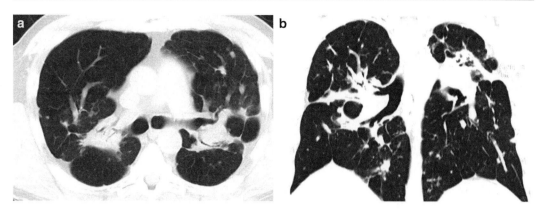

Fig. 2.17 Fibrotic sarcoidosis. Axial (**a**) and coronal (**b**) CT reconstructions demonstrate upper lobe predominant perihilar conglomerate masses associated with marked bronchovascular distortion

of UIP was made in only about 50% of cases. In other cases of histologically confirmed UIP, the CT features were not typical enough to make a confident diagnosis. Similar findings were reported in a study by Raghu et al. [38]. Other diseases in which a confident CT diagnosis is highly likely to be correct include lymphangitic carcinoma [8], Langerhans histiocytosis [39], lymphangiomyomatosis [39], and hypersensitivity pneumonitis (with micronodules) [40]. Advanced cases of sarcoidosis may also be diagnosed with confidence (see Fig. 2.17).

It must be clearly understood that even a confident CT diagnosis should be integrated with the available clinical information. Patients with discrepant findings on clinical evaluation and CT should usually undergo biopsy. Biopsy is also indicated in patients with nonspecific CT findings. HRCT can be valuable for predicting whether transbronchial biopsy would be helpful (in suspected sarcoidosis or lymphangitic carcinoma), and for identifying a suitable site for biopsy by the bronchoscopist or surgeon. When a biopsy is performed, it is important to review the biopsy in conjunction with the CT findings. Discrepancies between the CT pattern and the biopsy findings may be due to sampling of a nonrepresentative part of the lung.

CT of Specific Lung Diseases

Idiopathic Interstitial Pneumonias

UIP often has a characteristic appearance on CT [41]. The predominant CT pattern is usually either reticular abnormality, almost always associated with traction bronchiectasis, and frequently associated with honeycombing (see Figs. 2.7, 2.10, and 2.16) [42]. Pure ground-glass attenuation, if present, is usually sparse. The distribution of the abnormalities is basal predominant in most, but may be diffuse in the craniocaudal plane. Peripheral, subpleural predominance is present in over 90%. The fibrosis is asymmetric in up to 25% of cases [43]. In contrast to the homogenous appearance of nonspecific interstitial pneumonia (NSIP), the abnormalities of UIP often have a patchy distribution. As the disease progresses, it often appears to "creep" up the periphery of the lung, causing subpleural reticular abnormality in the upper lungs [37].

Multiple prospective and retrospective studies have shown that a confident or highly confident diagnosis of UIP, based on the CT features outlined earlier, has a specificity of over 90% for the pathologic diagnosis of UIP [33–35, 38, 40, 42]. Honeycombing in the lower lobes, and linear abnormality in the upper lobes, are the most reliable features for differentiating between UIP and its clinical mimics (see Fig. 2.10) [37]. In a study by Flaherty et al., the observation of honeycombing on HRCT indicated the presence of UIP with a sensitivity of 90% and specificity of 86% [44]. However, there is a substantial minority (30–50%) of cases with histologic UIP (without honeycombing) in whom a confident diagnosis of UIP cannot be made based on the CT appearances (see Fig. 2.7). In these patients, the CT appearances of UIP overlap with those of NSIP and chronic hypersensitivity pneumonitis, and the diagnosis can only be established by lung biopsy.

Published descriptions of the CT appearances of NSIP have varied quite widely [42, 45–52], probably because of differing pathologic diagnostic criteria. However, a multidisciplinary workshop identified a relatively typical CT appearance among 67 patients who received a clinical–radiologic–pathologic consensus diagnosis of NSIP [53]. In this group, the CT appearances were characterized by confluent, symmetric, basal predominant, ground-glass and reticular abnormality with traction bronchiectasis and lower lobe volume loss (see Fig. 2.9). In contrast to UIP, the subpleural lung is often spared.

Consolidation is the radiologic hallmark of cryptogenic organizing pneumonia, seen in about 80% of cases (see Fig. 2.2). It generally shows no craniocaudal predilection though some series have shown a basal predominance [54–56]. The consolidation may have a perilymphatic distribution [57–61]. Other suggestive features may include a perilobular pattern (poorly defined opacity along interlobular septa) and the reverse halo sign (ring-like opacity with central ground-glass abnormality) [62, 63].

Lymphoid interstitial pneumonia is characterized by ground-glass abnormality. Discrete cysts may be seen in two-thirds of cases [64], and may be the dominant or only finding. The cysts typically have a perilymphatic distribution and usually lower lung predominant. Mediastinal or hilar lymphadenopathy is often seen.

Table 2.4 Patterns of lung injury most commonly associated with specific collagen vascular diseases

Disease entity	Lung pattern
Diffuse scleroderma	Nonspecific interstitial pneumonia
	Pulmonary hypertension
Limited scleroderma	Pulmonary hypertension
Rheumatoid arthritis	Usual interstitial pneumonia
	Obliterative bronchiolitis
	Follicular bronchiolitis
Polymyositis/ dermatomyositis	Nonspecific interstitial pneumonia
	Organizing pneumonia
Sjögren's syndrome	LIP
	Follicular bronchiolitis
Systemic lupus erythematosus	Pulmonary hemorrhage

Collagen Vascular Disease

Involvement of the respiratory system in the collagen vascular diseases is common. Most of the parenchymal manifestations of collagen vascular disease are similar to those found in idiopathic interstitial pneumonias [65] and can be classified using the same system [66]. Although any pattern of lung injury may occur with any of the collagen vascular diseases, each specific collagen vascular disease tends to be associated with two or three specific patterns of injury, summarized in Table 2.4.

Sarcoidosis

The manifestations of sarcoidosis in the lung are diverse. However, the salient features are lymphadenopathy and nodules. Hilar and mediastinal lymphadenopathy is typically symmetric and may be partially calcified. The nodules are characteristically clustered in a perilymphatic distribution (see Fig. 2.3) [5], and often regress at least partially with treatment. Other potentially reversible findings in sarcoidosis include large nodular opacities, septal thickening ground-glass abnormality, and consolidation [67].

In fibrotic sarcoidosis, perihilar clustered nodules form conglomerate masses, associated with bronchovascular distortion (Fig. 2.17) [68]. While the size of these fibrotic masses may decrease with time, the associated bronchial distortion usually persists or increases. Honeycombing may also be seen [69].

Hypersensitivity Pneumonitis

Hypersensitivity pneumonitis may be diagnosed on CT with high confidence in the presence of either of the following findings:

- Profuse, diffuse, poorly defined centrilobular nodules of ground-glass attenuation (see Fig. 2.4).
- Ground-glass attenuation associated with widespread multilobular decreased lung attenuation and expiratory air trapping (see Fig. 2.14).

A proportion of subjects with chronic hypersensitivity pneumonitis have lung fibrosis, which may be difficult to distinguish from UIP or NSIP. Features that help to distinguish chronic fibrotic HP from UIP and NSIP include upper or midlung predominance, sparing of the extreme lung bases, and the presence of multiple lobules of decreased attenuation and air trapping [36, 70].

Smoking-Related Lung Diseases

Infiltrative lung diseases caused by cigarette smoking include respiratory bronchiolitis, respiratory bronchiolitis-interstitial lung disease, desquamative interstitial pneumonia, and pulmonary Langerhans cell histiocytosis (PLCH). On CT scanning, patients with asymptomatic respiratory bronchiolitis generally show mild centrilobular nodularity and small patches of ground-glass attenuation [71].

In RB-ILD, centrilobular nodularity and ground-glass attenuation are usually more extensive than in asymptomatic RB (Fig. 2.18) [72]. Emphysema, bronchial wall thickening, and areas

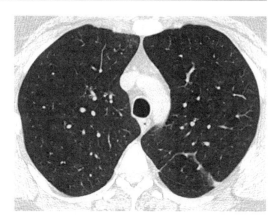

Fig. 2.18 Respiratory bronchiolitis interstitial lung disease in a patient with a 38 pack-year history of cigarette smoking. CT through the upper lungs shows marked airway wall thickening, with widespread poorly defined ground-glass attenuation, and smudgy centrilobular nodularity

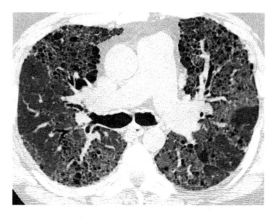

Fig. 2.19 Desquamative interstitial pneumonia in a cigarette smoker. CT through the mid-lungs shows diffuse ground-glass attenuation. Numerous cysts are seen within the areas of ground glass. In contrast to honeycomb cysts, these cysts do not show subpleural clustering

of decreased lung attenuation are commonly also present [73]. When patchy abnormalities of this type are present in heavy smokers with impaired pulmonary function, RB-ILD may be diagnosed with a high degree of confidence. The CT findings of RB-ILD are at least partially reversible in patients who stop smoking [73, 74].

Ground-glass attenuation is seen in all patients with DIP [46], with lower lobe predominance in about 75% of the patients (Fig. 2.19). Peripheral predominance is seen in about 60%.

Cysts are seen within areas of ground-glass attenuation in at least 50% of cases (Fig. 2.19).

Cystic Lung Diseases

The most common cystic lung diseases are PLCH, lymphangioleiomyomatosis (LAM), and lymphoid interstitial pneumonia. The combination of pulmonary nodules and cysts, predominating in the upper lungs is virtually diagnostic of PLCH (Fig. 2.20) [75–78]. The nodules may be well defined, poorly defined, or stellate, and may be cavitary. The cysts are often irregular or lobulated in outline. PLCH may be distinguished from LAM by the presence of nodules, by the irregular outline of the cysts, and by the sparing of the lung bases.

Cysts are the pathognomonic feature of LAM (see Fig. 2.11) [79–85]. The cysts are usually multiple and distributed in a uniform fashion in lung that is otherwise normal. Cysts are clearly demarcated by a thin even wall (1–2 mm thick) and are usually rounded. Vessels are often seen at

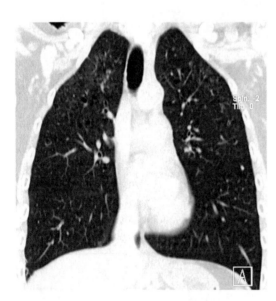

Fig. 2.20 Pulmonary Langerhans cell histiocytosis in a young cigarette smoker. Coronal CT shows poorly defined centrilobular nodules in the upper lungs associated with a few small cysts. The associated ground-glass attenuation may represent a component of respiratory bronchiolitis interstitial lung disease

the margins of the cysts. The cysts are usually 5–15 mm, but may range from 2 to 50 mm. The number of cysts varies widely, depending on the clinical presentation; cysts are usually extensive in those who present with symptoms of pulmonary impairment, but often quite sparse in those who present with complications such as pneumothorax, pleural effusion, etc. CT has enhanced awareness of the intra-abdominal manifestations of LAM. In addition to renal angiomyolipomas (found in 30–50% of patients), other manifestations include hepatic angiomyolipomas, lymphangiomyomas, and enlarged retroperitoneal lymph nodes [86, 87].

Cysts are often a salient feature of LIP, discussed earlier. The predominantly perilymphatic distribution of these cysts usually helps distinguish them from LAM and PLCH.

Small Airways Disease

Computed tomography has contributed substantially to our understanding of small airways diseases and offers a convenient method for classification of these diverse entities. A current CT-based classification of small airways disease is presented in Table 2.5.

In patients with constrictive bronchiolitis (see Fig. 2.13), the primary CT finding is dramatic decrease in lung density in affected lobules or subsegments, associated with narrowing of the pulmonary vessels. Such findings are identified in individuals with obliterative bronchiolitis related to prior infection, connective tissue disease, toxic fume inhalation, and transplantation [88–92]. Expiratory images are usually helpful in confirming air trapping.

Cellular bronchiolitis is characterized on CT by centrilobular nodularity with a tree-in-bud pattern (see Fig. 2.5). It is most commonly seen in patients with acute or chronic pulmonary infection. In the acute context, it is usually seen in patients with atypical pneumonia due to mycoplasma [93] or viruses. In those who are not acutely ill, the most common causes are mycobacterial infection and aspiration.

Table 2.5 CT-based classification of small airways diseases

Radiologic pattern	Characteristic radiologic features	Causes
Cellular bronchiolitis	Centrilobular nodularity	Acute or chronic infection (mycobacterial, fungal)
	Tree-in-bud pattern	Aspiration
		Hypersensitivity pneumonitis
Constrictive bronchiolitis	Diffuse or geographic air trapping/mosaic pattern	Rheumatoid disease
	Bronchial dilation	Chronic rejection
		Childhood viral/mycoplasma infection
		Prior toxic fume exposure
		Cryptogenic bronchiolitis obliterans
Panbronchiolitis	Tree-in-bud pattern	Diffuse panbronchiolitis
	Bronchiolectasis	Cystic fibrosis
	Bronchiectasis	Immune deficiency
		Nontuberculous mycobacterial infection
		Inflammatory bowel disease
Respiratory bronchiolitis	Poorly defined centrilobular nodules	Other inhalation exposures
	Patchy ground-glass attenuation	
Follicular bronchiolitis	Centrilobular nodules	Sjogren syndrome and other collagen vascular diseases
	Peribronchial nodules	Immunodeficiency
	Ground-glass opacity	

Adapted from Lynch DA. Imaging of diffuse parenchymal lung diseases. In: Schwarz M, King T, editors. Interstitial lung disease. 5th ed. McGraw Hill; 2011. p. 105–49

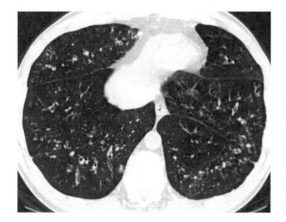

Fig. 2.21 Diffuse panbronchiolitis pattern in a patient with ulcerative colitis. CT through the lower lungs shows widespread cylindric bronchiectasis and multifocal tree-in-bud pattern. Differential diagnosis would include chronic infection

Panbronchiolitis, typically seen in Asian patients, is associated with tree-in-bud pattern associated with bronchiolar dilation, bronchiectasis, and patchy consolidation [94]. The abnormality is usually most marked in the lower lobes bilaterally. A similar pattern may be seen in individuals with inflammatory bowel disease (see Fig. 2.21).

CT-Based Strategy for Diagnosis of Diffuse Lung Disease

HRCT is now a pivotal modality in establishing the diagnosis of diffuse lung disease. Table 2.6 presents a proposed strategy for this purpose. A few points are important with regard to this table:

- The level of diagnostic confidence of the radiologic diagnosis is very important and should be specifically stated. A high-confidence diagnosis, based on typical features, is much more likely to be correct than a lower confidence diagnosis, particularly with IPF.
- Certain radiologic findings, particularly ground-glass abnormality, consolidation, and reticular abnormality are relatively nonspecific and will usually require further diagnostic evaluation.

Table 2.6 Diagnostic strategy in diffuse lung disease based on CT features

Category 1: No invasive procedures needed if clinical and CT features are typical

Usual interstitial pneumonia

Lymphangiomyomatosis

Langerhans histiocytosis

Hypersensitivity pneumonitis

Pneumoconiosis

Collagen vascular disease

Category 2: Bronchoalveolar lavage

Pulmonary alveolar proteinosis

Infection

Category 3: Transbronchial biopsy

Sarcoid

Lymphangitic carcinoma

Lymphoproliferative disorders

Category 4: Surgical lung biopsy

Nonspecific CT appearances (e.g., ground-glass abnormality, reticular abnormality), without a clinical explanation

Typical CT appearance of a condition, with atypical clinical features

Typical clinical features of a condition, with atypical CT

Adapted from Lynch DA. Imaging of diffuse parenchymal lung diseases. In: Schwarz M, King T, editors. Interstitial lung disease. 5th ed. McGraw Hill; 2011. p. 105–49

- CT may be helpful in identifying optimal sites for transbronchial or surgical biopsy.
- If clinical or imaging features are atypical, biopsy is still indicated.

References

1. Mayo JR. CT evaluation of diffuse infiltrative lung disease: dose considerations and optimal technique. J Thorac Imaging. 2009;24(4):252–9.
2. Hansell DM, Bankier AA, Macmahon H, McLoud TC, Müller NL, Remy J. Fleischner Society: glossary of terms for thoracic imaging. Radiology. 2008; 246(3):697–722.
3. Leung A, Miller R, Müller N. Parenchymal opacification in chronic infiltrative lung disease: CT-pathologic correlation. Radiology. 1993;188:209–14.
4. Austin J, Müller N, Friedman P, Hansell D, Naidich D, Remy-Jardin M, et al. Glossary of terms for CT of the lungs: recommendations of the nomenclature committee of the Fleischner Society. Radiology. 1996;200:327–31.
5. Remy-Jardin M, Beuscart R, Sault MC, Marquette CH, Remy J. Subpleural micronodules in diffuse infiltrative lung diseases: evaluation with thin-section CT scans. Radiology. 1990;177(1):133–9.
6. Gruden JF, Webb WR, Naidich DP, McGuinness G. Multinodular disease: anatomic localization at thin-section CT – multireader evaluation of a simple algorithm. Radiology. 1999;210(3):711–20.
7. Aberle DR, Gamsu G, Ray CS, Feuerstein IM. Asbestos-related pleural and parenchymal fibrosis: detection with high-resolution CT. Radiology. 1988;166:729–34.
8. Stein M, Mayo J, Müller N, Aberle D, Webb W, Gamsu G. Pulmonary lymphangitic spread of carcinoma: appearance on CT scans. Radiology. 1987; 162:371–5.
9. Müller NL, Miller RR, Webb WR, Evans KG, Ostrow DN. Fibrosing alveolitis: CT-pathologic correlation. Radiology. 1986;160(3):585–8.
10. Westcott JL, Cole SR. Traction bronchiectasis in end-stage pulmonary fibrosis. Radiology. 1986;161: 665–9.
11. Remy-Jardin M, Giraud F, Remy J, Copin MC, Gosselin B, Duhamel A. Importance of ground-glass attenuation in chronic diffuse infiltrative lung disease: pathologic-CT correlation. Radiology. 1993;189(3):693–8.
12. Meziane MA, Hruban RH, Zerhouni EA, Wheeler PS, Khouri NF, Fishman EK, et al. High resolution CT of the lung parenchyma with pathologic correlation. Radiographics. 1988;8(1):27–54.
13. Godwin J, Müller N, Takasugi J. Pulmonary alveolar proteinosis: CT findings. Radiology. 1988;169:609–13.
14. Tan RT, Kuzo RS. High-resolution CT findings of mucinous bronchioloalveolar carcinoma: a case of pseudopulmonary alveolar proteinosis. AJR Am J Roentgenol. 1997;168(1):99–100.
15. Laurent F, Philippe JC, Vergier B, Granger-Veron B, Darpeix B, Vergeret J, et al. Exogenous lipoid pneumonia: HRCT, MR, and pathologic findings. Eur Radiol. 1999;9(6):1190–6.
16. Murayama S, Murakami J, Yabuuchi H, Soeda H, Masuda K. "Crazy paving appearance" on high resolution CT in various diseases. J Comput Assist Tomogr. 1999;23(5):749–52.
17. Stern E, Swensen S, Hartman T, Frank M. CT mosaic pattern of lung attenuation: distinguishing different causes. AJR Am J Roentgenol. 1995;165:813–6.
18. Arakawa H, Webb WR, McCowin M, Katsou G, Lee KN, Seitz RF. Inhomogeneous lung attenuation at thin-section CT: diagnostic value of expiratory scans. Radiology. 1998;206(1):89–94.
19. Murata K, Khan A, Herman PG. Pulmonary parenchymal disease: evaluation with high-resolution CT. Radiology. 1989;170:629–35.
20. Noma S, Khan A, Herman PG, Rojas KA. High-resolution computed tomography of the pulmonary parenchyma. Semin Ultrasound CT MR. 1990;11: 365–79.
21. Webb W, Stein M, Finkbeiner W, Im J-G, Lynch D, Gamsu G. Normal and diseased isolated lungs: high resolution CT. Radiology. 1988;166:81–7.
22. Murata K, Itoh H, Todo G, Kanaoka M, Noma S, Itoh T, et al. Centrilobular lesions of the lungs: demonstration

by high-resolution CT and pathologic correlation. Radiology. 1986;161:641–5.

23. Staples CA, Gamsu G, Ray CS, Webb WR. High resolution computed tomography and lung function in asbestos-exposed workers with normal chest radiographs. Am Rev Respir Dis. 1989;139:1502–8.

24. Begin R, Ostiguy G, Fillion R, Colman N. Computed tomography in the early detection of silicosis. Am Rev Respir Dis. 1991;144:697–705.

25. Bergin C, Bell D, Coblentz C, et al. Sarcoidosis: correlation of pulmonary parenchymal pattern at CT with results of pulmonary function tests. Radiology. 1989;171:619–24.

26. Harrison NK, Glanville AR, Strickland B, Haslam PL, Corrin B, Addis BJ, et al. Pulmonary involvement in systemic sclerosis: the detection of early changes by thin section CT scan, bronchoalveolar lavage and 99mTc-DTPA clearance. Respir Med. 1989;83(5):403–14.

27. Schurawitzki H, Stiglbauer R, Graninger W, Herold C, Polzleitner D, Burghuber OC, et al. Interstitial lung disease in progressive systemic sclerosis: high-resolution CT versus radiography. Radiology. 1990;176(3):755–9.

28. Hansell D, Moskovic E. High-resolution computed tomography in extrinsic allergic alveolitis. Clin Radiol. 1991;43:8–12.

29. Silver S, Müller N, Miller R, Lefcoe M. Hypersensitivity pneumonitis: evaluation with CT. Radiology. 1989;173:441–5.

30. Aberle DR, Gamsu G, Ray CS. High-resolution CT of benign asbestos-related diseases: clinical and radiographic correlation. AJR Am J Roentgenol. 1988; 151(5):883–91.

31. Lynch DA, Rose CS, Way D, King TJ. Hypersensitivity pneumonitis: sensitivity of high-resolution CT in a population-based study. Am J Roentgenol. 1992;159: 469–72.

32. Mathieson JR, Mayo JR, Staples CA, Müller NL. Chronic diffuse infiltrative lung disease: comparison of diagnostic accuracy of CT and chest radiography. Radiology. 1989;171(1):111–6.

33. Swensen S, Aughenbaugh G, Myers J. Diffuse lung disease: diagnostic accuracy of CT in patients undergoing surgical biopsy of the lung. Radiology. 1997; 205:229–34.

34. Hunninghake GW, Zimmerman MB, Schwartz DA, King TE, Lynch J, Hegele R, et al. Utility of a lung biopsy for the diagnosis of idiopathic pulmonary fibrosis. Am J Respir Crit Care Med. 2001;164(2):193–6.

35. Tung KT, Wells AU, Rubens MB, Kirk JM, du Bois RM, Hansell DM. Accuracy of the typical computed tomographic appearances of fibrosing alveolitis. Thorax. 1993;48(4):334–8.

36. Lynch D, Newell J, Logan P, King T, Müller N. Can CT distinguish idiopathic pulmonary fibrosis from hypersensitivity pneumonitis? AJR Am J Roentgenol. 1995;165:807–11.

37. Hunninghake GW, Lynch DA, Galvin JR, Gross BH, Müller N, Schwartz DA, et al. Radiologic findings are strongly associated with a pathologic diagnosis of usual interstitial pneumonia. Chest. 2003;124(4):1215–23.

38. Raghu G, Mageto YN, Lockhart D, Schmidt RA, Wood DE, Godwin JD. The accuracy of the clinical diagnosis of new-onset idiopathic pulmonary fibrosis and other interstitial lung disease: a prospective study. Chest. 1999;116(5):1168–74.

39. Bonelli FS, Hartman TE, Swensen SJ, Sherrick A. Accuracy of high-resolution CT in diagnosing lung diseases. AJR Am J Roentgenol. 1998;170(6):1507–12.

40. Nishimura K, Izumi T, Kitaichi M, Nagai S, Itoh H. The diagnostic accuracy of high-resolution computed tomography in diffuse infiltrative lung diseases. Chest. 1993;104(4):1149–55.

41. Sumikawa H, Johkoh T, Ichikado K, Taniguchi H, Kondoh Y, Fujimoto K, et al. Usual interstitial pneumonia and chronic idiopathic interstitial pneumonia: analysis of CT appearance in 92 patients. Radiology. 2006;241(1):258–66.

42. Johkoh T, Müller NL, Cartier Y, Kavanagh PV, Hartman TE, Akira M, et al. Idiopathic interstitial pneumonias: diagnostic accuracy of thin-section CT in 129 patients. Radiology. 1999;211(2):555–60.

43. Sumikawa H, Johkoh T, Colby TV, Ichikado K, Suga M, Taniguchi H, et al. Computed tomography findings in pathological usual interstitial pneumonia: relationship to survival. Am J Respir Crit Care Med. 2008; 177(4):433–9.

44. Flaherty KR, Toews GB, Travis WD, Colby TV, Kazerooni EA, Gross BH, et al. Clinical significance of histological classification of idiopathic interstitial pneumonia. Eur Respir J. 2002;19(2):275–83.

45. Kim EY, Lee KS, Chung MP, Kwon OJ, Kim TS, Hwang JH. Nonspecific interstitial pneumonia with fibrosis: serial high-resolution CT findings with functional correlation. AJR Am J Roentgenol. 1999; 173(4):949–53.

46. Hartman TE, Primack SL, Swensen SJ, Hansell D, McGuinness G, Müller NL. Desquamative interstitial pneumonia: thin-section CT findings in 22 patients. Radiology. 1993;187(3):787–90.

47. Park JS, Lee KS, Kim JS, Park CS, Suh YL, Choi DL, et al. Nonspecific interstitial pneumonia with fibrosis: radiographic and CT findings in seven patients. Radiology. 1995;195(3):645–8.

48. Cottin V, Donsbeck A, Revel D, Loire R, Cordier J. Nonspecific interstitial pneumonia: individualization of a clinicopathologic entity in a series of 12 patients. Am J Respir Crit Care Med. 1998;158:1286–93.

49. Nagai S, Kitaichi M, Itoh H, Nishimura K, Izumi T, Colby TV. Idiopathic nonspecific interstitial pneumonia/fibrosis: comparison with idiopathic pulmonary fibrosis and BOOP. Eur Respir J. 1998;12(5):1010–9.

50. Johkoh T, Müller NL, Colby TV, Ichikado K, Taniguchi H, Kondoh Y, et al. Nonspecific interstitial pneumonia: correlation between thin-section CT findings and pathologic subgroups in 55 patients. Radiology. 2002;225(1):199–204.

51. Nishiyama O, Kondoh Y, Taniguchi H, Yamaki K, Suzuki R, Yokoi T, et al. Serial high resolution CT findings in nonspecific interstitial pneumonia/fibrosis. J Comput Assist Tomogr. 2000;24(1):41–6.

52. MacDonald S, Rubens M, Hansell D, Copley S, Desai S, du Bois R, et al. Nonspecific interstitial pneumonia and usual interstitial pneumonia: comparative appearances and diagnostic accuracy of high-resolution computed tomography. Radiology. 2001;221:600–5.

53. Travis WD, Hunninghake G, King Jr TE, Lynch DA, Colby TV, Galvin JR, et al. Idiopathic nonspecific interstitial pneumonia: report of an American Thoracic Society project. Am J Respir Crit Care Med. 2008; 177(12):1338–47.

54. Epler GR, Colby TV, McLoud TC, Gaensler EA, Carrington CB. Bronchiolitis obliterans organizing pneumonia. N Engl J Med. 1985;312(3):152–8.

55. Costabel U, Teschler H, Schoenfeld B, Hartung W, Nusch A, Guzman J, et al. BOOP in Europe. Chest. 1992;102(1 Suppl):14S–20S.

56. Izumi T, Kitaichi M, Nishimura K, Nagai S. Bronchiolitis obliterans organizing pneumonia. Clinical features and differential diagnosis. Chest. 1992;102(3):715–9.

57. Müller NL, Colby TV. Idiopathic interstitial pneumonias: high-resolution CT and histologic findings. Radiographics. 1997;17(4):1016–22.

58. Alasaly K, Müller N, Ostrow DN, Champion P, FitzGerald JM. Cryptogenic organizing pneumonia. A report of 25 cases and a review of the literature. Medicine. 1995;74(4):201–11.

59. Haddock JA, Hansell DM. The radiology and terminology of cryptogenic organizing pneumonia. Br J Radiol. 1992;65(776):674–80.

60. Bartter T, Irwin RS, Nash G, Balikian JP, Hollingsworth HH. Idiopathic bronchiolitis obliterans organizing pneumonia with peripheral infiltrates on chest roentgenogram. Arch Intern Med. 1989;149(2):273–9.

61. Müller NL, Staples CA, Miller RR. Bronchiolitis obliterans organizing pneumonia: CT features in 14 patients. AJR Am J Roentgenol. 1990;154:983–7.

62. Kim SJ, Lee KS, Ryu YH, Yoon YC, Choe KO, Kim TS, et al. Reversed halo sign on high-resolution CT of cryptogenic organizing pneumonia: diagnostic implications. AJR Am J Roentgenol. 2003;180(5):1251–4.

63. Polverosi R, Maffesanti M, Dalpiaz G. Organizing pneumonia: typical and atypical HRCT patterns. Radiol Med. 2006;111(2):202–12.

64. Johkoh T, Müller NL, Pickford HA, Hartman TE, Ichikado K, Akira M, et al. Lymphocytic interstitial pneumonia: thin-section CT findings in 22 patients. Radiology. 1999;212(2):567–72.

65. American Thoracic Society/European Respiratory Society international multidisciplinary consensus classification of the idiopathic interstitial pneumonias. Am J Respir Crit Care Med. 2002;165(2):277–304.

66. Kim EA, Lee KS, Johkoh T, Kim TS, Suh GY, Kwon OJ, et al. Interstitial lung diseases associated with collagen vascular diseases: radiologic and histopathologic findings. Radiographics. 2002;22(Spec No):S151–65.

67. Murdoch J, Müller N. Pulmonary sarcoidosis: changes on followup examination. Am J Roentgenol. 1992; 159:473–7.

68. Brauner M, Grenier P, Mompoint D, Lenoir S, deCremoux HP. Pulmonary sarcoidosis: evaluation with high resolution CT. Radiology. 1989;172:467–71.

69. Hennebicque AS, Nunes H, Brillet PY, Moulahi H, Valeyre D, Brauner MW. CT findings in severe thoracic sarcoidosis. Eur Radiol. 2005;15(1):23–30.

70. Silva CI, Müller NL, Lynch DA, Curran-Everett D, Brown KK, Lee KS, et al. Chronic hypersensitivity pneumonitis: differentiation from idiopathic pulmonary fibrosis and nonspecific interstitial pneumonia by using thin-section CT. Radiology. 2008;246(1):288–97.

71. Remy-Jardin M, Remy J, Gosselin B, Becette V, Edme JL. Lung parenchymal changes secondary to cigarette smoking: pathologic-CT correlations. Radiology. 1993;186(3):643–51.

72. Holt R, Schmidt R, Godwin J, Raghu G. High resolution CT in respiratory bronchiolitis-associated interstitial lung disease. J Comput Assist Tomogr. 1993; 1993:46–50.

73. Park JS, Brown KK, Tuder RM, Hale VA, King Jr TE, Lynch DA. Respiratory bronchiolitis-associated interstitial lung disease: radiologic features with clinical and pathologic correlation. J Comput Assist Tomogr. 2002;26(1):13–20.

74. Nakanishi M, Demura Y, Mizuno S, Ameshima S, Chiba Y, Miyamori I, et al. Changes in HRCT findings in patients with respiratory bronchiolitis-associated interstitial lung disease after smoking cessation. Eur Respir J. 2007;29(3):453–61.

75. Brauner MW, Grenier P, Mouelhi MM, Mompoint D, Lenoir S. Pulmonary histiocytosis X: evaluation with high-resolution CT. Radiology. 1989;172:255–8.

76. Moore AD, Godwin JD, Müller NL, Naidich DP, Hammar SP, Buschman DL, et al. Pulmonary histiocytosis X: comparison of radiographic and CT findings. Radiology. 1989;172(1):249–54.

77. Kulwiec E, Lynch D, Aguayo S, Schwarz M, King Jr TE. Imaging of pulmonary histiocytosis X. Radiographics. 1992;12:515–26.

78. Koyama M, Johkoh T, Honda O, Tsubamoto M, Kozuka T, Tomiyama N, et al. Chronic cystic lung disease: diagnostic accuracy of high-resolution CT in 92 patients. AJR Am J Roentgenol. 2003;180(3):827–35.

79. Bergin CJ, Coblentz CL, Chiles C, Bell DY, Castellino RA. Chronic lung diseases: specific diagnosis by using CT. AJR Am J Roentgenol. 1989;152(6):1183–8.

80. Lenoir S, Grenier P, Brauner MW, Frija J, Remy JM, Revel D, et al. Pulmonary lymphangiomyomatosis and tuberous sclerosis: comparison of radiographic and thin-section CT findings. Radiology. 1990;175(2):329–34.

81. Aberle DR, Hansell DM, Brown K, Tashkin DP. Lymphangiomyomatosis: CT, chest radiographic, and functional correlations. Radiology. 1990;176(2):381–7.

82. Müller NL, Chiles C, Kullnig P. Pulmonary lymphangiomyomatosis: correlation of CT with radiographic and functional findings. Radiology. 1990; 175(2):335–9.
83. Rappaport D, Weisbrod G, Herman S, Chanberlain D. Pulmonary lymphangioleiomyomatosis: high-resolution CT findings in four cases. AJR Am J Roentgenol. 1989;152:961–4.
84. Sherrier RH, Chiles C, Roggli V. Pulmonary lymphangioleiomyomatosis: CT findings. AJR Am J Roentgenol. 1989;153(5):937–40.
85. Templeton PA, McLoud TC, Müller NL, Shepard JA, Moore EH. Pulmonary lymphangioleiomyomatosis: CT and pathologic findings. J Comput Assist Tomogr. 1989;13(1):54–7.
86. Avila NA, Kelly JA, Chu SC, Dwyer AJ, Moss J. Lymphangioleiomyomatosis: abdominopelvic CT and US findings. Radiology. 2000;216(1):147–53.
87. Avila NA, Dwyer AJ, Rabel A, Moss J. Sporadic lymphangioleiomyomatosis and tuberous sclerosis complex with lymphangioleiomyomatosis: comparison of CT features. Radiology. 2007;242(1): 277–85.
88. Chang AB, Masel JP, Masters B. Post-infectious bronchiolitis obliterans: clinical, radiological and pulmonary function sequelae. Pediatr Radiol. 1998; 28(1):23–9.
89. Lynch D, Brasch R, Hardy K, Webb W. Pediatric pulmonary disease: assessment with high-resolution ultrafast CT. Radiology. 1990;176:243–8.
90. Lynch D, Hay T, Newell Jr JD, Divgi V, Fan L. Pediatric diffuse lung disease: diagnosis and classification by high-resolution CT. AJR Am J Roentgenol. 1999;173:713–8.
91. Padley SP, Adler BD, Hansell DM, Müller NL. Bronchiolitis obliterans: high resolution CT findings and correlation with pulmonary function tests. Clin Radiol. 1993;47(4):236–40.
92. Worthy SA, Park CS, Kim JS, Müller NL. Bronchiolitis obliterans after lung transplantation: high-resolution CT findings in 15 patients. AJR Am J Roentgenol. 1997;169(3):673–7.
93. Reittner P, Müller NL, Heyneman L, Johkoh T, Park JS, Lee KS, et al. Mycoplasma pneumoniae pneumonia: radiographic and high-resolution CT features in 28 patients. AJR Am J Roentgenol. 2000;174(1): 37–41.
94. Akira M, Higashihara T, Sakatani M, Hara H. Diffuse panbronchiolitis: follow-up CT examination. Radiology. 1993;189(2):559–62.

Bronchoalveolar Lavage

3

Marjolein Drent and Catharina F.M. Linssen

Abstract

Bronchoalveolar lavage (BAL) explores large areas of the alveolar compartment. After the introduction as a research tool, BAL has been appreciated extensively for clinical applications in the field of opportunistic infections and diffuse interstitial lung diseases (DILDs). It is considered as a safe, minimally invasive procedure. In selected cases, BAL has become an accepted technique for establishing or ruling out a diagnosis with only a low risk of incorrect diagnosis. BAL fluid (BALF) analysis can be very helpful in the differential diagnosis. A grouping of features, an elevated total cell count, predominantly lymphocytes, together with a nearly normal percentage of eosinophils and polymorphonuclear neutrophils and the absence of plasma cells, distinguishes the most likely diagnosis of sarcoidosis from the most common DILD, extrinsic allergic alveolitis (EAA), nonspecific interstitial pneumonia, and idiopathic pulmonary fibrosis (IPF). Knowledge about disease presentation or activity at the time the BAL is performed as well as the smoking status and possible history of occupational and/or environmental exposures is crucial for adequate interpretation of individual BALF analysis results. In contrast, the usefulness of BAL in the management and prediction of the prognosis of a certain disorder is, so far, rather controversial.

Keywords

Alveolitis • Bronchoalveolar lavage • Differential diagnosis • Interstitial lung diseases • Extrinsic allergic alveolitis • Hypersensitivity pneumonitis • Pulmonary fibrosis • Sarcoidosis

M. Drent (✉)
Respiratory Medicine, ild care consultancy,
Maastricht University Medical Centre (MUMC+),
Maastricht, The Netherlands
e-mail: ildcare@gmail.com

C.F.M. Linssen
Department of Medical Microbiology,
Maastricht University Medical Centre (MUMC+),
Maastricht, The Netherlands

R.P. Baughman and R.M. du Bois (eds.), *Diffuse Lung Disease: A Practical Approach*,
DOI 10.1007/978-1-4419-9771-5_3, © Springer Science+Business Media, LLC 2012

Introduction

Bronchoalveolar lavage (BAL) – an easily performed and well-tolerated procedure – can retrieve cells, solutes, and other substances from the lower respiratory tract which can aid in the assessment of the health status of the lung [1–4]. When applied according to standardized protocols and considered in the context of other information (gained from conventional ancillary diagnostic tests combined with a thorough clinical evaluation), BAL can be very useful in the diagnostic workup of diffuse infiltrative lung disease. In selected cases, BAL has the benefit of avoiding more invasive diagnostic procedures, such as tissue biopsies. Even when not diagnostic, BAL is often supportive of a specific diagnosis. Moreover, the analysis results may be inconsistent with the suspected diagnosis, and then focus attention on more appropriate, further investigations. In that case, a biopsy should be considered as the final diagnostic step. Pulmonary diseases including diffuse interstitial lung diseases (DILDs) have traditionally been evaluated by laboratory tests, lung function tests, imaging procedures, and tissue biopsies. Identifying the underlying disorder poses a significant challenging task for the clinician and requires a multidisciplinary approach with optimal resources. These disorders may be of infectious, noninfectious immunologic, malignant, environmental, or occupational etiology. To secure an accurate diagnosis a thorough history is essential as it may identify a potential etiological factor (e.g., drug reaction, environmental and/or occupational exposures). Lung parenchymal evaluation by high-resolution CT scanning (HRCT) of the chest may provide virtually diagnostic images in certain forms of DILDs. The differential diagnosis rests on the clinician's interpretation of the patient's history, additional tests including BAL and, if necessary, tissue sampling. Provided that its limitations are kept in mind, there appears to be a place for BAL in the evaluation of DILDs. The pattern of inflammatory cells may be helpful in narrowing the differential diagnosis [1–3]. In this chapter, the potential practical value of BAL in the diagnostic workup of DILD will be discussed.

Clinical Usefulness of BAL

In the diagnostic workup of specific DILDs, the additional usefulness of BAL fluid (BALF) analysis has been widely appreciated [1–3, 5]. BALF components can be obtained and these findings can be compared with those in blood. An advantage of using BALF (rather than blood) is the fact that the constituents in BALF are produced on site (within the lung) [1–3, 5] which makes it possible to reconstruct the actual situation within the alveoli. Furthermore, it was anticipated that the cellular components of BALF could be used in the prediction of therapy response and/or prognosis [6–8]. These possible uses of BAL are, however, controversial and the most critically discussed aspects of BAL.

Diagnostic Applications of BALF

Thorough clinical assessment should be considered as the key diagnostic procedure. Even when lung biopsy is performed, an accurate diagnosis is dependent on optimal usage of all available clinical information [9]. When evaluating a patient with suspected DILD the diagnostic approach should include:

- Full (medical) history including all available details about possible occupational and/or environmental exposures
- Physical examination, assessing whether the disorder is multisystemic (skin lesions, arthralgia, ocular inflammation)
- Lung function tests and evaluation of arterial blood gases
- Chest radiography and often a HRCT scan
- Selected blood tests where appropriate, including autoantibodies, precipitins, ANCA, angiotensin converting enzyme (ACE), lactate dehydrogenase (LDH), and interleukin (IL)-2R

If these do not establish a likely diagnosis, more invasive diagnostic tests are required and include:

- BAL
- Transbronchial lung biopsy
- Surgical lung biopsy

Bronchoalveolar Lavage Procedure and Confounding Factors

In general, BAL is a safe, noninvasive and generally well-tolerated procedure. Most of the reported side effects are closely related to the endoscopic procedure, volume, and temperature of the instilled fluid [1, 10]. Common complications or side effects associated with the lavage itself include coughing during the procedure, transient fever, chills, and marked malaise occurring some hours after the performance of the BAL. Although mortality has been associated with BAL, the overall complication rate of BAL was reported to be less than 3%, compared to 7% when combined with transbronchial biopsies [1, 10]. Various technical aspects of BAL are critical in obtaining representative samples [11]. Some intrinsic variability of the BAL procedure and results of the interpretation of the BALF profile can be limited by using a standard approach. The use of guidelines and recommendations for a standardized approach regarding the procedure as well as processing the material and use of central laboratories has reduced variations in obtaining samples and analyzing and interpreting data. Attempts have been made to set up a framework for the different steps of the procedure, such as the amount and temperature of fluid injected, the number of aliquots used (usually 4 of 50 or 60 ml), the "dwelling time," and aspiration pressure (low pressure wall suction (<60 mmHg)) [12]. The basic goal is to ensure that the injected fluid reaches the appropriate pathological area. In addition, the aspirate has to be a representative sample, containing cells and solutes, reflecting the pathophysiological process of the inflammation. In general, fluid obtained at one site is representative for the whole lung as inflammation in DILD is not limited to one site. While this is true, for example, in sarcoidosis, differences in lavage population have been reported in studies of patients with idiopathic pulmonary fibrosis (IPF). Several groups have made specific recommendations about the acquiring and handling of BAL [10–12]. Table 3.1 summarizes various aspects of the procedure which might influence the BALF analysis results. The position of the patient can affect the lavage, and gravity may impede lavage return from more gravity-dependent lung regions. From an anatomic point of view, the middle lobe or lingula is most convenient to access, and, therefore, routinely used. However, review of the chest CT scan may help in selecting the best areas

Table 3.1 Aspects affecting BAL fluid analysis results

Source of variability	US BAL cooperative [10]	ERS 1999 [11, 12]	ATS Statement 2011 [13]; in press
Disease process itself	Stated	State underlying disease	State underlying disease
Suction pressure during the procedure	"Gently" aspirate by handheld syringe	Keep to a minimum (25–100 mmHg)	Keep below 100 mmHg. Avoid visible airway collapse
Handling of fluid: filtered/ nonfiltered; concentrated	No comment	State technique specifically	No filtering with gauze
Volume instilled	240 ml	Instill at least 100 ml	Instill at least 100 ml
Handling of first aliquot recovered	Pooled all samples	Specify	Pool all samples unless specified
Number of aliquots	Four	Specify and standardize	Specify and standardize
Position of patient	Semirecumbent	Specify	Specify
Area that is lavaged	Right middle lobe/lingula	Specify	Specify
Number of areas lavaged	One	Specify	Specify
Variability of lavage return	Discontinued lavage if difference between instilled and aspirated was >100 ml	Report volume and percent of fluid returned. Establish minimal percent recovered	Report volume and percent of fluid returned. At least 5% of instilled volume must be recovered
Reporting acellular components	Report per ml of fluid recovered	Report per ml of fluid recovered	Report per ml of fluid recovered
Sample storage	Specified	Specify	Specify

to be lavaged. It has been shown that similar results for BAL are usually seen in different lobes in sarcoidosis patients but not in cases of pulmonary fibrosis [14]. For example, lavage performed in an area with extensive honeycombing will yield a smaller return of fluid and different cells than a lavage that is performed in an area of ground glass changes. In general, it is advisable to avoid areas of extensive honeycombing. This is similar to the logic of avoiding these end-stage areas when performing an open lung biopsy. In localized disease, however, such as malignant lesions and infectious lesions, lavage at the site of abnormality is mandatory [12].

Confounding Factors

The epithelial cell layer is vulnerable to trauma. Damage caused by insertion of the fiberoptic bronchoscope into the airways may result in a number of confounding aspects including an increase of the amount of erythrocytes in the BALF. Repeated lavage within a few days may reveal increased neutrophils as a result of the previous lavage. Some effects are simply due to the bronchoscopy itself, while others are more likely to occur as a result of the BAL or personal characteristics of the patient like smoking, age, and/or drug-use. Cigarette smoking influences the recovery of the fluid, the viability and quantity of the cells, as well as amount of solutes. Smoking has been shown to adversely affect the alveolar microenvironment both in health and disease. Smokers tend to have more alveolar macrophages (AMs) and neutrophils in their BALF. There are often 10- to 100-fold more macrophages retrieved in smokers compared to nonsmokers. Since the cellular BALF population is usually reported as a percentage of retrieved cells, this absolute increase in macrophages will lead to a proportional drop in the percentage of lymphocytes. These macrophages often contain pigmented material related to the inhaled smoke. The macrophages are often activated, releasing increased amounts of oxygen free radicals, for example. To date in extrinsic allergic alveolitis (EAA), the cellular profile in BALF was found to be related to the time between termination of antigen exposure and

the actual performance of BAL. The different phases of the immune responses involved in EAA are reflected in a varying composition of the cellular profile within the BALF.

Processing of BALF

The retrieved BALF is prepared for total and differential cell counts. Moreover, the obtained cells can be evaluated by cytological techniques and immunohistochemical procedures.

Cell Counting

Cell counts can be performed by a hemacytometer and should be performed on unconcentrated samples. For differential cell count, most laboratories prepare the slides using a cytocentrifuge. Since cytocentrifugation speed and duration can affect the mean lymphocyte and macrophage counts of BALF, a standardized protocol has been proposed using the following conditions: speed: 650 rpm, time: 10 min, acceleration rate: low [15]. Cytocentrifuge-prepared slides are usually stained with Wright's or May-Grünwald-Giemsa (MGG) stains [12] which are excellent for the identification of leukocytes and macrophages. However, both Wright and MGG stains render nuclear features in less detail as compared to Papanicolaou stains and are therefore less suitable for the detection of malignancy and viral inclusion bodies. Rapid substitutes are available, such as the Dif-Quik stain. This stain, however, is not able to stain mast cells [12]. In addition to the usual MGG staining, which allows enumeration of cells containing intracellular microorganisms, special stains and culture of BALF samples have increased the accuracy of diagnosing (opportunistic) infections [16].

Immunohistochemistry

The use of immunologic markers allows staining for cell markers. These are most commonly performed on lymphocytes. The T cell is the most common lymphocyte found in BALF. Studies of the CD4 and CD8 positive cells can be performed on cytocentrifuge-prepared slides. Another common method is performing flow cytometry, but this method usually requires at least a million cells for an adequate analysis. The most common application of the CD4:CD8 ratio has been in sarcoidosis and EAA. Initial reports concentrated on the increased CD4:CD8 ratio seen in sarcoidosis and the low ratio seen in EAA [17]. However, it is clear that many patients with sarcoidosis have normal or even reduced CD4:CD8 ratio [17]. In addition, some cases of EAA have been reported to have normal or elevated CD4:CD8 ratios [18]. While some feel that CD4:CD8 ratios add considerably to the diagnostic reliability of BAL [19], others feel that CD4:CD8 ratios can provide prognostic information [17]. In cases of possible lymphoma, B cell markers such as lambda and kappa surface membrane immunoglobulin can be performed. The presence of a high proportion of either kappa or lambda implies a monoclonal population, usually indicating lymphoma or leukemia in the lung [20]. Because of autofluorescence of macrophages, immunochemistry is less commonly used for markers of macrophages.

Cellular BALF Features

In healthy, nonsmoking controls, BALF samples contain 80–90% AMs, 5–15% lymphocytes (Lym), 1–3% polymorphonuclear neutrophils (PMNs), <1% eosinophils (Eos), and <1% mast cells (MC) [10]. Within the lung, all these cell populations can act as inflammatory cells. In patients with DILD, marked changes in cell yield and cell differentiation may occur (Table 3.2). The presence of squamous epithelial cells in BALF is an indication of oropharyngeal contamination [21],

Table 3.2 Cellular bronchoalveolar lavage fluid (BALF) profile characteristics of the most common (diffuse) lung diseases

Associated diseases	AMs	Lym	PMNs	Eos	PC	MC	RPII	CD4:CD8 ratio
Noninfectious diseases								
Sarcoidosis		+	=	=/+	0	=/+	0	=/+/–
Extrinsic allergic alveolitis	FAM	+	+	=/+	0/1	++	0/1	–/=
Drug-induced pneumonitis	FAM	++	+	+	0/1	++	0/1	–/=
Idiopathic pulmonary fibrosis		+	+/++	+	0	+	0/1	=
COP	FAM	+	+	+	0/1	=/+	0/1	–
Eosinophilic pneumonia		+	=	++	0/1	=/+	0/1	–
Alveolar proteinosis	FAM	+	=	=	0	=	0	+/=
Connective tissue disorders		+	=/+	=/+	0	=/+	0	=/+/–
Diffuse alveolar hemorrhage	Fe+++	=/+	+	=/+	0	=	0/1	=
Acute interstitial pneumonia	Fe++	=/+	++	=/+	0/1	=	0	=
ARDS	Fe+	+	++	+	0	=/+	0/1	–/=
Asthma		=	=	+	0	=	0	=
Malignancies								
Hematologic malignancies		+	+	=/+	0	=/+	0	–/=
Bronchus carcinoma		=	=	=	0	+/=	0	–/=
Lymphangitis carcinomatosa		+	+/=	+/=	0/1	+/=	0	+/=
Infectious diseases								
Ventilator-associated pneumonia	FAM	=	++	=	0	=	0/1	=
Pneumocystis pneumonia		=/+	+	+/–	0/1	=	0/1	=
Viral pneumonia		=	++	=	0	=	0/1	=/–
Aspiration pneumonia	FAM	=	++	=	–	=	0/1	=/–

+ and ++, increased; =, normal; –, decreased; 0, not present; 1, present; AMs, alveolar macrophages; ARDS, adult respiratory distress syndrome; COP, cryptogenic organizing pneumonia; Eos, eosinophils; Lym, lymphocytes; MC, mast cells; PC, plasma cells; PMNs, polymorphonuclear neutrophils; Fe, iron stain; RPII, reactive type II pneumocytes; FAM, foamy alveolar macrophages while the presence of, excessive amounts of, bronchial epithelial cells point towards bronchial contamination. In both cases, the differential cell count, the quantitative culture, and the sensitivity for detection of possible pathogenic microorganisms (for instance, *Pneumocystis jiroveci*) can be negatively influenced.

Alveolar Macrophages

The dominant cell type, in BALF of a healthy person, is the AMs. The cytoplasm of these cells is pale and may contain phagocytized material such as hemosiderin, cell fragments, carbon, or other foreign body material. Dust particles in AMs or elevated asbestos body counts in BALF and/or the presence of birefringent material or inclusion bodies point towards dust or fiber exposure that may cause illness [22]. In diffuse alveolar hemorrhage (DAH), for instance, BAL is the method of choice for diagnosing alveolar bleeding. BALF taken from these patients show free red blood cells and AMs which contain phagocytized hemosiderin (iron-positive macrophages) [23]. Foamy or "lipid-laden" AMs are macrophages that display clear and complete cytoplasm vacuolization. Although this finding usually is nonspecific, it might be indicative of EAA, hypersensitivity pneumonitis (HP), drug-induced pneumonitis, or lipoid pneumonia either caused by injection or inhalation of oil substrates. In pulmonary alveolar proteinosis, BALF analysis has a sensitivity approaching 100% making the need of biopsy obsolete in most cases. The macroscopic appearance of the fluid is milky and turbid. Light microscopy reveals acellular oval bodies, few and "foamy" macrophages, and a dirty background due to large amounts of amorphous debris [23]. Occasionally, especially in TH1-mediated disorders, multinucleated giant AMs can be found in BALF [1]. Macrophages retrieved by BAL may be activated and released among other cytokines and oxygen free radicals. However, these products of AMs and other airway cells have not proved to be useful in the differential diagnosis of DILD or in evaluating therapy.

Lymphocytes

Mature Lym are the smallest nucleated cells in BALF. They contain a relatively large nucleus and little cytoplasm. Activated Lym are larger than mature Lym and contain more cytoplasm. The percentage in Lym present in BALF can be increased in a number of DILD. Granulomatous lung inflammatory disorders such as sarcoidosis and EAA, associated either with a drug reaction or inhalation of antigens causing a host response, may display similarities in clinical presentation. However, these latter disorders demonstrate a different cellular profile in BALF [24]. Clinical manifestations of sarcoidosis depend on the intensity of the inflammation and organ systems affected. In BALF an increased number of Lym, predominantly activated T-helper cells are present. As microbial causes of sarcoidosis continue to be sought, BAL specimens are helpful in this pursuit [25]. Diseases with an increased number of Lym in BALF can be further differentiated into those with an elevated, normal, or decreased CD4:CD8 ratio. However, neither the number of Lym nor the CD4:CD8 ratio in BALF is specific features of any lung disease [6, 7, 19]. In a fresh wet mount BALF cell preparation, viewed under phase contrast microscopy, from a patient with active sarcoidosis, the appearance of Lym stuck to the surface of AMs – rosettes – is striking [2]. The cells adhere, do not fall off and are not phagocytized by the AM. In some cases, the alveolitis remains subclinical, whereas others present with pulmonary symptoms [26, 27]. This alveolitis reflects a local expression of a disseminated immunological reaction. Also, in case of extrathoracic manifestations such as ocular sarcoidosis and erythema nodosum features of an alveolitis suspected of sarcoidosis can be found, and, therefore, BALF analysis may be of additional diagnostic value. However, other DILD, such as Wegener's granulomatosis, as well as extrathoracic granulomatous diseases, such as Crohn's disease and primary biliary cirrhosis may demonstrate a (subclinical) lymphocyte alveolitis similar to sarcoidosis [28, 29]. There is no single cell type present in BALF that appears to be predictive for sarcoidosis or EAA. The combination of an elevated total cell count with predominantly Lym, together with a nearly normal percentage of Eos and PMNs and the absence of plasma cells in the BALF, points to sarcoidosis, rather than EAA, as the most likely diagnosis [30, 31]. In sarcoidosis, the majority of cases have an increased number of Lym and a normal amount of Eos and PMNs [24]. However, in severe cases of sarcoidosis, the number of PMNs can be increased as well [8]. In contrast, in BALF obtained from EAA patients not only the number of Lym but also the number of Eos and PMNs is increased substantially [24]. Moreover, the clinical manifestation of EAA shows considerable variation as it is related to the frequency and intensity of exposure to the causative agent. The cellular profile in BALF obtained from EAA patients is related to the time elapsed between termination of antigen exposure and the actual performance of BAL. The different phases of the immune responses involved in EAA are reflected in a varying composition of BALF samples [32]. Therefore, a model BALF cell profile does not exist in EAA. In the cellular variant of nonspecific interstitial pneumonia (NSIP), a lymphocytosis is observed [33]. However, an increase in Lym is quite rare in IPF, and other diseases or additional drug-induced reaction should then thoroughly be excluded [24].

Plasma Cells

Plasma cells, which have a similar appearance as Lym but with a nucleus which lies eccentric, are normally absent in BALF of healthy individuals. The presence of PC together with "foamy macrophages" and an increased number of Lym in BALF is very suggestive of the diagnosis of EAA or drug-induced HP [32]. Moreover, patients with plasma cells in BALF show signs of a more active alveolitis and a positive relation between the number of plasma cells and immunoglobulin levels in BALF. Other diseases that are associated with the presence of PC in BALF include bronchiolitis obliterans with organizing pneumonia (BOOP), cryptogenic organizing pneumonia (COP), chronic eosinophilic pneumonia (CEP), Legionella pneumonia, pneumocystis pneumonia (caused by *P. jiroveci*), and malignant non-Hodgkin's lymphoma [32].

Polymorphonuclear Neutrophils

The PMN has a characteristic segmented, multilobe nucleus, which contains densely clumped chromatin and no nucleoli, and the cytoplasm contains fine granules. Elevation of the BALF PMNs count may occur in several clinical conditions, such as IPF, asbestosis, adult respiratory distress syndrome (ARDS), Wegener's granulomatosis, and predominantly in pulmonary infections [10, 24, 33]. To date, the lavage profile alone is nonspecific in IPF [19, 33]. An increase in the number of PMNs in 70–90% of the cases, together with a mild increase in the number of Eos, and, sometimes an increase in Lym was reported [24]. However, the cellular BALF profile appeared to be quite different from the BALF profile assessed from patients suffering from disorders with similar clinical presentation, e.g., sarcoidosis or EAA [24]. The cellular profile of BALF samples from patients with a bacterial pneumonia generally differ significantly from samples of noninfectious etiology. The percentage PMNs present in BALF has been investigated as a potential marker to differentiate between infectious and noninfectious pulmonary diseases. Unfortunately, the various studies show discrepant results [34–36]. However, the general notion is that a BALF showing <50% PMNs excludes a bacterial pneumonia as the underlying diagnosis [34]. Notably, just one variable, namely the infected cell count was universally found to distinguish between bacterial infections and noninfectious disorders. Infected cells, also known as intracellular microorganisms or ICOs, are cells (mainly PMNs) that have phagocytized microorganisms. Various cutoff values have been proposed, varying from 25 to 1% [35, 36], the most commonly used cutoff value however is 2%. The extent of the increase of PMNs in BALF appears to be associated with severity and prognosis of several disorders [6, 8].

Eosinophils

Eosinophils show bilobed nuclei rather than the more complexly lobulated nuclei of PMNs. The most distinctive feature of Eos is the presence of orange colored cytoplasmatic granules. A predominant eosinophilia is indicative of an eosinophilic pneumonia, the Churg–Strauss syndrome, allergic bronchopulmonary aspergillosis, or a drug-induced eosinophilic lung reaction [37]. In addition, using monoclonal antibody techniques, pulmonary histiocytosis X can be identified by HRCT together with appropriate BALF analysis (CD1+ Langerhans cells >4% in 50% of patients) [2].

The diagnosis of lung eosinophilia can usually be made quickly and safely with BALF analysis (BALF differential with ≥25% Eos). An increased number of Eos can be seen in a variety of interstitial lung diseases, including EAA, IPF, collagen vascular disease-associated pulmonary fibrosis, and pneumocystis pneumonia [24, 33]. However, these conditions rarely include more than 10% Eos. Patients with a higher percentage of Eos most likely have an eosinophilic lung disease.

Mast Cells

Mast cells or basophils posses a single eccentrically located nucleus and membrane-bound (histamine-containing) cytoplasmatic granules, which stain brightly purple in a MGG stain. It has been suggested that lung MC play a role in the pathogenesis of lung inflammation, the stimulation of collagen deposition and fibrosis [38]. Release of mediators by MC may increase lung capillary permeability and allow increased access of inflammatory cells into the interstitium. These relatively large cells are found to be increased in BALF obtained from patients with EAA, especially in those cases suffering from the acute form [39]. Furthermore, increases in BALF MC have been reported in tuberculosis, malignant lymphomas, and IPF as well as asthma, and, although to a much lesser extent, in sarcoidosis. Moreover, the presence and raised levels of mediators released by MC was suggested to be indicative of more advanced or progressive disease.

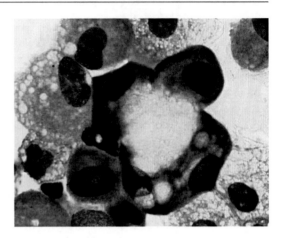

Fig. 3.1 This figure shows a cluster of reactive type II pneumocytes. The cells are already recognizable at low magnification since they are large cells with a small, *dark-colored* nucleus. They typically have *dark-colored* cytoplasm with large vacuoles and they often cluster together as shown in this figure. MGG stain, magnification ×1,000

Reactive Type II Pneumocytes

Type II pneumocytes are cells producing surfactant present at the inside of alveoli. Normally, these cells are not present in BALF or are indistinguishable from Ams. In case of serious pulmonary damage, they can be seen in BALF as reactive type II pneumocytes (RPII) (Fig. 3.1). RPII cells are large cells with a small, dark-colored nucleus. They have dark-colored cytoplasm which contains large vacuoles. They often cluster together giving them a gland-like appearance. These cells have been described in BALF from patients with ARDS [40], PCP [41], EAA, DAH, eosinophilic pneumonia, and bacterial pneumonia [41].

Additional Stain in DAH

DAH or the alveolar hemorrhage syndromes are associated with disorders such as Goodpasture's syndrome, Wegener's granulomatosis and other vasculitides, idiopathic pulmonary hemosiderosis, collagen vascular diseases, congestive heart failure, and drug reactions. As many syndromes may cause DAH, other clinical and laboratory features are required to establish the cause of the bleeding.

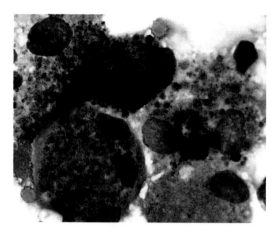

Fig. 3.2 The cells shown in this figure are alveolar macrophages which have phagocytized material (debris-loaded macrophages). This can be recognized by the *dark-colored* debris present within the cytoplasm. MGG stain, magnification ×1,000

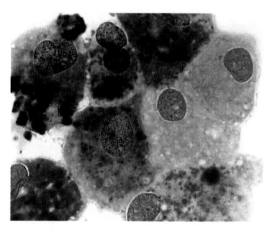

Fig. 3.3 This figure shows alveolar macrophages which stain positive in an iron stain (Perls' stain). To differentiate between debris and hemosiderin present in debris-loaded macrophages this stain can be useful. Macrophages which contain hemosiderin stain *bright blue* while the other cells remain *pink*. Perls' stain, magnification ×1,000

The occurrence of DAH can be established by BAL, even if the bleeding is occult by identifying numerous hemosiderin-laden AMs [29, 38], using an iron stain (Perls' stain, Figs. 3.2 and 3.3). The color of the BALF specimen obtained from these patients might change from light red (first fraction) to full red (last fraction). In contrast, in case of a proximal bleeding from the bronchi, the first fraction is dark red and the last one less intensive red.

In general, the differential cell count in BALF is not abnormal. However, many inclusion bodies representing fragmented red blood cells can be found in the AMs.

Disease-Specific Features in BALF

In a number of diseases such as alveolar proteinosis, pulmonary Langerhans cell histiocytosis, EAA and drug-induced pneumonitis, eosinophilic pneumonia, pulmonary hemosiderosis, occupationally induced diseases, and infections which can mimic diffuse lung disease, lavage can be diagnostic [1–3, 5, 42]. Lavage has proven its practical value in identifying infections such as bacterial pneumonia and opportunistic infections such as PCP, cytomegalovirus infections, fungal infections (*Cryptococcus neoformans, Aspergillus fumigatus*), and mycobacterial infections (*M. tuberculosis* and atypical mycobacteria). An additional value lies in differentiating these infectious disorders from alveolar hemorrhage, pulmonary involvement by an underlying malignancy, and drug-induced pneumonitis [21, 36, 42]. For some DILDs, abnormal BALF findings alone do not mean disease. Dairy farmers in Quebec with pulmonary symptoms, an abnormal chest roentgenogram, and a lavage showing increased Lym are felt to have HP [26, 27]. However, an asymptomatic farmer may have the same BALF findings, indicating focal lung sensitization [27]. These asymptomatic farmers do not necessarily progress to symptomatic disease, even after 6 years of follow-up [27]. The clinician therefore has to recognize that BALF findings are of limited prognostic value in this situation. In line with this, patients treated with amiodarone without pulmonary damage might have signs of a subclinical alveolitis demonstrated by the presence of "foamy alveolar macrophages" and a high amount of Lym and sometimes PC in their BALF. However, the early diagnosis of lung toxicity due to a certain drug such as amiodarone is crucial and mandates the immediate cessation of therapy with the drug and sometimes treatment with corticosteroids [43]. An early diagnosis of such pneumonitis is of interest because early drug cessation

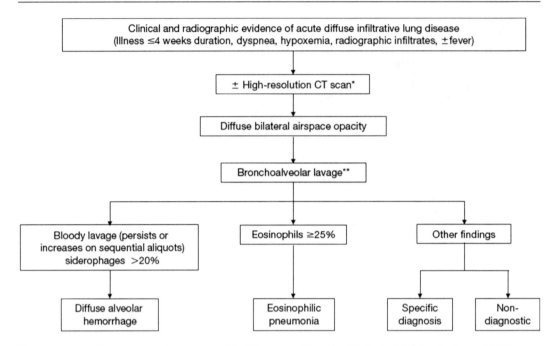

Fig. 3.4 Approach to a patient who presents with diffuse interstitial lung disease with less than 4 weeks of symptoms. The HRCT scan (*) may not be necessary but may be useful to identify the bronchoalveolar lavage (BAL) target area. In patients who can tolerate bronchoscopy, BAL (**; exclusion of infection mandated) should be performed

obviates installation of irreversible fibrosis. Moreover, it is important to consider each drug to be a potent agent, as not every drug is recognized to be liable to induce sudden and severe respiratory disorders [43]. The lavage profile alone is nonspecific in idiopathic interstitial pneumonias (IIP). However, the cellular BALF profile in IPF appears to be quite different from the profile assessed from patients suffering from disorders with similar clinical presentation, e.g., sarcoidosis or EAA. Moreover, signs of diffuse alveolar damage (DAD) and the presence of RPII indicative of more or less acute damage and acute interstitial pneumonia (AIP) can present in BALF [40, 41]. Distinguishing IPF from NSIP using the pattern of inflammatory cells in BALF is far more difficult. Patients with NSIP have a relative hypercellularity. A BAL lymphocytosis with a predominance of a suppressor subset of T Lym in BAL is more suggestive of NSIP, cellular variant than IPF [33]. In BALF obtained from a group of patients with the clinical features of IPF, Lym were no more frequent than in IPF. The clinical value of BALF analysis to stage or monitor

DILDs is of limited value. Increases in the number of PMNs and/or Eos have been associated with a worse prognosis, whereas a lymphocytosis in general has been noted to be associated with a better outcome and a greater responsiveness to corticosteroids. Given the value of BAL in diagnosing some specific diseases, bronchoscopy with lavage has often been recommended as part of the routine evaluation of interstitial lung disease [5]. The role of lavage in the evaluation of interstitial lung disease has recently been reviewed [4]. The evaluation is based on whether the presentation is acute or chronic. While in some cases, the duration of symptoms may not be clear, many patients with ILD have had gradually progressive symptoms over weeks or months. In patients with acute symptoms, one has to consider infection, pulmonary hemorrhage, and other conditions. This evaluation is shown in Fig. 3.4. For the usual patient with DILD, symptoms have been chronic. Figure 3.5 shows the proposed evaluation. There are several practical features included in this figure. For the patient with end-stage lung disease, invasive procedures may

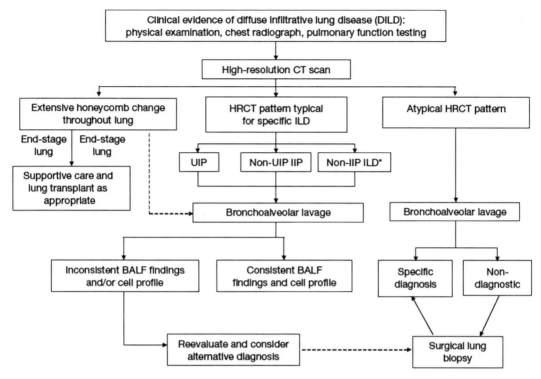

Fig. 3.5 Evaluation of a patient with chronic interstitial lung disease. In a patient with severe, advanced disease and extensive honeycombing, diagnostic procedures may be deemed too risky to perform. In other situations, the HRCT scan may be considered classic for a specific interstitial lung disease, such as idiopathic pulmonary fibrosis. Further evaluation, including bronchoalveolar lavage may be done to support the diagnosis and to rule out other processes. *Includes sarcoidosis, extrinsic allergic alveolitis (EAA), Langerhans' cell histiocytosis (LCH), eosinophilic pneumonia, etc. *BALF* bronchoalveolar lavage fluid, *IP* idiopathic interstitial pneumonia, *UIP* usual interstitial pneumonia

be of more risk than of potential benefit. In that case, further diagnostic procedures including bronchoscopy may not be performed [43].

References

1. Baughman RP, Drent M. Role of bronchoalveolar lavage in interstitial lung disease. Clin Chest Med. 2001;22:331–41.
2. Reynolds HY. Diagnostic and management strategies for diffuse interstitial lung disease. Chest. 1998;113:192–202.
3. Meyer KC. The role of bronchoalveolar lavage in interstitial lung disease. Clin Chest Med. 2004;25:637–49.
4. Reynolds HY. Present status of bronchoalveolar lavage in interstitial lung disease. Curr Opin Pulm Med. 2009;15:479–85.
5. American Thoracic Society. Idiopathic pulmonary fibrosis: diagnosis and treatment. International consensus statement. American Thoracic Society (ATS), and the European Respiratory Society (ERS). Am J Respir Crit Care Med. 2000;161:646–64.
6. Ward K, O'Connor C, Odlum C, et al. Prognostic value of bronchoalveolar lavage in sarcoidosis: the critical influence of disease presentation. Thorax. 1989; 44:6–12.
7. Fireman E, Vardinon N, Burke M, et al. Predictive value of response to treatment of T-lymphocyte subpopulations in idiopathic pulmonary fibrosis. Eur Respir J. 1998;11:706–11.
8. Drent M, Jacobs JA, de Vries J, et al. Does the cellular bronchoalveolar lavage fluid profile reflect the severity of sarcoidosis? Eur Respir J. 1999;13:1338–44.
9. du Bois RM. Diffuse lung disease: a view for the future. Sarcoidosis Vasc Diffuse Lung Dis. 1997;14:23–30.
10. Bronchoalveolar lavage constituents in healthy individuals, idiopathic pulmonary fibrosis, and selected comparison groups. The BAL Cooperative Group Steering Committee. Am Rev Respir Dis. 1990;141:S169–S202.
11. Haslam PL, Baughman RP. Report of ERS Task Force: guidelines for measurement of acellular components and standardization of BAL. Eur Respir J. 1999;14:245–8.

12. Klech H, Pohl WR. Technical recommendations and guidelines for bronchoalveolar lavage (BAL): report of the European Society of Pneumonology Task Group on BAL. Eur Respir J. 1989;2:561–85.

13. Meyer KC, Raghu G, Baughman RP, et al. The clinical utility of bronchoalveolar lavage cellular analysis in interstitial lung disease: an international consensus statement. Am J Respir Crit Care Med 2011; in press.

14. Garcia JG, Wolven RG, Garcia PL, et al. Assessment of interlobar variation of bronchoalveolar lavage cellular differentials in interstitial lung diseases. Am Rev Respir Dis. 1986;133:444–9.

15. De Brauwer EI, Jacobs JA, Nieman F, et al. Cytocentrifugation conditions affecting the differential cell count in bronchoalveolar lavage fluid. Anal Quant Cytol Histol. 2000;22:416–22.

16. De Brauwer E, Jacobs J, Nieman F, et al. Test characteristics of acridine orange, Gram, and May-Grunwald-Giemsa stains for enumeration of intracellular organisms in bronchoalveolar lavage fluid. J Clin Microbiol. 1999;37:427–9.

17. Drent M, Grutters JC, Mulder PG, et al. Is the different T helper cell activity in sarcoidosis and extrinsic allergic alveolitis also reflected by the cellular bronchoalveolar lavage fluid profile? Sarcoidosis Vasc Diffuse Lung Dis. 1997;14:31–8.

18. Ando M, Konishi K, Yoneda R, Tamura M, et al. Difference in the phenotypes of bronchoalveolar lavage lymphocytes in patients with summer-type hypersensitivity pneumonitis, farmer's lung, ventilation pneumonitis, and bird fancier's lung: report of a nationwide epidemiologic study in Japan. J Allergy Clin Immunol. 1991;87:1002–9.

19. Welker L, Jorres RA, Costabel U, et al. Predictive value of BAL cell differentials in the diagnosis of interstitial lung diseases. Eur Respir J. 2004;24:1000–6.

20. Keicho N, Oka T, Takeuchi K, et al. Detection of lymphomatous involvement of the lung by bronchoalveolar lavage. Application of immunophenotypic and gene rearrangement analysis. Chest. 1994;105:458–62.

21. Jacobs JA, De Brauwer EI, Ramsay G, et al. Detection of non-infectious conditions mimicking pneumonia in the intensive care setting: usefulness of bronchoalveolar fluid cytology. Respir Med. 1999;93:571–8.

22. Drent M, Mansour K, Linssen C. Bronchoalveolar lavage in sarcoidosis. Semin Respir Crit Care Med. 2007;28:486–95.

23. Costabel U, Guzman J, Bonella F, et al. Bronchoalveolar lavage in other interstitial lung diseases. Semin Respir Crit Care Med. 2007;28:514–24.

24. Drent M, Jacobs JA, Cobben NA, et al. Computer program supporting the diagnostic accuracy of cellular BALF analysis: a new release. Respir Med. 2001;95:781–6.

25. Drake WP, Newman LS. Mycobacterial antigens may be important in sarcoidosis pathogenesis. Curr Opin Pulm Med. 2006;12:359–63.

26. Cormier Y, Belanger J, LeBlanc P, et al. Bronchoalveolar lavage in farmers' lung disease: diagnostic and physiological significance. Br J Ind Med. 1986;43:401–5.

27. Laviolette M, Cormier Y, Loiseau A, et al. Bronchoalveolar mast cells in normal farmers and subjects with farmer's lung. Diagnostic, prognostic, and physiologic significance. Am Rev Respir Dis. 1991;144:855–60.

28. Camus P, Colby TV. The lung in inflammatory bowel disease. Eur Respir J. 2000;15:5–10.

29. Schnabel A, Reuter M, Gloeckner K, et al. Bronchoalveolar lavage cell profiles in Wegener's granulomatosis. Respir Med. 1999;93:498–506.

30. Drent M, van Velzen-Blad H, Diamant M, et al. Relationship between presentation of sarcoidosis and T lymphocyte profile. A study in bronchoalveolar lavage fluid. Chest. 1993;104:795–800.

31. Drent M, Wagenaar S, van Velzen-Blad H, et al. Relationship between plasma cell levels and profile of bronchoalveolar lavage fluid in patients with subacute extrinsic allergic alveolitis. Thorax. 1993;48:835–9.

32. Drent M, van Velzen-Blad H, Diamant M, et al. Differential diagnostic value of plasma cells in bronchoalveolar lavage fluid. Chest. 1993;103:1720–4.

33. Nagai S, Kitaichi M, Itoh H, et al. Idiopathic nonspecific interstitial pneumonia/fibrosis: comparison with idiopathic pulmonary fibrosis and BOOP. Eur Respir J. 1998;12:1010–9.

34. Cobben NA, Jacobs JA, van Dieijen-Visser MP, et al. Diagnostic value of BAL fluid cellular profile and enzymes in infectious pulmonary disorders. Eur Respir J. 1999;14:496–502.

35. Allaouchiche B, Jaumain H, Dumontet C, et al. Early diagnosis of ventilator-associated pneumonia. Is it possible to define a cutoff value of infected cells in BAL fluid? Chest. 1996;110:1558–65.

36. Chastre J, Fagon JY. Ventilator-associated pneumonia. Am J Respir Crit Care Med. 2002;165:867–903.

37. Newman Taylor A. Pulmonary eosinophilia: the eosinophilic pneumonias. In: Olivieri D, editor. Interstitial lung diseases. Sheffield: European Respiratory Monograph; 2000. p. 206–25.

38. Cordier JF. Pulmonary vasculitis. Rev Med Interne. 2002;23:547s–8.

39. Pesci A, Rossi GA, Bertorelli G, et al. Mast cells in the airway lumen and bronchial mucosa of patients with chronic bronchitis. Am J Respir Crit Care Med. 1994;149:1311–6.

40. Grotte D, Stanley MW, Swanson PE, et al. Reactive type II pneumocytes in bronchoalveolar lavage fluid from adult respiratory distress syndrome can be mistaken for cells of adenocarcinoma. Diagn Cytopathol. 1990;6:317–22.

41. Linssen KC, Jacobs JA, Poletti VE, et al. Reactive type II pneumocytes in bronchoalveolar lavage fluid. Acta Cytol. 2004;48:497–504.

42. Meyer KC. Bronchoalveolar lavage as a diagnostic tool. Semin Respir Crit Care Med. 2007;28:546–60.

43. Costabel U, Uzaslan E, Guzman J. Bronchoalveolar lavage in drug-induced lung disease. Clin Chest Med. 2004;25:25–35.

Pathology of Diffuse Lung Disease

4

Thomas V. Colby and Kevin O. Leslie

Abstract

The most important aspect of the pathologic evaluation of diffuse lung disease is correlation of the findings with the clinical and radiologic features. This is emphasized throughout the chapter and numerous examples are given. Clinical and radiologic correlation, particularly with HRCT, improves the overall clinical diagnostic accuracy, as well as helping to hone pathologic interpretation and differential diagnosis. Such correlation is important in all lung biopsy samples, including surgical lung biopsies and even transbronchial biopsies. While in general a surgical lung biopsy is more likely to give a diagnosis, there are a number of situations where transbronchial biopsies are useful and these are outlined.

This chapter includes general comments on the finding of fibrosis, interstitial inflammation, acute lung injury, and granulomatous inflammation. The following entities are discussed: sarcoidosis, idiopathic pulmonary fibrosis/usual interstitial pneumonia, nonspecific interstitial pneumonia, interstitial lung disease associated with the collagen vascular diseases, vasculitic syndromes, alveolar hemorrhage syndromes, hypersensitivity pneumonitis, pulmonary alveolar proteinosis, lymphangioleiomyomatosis, bronchiolitis, pneumoconiosis, and drug reactions.

Keywords

Interstitial lung disease • Pathology • Transbronchial biopsy • Surgical lung biopsy • Lung biopsy • Bronchiolitis

T.V. Colby (✉)
Mayo Clinic Scottsdale, Scottsdale, AZ, USA
e-mail: colby.thomas@mayo.edu

K.O. Leslie
Department of Pathology, Division of Anatomic
Pathology, Mayo Clinic College of Medicine;
Laboratory Medicine and Pathology,
Mayo Clinic Arizona, Scottsdale, AZ, USA

R.P. Baughman and R.M. du Bois (eds.), *Diffuse Lung Disease: A Practical Approach*,
DOI 10.1007/978-1-4419-9771-5_4, © Springer Science+Business Media, LLC 2012

Introduction

Diffuse lung disease is necessarily approached in an integrated fashion with correlation of clinical, radiologic, and pathologic features. Depending upon on the disease entity, a diagnosis may be reached in a variety of ways, not all of which are on the basis of tissue biopsy. Thus, pathology is not always needed.

High-resolution CT scanning in the evaluation and diagnosis of diffuse lung disease is now an established part of clinical practice. Briefly, HRCT allows evaluation of a number of features that are not apparent in a tissue biopsy, such as distribution of disease within the chest cavity and extent of changes globally in the lungs. In some cases, HRCT allows a specific diagnosis with a degree of accuracy that approaches that of tissue biopsy and thus obviates the need for biopsy. Tissue biopsies, even surgical lung biopsies, are subject to sampling error (since they represent only a tiny portion of the total lung tissue) and thus may not be the gold standard, especially in cases in which HRCT has suggested a disease spectrum not sampled in the biopsy. Biopsies become a relative gold standard, complemented by the findings from HRCT. In practice, HRCT modifies the biopsy interpretation by the pathologist and vice versa in situations in which the features on biopsy lead to reinterpretation of the radiologic findings by the radiologist.

Tissue Sampling

Lung tissue can be sampled by a variety of cytologic and histologic techniques in patients with diffuse lung disease. While cytologic preparations allow a specific diagnosis in a small percentage of diffuse lung diseases (such as some infections, some neoplasms, and a few miscellaneous conditions), for the most part histology is required. Histologic specimens include endobronchial biopsies (BrBx), transbronchial biopsies (TBBx), video-assisted thoracic surgical biopsies (VATS Bx), and traditional open lung biopsy (OLBx). The last two are considered surgical lung biopsies.

Depending on the specific disease, any of these biopsy techniques may allow a definitive diagnosis, however overall, one is most likely to get a specific tissue diagnosis with a surgical lung biopsy. In general, small (endobronchial or transbronchial) biopsies may be diagnostic in diseases in which the histologic changes are unique or sufficiently characteristic that they may be appreciated even in tiny specimens. In addition, conditions that follow lymphatic routes (e.g., sarcoidosis, lymphangitic carcinoma) are relatively accessible to TBBx. Examples include certain infections, neoplasms, and diseases with unique histologic features such as lymphangioleiomyomatosis (LAM), pulmonary Langerhans cell histiocytosis, pulmonary alveolar proteinosis (PAP), and some others (see Table 4.1).

Table 4.1 Why TBBx is useful in selected conditions

Disease entity	Unique/specific histology	Characteristic histology	Lymphangitic
Pulmonary Langerhans cell histiocytosis	X		
Lymphangioleiomyomatosis	X		
Sarcoidosis		X	X
Cellular phase of Silicosis	X		X
Eosinophilic pneumonia		X	
Pulmonary alveolar proteinosis		X	
Lymphangitic carcinoma	X		X
Diffuse lymphomas	X		X
Some infection	X		
Amyloidosis	X		
Hypersensitivity pneumonitis		X	

In diseases that show patterns of inflammation and fibrosis (which is true for most of the idiopathic interstitial pneumonias), TBBx are only occasionally helpful. The findings are frequently abnormal, but they are not specific. Surgical lung biopsies allow recognition of patterns of inflammation and fibrosis that comprise the idiopathic interstitial pneumonias, and when histologic diagnosis is needed in these cases, surgical lung biopsy is usually necessary.

The usefulness (or lack thereof) of these various tissue biopsy techniques will be discussed for each of the disease entities covered in this chapter.

General Comments Regarding Histologic Findings

"*Fibrosis*" used in histologic descriptions includes a variety of patterns recognized by the pathologist. "Fibrosis" has often been used to include proliferations of fibroblastic tissue within airspaces (airspace organization, organizing pneumonia) or in the interstitium. Relatively little collagen is laid down in these settings and the term "*organization*" is more appropriate since it does not imply an end-stage irreversible process. This kind of fibroblastic proliferation often take the appearance of *organizing pneumonia* in which the organization is seen as intraluminal (either in small airways or alveoli) rounded polyps of granulation tissue. It is typically seen in cases of relatively recent lung injury and is considered a nonspecific reaction pattern.

"*Fibrosis*" has also been used for lung injury where collagen is deposited in the interstitium (see Fig. 4.11). Interstitial fibrosis is not synonymous with organization and usually implies irreversible collagen deposition. With marked interstitial deposition of collagen there is a significant derangement of lung architecture which often results in *honeycombing* in which airspaces are simplified into large architecturally abnormal cystic spaces with thick fibrous septa between them (see Figs. 4.4 and 4.5). The spaces are often lined by metaplastic bronchiolar-type inflammation

and contain pools of mucus with inflammatory cells. Not all marked interstitial fibrosis produces honeycomb change. In some instances, the fibrosis is dense and diffuse and replaces airspaces. In such instances smooth muscle metaplasia (as distinct from the normal muscle associated with airways and vessels) may be quite marked.

Interstitial infiltrate is used to describe inflammatory cellular infiltrates within the interstitium. These are usually mononuclear and comprised primarily of lymphocytes and plasma cells. The term "cellular interstitial pneumonia" may sometimes be used to describe this finding.

Inflammation in the lung may also be alveolar. *Alveolar space inflammation* most commonly includes macrophages, eosinophils, and neutrophils. Eosinophils and neutrophils commonly have associated exudates, including edema fluid, or fibrin. The presence of eosinophils is not that common in biopsy material and often suggests a relatively small list of conditions including asthma, eosinophilic pneumonia and related conditions, and pulmonary Langerhans' cell histiocytosis. In some instances, airspace foam cells are a dominant feature.

Diffuse alveolar damage (DAD) is common reflection of severe acute lung injury: edema, exudate, and hyaline membranes in airspaces in the earliest phases, interstitial and airspace organization in later phases. DAD has a number of causes and is considered a nonspecific reaction pattern of the lung to injury.

Acute Lung Injury (ALI) is a term that may be used by pathologists; it refers to the two most common patterns of recent lung injury: DAD and organizing pneumonia.

Type 2 cell proliferation (metaplastic alveolar lining cells) is a common nonspecific response to lung injury and rarely of diagnostic usefulness.

Like the alveolar parenchyma, *small airways* may show an inflammatory reaction that has a cellular and a mesenchymal component. Acute or chronic inflammatory cells may be involved with acute inflammatory cells being luminal in airway disease and chronic inflammatory cells being mural. The mesenchymal reaction may take the form of collagen deposition in the submucosa (with luminal narrowing as in constrictive bronchiolitis) or in

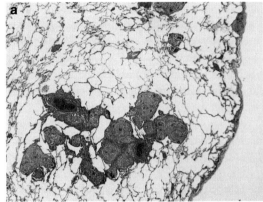

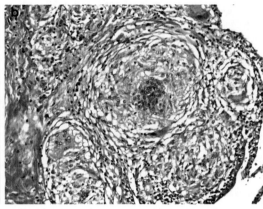

Fig. 4.1 Sarcoidosis. (**a**) There are coalescing, nonnecrotizing granulomas surrounding a bronchovascular bundle. Pleural granulomas are also noted (*upper right*). This represents a lymphatic distribution. (**b**) Higher power microscopy shows nonnecrotizing granulomatous inflammation surrounded by a cuff of fibrous tissue containing a modest numbers of lymphocytes

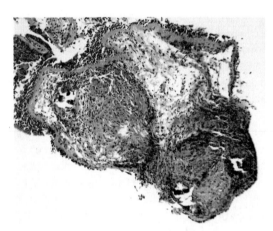

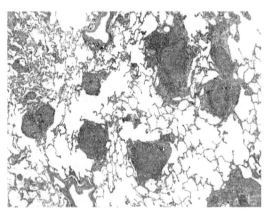

Fig. 4.2 Transbronchial biopsy in sarcoidosis. This endobronchial biopsy shows two granulomas in the bronchial submucosa. The *dark blue* material represents calcified Schaumann bodies, a common finding associated with sarcoid granulomas

Fig. 4.3 Disseminated *Mycobacterium avium* infection. There are scattered granulomas that do not show a distribution along lymphatic routes. They have a relatively prominent cuff of lymphocytes. The intervening lung tissue is relatively normal

the adventitial region (peribronchiolar scarring), or both. In the setting of asthma, smooth muscle proliferation may be a dominant finding.

A "*granuloma*" refers to an inflammatory structure containing epithelioid histiocytes. The best formed "classic" granulomas are seen in sarcoidosis and tuberculosis but less well-formed granulomas are encountered in a number of diffuse lung diseases (see Figs. 4.1–4.3), notably hypersensitivity pneumonitis (HP). In HP the granulomas are usually recognized as small relatively inconspicuous loose clusters of epithelioid histiocytes with or without associated giant cells (see Fig. 4.23). In some instances, the "granuloma" in HP manifests only as a loose cluster of giant cells.

Interpretation of Pathology Reports

Clinical practice settings differ in terms of the degree of interaction between clinicians and pathologists. In many situations, the clinician is confronted only with the pathology report and the case has not been discussed with the pathologist. The clinician is then faced with interpreting the report in light of the available clinical and radiologic data. Ideally the pathologist should have been apprised of these prior to completing the report.

When the clinician reads the pathology report, subtle clues are often picked up by the clinician that allows him/her to gauge the pathologist's confidence in the interpretation and diagnosis. Often the length of a pathology report is inversely proportional to the pathologist's confidence of diagnosis. A report that conveys only histologic findings (i.e., a descriptive diagnosis) rather than a definite pathologic of clinicopathologic diagnosis should also alert the clinician to the possibility that the pathologist may not be entirely confident of his/her interpretation. The confidence of the pathologist's interpretation plays a role in the issues discussed below.

There are a number of instances in which the pathology report is considered inadequate by the clinician and these should be dealt with on a case-by-case basis. When a histologic diagnosis (or the descriptive findings in the pathology report) does not fit with the clinical impression(s), the first thing to do is to make sure that the pathologist is aware of the history and what the specific questions are to be addressed in histologic interpretation. This may allow resolution of the problem with reassessment of the biopsy by the pathologist. Ideally the pathologist will make a histologic interpretation that ties together the histologic findings with the clinical and radiologic findings and suggest a clinicopathologic diagnosis that would then be confirmed by the clinician.

If the pathologist is clearly not conversant with the clinical conditions being considered and the pathology report does not allow the clinician to correlate the histologic findings with the clinical and radiologic findings, the clinician should consider getting additional histologic opinions. Additional opinions may also be needed in cases in which a histologic diagnosis that has been re-reviewed (and reconfirmed) still does not fit with the clinical findings.

Additional histologic opinions should also be considered when the clinical course does not fit with the expected clinical course for the clinicopathologic diagnosis that has been rendered.

Specific Entities

Sarcoidosis

Histologic Findings (Figs. 4.1 and 4.2)
- Coalescing nonnecrotizing granulomas along lymphatic routes in the pleura, septa, and along bronchovascular bundles.
- Vascular or airway involvement/invasion common. Bronchial mucosal involvement (seen on BrBx).
- Central fibrinoid necrosis of the granulomas in approximately 20% of the cases.
- Large lesions may hyalinize.
- Intervening lung tissue relatively normal.
- Granulomas may be surrounded by a variable degree of lamellar densely eosinophilic collagen with inconspicuous lymphocytic infiltrate.

Differential Diagnosis
Berylliosis, miliary granulomatous infections (including *Mycobacterium avium-intracellulare* in normal hosts – Fig. 4.3), HP, and miscellaneous conditions (drug reactions, neoplasms associated with granulomas, IV drug abuse, Sjogrens syndrome, pulmonary veno-occlusive disease, Churg–Strauss syndrome, bronchocentric granulomatosis, Wegener's granulomatosis).

Biopsy Diagnosis
BrBx useful, particularly if gross lesions apparent at bronchoscopy; transbronchial biopsy also useful; the full histologic features are best appreciated in open lung biopsies (note: BrBx/TBBx positive in up to 80% of cases with multiple biopsy samples).

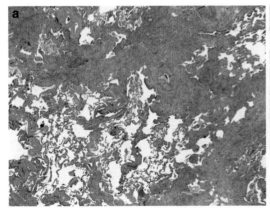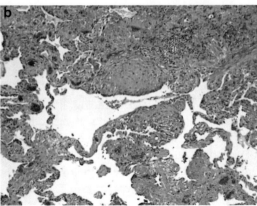

Fig. 4.4 Usual interstitial pneumonia. (**a**) There is a patchy fibrotic process with some regions of uninvolved lung tissue and some regions entirely destroyed by *dense pink* fibrous tissue. In some foci, paler bluish fibroblast foci are identified (see **b**). (**b**) Fibroblast foci (*center*) are recognizable by their convex shape and the presence of fibroblasts and increased mucopolysaccharide matrix imparting a *bluish* appearance

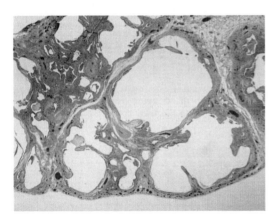

Fig. 4.5 Honeycomb change. The lung architecture is entirely destroyed by large abnormal airspaces lined by thick fibrous walls. No normal lung tissue is present

The presence of a solitary granuloma in biopsy material is much less specific than multiple granulomas showing the typical distribution and/or coalescence of sarcoidosis.

Caveats Regarding the Histology of Sarcoidosis

- Necrosis may be present in sarcoidosis.
- Miliary infections may lack necrosis.
- Polarizable birefringent calcium oxalates commonly present in sarcoid granulomas.
- Sampling error is an issue in BrBx and TBBx (20% or more of TBBx may miss the lesions).

- HRCT may be distinctive and complement the histologic identification of granulomas.
- Necrotizing sarcoid is very rare and a diagnosis usually made in retrospect after cultures are negative.

Idiopathic Pulmonary Fibrosis

Histologic Findings (Figs. 4.4 and 4.5)

- By current definition IPF shows usual interstitial pneumonia (UIP).
- Patchy fibrosis with tendency for subpleural and paraseptal location.
- Chronic scarring with architectural alteration (usually in the form of honeycombing).
- More active scarring in the form of fibroblast foci.
- Intervening lung tissue is commonly normal or shows minimal changes.
- Fibroblast foci distinct from airspace organization.

Differential Diagnosis

Many lung diseases are associated with fibrosis and thus the differential is broad. The main condition to be distinguished from UIP is nonspecific interstitial pneumonia (NSIP) which tends to lack the patchy involvement of the parenchyma seen in UIP and tends to have pathologic changes that are of similar age in contrast to the temporal heterogeneity (old scarring and more recent fibroblast foci) that characterize UIP.

Many other conditions may show some degree of interstitial fibrosis and honeycombing (with or without other histologic changes) including desquamative interstitial pneumonia, lymphocytic interstitial pneumonia, collagen vascular diseases (CVDs), drug reactions, pneumoconioses, sarcoidosis, pulmonary Langerhans' cell histiocytosis, chronic granulomatous infections, chronic aspiration, chronic HP, organized chronic eosinophilic pneumonia, organized DAD, chronic interstitial pulmonary edema/passive congestion, radiation, healed infectious pneumonias, pulmonary veno-occlusive disease, late stages of cryptogenic organizing pneumonia, and bronchiolar scarring. Some lesions with spindle cells may be confused with fibrosis (e.g., LAM, spindle cell tumors).

Biopsy Diagnosis

A surgical lung biopsy is required for the *histologic* identification of UIP (but may not be necessary for the clinical diagnosis of IPF if classic HRCT changes are present). TBBx are frequently abnormal but the findings are usually nonspecific.

Caveats Regarding UIP

- Biopsy should show a clear tendency to fibrosis and architectural destruction.
- Sampling error is an issue because of the patchy nature of the process.
- Since the scarring is worse in subpleural regions, wedges that do not go deep enough may show only honeycomb change.
- Biopsies, or portions thereof, may resemble NSIP.
- Some cases may show honeycombing/"end-stage lung" only (in which the pathologic diagnosis may be "honeycombing consistent with UIP").
- HRCT augments biopsy interpretation by showing extent of fibrosis and confirming presence of honeycombing.

- In UIP fibrosis far overshadows inflammation; UIP generally shows relatively little mononuclear cell infiltrate.
- In acute exacerbation of IPF, DAD or organizing is superimposed on the background fibrosis.

Nonspecific Interstitial Pneumonia

Histologic Findings (Figs. 4.6 and 4.7)

- Cellular variant of NSIP is characterized by diffuse mononuclear cell infiltrates of mild to moderate degree without centrilobular accentuation and without associated interstitial fibrosis.
- Fibrotic variant of NSIP shows interstitial fibrosis that is relatively diffuse and of uniform age with little or no honeycombing or fibroblast foci and variable cellular infiltrates.
- Focal airspace organization (organizing pneumonia) may be present.
- Granulomas, marked eosinophil infiltrate, extensive organization, and extensive honeycombing are strongly against the diagnosis of NSIP.

Differential Diagnosis

From the *clinical point of view* the histologic pattern of NSIP may be seen in drug reactions,

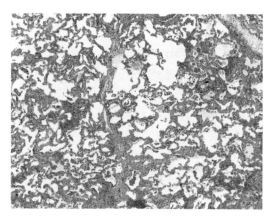

Fig. 4.6 Nonspecific interstitial pneumonia (NSIP). This example of cellular NSIP shows a diffuse mild interstitial mononuclear cell infiltrate without appreciable architectural distortion or fibrosis

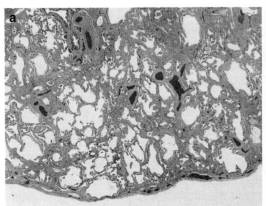

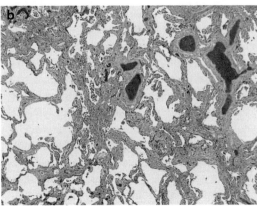

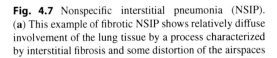

Fig. 4.7 Nonspecific interstitial pneumonia (NSIP). (**a**) This example of fibrotic NSIP shows relatively diffuse involvement of the lung tissue by a process characterized by interstitial fibrosis and some distortion of the airspaces without frank honeycomb change. (**b**) Higher power evaluation of the case shown in (**a**) shows the presence of interstitial fibrosis without marked architectural distortion

CVDs, HP, and as an idiopathic interstitial pneumonia.

Histologically the presence of inflammation and variable degrees of fibrosis lead to a differential diagnosis of UIP (when there is prominent fibrosis), organizing pneumonia (when airspace organization is prominent), HP without granulomas (in which case centrilobular accentuation of the inflammation may be present), and LIP (when the cellular infiltrate is dense). The features of NSIP overlap with many other conditions, including those listed in the differential diagnosis for UIP in the IPF section.

Biopsy Diagnosis

- The diagnosis of NSIP requires a surgical lung biopsy.

Caveats Regarding NSIP

- Sampling may be an issue since some portions of the lung tissue (or biopsy of other lobes) from patients with UIP may show NSIP.
- Diagnostic criteria for NSIP have been variable and have yet to be uniformly agreed upon.
- The diagnosis of NSIP has been used in a number of ways and one must know the source and context of the diagnosis.

Collagen Vascular Diseases

Histologic Findings

As a group, CVDs are associated with a variety of histologic changes in the lung that can be broadly grouped as diffuse parenchymal lung disease (Figs. 4.8–4.12), airway disease (Figs. 4.13 and 4.14), vascular disease (Fig. 4.15), pleural disease, nodular disease (Fig. 4.16), and (quite frequently) mixtures of these. Indirect respiratory effects and neoplasms also are recognized (see Table 4.1).

In contrast to idiopathic interstitial pneumonias, interstitial lung diseases in the CVDs are more likely to show lymphoid hyperplasia, prominent plasma cells, and to be difficult to classify (into a single pattern similar to an IIP) since they tend to show a mixture of patterns (e.g., both airway lesions and interstitial lesions together). The patterns encountered include: UIP, NSIP, DAD, organizing pneumonia, eosinophilic pneumonia, PAP, diffuse alveolar hemorrhage, diffuse lymphoid hyperplasia, lymphocytic interstitial pneumonia, amyloidosis, aspiration pneumonia, nodules, and apical fibrobullous disease.

Differential Diagnosis

- Depends on clinical and histologic findings (see Table 4.2).

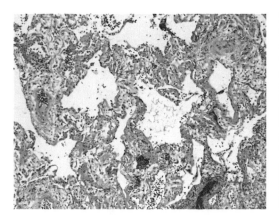

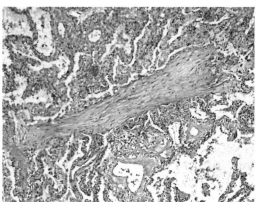

Fig. 4.8 Diffuse alveolar damage in SLE. The alveolar walls are edematous (*center*) and many are lined by a thin eosinophilic hyaline membrane. Some flocculant edema fluid is present in the alveolar spaces

Fig. 4.9 Organizing pneumonia in RA. There is edematous polypoid fibroblastic tissue cut longitudinally in an alveolar duct. The surrounding alveolar walls show non-specific mild inflammation, type 2 cell metaplasia, and some increase in alveolar macrophages

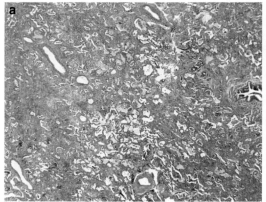

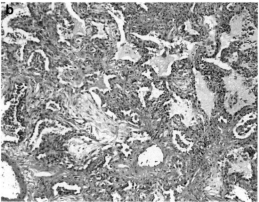

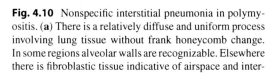

Fig. 4.10 Nonspecific interstitial pneumonia in polymyositis. (**a**) There is a relatively diffuse and uniform process involving lung tissue without frank honeycomb change. In some regions alveolar walls are recognizable. Elsewhere there is fibroblastic tissue indicative of airspace and interstitial organization. (**b**) Higher power evaluation of the case shown in (**a**) shows alveolar septal infiltrate by mononuclear cells, some widening and type 2 cell metaplasia, and foci of airspace organization/organizing pneumonia (*lower left center*, *upper right center*)

Biopsy Diagnosis

Interpretation of biopsies in CVDs depends on the clinical circumstances and what the question is. Clinical considerations may include CVD-associated thoracic disease, drug reaction, infection, or some other process. Surgical lung biopsy is necessary for pattern recognition in the case of CVD-associated ILD. Transbronchial biopsy (with or without bronchoalveolar lavage) may be adequate in cases in which infection must be excluded. Drug reactions are rarely proven or disproven histologically, and biopsies done to diagnose a drug reaction are rarely definitive.

Caveats

The clinical history and radiologic findings are the key to histologic interpretation of lung biopsies in the CVDs.

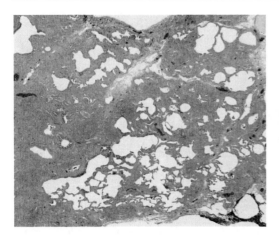

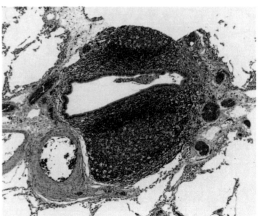

Fig. 4.11 Usual interstitial pneumonia occurring in the setting of systemic lupus erythematosis. There is marked fibrous distortion of lung architecture, worst in the *left side* of the figure. Some relatively preserved alveoli are present (*lower center*). An occasional lymphoid follicle is present (*left center*)

Fig. 4.13 Rheumatoid arthritis with associated follicular bronchiolitis. A small bronchiole is cuffed by lymphoid follicles containing prominent germinal centers

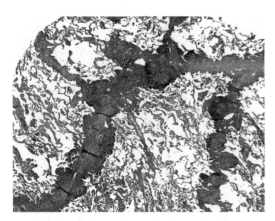

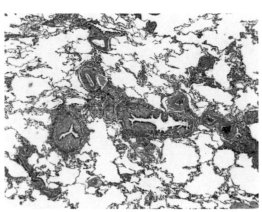

Fig. 4.14 Constrictive bronchiolitis in rheumatoid arthritis. Sections of two bronchioles show marked luminal narrowing by subepithelial collagen deposition. One of the bronchioles is cut in cross section (9 o'clock) whereas the other (*center*) is cut longitudinally and shows how the subepithelial scarring in constrictive bronchiolitis can be a focal change in an individual airway

Fig. 4.12 Diffuse lymphoid hyperplasia in rheumatoid arthritis. There is a proliferation of lymphoid follicles with germinal centers distributed along interlobular septa

In patients with CVD on drugs known to cause lung disease, a drug reaction may be an issue and histologically it is rarely possible to separate drug-induced pathology from CVD-associated pathology.

Many of the drugs that patients with CVDs are on lead to immunosuppression and infection is an issue that should be addressed with cultures and special stains.

Vasculitis

Histologic Findings

The ANCA-associated vasculitides are the most common forms of vasculitis to affect the lung. Among these, Wegener's granulomatosis is more common than microscopic polyangiitis which in turn is more common than Churg–Strauss disease in biopsy material.

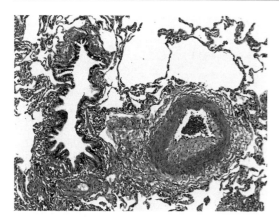 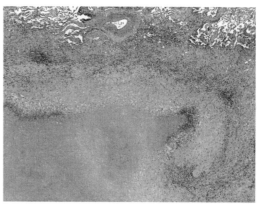

Fig. 4.15 Pulmonary hypertension in progressive systemic sclerosis. A small pulmonary artery shows marked medial hypertrophy with some eccentric intimal thickening

Fig. 4.16 Rheumatoid nodule. Adjacent to a small bronchiole and its accompanying pulmonary artery (*top center*) there is a large necrobiotic nodule with central fibrinoid necrosis and surrounding palisaded histiocytes characteristic of a rheumatoid nodule

Table 4.2 Patterns of lung disease in connective tissue disorders

Lesions	Conditions							
	RA	SLE	Scleroderma	PM/DM	SS	MCTD	AS	PC
Pleural disease								
Pleuritis +/− effusion	+	+	+	+	+	+	+	
Pleural fibrosis	+	+	+	+	+	+	+	
Sterile or septic empyema	+			+			+	
Spontaneous pneumothorax							+	
Interstitial/parenchymal lesions								
Usual interstitial pneumonia (IP)	+	+	+	+	+	+	+	
Diffuse alveolar damage	+	+	+	+	+	+	+	
Nonspecific IP	+	+	+	+	+	+	+	
Organizing pneumonia	+	+	+	+	+	+		
Lymphocytic IP/LH	+	+	+	+	+	+		
Granulomatous IP	+	+			+	+		
Apical fibrobullous disease	+					+		
Aspiration pneumonia	+					+		
Necrobiotic rheumatoid nodule	+					+		
+/− rupture	+					+		
Amyloid deposits								
Alveolar lesions								
Diffuse hemorrhage	+	+	+	+		+		
Eosinophilic pneumonia	+			+		+		
Alveolar proteinosis						+		
Vascular lesions								
Vasculitis	+	+	+	+	+	+		
Pulmonary hypertension	+	+	+	+	+	+		
Thromboembolism		+						
Airway lesions								
Bronchiolitis +/− fibrosis	+	+		+	+	+		+
Follicular bronchiolitis	+	+			+	+		
Constrictive bronchiolitis	+					+		
Bronchiectasis	+					+		

(continued)

Table 4.2 (continued)

Lesions	Conditions							
	RA	SLE	Scleroderma	PM/DM	SS	MCTD	AS	PC
Xerotrachea	+	+			+		+	
Bronchocentric granulomatosis	+							
Diffuse panbronchiolitis								
Indirect respiratory effects								
Diaphragmatic or respiratory	+	+		+	+	+	+	
muscle dysfunction		+		+			+	
Thoracic cage immobility								
Atelectasis (shrinking)								
Neoplasms								
Lung cancer		+	+		+	+	+	
Lymphoma		+				+		
Kaposi's sarcoma								

RA rheumatoid arthritis, *SLE* systemic lupus erythematosus, *PM/DM* polymyositis/dermatomyositis, *SS* Sjogren's syndrome, *MCTD* mixed connective tissue disease, *AS* ankylosing spondylosis, *PC* polychondritis, *LH* lymphoid hyperplasia
Modified from Travis WD, Colby TV, Koss MN, Rosado de Christiansen M, Muller N, King TE. Non-neoplastic disorders of the lower respiratory tract. Atlas of nontumor pathology, vol. 2. Washington, DC: Armed Forces Institute of Pathology and American Registry of Pathology; 2002

Wegener's Granulomatosis (Figs. 4.17 and 4.18)

- Components of vasculitis, necrotizing granulomatous inflammation (without sarcoid-like granulomas), and inflammatory consolidation of the lung tissue all of which vary in extent from case to case.
- Vasculitis involves small and medium size arteries and veins often with an eccentric mural infiltrate of inflammatory cells dominated by monocyte-like cells within which microabscesses may form and ultimately enlarge into a necrotic granuloma in the vessel wall.
- Capillaritis and/or hemorrhage may be present and are the only findings in some cases.
- Necrotizing granulomatous features characterized by geographic basophilic necrosis (often unrelated to the vasculitis) arises from coalescence of microabscesses.
- Involved lung tissue tends to show an "inflammatory background" with fibrosis, organization, and acute and chronic inflammation, and scattered giant cells.
- Alveolar hemorrhage (acute or chronic with or without capillaritis) may be present and is the only finding in some cases.

Microscopic Polyangiitis (Fig. 4.19)

- Vasculitis of small- to medium-sized arteries and veins; capillaritis
- Lacks granulomatous features and lacks large zones of confluent necrosis.
- Giant cells are lacking.
- Alveolar hemorrhage (with or without capillaritis) is commonly present and may be the only finding present.

Churg–Strauss Syndrome (Fig. 4.20)

- Classically vasculitis, tissue eosinophil infiltrates, and extravascular necrotizing granulomas; these features are rarely seen all together in a lung biopsy.
- Changes of asthma in the airways.
- Eosinophilic pneumonia, scattered nonnecrotizing granulomas, vasculitis, extravascular necrosis may also be seen.

Differential Diagnosis

Although Wegener's granulomatosis has subtle histologic differences from granulomatous infections, infection is at the top of the differential diagnosis and cultures and special stains should be performed. Among the granulomatous infections,

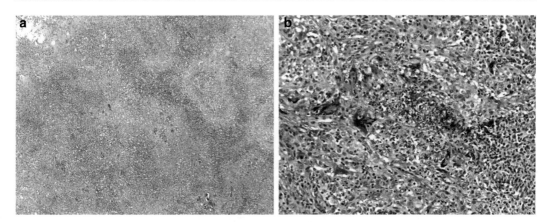

Fig. 4.17 Wegener's granulomatosis. (**a**) There is geographic necrosis identifiable at low power as irregular basophilic zones of necrosis surrounded by the less basophilic and more eosinophilic viable tissue. (**b**) Higher power evaluation shows a region of microabscess formation (*center*) with surrounding cuff of multinucleated giant cells without accompanying nonnecrotizing sarcoid-like granulomas

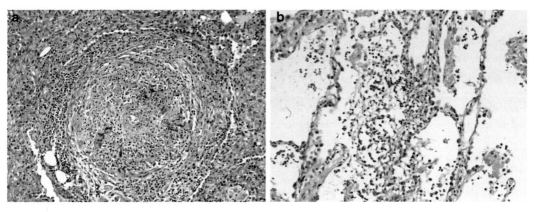

Fig. 4.18 Vasculitis in Wegener's granulomatosis. (**a**) There is a small artery with transmural inflammatory infiltrate including occasional giant cells (7 o'clock). (**b**) Involvement of capillaries is termed capillaritis and is associated with neutrophilic infiltrates in the alveolar septum, sometimes with destruction of the septum (*center*)

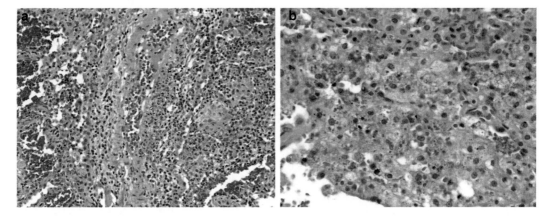

Fig. 4.19 Microscopic polyangiitis. (**a**) A small artery shows an inflammatory infiltrate involving the adventitia and media (*right center*). The surrounding lung shows hemorrhage and interstitial neutrophils consistent with associated capillaritis. (**b**) There is evidence of old hemorrhage with numerous hemosiderin-laden macrophages

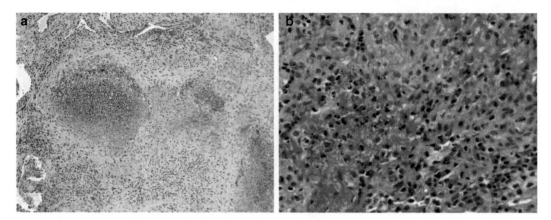

Fig. 4.20 Churg–Strauss syndrome. (**a**) There is a region of parenchymal necrosis that is somewhat eosinophilic in character. (**b**) The lung tissue in Churg–Strauss syndrome typically shows a marked infiltrate of eosinophils

mycobacterial infection is the one most likely to simulate Wegener's granulomatosis. Microscopic polyangiitis is distinguished from Wegener's granulomatosis primarily on the basis of the absence of granulomatous features. Churg–Strauss disease requires the presence of asthma and peripheral eosinophilia in addition to clinical or histologic evidence of systemic vasculitis.

In cases with alveolar hemorrhage, other causes of alveolar hemorrhage syndromes especially CVDs and antiglomerular basement membrane antibody disease should be excluded.

Biopsy Diagnosis

The features of these forms of vasculitis may sometimes be recognized in TBBx, but larger biopsies are usually needed and surgical lung biopsy is often undertaken in this clinical setting. The histologic findings should be interpreted in the context of the clinical (what organ systems are affected) and the serologic (ANCA tests, anti-GBM antibodies, ANA, etc.) findings. Churg–Strauss disease may be diagnosed on the basis of clinical findings making histologic evaluation unnecessary. In cases with extensive clinical and serologic data that point toward one diagnosis, the findings in a transbronchial biopsy may be nonspecific but considered "consistent with" the clinically suspected diagnosis.

Caveats

The diagnosis of vasculitic syndromes requires give and take between the pathologist and the clinician, and the histologic findings may be reinterpreted in light of additional clinical information as it becomes available (and vice versa).

Wegener's granulomatosis commonly includes an inflammatory background that is histologically nonspecific and an inflammatory infiltrate without vasculitis or necrosis does not exclude a diagnosis of WG.

The diagnosis of Churg–Strauss disease cannot be made by biopsy alone; clinical findings (including evidence of systemic vasculitis) are necessary.

Alveolar Hemorrhage Syndromes

Histologic Findings (Figs. 4.21 and 4.22)

- Basic histologic response to alveolar hemorrhage is similar for most syndromes.
- Fresh hemorrhage is often associated with fibrin and followed by organization and hemosiderin-filled macrophages.
- Capillaritis may or may not be present in acute alveolar hemorrhage.
- With chronicity there is interstitial and airspace accumulation of hemosiderin, increased alveolar macrophages, and mild interstitial fibrosis.

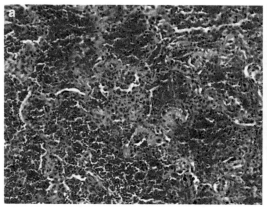
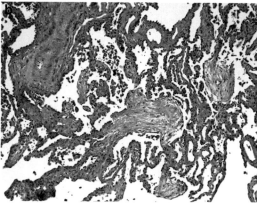

Fig. 4.21 (**a**) Diffuse alveolar hemorrhage. The airspaces are filled with fibrin and there is an increase in neutrophils in the interstitium (*center*) typical of capillaritis. (**b**) Organizing alveolar hemorrhage. In addition to the intraluminal polyps of organizing fibroblastic tissue there are pigmented hemosiderin-laden macrophages in the alveoli (*upper left center*) indicative of old hemorrhage

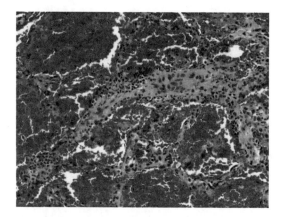

Fig. 4.22 Capillaritis in diffuse alveolar hemorrhage. There are prominent interstitial neutrophils along a small vessel and in the interstitium (*center*). The surrounding alveoli show recent hemorrhage

- Iron encrustation of the elastic vessels may be identified in chronic hemorrhage.
- Alveolar hemorrhage due to WG is the only form of alveolar hemorrhage that may be histologically diagnosed in biopsy material if the characteristic features of Wegener's are also present (scattered giant cells, microabscess formation, basophilic necrosis, and vasculitis).

Differential Diagnosis
- Fresh traumatic hemorrhage from the biopsy procedure itself; this is the most common cause of red cells in alveolar spaces in surgical lung biopsies.
- Cigarette smoking (an extremely common cause of Prussian blue positive macrophages in the airspaces).
- Biopsy related margination of neutrophils in subpleural vessels mimics capillaritis.
- Infection-related capillaritis (particularly viral infections in immunosuppressed patients).
- Hemosiderosis from cardiac disease or siderosis from exposure (e.g., welders)

Biopsy Diagnosis
The above features of alveolar hemorrhage may be identified in either transbronchial or surgical lung biopsies. In TBBx careful clinicopathologic correlation is indicated.

Caveats
- Capillaritis is not specific and seen in many of the causes of alveolar hemorrhage.
- Capillaritis is transitory and its absence does not exclude an alveolar hemorrhage syndrome.
- Smoking and left heart failure are common causes of Prussian Blue positive macrophages (i.e., "hemosiderosis") in airspaces.
- Traumatic hemorrhage is the most common cause of alveolar red blood cells in lung biopsy material.

- Pulmonary siderosis deposition may be the result of an occupational exposure (such as welding).

Hypersensitivity Pneumonitis

Histologic Findings (Fig. 4.23)
- Centrilobular inflammatory process (affecting bronchioles and alveolar duct regions preferentially).
- Inflammation generally overshadows fibrosis.
- Cellular inflammation most prominent along bronchioles and alveolar ducts and less prominent toward the periphery of the lobule.
- Scattered nonnecrotizing small loose granulomas.

- Giant cells, singly or in clusters; sometimes contain cholesterol clefts.
- Airspace foam cells.
- Airspace organization may or may not be present.

Differential Diagnosis
- Sarcoidosis: Granulomas are the dominant finding; in HP the granulomas tend to be relatively inconspicuous compared to the airway-centered inflammation.
- Miliary granulomatous infections: Granulomas tend to be the dominant feature; necrosis may or may not be present.
- Sjogren's syndrome: Lymphoid hyperplasia with germinal centers tends to be more prominent than in HP.

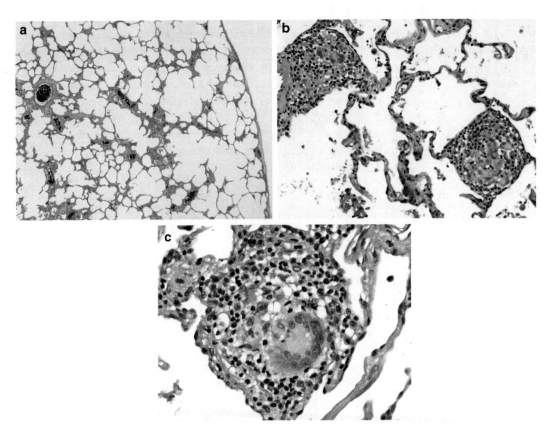

Fig. 4.23 Hypersensitivity pneumonitis. (**a**) There is an inflammatory process without appreciable fibrosis. The process is most prominent in the centrilobular regions (*center*). The lung architecture is relatively preserved. (**b, c**) The granulomas in hypersensitivity pneumonitis tend to be small and scattered and sometimes composed of small clusters of epithelioid cells or occasional giant cells

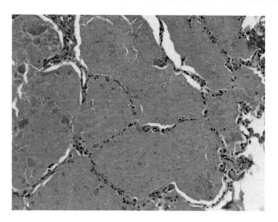

Fig. 4.24 Pulmonary alveolar proteinosis. The airspaces are filled by granular eosinophilic material that contains eosinophilic globules and shows some cracking artifact with separation from alveolar walls

Caveats
- Some cases of HP have a nearly classical HRCT appearance which may support (or be against) the histologic findings.
- Diffuse *Mycobacterium avium* infection in normal hosts may mimic HP ("hot tub lung").
- Most cases of HP do not look anything like sarcoidosis or infection; the granulomas are relative few and inconspicuous.

Pulmonary Alveolar Proteinosis

Histologic Findings (Fig. 4.24)
- Granular eosinophilic material flooding airspaces.
- Little change in the alveolar interstitium.
- Cholesterol clefts and hyaline globs in the alveolar spaces.
- Intra-alveolar material is PAS positive and diastase resistant (a nonspecific finding) and stains for surfactant apoprotein.

Differential Diagnosis
The eosinophilic intra-alveolar material of proteinosis may be mimicked by (but is histologically separable from) the alveolar foamy material in *Pneumocystis carinii* pneumonia, edema fluid, fibrin, and hyaline membranes. A focal proteinosis reaction (histologically identical to idiopathic PAP) may be seen in regions of chronic fibrosis,

as a reaction associated with infection, and around some mass lesions.

Biopsy Diagnosis
Transbronchial biopsy or surgical lung biopsy may suffice to identify the distinctive intra-alveolar material. It is also recognizable in bronchoalveolar lavage smears (and sometimes grossly at the time of bronchoscopy) and in cell block preparations from BAL fluid.

Caveats
- PAP is distinctive and histologically distinguishable from other causes of intra-alveolar eosinophilic material.
- PAP may be associated with secondary infections (most notably nocardia).
- A PAP-like reaction may be a focal finding in a number of conditions.

Lymphangioleiomyomatosis

Histologic Findings (Fig. 4.25)
- Cystic change in the lung parenchyma.
- Fascicles of spindle cells resembling smooth muscle cells, usually in the cyst walls; these cells are positive for smooth muscle markers as well as HMB-45.
- The degree of cystic change and the degree of smooth muscle proliferation may be independent of one another and vary in extent from case to case.
- Evidence of prior hemorrhage with hemosiderin-filled macrophages.
- Some patients with LAM also have multifocal micronodular pneumocyte hyperplasia as an additional finding: small nodular proliferations of polygonal type 2 cells that are considered a hamartomatous proliferation.

Differential Diagnosis
The cystic change must be differentiated from emphysema, bullae, honeycombing, pulmonary Langerhans cell histiocytosis, Sjogren's syndrome, and cystic spindle cell neoplasms.

The spindle cell fascicles must be differentiated from fibrosis and other causes of smooth

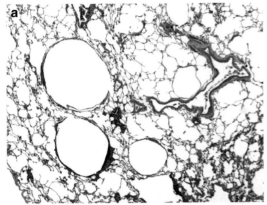
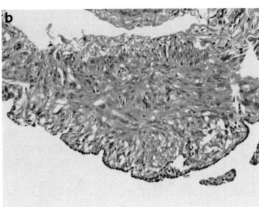

Fig. 4.25 Lymphangioleiomyomatosis (LAM). Low power shows cystic change (**a**). The cystic spaces have a definite rounded character and in some of them a thin eosinophilic fascicles of tissue is apparent indicative of the smooth muscle proliferation of LAM. The proliferating spindle cell resemble smooth muscle cells (**b**) but have distinctive staining characteristics showing evidence of melanocytic differentiation with positivity for HMB-45

muscle proliferation, particularly that associated with airway disease (especially alveolar duct smooth muscle proliferation in smokers) and metaplastic smooth muscle in fibrotic diseases. The smooth muscle in these situations is HMB-45 negative. LAM should also be distinguished from lymphangiomas and lymphangiomatosis.

Biopsy Diagnosis

The histologic features of LAM are unique and if sought may be identified by TBBx as well surgical lung biopsies. (Note: Some cases are diagnosed on the basis of HRCT without tissue biopsy).

Caveats

- HMB-45 positivity is variable and in some cases only a few cells stain.
- The spindle cell fascicles may be focal and inconspicuous.
- The histology of LAM is unique and thus recognizable in tiny biopsy specimens.

Bronchiolitis

The term bronchiolitis is used to encompass a spectrum of inflammatory and fibrotic changes in the small airways. These reactions typically include a cellular response (acute and or chronic inflammatory cells) and a mesenchymal response (fibrosis) that may involve different compartments of the airway. The interplay of the cellular reaction and the mesenchymal reaction determines the precise clinical and radiologic features in a given case of bronchiolitis. For example, some forms of bronchiolitis do not compromise the airway lumen, and airflow obstruction is not a clinical or radiologic feature. This spectrum of changes can be grouped as follows:

- Asthmatic type changes (eosinophil infiltrates, basement membrane thickening, smooth muscle hyperplasia, goblet cell metaplasia, mucus plugging).
- Cellular bronchiolitis (acute and or chronic inflammatory cellular infiltrates, +/− luminal exudate), follicular hyperplasia in the case of follicular bronchiolitis (Fig. 4.26).
- Bronchiolitis obliterans with intraluminal polyps (a change commonly seen in association with organizing pneumonia).
- Constrictive bronchiolitis (airway luminal narrowing or complete obliteration due to subepithelial collagen deposition (Fig. 4.27)).
- Peribronchiolar fibrosis with bronchiolar metaplasia (scarring around the airway with relative preservation of the airway lumen).
- Mixtures of the above.

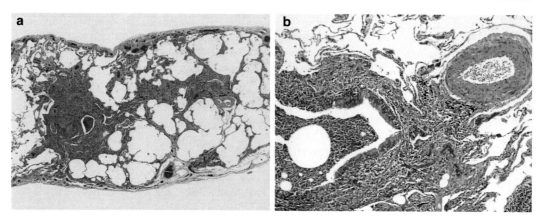

Fig. 4.26 Chronic cellular bronchiolitis. There is an inflammatory process centered on the small airways in the centrilobular regions of this wedge lung biopsy (**a**). Higher power evaluation (**b**) shows chronic inflammation in the walls of the bronchioles with a central luminal exudate containing neutrophils

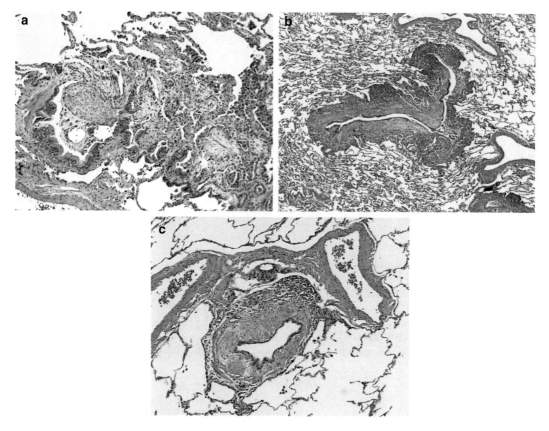

Fig. 4.27 (**a**) Bronchiolitis obliterans with intraluminal polyps. For cases in which there are intraluminal polyps of organizing connective tissue in the bronchioles (*left center*). This is associated with the organization extending into the surrounding lung tissue (termed organizing pneumonia) to the *right* of the bronchiole. (**b, c**) Constrictive bronchiolitis. The term bronchiolitis obliterans has also been used for cases showing features of constrictive bronchiolitis. The bronchiole cut longitudinally (**b**) shows marked fibrous thickening of the subepithelial region of the bronchiole leading to appreciable luminal compromise. Cross section evaluation (**c**) also highlights the scarring and luminal narrowing

The term "bronchiolitis obliterans" has been used in a variety of ways: to refer to the *pathologic* finding of intraluminal polyps in the small airways (bronchiolitis obliterans with intraluminal polyps) and to the lesion currently called constrictive bronchiolitis (with luminal narrowing). As a clinical syndrome, "bronchiolitis obliterans" refers to obstructive lung disease due to the pathology in the small airways; in the setting of transplantation the term "obliterative bronchiolitis" (OB) is generally used to refer to small airway airflow obstruction developing after transplantation and the pathologic correlate of both of these is constrictive bronchiolitis.

The concept of "end-stage bronchiolitis" is useful for cases in which irreversible scarring and architectural remodeling in the small airways are present, and the etiology may no longer be apparent (or even relevant). These cases often show acute and chronic cellular bronchiolitis, constrictive bronchiolitis, ectasia with mucostasis and luminal exudate, and variable degrees of peribronchiolar scarring and bronchiolar metaplasia. "End-stage bronchiolitis" is analogous to the concept of bronchiectasis involving the larger airways.

Differential Diagnosis for Bronchiolitis

- Hypersensitivity pneumonitis
- Bronchiolar changes in interstitial pneumonias
- Secondary bronchiolar changes distal to bronchiectasis
- Lymphoreticular infiltrates along bronchioles (including diffuse lymphoid hyperplasia and lymphoma/leukemia).

Biopsy Diagnosis
Surgical lung biopsy is generally needed for histologic diagnosis of bronchiolitis. Bronchiolar abnormalities may be apparent in a transbronchial biopsy and sometimes, with HRCT correlation, a clinicopathologic diagnosis can be rendered.

Caveats
- The histologic spectrum of bronchiolitis is associated with a broad clinical spectrum of disease (including obstructive *and* restrictive diseases).

- HRCT is useful in recognizing bronchiolar pathology and may aid histologic diagnosis.
- Careful clinical–radiologic–pathologic correlation is necessary to interpret bronchiolitis, particularly in cases where the bronchiolar changes are subtle.

Pneumoconioses

Pneumoconioses are lung disease caused by exposure to exogenous agents, typically inorganic dusts. The pathologic findings are quite variable, and the key features of some of the well-known forms of pneumoconiosis are shown below:

Coworkers Pneumoconiosis
Histiocytic dust macules with large amounts of anthracotic pigment centering primarily on alveolar ducts; some associated fibrosis may be present if there is co-exposure to appreciable amounts of silica.

Silicosis/Silicatosis
Macules of dust-filled histiocytes along small airways and lymphatic routes (as the dust is cleared through the lymphatic routes) in the septa and pleura; nodular fibrosis (silicotic type nodules) develop over time and with increased exposure (Figs. 4.28 and 4.29).

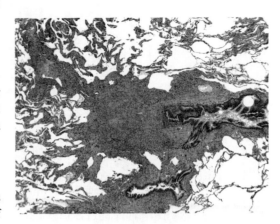

Fig. 4.28 Silicosis. There is a cuff of dust-filled histiocytes around a small bronchiole

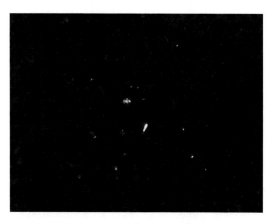

Fig. 4.29 Silicosis. Polarization of the histiocytes in Fig. 4.28 shows weakly birefringent silica particles and more brightly birefringent silicate particles

Table 4.3 Diffuse lung disease associated with drugs

Edema
Hemorrhage
Alveolar proteinosis
Lymphoid hyperplasia
Diffuse alveolar damage
Usual interstitial pneumonia
Nonspecific interstitial pneumonia
Lymphocytic interstitial pneumonia
Giant cell interstitial pneumonia
Granulomatous interstitial pneumonia
Organizing pneumonia
Eosinophilic pneumonia
Emphysema
Calcification
Airway disease/bronchiolitis
Pulmonary vascular disease/hypertension

Asbestosis

The presence of asbestos bodies (ferruginated asbestos fibers) with associated interstitial fibrosis which appears to start along small airways where the fibers are initially deposited; late in its course asbestosis may resemble UIP.

Berylliosis

The immunologic reaction to beryllium in susceptible patients results in a granulomatous inflammation which may closely mimic sarcoidosis, or NSIP.

Cobalt/Hard Metal Pneumoconiosis

Produces "giant cell interstitial pneumonia" with a bronchiolocentric inflammatory process with interstitial inflammation and peribronchiolar airspaces containing large numbers of multinucleated giant cells.

Caveats

Small amounts of silica/silicates are present in virtually any adult lung, particularly that of an individual who is or has been a smoker.

Pneumoconiosis is a clinical–radiologic–pathologic diagnosis and the presence of exogenous dust in the lung tissue needs to be associated with identifiable radiologic and/or clinical findings.

Drug Reactions

The clinical and pathologic spectrum of abnormalities associated with drug toxicity in the lung spans virtually all of clinical pulmonary disease as well as virtually all pathologic patterns of diffuse lung disease. Clinical patterns are summarized elsewhere in this book. Pathologic patterns of diffuse lung disease associated with drug reactions are given in Table 4.3. The role of pathologic evaluation of lung tissue in putative drug reactions is twofold. The possibility of other causes of the lung disease, particularly infection, need to be addressed with appropriate studies (special stains for microorganisms, etc.), and the reaction pattern that is present needs to be defined and then correlated with the known reactions associated with the suspected drug(s) (Fig. 4.30).

Drug reactions can broadly be divided into those that are dose related (e.g., many cases of amiodarone toxicity), and those that are idiosyncratic representing a unique interaction between the patient and the given drug. In some cases both of these mechanisms may be at play.

Caveats

- A drug reaction in the lung is nearly always a diagnosis of exclusion of other causes of that reaction pattern/clinical pulmonary disease.

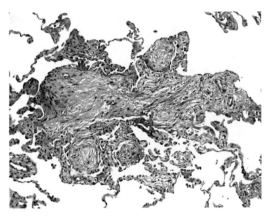

Fig. 4.30 Fludarabine reaction. There is focus of organizing pneumonia. After clinical pathologic correlation this nonspecific finding was attributed to fludarabine

• A given drug might be associated with a number of pathologic patterns.
• A given pathologic pattern may be associated with many drugs.
• Some drug reactions may be associated with relatively localized lung disease (e.g., nodules/patchy infiltrates).

• The effects of drug toxicity may take many years to manifest (e.g., BCNU-related fibrosis many years after the drug was received).

Further Reading

American Thoracic Society/European Respiratory Society international multidisciplinary consensus classification of the idiopathic interstitial pneumonias. Am J Respir Crit Care Med. 2002;165:277–304.

Colby TV, Carrington CB. Interstitial lung disease. In: Thurlbeck WM, Churg AM, editors. Pathology of the lung. 2nd ed. New York: Thieme Medical; 1995. p. 589–739. Chapter 25.

Katzenstein AL. Katzenstein and Askin's surgical pathology of non-neoplastic lung disease. 4th ed. Philadelphia: WB Saunders; 2006.

Leslie KO, Colby TV, Swensen SJ. Histopathologic patterns of interstitial lung disease. In: Schwartz M, King TE, editors. interstitial lung disease. 4th ed. Hamilton: B.C. Decker; 2003. p. 31–53. Chapter 2.

Travis WD, Colby TV, Koss MN, Rosado de Christiansen M, Muller N, King TE. Non-neoplastic disorders of the lower respiratory tract. Atlas of nontumor pathology. 2nd ed. Washington, DC: Armed Forces Institute of Pathology and American Registry of Pathology; 2002.

Pulmonary Function Testing

5

Athol U. Wells, Simon Ward,
and Derek Cramer

Abstract

Pulmonary function tests (PFT) remain the most accurate means of quantifying the severity of diffuse lung disease. PFT are an essential aide to the identification or exclusion of early diffuse lung disease in high-risk groups and when there is unexplained exercise intolerance. Individual diffuse lung disorders have typical patterns of pulmonary function impairment and, thus, pulmonary function estimation may refine the differential diagnosis. However, the two major utilities of PFT estimation are to stage disease severity and to identify serial change in disease severity. In the staging of disease severity, the most difficult challenge is to deconstruct the pulmonary function profile when more than one disorder is present and this requires the reconciliation of PFT, imaging findings and clinical information.

In the detection of serial changes in disease severity, the most difficult challenge is to distinguish between genuine change and spurious change due to measurement variation. This problem is addressed by robust quality assurance and quality control procedures, to ensure technical accuracy and to minimise measurement variability. Repeated assessment of biological controls at frequent intervals is an integral part of this process.

Keywords

Pulmonary function tests • Detection of early disease • Staging disease severity • Identifying serial change in severity • Quality assurance • Biological controls

A.U. Wells (✉)
Interstitial Lung Disease Unit, Royal Brompton
Hospital, London, UK
e-mail: Athol.Wells@rbht.nhs.uk

S. Ward • D. Cramer
Lung Function Department, Royal Brompton
Hospital, London, UK

R.P. Baughman and R.M. du Bois (eds.), *Diffuse Lung Disease: A Practical Approach*,
DOI 10.1007/978-1-4419-9771-5_5, © Springer Science+Business Media, LLC 2012

Introduction

In diffuse lung disease (DLD), it has long been recognised that pulmonary function tests (PFT) better reflect the histological severity of the underlying disease process than plain chest radiography or symptoms [1]. Based on this widespread view, the measurement of PFT has had a central role in the management of ILD over many decades, but a role that has evolved. Early expectations are often over-optimistic with the clinical application of any test, before realism wins the day. It was argued by some that the degree of impairment of individual PFT, including exercise variables, might be linked selectively to the histological severity of inflammation at surgical biopsy. A reliable non-invasive surrogate for inflammation in DLD remains an unmet need to the present day. In historical series, conflicting findings emerged from functional–morphologic correlations in several small populations containing a mixture of diffuse lung disorders. Eventually, it was concluded from a larger study of idiopathic interstitial pneumonia that pulmonary function variables provided no useful selective linkage to the severity of inflammation, but only to the overall morphologic severity of disease [2].

Thus, the cardinal roles of pulmonary function estimation, highlighted in this chapter, are to quantify disease severity at baseline and in the detection of serial change. Also covered is the use of PFT to detect the presence of disease in certain clinical contexts, the range of pattern of functional impairment in DLD, the problem of complex pulmonary function impairment due to coexistent disease processes and issues related to quality assurance and fitness to fly tests.

A glossary of abbreviations for routine PFT is given in Table 5.1.

Table 5.1 A glossary of abbreviations for routine pulmonary function variables

FEV1	Forced expiratory volume in 1 s
FVC	Forced vital capacity
TLC	Total lung capacity
VA	Alveolar volume
DLco	Carbon monoxide diffusing capacity
Kco	Carbon monoxide transfer coefficient
MEF25	Maximum expiratory flow at 25% forced vital capacity

The Use of PFT to Detect or Exclude Early DLD

By the time that DLD is sufficiently severe to cause exercise limitation, abnormalities are almost always evident on high-resolution computed tomography (HRCT) and overt pulmonary function impairment is usual. However, PFT estimation also has an important ancillary role in detecting or excluding early DLD in high-risk populations and, with the demonstration of normal values, in establishing in individual cases that DLD is an implausible cause of unexplained dyspnoea.

The use of PFT to detect very early DLD is not a realistic goal in unselected populations, given the moderately low prevalence of DLD in the community. However, with increasing recognition that DLD, with or without pulmonary hypertension, has become the most frequent cause of death in some connective tissue diseases, it is argued by some that PFT should be performed as a part of routine baseline staging in these disorders. In several historical series, the prevalence of PFT impairment was explored in moderately large patient cohorts with systemic sclerosis (SSc) and rheumatoid arthritis (RA). In general, carbon-monoxide diffusing capacity (DLco) is the most sensitive test, with reduction in a majority or large minority of cases in these diseases. Reductions in volumes are less sensitive and seldom occur without concurrent reductions in DLco levels.

However, minor reductions in DLco or spirometric volumes do not, in themselves, establish that DLD is either present or clinically significant [3]. Measures of gas transfer are highly nonspecific, being influenced alike by interstitial processes and pulmonary vasculopathy, including sub-clinical pulmonary vasculopathy which may be common in SSc, explaining a shift in the whole population range of DLco levels in that disease, even when DLD is not apparent. Lung volumes, including total lung capacity (TLC) and forced vital capacity (FVC) are more specific to interstitial disease, but the interpretation of minor reductions is hampered by the wide range in normal values (generally 80–120% of predicted values based on age, gender and height) [4]. Thus, without knowledge of pre-morbid values (before the onset of CTD), an initial FVC value of 78% of predicted cannot be interpreted as either minimally reduced (if, for example, the premorbid value was 81%) or substantially reduced (e.g. premorbid value 115% and, thus, a reduction of 30% from baseline).

Despite these constraints, routine baseline PFT are warranted in systemic diseases in which there is a high prevalence of interstitial involvement (sarcoidosis, SSc, polymyositis/dermatomyositis). PFT should also be performed in CTD before the institution of therapies with a significant likelihood of pulmonary toxicity (e.g. methotrexate therapy in RA). Knowledge of baseline values accounts for the confounding effect of the normal range, in the interpretation of subsequent minor functional impairment. In this way, trends within the normal range can be interpreted and the likely significance of mild reductions in PFT below the normal range can be better understood, when PFT are repeated for clinical reasons. In "multicompartment disorders" with the potential for separate vascular and interstitial disease (including SSc and sarcoidosis), a minimal baseline protocol should include spirometric volumes and DLco.

PFT are also useful in evaluating the common scenario of unexplained exercise intolerance. The presence of dyspnoea is a particularly unreliable indicator of lung disease in systemic disorders. In connective tissue diseases, exertional dyspnoea is often due to musculoskeletal limitation (myopathy or arthropathy) which, by reducing the efficiency of locomotion, increases the respiratory work load of normal daily activity. In these disorders, cardiac involvement, anaemia and loss of fitness due to systemic morbidity may also contribute to exertional dyspnoea. In general, the absence of PFT abnormalities effectively excludes clinically significant DLD in the context of chronic exertional dyspnoea. In part, this reflects the existence of normal pulmonary function reserve: even vigorous normal daily activities will not be compromised by minor reductions in PFT. Moreover, in slowly progressive diseases, a natural process of physiological adaptation may occur, such that exercise limitation may not be apparent until DLco levels fall below 60% of predicted normal values. A normal DLco level is a particularly

helpful negative finding when DLD is suspected, given the sensitivity of the test. However, less weighting should be given to the negative predictive value of "normal" PFT when dyspnoea is recent in onset: a rapid fall in PFT to the lower end of the normal range, without sufficient time for adaptation to occur, may result in awareness of respiratory compromise.

Typical Patterns of Pulmonary Function Impairment

In DLDs, a wide variety of patterns of pulmonary function impairment is encountered, reflecting the heterogeneous pathological processes in these disorders. Restrictive ventilatory defects and airflow obstruction may occur in isolation or as components of a mixed ventilatory defect. Moreover, the clinical interpretation of PFT in DLD requires a working knowledge of the functional profiles of other respiratory diseases, due to the frequency with which they coexist with DLD.

A restrictive ventilatory defect (reduced TLC and FVC; increased FEV1/FVC ratio) is characteristically seen in the idiopathic interstitial pneumonias, in association with a reduction in DLco [5] which is usually significantly greater (expressed as a percentage of normal predicted values) than the falls in lung volumes. Arterial oxygen levels in restrictive lung disease tend to be well preserved until interstitial lung disease is advanced, unless there is coexisting pulmonary hypertension, reflecting the redistribution of pulmonary blood to well-ventilated lung by arterial hypoxic vasoconstriction. By contrast, the alveolar–arterial oxygen gradient tends to widen earlier in the course of disease. This functional profile applies to many fibrosing DLDs, including hypersensitivity pneumonitis and occupational diseases such as asbestosis and is seldom diagnostically helpful. However, cryptogenic organising pneumonia may present with disproportionate hypoxia due to shunting of blood through dilated vessels within consolidated lung tissue [6].

Airflow obstruction in DLD, typically seen in lymphangioleiomyomatosus and Langerhans cell histiocytosis, is indistinguishable from the ventilatory defect of intrinsic airways disease and smoking-related emphysema. There is an obstructive ventilatory defect, as shown by a disproportionate reduction in FEV1, a reduction in the FEV1/FVC ratio, an increase in TLC, a reduction in airflow at low lung volumes (MEF25) and an obstructive pattern in the expiratory limb of the flow–volume curve. However, measures of gas transfer distinguish usefully between intrinsic airways disease and other obstructive disorders. DLco and Kco levels are strikingly reduced in advanced emphysema [7], lymphangioleiomyomatosus and Langerhans cell histiocytosis but are preserved in isolated intrinsic airways diseases such as constrictive bronchiolitis until the FEV1 falls below 1 L, at which point, reduction in DLco levels can be expected [8]. Kco levels tend to remain normal, even in end-stage bronchiolar disorders.

A mixed ventilatory defect is frequent in diseases in which there is an airway component, including sarcoidosis, hypersensitivity pneumonitis and rheumatoid lung and may also be indicative of the co-existence of disease processes (e.g. emphysema and idiopathic pulmonary fibrosis). In a predominantly restrictive defect, the presence of airflow obstruction may be disclosed by an elevated RV/TLC ratio [9] or by evidence of an obstructive component on perusal of flow–volume curves.

The presence of concurrent pulmonary vascular disease in DLD results in a disproportionate fall in gas transfer [10]. Importantly, major reductions in pulmonary vascular reserve may occur before pulmonary hypertension becomes apparent, as a result of the considerable normal pulmonary vascular reserve. The likelihood of underlying pulmonary hypertension is increased when a disproportionate reduction in gas transfer is associated with severe resting hypoxia or major arterial oxygen desaturation with minor exertion). In generally, patterns of lung function impairment do not discriminate between individual pulmonary vascular disorders. However, in diffuse alveolar haemorrhage syndromes, DLco and Kco levels, measured using single breath testing, may increase substantially to, for example, levels 200–300% above the upper limit of normal, due to uptake of carbon-monoxide by intra-alveolar haemoglobin [11]. This finding is rarely diagnostically helpful as it persists for only 24–36 h following alveolar haemorrhage.

The restrictive ventilatory defect of extra-pulmonic restriction [12] is largely indistinguishable from that of interstitial fibrosis, apart from the frequent finding of relative preservation of RV (i.e. an increased RV/TLC ratio) in pleural disease [13]. The most reliable discriminatory feature is that in extra-pulmonic restriction, DLco levels fall only slightly, and Kco levels rise to supra-normal values [14] (as blood volume within ventilated lung changes little, even in major extra-pulmonic restriction). In the absence of alveolar haemorrhage, a major increase in Kco is a reliable indicator of extra-pulmonary restriction. In severe extra-pulmonary restriction, and especially in severe respiratory muscle weakness, arterial gases may disclose alveolar hypoventilation (i.e. hypoxia in association with hypercapnia and a normal calculated alveolar–arterial oxygen gradient) [15].

In severe respiratory muscle weakness, the effort-dependent early part of the expiratory flow–volume curve may be selectively affected, resulting in disproportionate reductions in peak flow [16]. However, standard PFT are insensitive to muscle weakness, with a decrease in muscle strength of at least 50% required to produce reductions in lung volumes [17]. Muscle weakness can be distinguished from sub-maximal effort (as in advanced disease) by the characteristic failure to sustain expiration in sub-maximal effort, resulting in reductions in FVC in association with an increase in residual volume.

Historically, patterns of pulmonary function impairment were diagnostically useful in DLD but have been largely supplanted, in this regard, by HRCT. However, the presence of a mixed ventilatory defect is occasionally useful in increasing the diagnostic likelihood of hypersensitivity pneumonitis or sarcoidosis (as opposed to an idiopathic interstitial pneumonia).

Patterns of Pulmonary Function Impairment in Sarcoidosis

Although sarcoidosis is widely viewed as an interstitial lung disease, characterised by the clustering of non-caseating granulomas in the alveolar walls, small lymphatic channels, perivascular and peribronchiolar regions, the larger airways and respiratory muscles may also be involved. Patterns of pulmonary function abnormalities are highly heterogeneous, with air-flow obstruction, lung restriction, a mixed obstructive/restrictive ventilatory effect and disproportionate reduction in gas transfer (suggestive of a pulmonary vasculopathy) occurring in sizeable patient sub-groups.

Lung restriction, which may be prominent, is the most prevalent pattern in severe parenchymal lung disease, especially in patients with chest radiographic stages III and IV [18]. Even in apparently mild disease, a restrictive defect may be present, with reductions in FVC of 15–25% and reductions in DL_{CO} of 25–50% reported in patients with radiological stage 0 disease [19]. Reduced DL_{CO} levels are seen in up to 50% of patients with sarcoidosis, although usually less severe than in patients with idiopathic pulmonary fibrosis [20].

Airflow obstruction occurs in up to 60% of patients with pulmonary sarcoidosis and was the most frequent physiologic abnormality in one longitudinal study, occurring in all radiographic stages of disease and increasing in prevalence with increasing chest radiographic stage [21]. Fibrotic reticular abnormalities, peribronchial thickening and mosaic attenuation are the HRCT morphologic determinants of airflow obstruction [22, 23] which does not, in most cases, reverse with treatment. Morphologic abnormalities responsible for airflow obstruction include peribronchiolar fibrosis, airway narrowing from endobronchial granulomatous lesions or their resultant fibrotic scarring, distortion due to surrounding parenchymal fibrosis and compression by enlarged lymph nodes.

The Staging of Disease Severity and Prognostic Evaluation

Key points in the staging of disease severity and prognostic evaluation are listed in Table 5.2. In established DLD, the main purposes of pulmonary function estimation are to quantify the initial functional severity of disease, and to detect changes in severity with time. The large number

Table 5.2 Key points in the use of PFT to stage disease severity

1. In fibrosing lung disease, DLco levels best reflect morphologic severity
2. In fibrosing lung disease, lung volumes and arterial oxygen levels correlate poorly with morphologic severity
3. In pulmonary sarcoidosis, patterns of pulmonary function impairment are highly heterogeneous
4. In fibrosing lung disease, DLco is the resting variable that best predicts mortality
5. In idiopathic pulmonary fibrosis, oxygen desaturation to <88% during a 6-min walk test is associated with increased mortality
6. In interstitial lung disease, maximal exercise testing has no role in routine prognostic evaluation

of resting and exercise variables that can be measured routinely prompted attempts to identify PFT variables correlating most strongly with the underlying morphological severity of disease. Historical attempts to link pulmonary function variables to the histological severity of disease at surgical biopsy were constrained by low numbers of patients and the fact that the severity of disease in biopsy tissue is not necessarily indicative of disease severity throughout the lung. The search for a pulmonary function variable correlating selectively with the histological severity of inflammation also proved fruitless. However, the advent of HRCT provided, for the first time, a means of examining individual pulmonary function variables against the global morphologic severity of DLD.

Functional–morphologic correlations, based on the extent of disease on HRCT, have largely been evaluated in the historical entity of "idiopathic pulmonary fibrosis" [24, 25], prior to the reclassification of the idiopathic interstitial pneumonias, although it appears that the findings apply equally to patients with idiopathic pulmonary fibrosis, diagnosed using current criteria [26]. Amongst resting pulmonary function variables, DLco levels consistently reflect disease extent on HRCT more accurately than other functional indices. Lung volumes, including FVC and TLC, correlate surprisingly poorly with the morphologic extent of disease. Based on these observations, it can be concluded that disease severity in the idiopathic interstitial pneumonias is not adequately staged by spirometric volumes but requires gas transfer estimation. It appears that all of these observations apply equally to pulmonary fibrosis associated with SSc (in which nonspecific interstitial pneumonia is the usual histologic pattern), based on correlations between PFT and HRCT disease extent [27].

Arterial hypoxaemia at rest is associated with extensive disease on HRCT in idiopathic interstitial pneumonias but arterial oxygen levels do not correlate well with disease extent across the whole spectrum of disease severity. Maximal exercise testing has been advocated as a means of staging the severity of fibrosing lung disease. However, the amplitude of desaturation on exercise, with or without adjustment for respiratory work, has a lower correlation with the extent of disease on HRCT than DLco levels in both idiopathic interstitial pneumonia [26] and interstitial lung disease in scleroderma [27], although superior to lung volumes. Sub-maximal exercise data, including 6-min walk test variables, have not been compared formally with maximal exercise testing in their correlation with HRCT disease extent.

The prognostic value of PFT has been widely examined in the idiopathic interstitial pneumonias, grouped together and in patients with idiopathic pulmonary fibrosis or non-specific interstitial pneumonia, diagnosed using modern criteria. Overall, the prognostic value of baseline PFT has mirrored correlations between PFT and the extent of disease on HRCT, with DLco levels most consistently predictive of mortality. However, findings have varied widely with the nature of the populations studied, with resting arterial oxygen levels associated with a high mortality when disease is advanced but less useful as a prognostic marker across the whole range of disease severity. Lung volumes have generally been less predictive of outcome in the IIPs than DLco levels, in part because of the confounding effects of concurrent emphysema. In some younger biopsied cohorts, presumably with a lower prevalence of emphysema, FVC levels have been more strongly predictive of mortality.

Maximal exercise test variables have also had prognostic value [26, 28] but have not been shown to surpass DLco levels in this regard [26] and do not have a routine role in predicting overall survival in IPF or other fibrosing diseases. By contrast, desaturation below 88% during a 6-min walk test has provided powerful prognostic information in fibrotic idiopathic interstitial pneumonia in two studies [29, 30]. It remains uncertain whether this finding reflects more accurate quantification of the severity of lung fibrosis or, as seems more likely, the identification of a subset of patients with pulmonary hypertension at rest or on exercise. Interestingly, the 6-min walk distance, a cardinal variable in the evaluation of pulmonary hypertension, has little or no prognostic significance when evaluated as a continuous variable.

Composite indices have been developed in an attempt to refine prognostic evaluation. The clinical/radiological/physiological (CRP) score, first reported by Waters [28], has been refined as a relatively simplified score, the new CRP score [31], but both CRP scores suffer from the need to combine many variables, including ILO scoring of the chest radiograph and maximal exercise data. Both forms of the CRP score have been used in clinical studies but are not readily applicable to routine practise. By contrast, the composite physiologic index (CPI) has the advantage of containing only spirometric volumes and DLco levels and appears to predict mortality more strongly than individual lung function indices [26]. The CPI was derived, using stepwise regression, as the best fit of routine PFT against disease extent on HRCT in a mixed population of IPF and fibrotic NSIP: it is calculated by the formula: $CPI = 92.1 - (0.68 \times$ % predicted DLco$) - (0.53 \times$ % predicted FVC$) + (0.35 \times$ % predicted FEV1$)$. This accessible index quantifies functional impairment ascribable to interstitial disease, whilst excluding functional impairment due to emphysema [26, 32].

The advantages of DLco in staging severity in fibrosing interstitial diseases are less applicable in diseases with a significant airway component. In sarcoidosis, as discussed earlier, there are separate patient sub-groups with predominant restriction, predominant or isolated airflow obstruction and disproportionate reductions in DLco and no single variable can be used to stage severity: in predominantly obstructive disease, DLco levels are often well preserved and do not reflect the severity of disease. Thus, in diseases with heterogeneous patterns of lung function impairment, and especially in sarcoidosis, it is important to evaluate in each patient which PFT provides the most abnormal signal and to take note of this, both in prognostic evaluation and in selecting which variables to focus on in serial monitoring.

All of the variables discussed above suffer from the fact that, as continuous variables, they fail to identify discrete patient groups at lower and higher risk of a bad outcome. Such distinctions are needed in clinical practise as treatment decisions are dichotomous. It can be argued that in DLD, a staging approach is required, analogous to staging in malignant disease. A simple division between limited and extensive disease has been proposed in IPF, using a DLco threshold of 40% of predicted normal [33]. More recently, a staging system has recently been developed in interstitial lung disease in SSc (Fig. 5.1) [34]. With the use of rapid semi-quantitative HRCT evaluation and the application of a percentage predicted FVC threshold value of 70%, prognostically useful distinctions can be rapidly and reproducibly made between "mild" and "severe" interstitial disease. It is likely that similar systems, integrating PFT and HRCT data, will be developed in other DLDs in the reasonably near future.

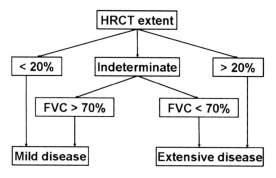

Fig. 5.1 A simple staging system for scleroderma lung [34]

Deconstructing Complex Patterns of Functional Impairment

Because pathological processes commonly coexist in DLD, patterns of functional impairment are often complex. Typical patterns of functional impairment associated with the more frequent combinations of disease processes are shown in Table 5.3. This problem applies most frequently in three specific scenarios: the mixture of emphysema and interstitial lung disease, the development of pulmonary hypertension in interstitial lung disease, and the mixture of disease processes that occur in connective tissue diseases.

As discussed earlier, smoking-related emphysema is often mixed with interstitial fibrosis in the idiopathic interstitial pneumonias and in rheumatoid lung, resulting in disproportionate reductions in DLco and Kco levels. This profile applies equally to the combination of interstitial fibrosis and pulmonary hypertension, also discussed earlier, and is especially prevalent in

Table 5.3 Typical patterns of pulmonary function impairment seen in association with selected combinations of disease processes

Pulmonary fibrosis Centrilobular emphysema	Normal lung volumes/mild restrictive or obstructive defect. Disproportionate reduction in DLco/severe reduction in Kco. Hypoxia frequent at rest or on exercise
Pulmonary fibrosis Pulmonary hypertension	Restrictive lung volumes. Disproportionate reduction in DLco, severe reduction in Kco, elevated FVC/DLco ratio. Hypoxia frequent at rest or on exercise
Pulmonary fibrosis Extra-pulmonary restriction	Restrictive ventilatory defect, often severe. DLco less severely impaired than expected, Kco normal or increased. Alveolar–arterial oxygen gradient may be normal
Pulmonary hypertension Extra-pulmonary restriction	Variable restrictive defect. DLco reduced, Kco reduced, normal or increased depending upon relative severity of disease processes. Hypoxia frequent at rest or on exercise

advanced DLD. In both scenarios, a reliance on spirometric volumes, alone, to stage disease severity and to monitor change may be highly misleading, underlining the importance of routine DLco estimation.

The detection of pulmonary vascular disease in the presence of interstitial lung disease causes particular difficulty. As in isolated pulmonary vascular disease, a disproportionate reduction in DLco, relative to lung volumes, should prompt further investigation for pulmonary hypertension [10], although not distinguishing between a primary pulmonary vasculopathy and secondary pulmonary hypertension. Historically, Kco levels (the DLco/VA ratio) has been used to quantify disproportionate reductions in DLco. More recently, a rising FVC/DLco ratio [35, 36] has been indicative of a higher likelihood of pulmonary hypertension. In reality, the two ratios can be viewed as approximately equivalent but a direct comparison is needed in future studies: in principle, the FVC/DLco ratio should be less reproducible as it incorporates the variability of both measurement techniques, whereas Kco is measured with a single manoeuvre.

The interpretation of patterns of functional impairment is even more problematic in the connective tissue diseases, in which pathological processes variably coexist in the interstitium, airways, pulmonary vasculature, pleura and respiratory muscles [3]. The combination of interstitial fibrosis and pulmonary hypertension may occur in any of the connective tissue diseases and is especially prevalent in SSc. In polymyositis/dermatomyositis, pulmonary hypertension is relatively infrequent and complex functional impairment more often arises from the combination of interstitial disease and respiratory muscle weakness. In Sjogrens Syndrome, lymphocytic interstitial infiltration may coexist with lymphocytic bronchiolitis, resulting in a mixed ventilatory defect. Rheumatoid arthritis (interstitial disease, airway disease, pleural disease, smoking-related emphysema and, less frequently, pulmonary vasculitis) and systemic lupus erythematosus (pleural disease, pulmonary vasculopathy, airway disease, respiratory muscle weakness and, less frequently, interstitial disease) are both notorious

for a wide range of possible combinations of disease processes.

In general, the deconstruction of complex patterns of functional impairment requires the integration of ancillary tests, especially HRCT, echocardiography and tests of respiratory muscle function. HRCT has a particularly important role in detecting concurrent emphysema, pleural processes and airway disease, because in experienced hands, an approximate assessment can be made as to whether PFT reductions are broadly appropriate for the observed extent of interstitial disease. Without the integration of HRCT findings and PFT, complex functional impairment is often difficult to rationalise.

PFT in the Monitoring of Change (See Table 5.4)

It has long been recognised that good discriminatory variables are not always good evaluative variables. A test which performs well at a single point in time does not always perform well in identifying serial change. Specifically, although DLco levels have the greatest prognostic utility at baseline evaluation in IPF, changes in disease severity are more accurately quantified by FVC trends (although no formal comparison has been made with other lung volumes, including slow VC). This insight comes from a number of IPF

Table 5.4 Key points in the use of PFT to monitor change in disease severity in idiopathic pulmonary fibrosis

1. In fibrosing lung disease, serial FVC trends predict mortality better than trends in other PFT
2. "Significant" change is defined as a 10% change in FVC or a 15% change in DLco, from *baseline* values
3. FVC and DLco levels should both be measured, to improve the accuracy of monitoring
4. Confounding from measurement variation is a relatively more frequent cause of apparent decline in slowly progressive disease
5. Serial DLco trends are more sensitive to change than serial FVC trends when emphysema is admixed with interstitial fibrosis
6. Neither maximal exercise testing nor 6-min walk testing has a routine role in measuring changes in disease severity

studies in which lung function trends at 6 months or at 1 year have been examined against survival [37–40]. In all these studies, serial FVC trends have strongly predicted mortality and have, in almost all analyses, been superior to DLco in this regard. The advantage of FVC over DLco is due, in part, to variability in DLco estimation. As discussed later, "drift" in gas transfer estimation can be dealt with by calibrating lung function equipment daily against normal biological controls such as staff members.

It should be stressed that the optimal mode of quantifying change in FVC has not been formally established. FVC trends can be stated as percentage change from baseline values or percentage change in predicted normal values. However, percentage change from baseline values has been used historically and has been proven to predict survival in the studies cited above. Thresholds for "significant" changes in PFT (FVC = 10% change from baseline; DLco = 15% change from baseline), derived from reproducibility data, are selected in order to exclude confounding from measurement variation. The designation of a 10% FVC threshold for change reflects the fact that on short-term repeat measurement, FVC values differ by less than 10% in 95% of normal subjects (i.e. within two standard deviations of change). Thus, measurement variation will result in an apparently significant change in FVC values during monitoring in 5% of patients, with spurious decline, thus, seen in 2.5% of cases. A 10% change in FVC corresponds to a fall from 2 to 1.8 L. Short-term PFT trends should be computed using absolute values rather than percentage predicted levels (which are inappropriately influenced by the timing of patient birthdays within or outside the monitored time period).

The primacy of serial FVC trends should not obscure the value of combining trends in FVC, TLC and DLco. Measurement variation is equally likely to result in the over-statement and the *understatement* of the degree of change. By evaluating separate measurement techniques (e.g. spirometry and estimation of gas transfer), the clinician can feel reassured that a uniform overall trend is unlikely to be spurious, even when "significant change" is not seen in all variables. This may be especially important in considering change in DLco, which is sometimes due to pulmonary vascular damage rather than progression of pulmonary fibrosis. The association of a "marginal" reduction in FVC (5–10% of baseline values) with a significant decline in DLco provides useful support for the latter. Recent data suggest that marginal reductions in FVC of 5–10% in IPF are associated with a worse outcome when compared to patients with stable FVC values [41].

The value of evaluating more than one PFT variable is especially important on Bayesian grounds, in more slowly progressive disease. In fibrotic non-specific interstitial pneumonia or sarcoidosis, for example, a change in disease severity is much less prevalent than in idiopathic pulmonary fibrosis, and measurement variation is a proportionately greater confounder. If the pre-test probability of "significant" change due to disease progression approximates 10% in less progressive disease, and the probability of spurious decline due to measurement variation approximates 2.5% (as discussed above), a 10% decline in FVC will represent true decline in only 80% of cases (i.e. a likelihood ratio of 10%:2.5% or 4:1). A concurrent change in DLco of 15% will increase the likelihood of true decline to 16:1 (over 95%). In IPF, by contrast, a disease in which pulmonary function decline can be expected in over a third of cases at 1 year [42], a 10% decline in FVC will represent true decline in 90–95% of patients. Thus, the designation of standard thresholds for change, irrespective of the progressiveness of the underlying disease or the time interval of monitoring, is a major over-simplification which needs to be confronted in future recommendations.

Similarly, the time interval of monitoring must be tailored to the underlying diagnosis, disease severity, changes in management and the observed rapidity of disease progression. In the absence of a specific clinical indication (such as increasing dyspnoea), it is not helpful to repeat PFT more frequently than three monthly in chronic DILD as there is not sufficient time for pulmonary function trends to reach thresholds for "significant" change. In idiopathic pulmonary fibrosis, it is usual to repeat measurement of FVC and DLco three to six monthly, with the exact time interval influenced by the likelihood that observed decline will result in a change in management (such as referral for lung transplantation). In other DILDs, including sarcoidosis, similar time intervals are appropriate initially. However, the frequency of monitoring must then be modulated according to the likelihood of disease progression, disease severity, observed progressiveness/stability during initial observation and the evaluation of regression or relapse of disease with changes in treatment.

The evaluation of multiple variables is also important when there is disease in more than one lung compartment, as in connective tissue disease or sarcoidosis. In isolation, change in any single variable may not clearly establish the site and severity of change. For example, in a patient with severe airflow obstruction, disease progression or regression is more likely to be captured by FEV1 trends. Thus, in mixed disease, no single PFT can be regarded as the primary measure of change in all patients. The need to integrate pulmonary function trends creates obvious difficulties in pharmaceutical studies, in which a single primary end-point is required. Monitoring disease is not straightforward in multi-compartment disease and requires a careful two-stage evaluation. At baseline, the lung function profile should be carefully deconstructed as discussed earlier – by integrating all lung function information, HRCT findings, clinical information, echocardiographic data and, in selected cases, respiratory muscle function testing, it is generally possible to assign approximate functional significance to each disease process [3]. Multidisciplinary appraisal should then be repeated when serial PFT show significant change, with the reconciliation of PFT trends in more than one variable, symptomatic change, chest radiographic findings and, when appropriate, HRCT evaluation. Two scenarios of mixed disease deserve particular mention.

The combination of emphysema and pulmonary fibrosis is common in IPF and results in the relative preservation of lung volumes and a marked reduction in DLco (which is affected by both disease processes) [26, 32, 43]. In some patients with end-stage disease, lung volumes remain normal when coexistent emphysema is severe. It follows logically that serial measurement of FVC may fail completely to demonstrate major progression of pulmonary fibrosis. In this scenario, serial reduction in DLco tends to be more sensitive. In reality, in most patients with both diseases, there is a point at which the extent of fibrosis greatly exceeds that of emphysema and FVC levels begin to decline and can be used to monitor progression. However, serial DLco trends should probably be given more weighting in this particular scenario. The combination of pulmonary fibrosis and pulmonary hypertension is also a difficult monitoring scenario. This may explain the observation that in advanced IPF, serial DLco trends predict mortality more strongly than serial FVC trends, in striking contrast to less advanced disease [44].

These considerations lie behind recommendations in forthcoming guidelines for the diagnosis and management of IPF that FVC and DLco levels should both be monitored. It is argued that in the absence of an alternative explanation, a 10% decline in FVC, with or without a concurrent change in DLco, and a 15% decline in DLco, with or without a concurrent change in FVC, should both be regarded as indicative of disease progression and as surrogates for mortality in trials of therapies in this disease.

There is no current evidence that serial maximal exercise testing provides useful prognostic information in fibrosing lung disease, over and above serial DLco trends. Furthermore, it appears that in fibrotic idiopathic interstitial pneumonia (IPF or fibrotic NSIP), maximal exercise variables are very poorly reproducible [30] and are, thus, poorly suited to the accurate identification of disease progression. By contrast, the 6-min walk distance is highly reproducible in the short term in fibrotic idiopathic interstitial pneumonia [30] and in the pulmonary fibrosis of SSc [45] and was considered, in principle, to be a good variable with which to monitor change, based on the precedence established in PAH. However, short-term evaluation takes no account of changes in the 6-min walk distance due to musculoskeletal factors, deconditioning, rehabilitation and changes over time in the pattern of ventilation to reduce respiratory work. It has now been shown in IPF treatment trials that striking changes in both directions often occur in the 6-min walk distance, when evaluated as a continuous variable, in the absence of change in PFT or other specific measures of the severity of pulmonary fibrosis [46, 47]. The prognostic utility of categorical change (i.e. to designated thresholds) in the 6-min walk distance has yet to be evaluated. However, at present the 6-min walk testing has no routine role at present in serial monitoring of changes in disease severity, although it may play a useful role in the reappraisal of indications for supplementary ambulatory oxygen.

The Accuracy and Reproducibility of PFT: Quality Assurance

Given the use of PFT threshold values to designate "significant" change, thorough quality control and quality assurance procedures in lung function laboratories are essential, to ensure technical accuracy and to minimise measurement variability. Quality control and quality assurance procedures should be documented and rigorously checked to ensure they meet recognised standards [48, 49]. The ATS/ERS standards specify details and guidelines pertaining to quality control and quality assurance relevant to routine lung function tests, including information relating to calibration and verification of equipment.

The importance of biological control data has been emphasised [50, 51]. Trend analyses on biological control data, produced by the performance of PFT by "normal" staff members, should be carried out frequently. Biological data should be obtained on a regular basis. In some laboratories, including the laboratory in our institution, staff members perform PFT at the start of every day, with a view to recalibrating equipment as necessary: our own experience leaves us in no doubt that this exercise is worthwhile, especially with regard to measures of gas transfer, which are less reproducible than lung volumes. It is acknowledged that this meticulous approach cannot always be reconciled with the demands of routine practise, but if so, the weekly acquisition of biological control data is strongly recommended (although this is a more stringent recommendation than

made in some guideline statements). Some current protocols for PFT obtained in pharmaceutical trials in IPF recommend the monthly acquisition of biological control data: it can be argued that this is insufficiently rigorous, especially with regard to variables such as FVC and DLco, often designated as primary or co-primary end-points. Trend analyses are especially useful in the identification of equipment malfunction, which is often undetected by routine calibration.

Cotes states that a coefficient of variation, defined as (standard deviation/mean)$\times 100$ of 4–8%, should be expected in pulmonary function laboratories with "high standards" [51]. However, with stringent monitoring of performance, quality assurance, quality control and test results, based on daily biological control data, a coefficient of variation of between 2 and 4% can be obtained for routine tests (spirometric volumes, TLC, measures of gas transfer). In our own institution, the performance of daily biological control tests for over two decades has been associated with a root mean square coefficient of variation (RMSCV) of less than 4% for all routine lung function parameters. This may account for the fact that in fibrotic idiopathic interstitial pneumonia (IPF, fibrotic NSIP), serial trends in DLco have had more prognostic significance in our population [39] than in other cohorts [37, 38, 40], in which serial FVC trends have had relatively greater prognostic accuracy. FVC estimation is less intrinsically variable, but rigorous quality assurance remains pivotal, given the recent observation that in IPF patients without a significant fall in FVC, "marginal" declines of 5–10% from baseline values are predictive of increased mortality.

Even with rigorous quality assurance, the reproducibility of MEF25 and RV is significantly lower than that of the other variables discussed above. MEF25 values are usually very low (<2 L/s), increasing relative measurement "noise" and the attendant coefficient of variation. The RV is derived from two measured parameters (functional residual capacity and expiratory reserve volume) and the increased coefficient of variation reflects a summation of the intrinsic variability of two measured parameters. Thus, neither variable is suited to the detection of significant functional change in routine practise.

Inter-laboratory variability is a further important consideration, especially at referral centres when PFT are compared to those performed previously at local laboratories. Plainly, inter-laboratory variability will be minimised by rigorous quality assurance, which results in only minor discrepancies in FVC values. However, DLco measurement is notoriously inconsistent between laboratories, despite quality assurance, due to the many technical variations that occur in gas transfer estimation. Thus, significant gas transfer trends, based upon measurements at separate laboratories, should be viewed with scepticism when spirometric values are stable.

The acquisition of biological control data is an important addition to other quality control procedures in the performance of cardiopulmonary exercise tests, and it has proved practicable to obtain exercise data from normal staff members on a weekly basis [52]. Based on published data, coefficients of variation should be less than 7% for peak oxygen uptake [52], less than 5% for peak oxygen uptake and peak carbon dioxide production and less than 7% for peak ventilation [53].

Fitness to Fly Tests

In patients with minor hypoxaemia who wish to travel by aeroplane, a hypoxic inhalation test (fitness to fly test) should be performed. Hypobaric hypoxaemia reflects the inverse relationship between oxygen partial pressure and altitude. This occurs during travel in a pressurised aircraft cabin as ambient pressure is decreased during ascent. Commercial aircraft typically cruise at 12,000 m. Engineering and financial constraints preclude sea-level pressurisation. Aircraft cabin is pressurised to a maximum altitude of approximately 2,500 m, which equates to breathing 15% oxygen at sea level [54]. In healthy individuals, the partial pressure of arterial blood (PaO_2) at this altitude depends, in part, on age and minute ventilation, but will generally fall to between 8.0 and 10.0 kPa (SpO_2 90–94%) [55]. The wide variation in the individual response to the hypobaric environment is not well understood [56]. Thus,

the British Thoracic Society (BTS) recommends a low threshold for performing pre-flight assessments in patients with respiratory disease [57, 58]. In this regard, severe lung function impairment and major exercise intolerance should prompt pre-flight assessment, even in the absence of minor hypoxaemia, as some patients with a normal PaO_2 at sea level may become significantly hypoxaemic when breathing 15% oxygen.

Hypobaric chambers, the "gold standard" means of in-flight assessment, are expensive and cumbersome and, thus, not widely available. Alternative methods include hypoxic inhalation tests and predictive equations. The hypoxic inhalation test is the preferred option as the level of hypoxaemia, on breathing 15% oxygen, exhibits considerable individual variability: predictive equations often considerably overestimate the need for in-flight oxygen [59]. During the hypoxic inhalation test, cabin altitude is simulated at sea level with a gas mixture containing 15% oxygen in nitrogen. Subjects breathe the hypoxic gas mixture from a Douglas bag for 20 min, with monitoring of oxygen saturation (SpO_2) and ECG throughout and the measurement of arterial gases at the beginning and end. The results can then be used to determine the flow rate of supplemental oxygen, if required. If the PaO_2 is less than 6.6 kPa (83% SpO_2), in-flight oxygen is needed (usually at 2 L/min via nasal prongs). An important caveat is that short-term hyperventilation during the test (as judged by $PaCO_2$ levels) may mask hypoxaemia and this should be taken into account, especially for long haul flights.

An alternative technique is to seat the patient in the body plethysmograph and to reduce oxygen concentration within the body box to 15% (FiO_2: 0.15) [55], allowing oxygen requirements to be titrated accurately using nasal prongs.

References

1. Keogh BA, Crystal RG. Pulmonary function testing in interstitial pulmonary disease. What does it tell us? Chest. 1980;78:856–964.
2. Cherniack RM, Colby TV, Flint A, et al. Correlation of structure and function in idiopathic pulmonary fibrosis. Am J Respir Crit Care Med. 1995;151:1180–8.

3. Wells AU. Pulmonary function tests in connective tissue disease. Semin Respir Crit Care Med. 2007; 28:379–88.
4. Quanjer PH. Standardised lung function testing. Clin Respir Physiol. 1983;19(Suppl):1–95.
5. Gibson GJ. Clinical tests of respiratory function. London: Chappell and Hall; 1996. p. 223–4.
6. Cordier J-F. Organising pneumonia. Thorax. 2000;55: 318–28.
7. Gould GA, Redpath AT, Ryan M, et al. Lung CT density correlates with measurements of airflow limitation and the diffusing capacity. Eur Respir J. 1991;4:141–6.
8. Hansell DM, Rubens MB, Padley SPG, Wells AU. Obliterative bronchiolitis: individual CT signs of small airways disease and functional correlation. Radiology. 1997;203:721–6.
9. Gibson GJ. Clinical tests of respiratory function. 3rd ed. London: Macmillan; 2009. p. 47, 48.
10. Burke CM, Glanville AR, Morris AJR, et al. Pulmonary function in advanced pulmonary hypertension. Thorax. 1987;42:151–5.
11. Lipscomb DJ, Patel K, Hughes JM. Interpretation of increases in the transfer coefficient for carbon monoxide (TLCO/VA or KCO). Thorax. 1978;33:728–33.
12. Broderich A, Fuortes LJ, Merchant JA, Galvin JR, Shwartz DA. Pleural determinants of restrictive lung function and respiratory symptoms in an asbestos-exposed population. Chest. 1992;101:684–91.
13. Colp C, Reichel J, Park SS. Severe pleural restriction: the maximum static pulmonary recoil pressure as an aide in diagnosis. Chest. 1975;67:658–64.
14. Wright PH, Hansen A, Kreel L, Capel LH. Respiratory function changes after asbestos pleurisy. Thorax. 1980; 35:31–6.
15. Gibson GJ, Pride NB, Newsom-Davis J, Loh LC. Pulmonary mechanics in patients with respiratory muscle weakness. Am Rev Respir Dis. 1977;115:389–95.
16. Vincken WG, Elleker MG, Cosio MG. Flow-volume loop changes reflecting respiratory muscle weakness in chronic neuromuscular disorders. Am J Med. 1987;83:673–80.
17. Braun NM, Arora NS, Rochester DF. Respiratory muscle and pulmonary function in polymyositis and other proximal myopathies. Thorax. 1983;38:616–23.
18. Neville E, Walker A, James DG. Prognostic factors predicting outcome of sarcoidosis: an analysis of 818 patients. QJ Med. 1983;2(208):525–33.
19. Alhamad EH, Lynch 3rd JP, Martinez FJ. Pulmonary function tests in interstitial lung disease: what role do they have? Clin Chest Med. 2001;22:715–50.
20. Lynch 3rd JP, Kazerooni EA, Gaye SE. Pulmonary sarcoidosis. Clin Chest Med. 1997;18:755–85.
21. Harrison BD, Shaylor JM, Stokes TC, Wilkes AR. Airflow limitation in sarcoidosis: a study of pulmonary function in 107 patients with newly diagnosed disease. Respir Med. 1991;85:59–64.
22. Gleeson FV, Traill ZC, Hansell DM. Evidence of expiratory CT scans of small-airway obstruction in sarcoidosis. AJR Am J Roentgenol. 1996;166:1052–4.
23. Hansell DM, Milne DG, Wilsher ML, Wells AU. Pulmonary sarcoidosis: morphologic associations of airflow obstruction on thin section computed tomography. Radiology. 1998;209:697–704.
24. Staples CA, Muller NL, Vedal S, Abboud R, Ostrow DN, Miller RR. Usual interstitial pneumonia: correlation of CT with clinical, functional and radiologic findings. Radiology. 1987;162:377–81.
25. Wells AU, King AD, Rubens MB, Cramer D, du Bois RM, Hansell DM. Lone CFA: a functional-morphological correlation based on extent of disease on thin-section computed tomography. Am J Respir Crit Care Med. 1997;155:1367–75.
26. Wells AU, Desai SR, Rubens MB, et al. Idiopathic pulmonary fibrosis: a composite physiologic index derived from disease extent observed on computed tomography. Am J Respir Crit Care Med. 2003;167:962–9.
27. Wells AU, Hansell DM, Rubens MB, et al. Fibrosing alveolitis in systemic sclerosis: indices of lung function in relation to extent of disease on computed tomography. Arthritis Rheum. 1997;40:1229–36.
28. Watters LC, King TE, Schwarz MI, Waldron JA, Stanford RE, Cherniack RM. A clinical, radiographic and physiologic scoring system for the longitudinal assessment of patients with idiopathic pulmonary fibrosis. Am Rev Respir Dis. 1986;133:97–103.
29. Lama VN, Flaherty KR, Toews GB, et al. Prognostic value of desaturation during a six-minute walk test in idiopathic interstitial pneumonia. Am J Respir Crit Care Med. 2003;168:1084–90.
30. Eaton T, Young P, Milne D, Wells AU. Six-minute walk, maximal exercise tests: reproducibility in fibrotic interstitial pneumonia. Am J Respir Crit Care Med. 2005;171:1150–7.
31. King TE, Tooze JA, Schwarz MI, Brown KR, Cherniack RM. Predicting survival in idiopathic pulmonary fibrosis: scoring system and survival model. Am J Respir Crit Care Med. 2001;164:1171–81.
32. Mura M, Zompatori M, Pacilli AM, Fasano L, Schiavina M, Fabbri M. The presence of emphysema further impairs physiologic function in patients with idiopathic pulmonary fibrosis. Respir Care. 2006;51:257–65.
33. Egan JJ, Martinez FJ, Wells AU, Williams T. Lung function estimates in idiopathic pulmonary fibrosis: the potential for a simple classification. Thorax. 2005; 60:270–3.
34. Goh NS, Desai SR, Veeraraghavan S, et al. Interstitial lung disease in systemic sclerosis: a simple staging system. Am J Respir Crit Care Med. 2008;177(11): 1248–54.
35. Nathan SD, Shlobin OA, Ahmad S, Urbanek S, Barnett SD. Pulmonary hypertension and pulmonary function testing in idiopathic pulmonary fibrosis. Chest. 2007;131:657–63.
36. Steen VD, Graham G, Conte C, Owens G, Medsger TA. JR. Isolated diffusing capacity reduction in systemic sclerosis. Arthritis Rheum. 1992;35:765–70.
37. Collard HR, King Jr TE, Bartelson BB, Vourlekis JS, Schwarz MI, Brown KK. Changes in clinical and physiologic variables predict survival in idiopathic pulmonary fibrosis. Am J Respir Crit Care Med. 2003;168:538–42.
38. Flaherty KR, Mumford JA, Murray S, et al. Prognostic implications of physiologic and radiographic changes

in idiopathic interstitial pneumonia. Am J Respir Crit Care Med. 2003;168:543–8.

39. Latsi PI, du Bois RM, Nicholson AG, et al. Fibrotic idiopathic interstitial pneumonia: the prognostic value of longitudinal functional trends. Am J Respir Crit Care Med. 2003;168:531–7.

40. King Jr TE, Safrin S, Starko KM, Brown KK, Noble PW, Raghu G, et al. Analyses of efficacy end points in a controlled trial of interferon-gamma1b for idiopathic pulmonary fibrosis. Chest. 2005;127: 171–7.

41. Zappala CJ, Latsi PI, Nicholson AG, et al. Marginal decline in forced vital capacity is associated with a poor outcome in idiopathic pulmonary fibrosis. Eur Respir J. 2010;35:830–6.

42. Demedts M, Beh J, Buh R, Costabel U, Dekhuijen R, Jansen HM, et al. High dose acetylcysteine in idiopathic pulmonary fibrosis. N Engl J Med. 2006;353: 2229–42.

43. Cottin V, Nunes H, Brillet PY, et al. Combined pulmonary fibrosis and emphysema: a distinct underrecognised entity. Eur Respir J. 2005;26:586–93.

44. Flaherty KR, Andrei AC, Murray S, et al. Idiopathic pulmonary fibrosis: prognostic value of changes in physiology and six-minute-walk test. Am J Respir Crit Care Med. 2006;174:803–9.

45. Buch MH, Denton CP, Furst DE, et al. Submaximal exercise testing in the assessment of interstitial lung disease secondary to systemic sclerosis: reproducibility and correlations of the 6-min walk test. Ann Rheum Dis. 2007;66:169–73.

46. King Jr TE, Behr J, Brown KK, et al. BUILD-1: a randomized placebo-controlled trial of bosentan in idiopathic pulmonary fibrosis. Am J Respir Crit Care Med. 2008;177:75–81.

47. Raghu G, Brown KK, Costabel U, et al. Treatment of idiopathic pulmonary fibrosis with etanercept: an exploratory, placebo-controlled trial. Am J Respir Crit Care Med. 2008;178:948–55.

48. Brusasco V, Crapo R, Viegi G. General considerations for lung function. Eur Respir J. 2005;26:153–61. Series "ATS/ERS Task Force: Standardisation of lung function testing".

49. Brusasco V, Crapo R, Viegi G. Standardisation of the single breath determination of carbon monoxide uptake in the lung. Eur Respir J. 2005;26:720–35. Series "ATS/ERS Task Force: Standardisation of lung function testing".

50. ARTP Working Groups on Standards of Care and Recommendations for Lung Function Departments. Quality assurance for lung function laboratories. 2006. http://www.ARTP.org.uk/.

51. Cotes JE, Chinn DJ, Miller MR. Lung function. 6th ed. Oxford: Blackwell; 2006. p. 79. ISBN 13:978-0-6320-6493-9.

52. Roca J, Whipp BJ, et al. Clinical exercise testing with reference to lung diseases: indications, standardization and interpretation strategies. ERS Task Force on Standardization of Clinical Exercise Testing. Eur Respir J. 1997;10:2662–89.

53. Reville SM, Morgan M. Biological quality control for exercise testing. Thorax. 2000;55:63–6.

54. Seccombe LM, Kelly PT, Wong CK, Rogers PG, Lim S, Peters MJ. Effect of simulated commercial flight on oxygenation in patients with interstitial lung disease and chronic obstructive pulmonary disease. Thorax. 2004;59:966–70.

55. Cramer D, Ward S, Geddes D. Assessment of oxygen supplementation during air travel. Thorax. 1996;51: 202–3.

56. Ernsting J, Nicholson AN, Rainford DJ, editors. Aviation medicine. 3rd ed. Oxford: Butterworth-Heinmann; 2000.

57. British Thoracic Society Standards of Care Committee. Managing passengers with respiratory disease planning air travel: British Thoracic Society recommendations. Thorax. 2002;57:289–304.

58. British Thoracic Society Standards of Care Committee. Managing passengers with respiratory disease planning air travel: Summary for primary care. 2004. http://www.brit-thoracic.org.uk/c2/uploads/FlightPCsummary04.pdf.

59. Martin SE, Bradley JM, Buick JB, Bradbury I, Elborn JS. Flight assessment in patients with respiratory disease: hypoxic challenge testing vs. predictive equations. Q J Med. 2007;100:361–7.

Diffuse Lung Disease: Classification and Evaluation

6

Harold R. Collard and Talmadge E. King Jr.

Abstract

There are more than 200 clinical forms of diffuse lung disease (DLD) with a wide variety of causes and associations. The physician faced with a suspected case of DLD must therefore have an organized and systematic approach to the diagnostic evaluation. One such approach is to divide these processes into five broad clinical categories. These are: primary disease related, environmental exposure related, drug induced, collagen-vascular associated, and the idiopathic interstitial pneumonias. The history and physical examination is of critical importance in identifying possible exposures to occupational and environmental substances known to cause DLD, documenting drug exposures, and eliciting symptoms and signs of collagen-vascular disease or other primary diseases. Radiographic, physiologic, and laboratory evaluation can often confirm the presumptive diagnosis. Importantly, a minority of patients will have no identifiable cause of DLD after careful clinical evaluation. These patients are considered to have idiopathic DLD, termed idiopathic interstitial pneumonias. The current ATS/ERS classification schema for the idiopathic interstitial pneumonias includes seven distinct subgroups associated with distinctive histopathological patterns of injury and repair: idiopathic pulmonary fibrosis (IPF), nonspecific interstitial pneumonia, acute interstitial pneumonia, cryptogenic organizing pneumonia, lymphocytic interstitial pneumonia, respiratory bronchiolitis-associated interstitial lung disease, and desquamative interstitial pneumonia.

H.R. Collard • T.E. King Jr. (✉)
Department of Medicine, University of California
San Francisco, San Francisco, CA, USA
e-mail: tking@medicine.ucsf.edu

R.P. Baughman and R.M. du Bois (eds.), *Diffuse Lung Disease: A Practical Approach*,
DOI 10.1007/978-1-4419-9771-5_6, © Springer Science+Business Media, LLC 2012

Keywords

Surgical lung biopsy • Environmental exposure • High-resolution CT scan
• Drug-induced lung disease • Collagen vascular disease • Idiopathic pulmonary fibrosis • Nonspecific interstitial pneumonia • Acute interstitial
pneumonia • Cryptogenic organizing pneumonia • Lymphocytic interstitial pneumonia • Respiratory bronchiolitis-associated interstitial lung disease • Desquamative interstitial pneumonia

Introduction

For over 100 years, physicians have recognized
diffuse lung disease (DLD) as a clinical entity.
There are now over 200 clinical forms of DLD
described in the literature with a wide variety of
causes and associations [1]. The physician faced
with a suspected case of DLD must therefore
have an organized and systematic approach to the
diagnostic evaluation.

Classification of DLD

DLD is generally divided into five broad clinical
categories (Table 6.1). These are: primary disease
related, environmental exposure related, drug
induced, collagen-vascular associated, and the
idiopathic interstitial pneumonias (IIPs). The history and physical examination is of critical importance in identifying possible exposures to
occupational and environmental substances known
to cause DLD, documenting drug exposures, and
eliciting symptoms and signs of collagen-vascular
disease or other primary diseases. Radiographic,
physiologic, and laboratory evaluation can often
confirm the presumptive diagnosis. A detailed
approach to the diagnosis of many of these conditions is found elsewhere in this text. A sizable
minority of patients, however, will have no identifiable cause of DLD after careful clinical evaluation. These patients are considered to have
idiopathic DLD, termed IIP.

Primary Disease-Related DLD

There are many primary diseases, both systemic
and organ specific, that are associated with DLD

Table 6.1 Classification of diffuse lung disease

Primary disease-related DLD
  Amyloidosis
  Chronic aspiration
  Chronic infection
  Eosinophilic pneumonia
  Inflammatory bowel disease
  Langerhans cell granulomatosis
  Lipoid pneumonia
  Lymphangioleiomyomatosis
  Malignancy (lymphoma, metastatic)
  Primary biliary cirrhosis
  Pulmonary alveolar proteinosis
  Sarcoidosis
  Viral hepatitis

Environmental exposure-related DLD (selected)
  Pneumoconiosis (inorganic substances)
    Asbestos
    Beryllium
    Hard metals
    Polyvinyl chloride
    Silica
  Hypersensitivity pneumonitis (organic substance)
    Bagassosis
    Bird fancier's lung
    Ceramic tile lung
    Chicken handler's lung
    Detergent worker's lung
    Farmer's lung
    Fishmeal worker's lung
    Goose down lung
    Humidifier lung
    Miller's lung
    Mushroom worker's lung
    Wood worker's lung

Drug-induced DLD (selected)
  Amiodarone
  Angiotensin Converting Enzyme Inhibitors
  Antibiotics (cephalosporins, nitrofurantoin, ethambutol)
  Chemotherapeutic Agents (bleomycin, alkylating
    agents, methotrexate)
  Cocaine
  Dilantin
  Monoclonal antibodies (antitumor necrosis factor,
    anti-CD20)
  NSAIDs
  Radiation
  Statins

(continued)

Table 6.1 (continued)

Connective tissue disease-associated DLD
  Ankylosing spondylitis
  Polymyositis/dermatomyositis
  Rheumatoid arthritis
  Systemic sclerosis (scleroderma)
  Sjögren's syndrome
  Systemic lupus erythematosus
  Undifferentiated connective tissue disease

Idiopathic interstitial pneumonia
  Acute interstitial pneumonia
  Cryptogenic organizing pneumonia
  Desquamative interstitial pneumonia
  Idiopathic pulmonary fibrosis
  Lymphocytic interstitial pneumonia
  Nonspecific interstitial pneumonia
  Respiratory bronchiolitis-associated interstitial lung
    disease

(see Table 6.1). It is important that the clinician evaluating patients with suspected DLD be aware of the potential for such diverse conditions as amyloidosis, inflammatory bowel disease, chronic infection (e.g., tuberculosis, histoplasmosis), and malignancy to cause DLD. Sarcoidosis is the most common systemic disease to cause DLD, and should be considered in all patients. Less common conditions such as Langerhans cell granulomatosis (also known as eosinophilic granuloma or histiocytosis X), lymphangioleiomyomatosis, pulmonary alveolar proteinosis, and eosinophilic pneumonia should also be considered in the right clinical context. Most of these conditions have characteristic historical, physical, and radiographic presentations as discussed in detail elsewhere in this text.

Environmental Exposure-Related DLD

There are an ever-growing number of environmental exposures associated with DLD (Table 6.1). Clinically these are divided into two groups, based on the presumed causative substance. DLD related to exposure to inorganic substances is categorized as "pneumoconiosis." DLD related to exposure to organic substances is categorized as "hypersensitivity pneumonitis." A careful environmental exposure history is essential in all patients presenting with DLD, as serological testing for circulating antigen-specific antibodies (i.e., serum

precipitins) is neither sensitive nor specific. Specific questioning about past and present occupation, residence, travel, hobbies, and pets (in particular birds) should be universally performed. Unless removed from the causative exposure, patients with environmental exposure-related DLD generally suffer progressive disability. Identifying an environmental cause for DLD therefore has significant clinical implications.

Drug-Induced DLD

Drugs can cause both acute and chronic DLD. A careful medication history should be taken in all patients presenting with DLD. This includes prescribed medications, over-the-counter drugs, and any nontraditional therapies. Several commonly used drugs are associated with a significant risk of DLD including amiodarone, methotrexate, and certain antibiotics (see Table 6.1). Although there is often a temporal relationship between starting the causative medication and the development of DLD, some cases may occur after years of therapy. Patients with a history of thoracic radiation can also develop DLD, often years after the causative exposure.

Connective Tissue Disease-Associated DLD

The association between connective tissue disease and DLD is well established (see Table 6.1). Pulmonary disease may be the first presentation in some cases, so a careful history, physical exam, and (in some cases) serological evaluation looking for evidence of connective disease is important. Many patients with connective tissue disease-associated DLD will have clinical, radiographic, and histopathologic manifestations indistinguishable from IIP.

IIP (Idiopathic DLD)

Up to 40% of patients presenting with DLD will have no identifiable primary disease, environmental exposure, drug history, or connective tissue disease after a thorough clinical evaluation. These patients are generally considered to have idiopathic DLD, or IIP (see Table 6.1). The classification of IIP is discussed later.

IIP: Current Clinicopathologic Classification

The current ATS/ERS classification schema for IIP includes "seven" distinct subgroups associated with distinctive histopathological patterns of injury and repair (Table 6.2) [2].

Idiopathic Pulmonary Fibrosis

Idiopathic pulmonary fibrosis (IPF), historically also called cryptogenic fibrosing alveolitis, is the most common form of IIP making up close to 60% of cases (Fig. 6.1). Until the late 1990s, the term IPF was commonly used to refer to any form of IIP. The ATS/ERS definition published in the year 2000 was much narrower, requiring the presence of usual interstitial pneumonia (UIP) pattern on surgical lung biopsy [3]. This redefinition was important, as IPF (as defined by the presence of UIP) has a poor response to traditional therapy and a poor prognosis when compared to other forms of IIP [4].

Clinical Presentation

Patients with IPF typically present with chronic progressive dyspnea (over months to years) and a chronic nonproductive cough. It is a disease of older age, generally diagnosed in the 6th and 7th decades of life; it is distinctly uncommon under the age of 50. There seems to be a slight male predominance, and most patients have a history of cigarette smoking. Physical examination often reveals fine, high-pitched bibasilar inspiratory crackles and digital clubbing. Pulmonary function testing commonly reveals restrictive lung disease (reduced TLC, FRC, and RV, decreased FEV_1 and FVC, and normal or increased FEV_1/

FVC ratio) and abnormal gas exchange (decreased DLCO and resting or exercise hypoxemia).

High-resolution computed tomography (HRCT) scanning generally reveals basilar-predominant, subpleural reticular abnormalities, traction bronchiectasis, and honeycombing. Extensive ground-glass abnormality is unusual and should suggest an alternative diagnosis. Nodularity and prominent hilar or mediastinal lymphadenopathy is also unusual.

Histopathology

By definition, patients with IPF have UIP pattern on histopathology. UIP pattern is characterized by areas of end-stage fibrosis and "honeycombing" (thickened collagenous septae surrounding airspaces lined by bronchial epithelium) proximate to areas of normal lung. The fibrosis is predominantly subpleural in distribution. Discrete areas of acute fibroblastic proliferation and collagen deposition, termed "fibroblastic foci," are essential to the histopathologic diagnosis of UIP pattern. These lesions may represent the site of ongoing disease activity, as increased numbers of fibroblastic foci appear to correlate with worse survival in some studies [5, 6]. There is generally minimal interstitial inflammation and absent granulomas.

Nonspecific Interstitial Pneumonia

The term "nonspecific interstitial pneumonia" (NSIP) originated as a histopathologic categorization that was reserved for surgical lung biopsies that did not demonstrate a clearly identifiable pattern (e.g., UIP) [7, 8]. The clinical diagnosis of NSIP likely represents a heterogeneous group of conditions; however, a recent consensus statement describes a distinct clinical phenotype [9]. Importantly, NSIP pattern is seen with a number of known causes of DLD including hypersensitivity pneumonitis, collagen-vascular disease, drug exposure, and infection [10–13]. The identification of NSIP pattern should prompt a careful search for these conditions, with the clinical diagnosis of NSIP being one of exclusion.

Table 6.2 Current classification schema for idiopathic interstitial pneumonia: an overview

Subgroup	Demographic	History and physical	High-resolution CT	Histology
IPF	Age: 55–75 years; Gender: M>F; Smoking: current or former history common	Chronic, progressive dyspnea over 6–12 months, dry cough, lower lobe inspiratory crackles, frequent clubbing	Bilateral, lower lobe, predominantly subpleural reticular abnormalities, traction bronchiectasis, minimal or no ground-glass opacities, honeycombing	UIP pattern: temporal heterogeneity of fibrosis, subpleural distribution, minimal inflammation, areas of focal myofibroblast proliferation and collagen deposition ("fibroblastic foci")
NSIP	Age: 45–55 years; Gender: M=F; Smoking: current or former history common	Chronic, progressive dyspnea over 6 months, dry cough, lower lobe inspiratory crackles, occasional clubbing	Bilateral, lower lobe reticular abnormalities, variable traction bronchiectasis, variable ground-glass opacities and consolidation, rare honeycombing	NSIP pattern[a]: temporal homogeneity of fibrosis, variable inflammation, rare fibroblastic foci
COP	Age: all ages (mean 50 years); Gender: M=F; Smoking: no association	Acute to subacute dyspnea and cough, fever, and diffuse inspiratory crackles common, clubbing absent	Patchy or nodular ground-glass opacities or consolidation, minimal reticular abnormality, traction bronchiectasis and honeycombing absent	OP pattern: patchy areas of myofibroblast aggregation and collagen deposition in the alveoli and distal bronchioles, minimal interstitial inflammation
AIP	Age: all ages (mean 50 years); Gender: M=F; Smoking: no association	Acute to subacute dyspnea and cough, occasional fever, diffuse inspiratory crackles common, clubbing absent	Diffuse bilateral ground-glass opacities or consolidation, minimal reticular abnormality, traction bronchiectasis (late), honeycombing absent	DAD pattern: diffuse hyaline membrane deposition, interstitial inflammation, type II pneumocyte hyperplasia, organizing fibrosis (late)
RBILD	Age: 30–55 years; Gender: M=F; Smoking: almost universal	Chronic, progressive dyspnea over 6 months, dry cough, lower lobe inspiratory crackles common, clubbing absent	Scattered bilateral, lower lobe ground glass, centrilobular nodules, bronchial wall thickening, traction bronchiectasis and honeycombing absent	RB pattern: bronchiolocentric pigmented macrophage accumulation, mild interstitial inflammation
DIP	Age: 40–55 years; Gender: M=F; Smoking: almost universal	Chronic, progressive dyspnea over 6 months, dry cough, lower lobe inspiratory crackles, rare clubbing	Diffuse bilateral, lower lobe predominant ground-glass opacities, variable reticular abnormality, traction bronchiectasis and honeycombing absent	DIP pattern: diffuse alveolar and distal bronchiolar pigmented macrophage accumulation, variable interstitial inflammation, mild septal fibrosis
LIP	Age: 30–55 years; Gender: F>M; Smoking: no association	Chronic, progressive dyspnea over 3–6 months, dry cough, lower lobe inspiratory crackles common, clubbing absent, occasional lymphadenopathy	Patchy ground-glass opacities, septal and bronchovascular thickening, centrilobular nodules, occasional thin-walled cysts, traction bronchiectasis and honeycombing absent	LIP pattern: Diffuse interstitial lymphocytic infiltration, type II cell hyperplasia, occasional lymphoid follicles

IPF idiopathic pulmonary fibrosis, *NSIP* nonspecific interstitial pneumonia, *DIP* desquamative interstitial pneumonia, *RBILD* respiratory bronchiolitis-associated interstitial lung disease, *LIP* lymphocytic interstitial pneumonia, *AIP* acute interstitial pneumonia, *COP* cryptogenic organizing pneumonia, *UIP* usual interstitial pneumonia, *RB* respiratory bronchiolitis, *DAD* diffuse alveolar damage, *OP* organizing pneumonia

[a]NSIP has a variety of histologic appearances and is typically divided into "cellular NSIP pattern" where interstitial inflammation is the predominant finding, and "fibrotic NSIP pattern" where interstitial fibrosis is the predominant finding. Fibrotic NSIP pattern and UIP pattern are often difficult to distinguish from one.

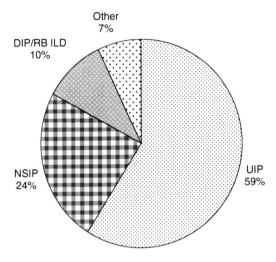

Other
7%

DIP/RB ILD
10%

NSIP
24%

UIP
59%

Fig. 6.1 Relative frequency of clinicopathologic sub-groups in idiopathic interstitial pneumonia (IIP). Figure based on summary data from five major retrospective reviews of surgical lung biopsy specimens from patients diagnosed with IIP. *UIP* usual interstitial pneumonia, *NSIP* nonspecific interstitial pneumonia, *DIP* desquamative interstitial pneumonia, *RBILD* respiratory bronchiolitis-associated interstitial lung disease

Clinical Findings

Like IPF, NSIP typically presents with chronic dyspnea and nonproductive cough, although the duration of symptoms is generally shorter. Patients are also generally younger than those with IPF, typically presenting between age 40 and 50, and more commonly female. They are less commonly smokers and have an increased incidence of positive autoimmune serologies. Hypoxemia, fever, and finger clubbing may occur, and fine, high-pitched bibasilar inspiratory crackles are common. Pulmonary function testing shows a restrictive pattern, similar to that seen in IPF.

HRCT scanning reveals variable degrees of ground-glass abnormality, most commonly bilateral and subpleural in distribution. Patchy areas of airspace consolidation, reticular abnormalities, and traction bronchiectasis may be present, but honeycombing is unusual. As discussed later, there is a continuum of findings in NSIP, with some cases radiographically indistinguishable from IPF [14, 15].

Histopathologic Findings

NSIP pattern is characterized by varying degrees of inflammation and fibrosis, with a minority of biopsies showing a predominantly lymphocytic interstitial inflammatory infiltrate ("cellular NSIP pattern"). The majority demonstrate a predominantly fibrotic interstitial process ("fibrotic NSIP pattern"), with varying degrees of overlying cellularity [7, 8]. Fibrosis in NSIP pattern is temporally uniform (i.e., all interstitial spaces are equally involved), an important distinction from UIP. Fibroblastic foci and honeycombing, if present, are rare. Nonetheless, fibrotic NSIP pattern can be difficult to distinguish from UIP pattern, and there is significant variability in interpretation of these biopsies even among expert pathologists.

Cryptogenic Organizing Pneumonia

Cryptogenic organizing pneumonia (COP) is an idiopathic lung disease characterized by proliferation of granulation tissue (i.e., organizing pneumonia) in the alveolar spaces, alveolar ducts and bronchioles, with minimal interstitial involvement. Organizing pneumonia can be found on surgical lung biopsy in association with a number of diseases (e.g., postinfectious, drug related, connective tissue disease related, posttransplant) [16–18]. It is also commonly seen accompanying other histopathologic patterns (e.g., UIP), in which case it is considered a secondary phenomenon. The diagnosis of COP is reserved for patients with isolated organizing pneumonia on surgical lung biopsy and a clinical history suggestive of IIP [2, 19].

Clinical Findings

COP typically presents with acute (days) to subacute (weeks) dyspnea and cough. Fever is relatively common, and COP is often misdiagnosed as community-acquired pneumonia. Patients with COP present at any age, with the mean age of approximately 50 years. Hypoxemia and inspiratory crackles are common. Finger clubbing is rare. Pulmonary function testing shows a mild-to-moderate restrictive pattern.

HRCT scanning demonstrates bilateral, often focal consolidation with variable ground glass, most commonly peribronchial in distribution. Peribronchovascular nodules and irregular lines are also seen. Honeycombing is rarely, if ever, present.

Histopathologic Findings

Organizing pneumonia pattern demonstrates serpentine areas of intraluminal myofibroblast proliferation in the bronchioles, alveolar ducts, and alveoli. These focal areas of fibrosis are temporally uniform. Mild interstitial inflammation and fibrosis may be present. The interstitial structures are generally well preserved, and honeycombing is not described.

Acute Interstitial Pneumonia

Acute interstitial pneumonia (AIP), also called Hamman–Rich disease, is an acute form of IIP generally characterized by rapid progression to respiratory failure. A few cases of AIP may be more indolent, with recurrent episodes over a period of weeks to months [20, 21]. AIP must be distinguished from acute exacerbation of chronic DLD such as IPF, which may mimic the clinical, radiographic, and even histopathologic presentation.

Clinical Findings

AIP can occur at any age, with the mean age at presentation being 50 years. Patients generally present with dyspnea and cough developing over a few days to weeks. Fever is occasionally present. Many patients report a viral prodrome consisting of myalgias and upper respiratory symptoms. Hypoxemia and diffuse inspiratory crackles are common. Clubbing is not observed. Pulmonary function testing shows a restrictive pattern.

HRCT scanning reveals ground-glass abnormality and consolidation, predominantly basilar but often located throughout all lung fields. Early stages of AIP may have patchy involvement while more advanced cases show diffuse abnormality. Traction bronchiectasis and honeycombing are rarely seen, but may be present in advanced cases.

Histopathologic Findings

Histopathology reveals diffuse alveolar damage (DAD). DAD is a common histopathologic pattern of acute lung injury, and is the typical finding in patients with Acute Respiratory Distress Syndrome. There are two histopathologic stages to DAD. In the acute, or exudative stage, edema, epithelial necrosis and sloughing, fibrinous exudates in air spaces, and hyaline membrane formation are characteristic findings. The process is usually widespread and temporally uniform. In the second, or organizing stage, proliferation of type II pneumocytes, resolution of hyaline membranes and alveolar exudates, and fibroblastic proliferation occurs. With time, end-stage fibrosis can develop and large cystic airspaces form resembling honeycombing. These cystic spaces, however, are lined with alveolar epithelium, in contrast to the bronchial epithelium seen in the honeycomb spaces associated with UIP pattern.

Respiratory Bronchiolitis-Associated Interstitial Lung Disease and Desquamative Interstitial Pneumonia

Respiratory bronchiolitis-associated interstitial lung disease (RBILD) and desquamative interstitial pneumonia (DIP) are arguably different clinical manifestations of the same smoking-related pathophysiologic condition. Although they are discussed together in this chapter, RBILD and DIP are still considered distinct clinical diagnoses.

Clinical Findings

Both RBILD and DIP present with chronic, progressive dyspnea and cough. Patients are typically younger, between 30 and 50 years old. The vast majority of patients with either condition has a smoking history or has had exposure to passive cigarette smoke [22, 23]. Physical exam may reveal hypoxemia and bibasilar inspiratory crackles. Clubbing is occasionally present in DIP. Pulmonary function testing is usually normal or mildly obstructive in RBILD, likely due to concomitant chronic obstructive pulmonary disease. A restrictive pattern is generally seen in DIP.

In patients with RBILD, HRCT often reveals bronchial wall thickening (proximal to sub-segmental bronchi), centrilobular nodules, and ground-glass opacity. Areas of hypoattenuation, pronounced on expiratory images, are also seen, suggestive of focal air trapping. DIP demonstrates more diffuse, predominantly lower lobe ground-glass abnormality, often peripheral in distribution. This is often accompanied by small cysts, which may represent areas of overlying emphysema. Honeycombing can be seen but is uncommon.

Histopathologic Findings

Both RBILD and DIP demonstrate accumulation of pigment-laden macrophages (dusty brown cytoplasm that may be positive for iron stains). The pigmented macrophages were originally, and incorrectly, thought to be "desquamated" epithelial cells, thus the name "desquamative" interstitial pneumonia. This finding is a common histopatho-logic pattern seen in smokers called respiratory bronchiolitis. The alveolar septae are mildly thickened by inflammatory infiltrate in both conditions. In patients with suspected IIP, surgical lung biopsy demonstrating respiratory bronchi-olitis pattern is consistent with the diagnosis of RBILD. DIP pattern reveals more widespread alveolar macrophage accumulation.

Lymphocytic Interstitial Pneumonia

The clinical and histopathologic findings of lym-phocytic interstitial pneumonia (LIP) are often the presenting signs of underlying autoimmunity (e.g., RA and Sjögren's syndrome), immunodefi-ciency (e.g., common variable immunodeficiency), or lymphoproliferative disorder [24]. However, a small minority of cases appears idiopathic.

Clinical Findings
Patients with LIP tend to be between 30 and 50 years old, and are predominantly female. Symptoms are generally slowly progressive, with dyspnea and cough most prominent. Hypoxemia may occur and bibasilar crackles are common.

Lymphadenopathy is occasionally present. Pul-monary function generally reveals restriction.

HRCT commonly shows variable degrees of diffuse ground-glass abnormality, poorly defined centrilobular nodules, thickened bronchovascular bundles, lymph node enlargement, and thin-walled cysts.

Histopathologic Findings
Surgical lung biopsy reveals a dense interstitial lymphocytic infiltrate. The infiltrates are mostly comprised of T lymphocytes, plasma cells, and macrophages. There is often associated type II pneumocyte hyperplasia. Lymphoid follicles are commonly observed.

Unclassifiable IIP

A few cases of IIP will not fit into the above clini-copathologic subgroups and are considered unclassifiable [2]. This may be because of inade-quate or missing clinical information, major discrepancies in clinical, radiographic, and histopathologic findings, or an inadequate or nondiagnostic biopsy. Occasionally, more than one histopathologic appearance can be seen in a single surgical biopsy, often when multiple lobes have been sampled. In patients with both UIP pattern and NSIP pattern, clinical behavior is similar to patients with IPF [25]. In other cases with multiple patterns on surgical lung biopsy, the diagnosis should be made based on the most specific clinicopathologic findings. Often when multiple patterns are present in a single biopsy one should consider hypersensitivity pneumonitis, drug-induced lung injury, or connective tissue disease.

Diagnostic Approach to DLD

The patient with suspected DLD presents a formi-dable diagnostic challenge to physicians, and an organized approach is critical (Fig. 6.2). There have been several excellent reviews of the general

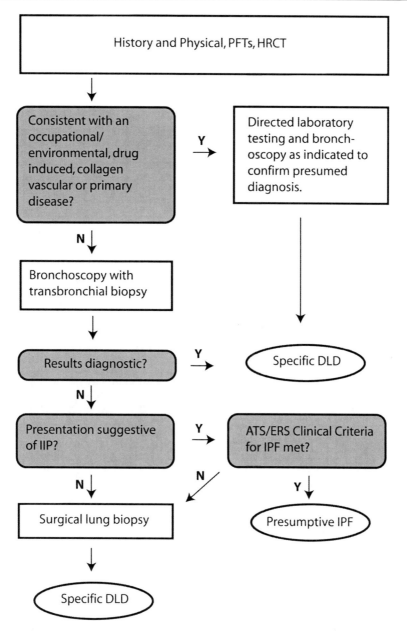

Fig. 6.2 Diagnostic approach to the diagnosis of DLD. The algorithm above is a basic overview, not a step-by-step guide to the clinical evaluation of patients with suspected DLD. In general, all patients should undergo an extensive history and physical examination, pulmonary function testing, and high-resolution CT scanning of the chest. In many cases, this initial evaluation will suggest a likely environmental exposure-related condition, a drug-induced condition, a connective tissue disease, or other primary disease, which will dictate further testing. Bronchoscopy with transbronchial biopsy may help identify a diagnosis in some of the remaining patients. A sizable minority of cases will require consideration of surgical lung biopsy. In patients whose clinical and radiographic evaluation meets the clinical criteria for the diagnosis of idiopathic pulmonary fibrosis, a presumptive diagnosis may be made. In all others, surgical lung biopsy should be pursued. *PFT* pulmonary function testing, *HRCT* high-resolution computed tomography scan, *DLD* diffuse lung disease, *IIP* idiopathic interstitial pneumonia, *IPF* idiopathic pulmonary fibrosis

approach to the diagnosis of DLD published previously [26]. A careful history and physical examination, pulmonary function testing, and HRCT scanning of the chest should be performed on all patients. The utility of the clinical and radiographic evaluation in DLD is detailed in other chapters. Often, an accurate diagnosis of DLD requires close collaboration between the clinician, radiologist, and pathologist, and every effort should be made to include a multidisciplinary discussion of cases in the diagnostic approach [27]. Below is a brief summary of each component with particular attention paid to their usefulness in the diagnosis and subclassification of IIP.

Clinical Characteristics

The role of the history, physical examination, and pulmonary function testing in the diagnosis of specific DLD is reviewed in depth in earlier chapters. An extensive history should be taken from all patients with suspected DLD. Special attention should be paid to potential environmental exposures, medications, and symptoms suggestive of connective tissue or other systemic diseases. The physical examination should look for evidence of adventitial breath sounds (particularly inspiratory crackles), digital clubbing, and other signs of disorders suggested by the patient's history. Pulmonary function testing will generally show restriction (decreased FVC and TLC) and abnormal gas exchange (decreased DLCO and resting or exercise hypoxemia), although some disorders will show airflow limitation. Progressive dyspnea over several months, dry cough, hypoxemia, inspiratory crackles, clubbing, and restrictive physiology are common findings in patients with IIP. None of these findings, however, are specific to IIP or its subgroups.

Bronchoscopy

The role of bronchoscopy in the diagnosis of specific DLD is reviewed in depth in earlier chapters. Bronchoscopy can be diagnostic in a number of

DLDs (e.g., sarcoidosis, eosinophilic pneumonia) and is useful in identifying chronic infection and malignancy. It is also helpful in suggesting certain diagnoses (e.g., hypersensitivity pneumonitis, DIP). There are, unfortunately, no bronchoscopic findings specific to IIP. Using the cellular constituency of the bronchoalveolar lavage fluid from patients with IIP to predict the underlying histopathology has been largely unsuccessful. Transbronchial biopsy is limited by the small size of the biopsy obtained and the lack of histological preservation due to mechanical crushing of the tissue. Because of these factors, transbronchial biopsy specimens have poor diagnostic accuracy for IIP. Accurate histopathologic evaluation generally requires larger tissue samples only obtainable through surgical lung biopsy.

Radiology

The role of radiology in the diagnosis of specific DLD is reviewed in depth in other chapters. The conventional chest radiograph lacks accuracy and reliability in DLD, with a correct diagnosis made in less than 50% of cases and only a 70% interobserver agreement. Further, up to 10% of patients with histopathologically confirmed DLD have normal chest radiographs. HRCT scanning is significantly more sensitive and specific for the diagnosis of DLD and has replaced conventional chest radiography as the preferred imaging method. Supine and prone inspiratory images, as well as expiratory images should be obtained to maximize the diagnostic sensitivity and specificity of HRCT.

HRCT scanning can be diagnostic in a number of DLDs (e.g., sarcoidosis, lymphangioleiomyomatosis, Langerhans cell histiocytosis, asbestosis). It can also be quite useful in distinguishing among the subgroups of IIP [2]. The ability of HRCT scanning to diagnose IPF has been widely investigated. Most studies of HRCT have reported sensitivities of 50–75% and specificities of greater than 90% for the diagnosis of IPF [28]. In the proper clinical setting, therefore, IPF can be reliably diagnosed by HRCT.

Histopathology

Surgical lung biopsy is the gold standard for the diagnosis of many forms of DLD. The role of histopathology in the diagnosis of specific DLD is reviewed in depth in other chapters. In the 1950s and 1960s, surgical lung biopsy was used frequently in the diagnosis of DLD. Today, it is less frequently used, as more disorders can be accurately diagnosed with less invasive methods such as HRCT.

In 1980, the largest retrospective review of open lung biopsy for DLD reported a diagnostic yield of 92% and an overall morbidity and mortality of 2.5% and 0.3%, respectively [29]. More recent studies have confirmed the diagnostic yield of open lung biopsy using a limited thoracotomy to be greater than 90% [30]. Thoracoscopic lung biopsy was introduced in the early 1980s as a potential alternative to thoracotomy. Studies comparing thoracoscopic and open surgical lung biopsy have consistently found thoracoscopy to have equivalent diagnostic yield, equal or lower morbidity, and decreased length of stay [30].

IIP: The Role of Surgical Lung Biopsy

The diagnosis of IIP can be made in the majority of cases without histopathology. Clinicopathologic subclassification of IIP is more difficult, however, and surgical lung biopsy has long been the gold standard for diagnosis. This section aims to address the clinical importance of clinicopathologic subclassification, and review the diagnostic accuracy of a nonhistopathologic approach to subclassification in IIP.

Importance of Clinicopathologic Subclassification of IIP

For the clinicopathologic subclassification of IIP to be clinically relevant, treatment approach, response to treatment, and/or prognosis must be influenced. If there is no difference in choice of therapy, response to therapy, or survival among the various subgroups, subjecting patients to a

morbid surgical procedure is hard to justify. Recent data clearly demonstrate that patients with IPF have a uniquely poor response to traditional therapy and prognosis compared to the other clinicopathologic subgroups of IIP, and that novel therapies for IPF may provide some benefit.

Response to Treatment

A review of published clinical trials looking at response to therapy in patients with IPF/UIP (defined using the ATS/ERS consensus criteria) suggests that IPF responds poorly, if at all, to corticosteroid or cytotoxic therapy [31]. Recently, several randomized, placebo-controlled trials of novel therapies for IPF have been conducted with mixed results (Table 6.3). Reviews of NSIP, COP, RBILD, DIP, and LIP have suggested better responsiveness to corticosteroids in these conditions [43–45]. Unfortunately, there are no prospective randomized placebo-controlled trials of therapy in these histopathologic subgroups of IIP. Most studies are retrospective reviews of patients who almost all received corticosteroid therapy.

Interpretation of the literature on response to therapy in IIP is further confounded by the constantly changing nomenclature. Many older studies of "IPF" that have reported marginal benefit to corticosteroid and/or cytotoxic therapy almost surely included patients with other forms of IIP and DLD, especially fibrotic NSIP [46, 47].

Based on the data available, there appears to be a difference in response to corticosteroid and cytotoxic therapy between IPF, as defined by the histopathologic presence of UIP pattern, and other subgroups of IIP.

Survival

Survival in IPF is uniquely poor (Fig. 6.3). There are several excellent retrospective studies comparing survival between histopathologic subgroups of IIP. A representative study found a significantly worse 5-year survival for patients with UIP (20%) compared to NSIP (70%) and DIP/RB-ILD (80%) [45]. The dramatic difference in survival between UIP and the other histopathologic subgroups has been substantiated by several other cohorts [8, 44]. The further classification of NSIP into cellular and

Table 6.3 Results of randomized, placebo-controlled trials in idiopathic pulmonary fibrosis

Study	Therapy	Primary outcome
Raghu et al. [32]	Interferon gamma 1-b and low dose prednisone	No difference in progression-free survival
Demedts et al. [33]	Acetylcysteine, prednisone, and azathioprine	Significant reduction in rate of decline in FVC
Azuma et al. [34]	Pirfenidone	No difference in lowest oxygen saturation during walk testing
Kubo et al. [35]	Warfarin	Significant reduction in mortality
King et al. [36]	Bosentan	No difference in disease worsening or mortality
Raghu et al. [37]	Etanercept	No difference in change in pulmonary function
King et al. [38]	Interferon gamma 1b	No difference in mortality
Taniguchi et al. [39]	Pirfenidone	Significant reduction in rate of decline in VC
CAPACITY-1 [41]	Pirfenidone	No difference in rate of decline in FVC
CAPACITY-2 [41]	Pirfenidone	Significant reduction in rate of decline in FVC
Daniels et al. [40]	Gleevec	No difference in progression-free survival
Zisman et al. [41]	Sildenafil	Differences in arterial oxygenation, DLCO, dyspnea, and QOL

DLCO = carbon monoxide diffusion capacity; QOL = quality of life

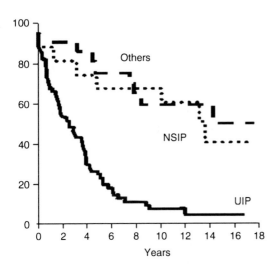

Fig. 6.3 Survival in clinicopathologic subgroups in idiopathic interstitial pneumonia. The survival difference between patients with UIP pattern and all others was statistically significant ($p<0.001$). *UIP* usual interstitial pneumonia, *NSIP* nonspecific interstitial pneumonia. From Bjoraker et al. Prognostic significance of histopathologic subsets in idiopathic pulmonary fibrosis. Am J Respir Crit Care Med 1998;157:199–203. Reprinted with permission of the American Thoracic Society. Copyright © American Thoracic Society

fibrotic subgroups appears to be important prognostically as well, with cellular NSIP having a significantly better prognosis than fibrotic NSIP.

Based on the above data, histopathologic subclassification of IIP is clinically relevant because it

affects the choice of therapy and prognosis, primarily through identifying patients with IPF. Accurately identifying patients with IPF allows for more informed consideration of the risks and benefits of therapy and more accurate prognostication. Because of their poor prognosis, patients with IPF should be referred for transplantation early, as it has been shown to prolong survival [48]. Lastly, patients with IPF should be considered for enrollment in clinical trials of investigational agents aimed at halting the fibroproliferative process central to this disease.

Accuracy of the Clinical Diagnosis of IPF

The ATS/ERS has recently published an evidence-based guideline on the diagnosis and management of IPF [49]. The diagnostic criteria for IPF focuses on the importance of a multidisciplinary review, and allow for the diagnosis of IPF based on clinical history and HRCT alone in certain cases (Table 6.4 and 6.5). The accuracy of a combined clinical/radiological diagnosis in the other clinicopathological subgroups of IIP remains unknown.

Three studies have shown the clinical diagnosis of IPF to be quite specific (i.e., very few false positive diagnoses) [50–52]. The sensitivity of the diagnosis was poorer, between 50 and 75%. In these studies, clinicians were blinded to the results of surgical lung biopsy, which was used as the

Table 6.4 Diagnostic Criteria for idiopathic pulmonary fibrosis

Criterion	Description
1	Exclusion of other known causes of interstitial lung disease (e.g. domestic and occupational environmental exposures, connective tissue disease, and drug toxicity).
2	The presence of a UIP pattern on high resolution computed tomography (HRCT) in patients not subjected to surgical lung biopsy.
3	Specific combinations of HRCT and surgical lung biopsy pattern in patients subjected to surgical lung biopsy.

Adapted from: Raghu G, et al. An Official ATS/ERS/JRS/ALAT Statement: Idiopathic Pulmonary Fibrosis: Evidence-based Guidelines for Diagnosis and Management. Am J Crit Care Med. 2011;183:788–824

Table 6.5 Combination of HRCT and surgical lung biopsy for the diagnosis of IPF

High-resolution computed tomography Pattern	Surgical Lung Biopsy Pattern (when performed)	Diagnosis of IPF?
UIP	UIP	YES
	Probable UIP	
	Possible UIP	
	Non-classifiable fibrosis *	
	Not UIP	No
Possible UIP	UIP	YES
	Probable UIP	
	Possible UIP	Probable †
	Non-classifiable fibrosis	
	Not UIP	No
Inconsistent with UIP	UIP	Possible
	Probable UIP	No
	Possible UIP	
	Non-classifiable fibrosis	
	Not UIP	

Adapted from: Raghu G, et al. An Official ATS/ERS/JRS/ALAT Statement: Idiopathic Pulmonary Fibrosis: Evidence-based Guidelines for Diagnosis and Management. Am J Crit Care Med. 2011;183:788–824
*Biopsies that reveal a pattern of fibrosis that does not meet the criteria for UIP pattern and the other idiopathic interstitial pneumonias.
†The accuracy of the diagnosis of IPF increases with multidisciplinary discussion

gold standard for diagnosis. These results argue that, when the clinical diagnosis appears secure, IPF can be confidently diagnosed. Importantly, these studies were performed by clinicians and radiologists experienced in the diagnosis of IIP. It is unclear how well these clinical criteria perform in more general practice settings.

It is important to pursue surgical lung biopsy in patients with suspected IPF who do not meet the clinical and radiological criteria for diagnosis,

and in whom the surgical risk is considered acceptable. Patient with severe gas exchange abnormalities (e.g., those on long-term oxygen supplementation) or substantial comorbidities (e.g., cardiac disease, obesity) may be at higher risk for complications from surgical lung biopsy, and these risks should be carefully considered. In patients who fit the clinical criteria for the diagnosis of IPF, the decision to forego surgical lung biopsy depends largely on the experience and confidence of the physicians involved. Regardless of experience, an integrated multidisciplinary approach is critical to achieving an accurate diagnosis.

Summary

The patient with suspected DLD presents a formidable diagnostic challenge to the clinician and an organized evaluation is essential. DLD is generally classified into five clinical categories: primary disease related, environmental exposure related, drug induced, connective tissue associated, and IIP. Careful attention must be paid to the history and physical examination looking for evidence to suggest a specific diagnosis. All patients with suspected DLD should have pulmonary function testing and HRCT performed. A sizable minority of patients will have no clear diagnosis after the above evaluation is complete. These patients most commonly have IIP.

In clinical practice today, patients with IIP are frequently treated with corticosteroids and cytotoxic therapy with the hope that they may be among the minority of patients who respond. Clinicopathologic subclassification may not be pursued. Based on currently available data, careful histopathologic subclassification clearly identifies a group of patients (i.e., those with IPF) who do not respond to these therapies and have a uniquely poor prognosis. The identification of patients with IPF, as currently defined by the presence of UIP, allows for more accurate prognostication, a more educated assessment of the potential risks and benefits of therapy, enrollment in clinical trials of novel therapies, and early referral for transplantation.

References

1. Schwarz MI, King Jr TE. Interstitial lung diseases. 5th ed. People's Medical Publishing House–USA, Shelton, CT; 2011.
2. American Thoracic Society/European Respiratory Society International Multidisciplinary Consensus Classification of the Idiopathic Interstitial Pneumonias. Am J Respir Crit Care Med. 2002;165:277–304.
3. American Thoracic Society. Idiopathic pulmonary fibrosis: diagnosis and treatment. International consensus statement. American Thoracic Society (ATS), and the European Respiratory Society (ERS). Am J Respir Crit Care Med. 2000;161:646–64.
4. Katzenstein AL, Myers JL. Idiopathic pulmonary fibrosis: clinical relevance of pathologic classification. Am J Respir Crit Care Med. 1998;157:1301–15.
5. King Jr TE, Schwarz MI, Brown K, et al. Idiopathic pulmonary fibrosis. Relationship between histopathologic features and mortality. Am J Respir Crit Care Med. 2001;164:1025–32.
6. Nicholson AG, Fulford LG, Colby TV, et al. The relationship between individual histologic features and disease progression in idiopathic pulmonary fibrosis. Am J Respir Crit Care Med. 2002;166: 173–7.
7. Katzenstein AL, Fiorelli RF. Nonspecific interstitial pneumonia/fibrosis. Histologic features and clinical significance. Am J Surg Pathol. 1994;18:136–47.
8. Travis WD, Matsui K, Moss J, Ferrans VJ. Idiopathic nonspecific interstitial pneumonia: prognostic significance of cellular and fibrosing patterns: survival comparison with usual interstitial pneumonia and desquamative interstitial pneumonia. Am J Surg Pathol. 2000;24:19–33.
9. Travis WD, Hunninghake G, King Jr TE, et al. Idiopathic nonspecific interstitial pneumonia: report of an American Thoracic Society project. Am J Respir Crit Care Med. 2008;177:1338–47.
10. Kim DS, Yoo B, Lee JS, et al. The major histopathologic pattern of pulmonary fibrosis in scleroderma is nonspecific interstitial pneumonia. Sarcoidosis Vasc Diffuse Lung Dis. 2002;19:121–7.
11. Lantuejoul S, Brambilla E, Brambilla C, Devouassoux G. Statin-induced fibrotic nonspecific interstitial pneumonia. Eur Respir J. 2002;19:577–80.
12. Sattler F, Nichols L, Hirano L, et al. Nonspecific interstitial pneumonitis mimicking Pneumocystis carinii pneumonia. Am J Respir Crit Care Med. 1997;156:912–7.
13. Vourlekis JS, Schwarz MI, Cool CD, et al. Nonspecific interstitial pneumonitis as the sole histologic expression of hypersensitivity pneumonitis. Am J Med. 2002; 112:490–3.
14. Park CS, Jeon JW, Park SW, et al. Nonspecific interstitial pneumonia/fibrosis: clinical manifestations, histologic and radiologic features. Korean J Intern Med. 1996;11:122–32.
15. MacDonald SL, Rubens MB, Hansell DM, et al. Nonspecific interstitial pneumonia and usual interstitial pneumonia: comparative appearances at and diagnostic accuracy of thin-section CT. Radiology. 2001; 221:600–5.
16. Lee KS, Kullnig P, Hartman TE, Muller NL. Cryptogenic organizing pneumonia: CT findings in 43 patients. AJR Am J Roentgenol. 1994;162:543–6.
17. Lazor R, Vandevenne A, Pelletier A, et al. Cryptogenic organizing pneumonia. Characteristics of relapses in a series of 48 patients. The Groupe d'Etudes et de Recherche sur les Maladies "Orphelines" Pulmonaires

(GERM"O"P). Am J Respir Crit Care Med. 2000;162:571–7.

18. Nagai S, Kitaichi M, Itoh H, et al. Idiopathic nonspecific interstitial pneumonia/fibrosis: comparison with idiopathic pulmonary fibrosis and BOOP. Eur Respir J. 1998;12:1010–9.

19. King Jr TE, Mortenson RL. Cryptogenic organizing pneumonia. The North American experience. Chest. 1992;102:8S–13.

20. Bouros D, Nicholson AC, Polychronopoulos V, du Bois RM. Acute interstitial pneumonia. Eur Respir J. 2000;15:412–8.

21. Vourlekis JS, Brown KK, Cool CD, et al. Acute interstitial pneumonitis: case series and review of the literature. Medicine. 2000;79:369–78.

22. Portnoy J, Veraldi KL, Schwarz MI, et al. Respiratory bronchiolitis-interstitial lung disease: long tern outcome. Chest. 2007;131(3):664–71.

23. Ryu JH, Myers JL, Capizzi SA, et al. Desquamative interstitial pneumonia and respiratory bronchiolitis-associated interstitial lung disease. Chest. 2005;127:178–84.

24. Swigris JJ, Berry GJ, Raffin TA, Kuschner WG. Lymphoid interstitial pneumonia: a narrative review. Chest. 2002;122:2150–64.

25. Flaherty KR, Travis WD, Colby TV, et al. Histopathologic variability in usual and nonspecific interstitial pneumonias. Am J Respir Crit Care Med. 2001;164:1722–7.

26. British Thoracic Society. The diagnosis, assessment and treatment of diffuse parenchymal lung disease in adults. Thorax. 1999;54 Suppl 1:S1–28.

27. Flaherty KR, King Jr TE, Raghu G, et al. Idiopathic interstitial pneumonia: what is the effect of a multidisciplinary approach to diagnosis? Am J Respir Crit Care Med. 2004;170:904–10.

28. Collard HR, King Jr TE. Demystifying idiopathic interstitial pneumonia. Arch Intern Med. 2003;163:17–29.

29. Toledo-Pereyra LH, DeMeester TR, Kinealey A, et al. The benefits of open lung biopsy in patients with previous non-diagnostic transbronchial lung biopsy. A guide to appropriate therapy. Chest. 1980;77:647–50.

30. Bensard DD, McIntyre Jr RC, Waring BJ, Simon JS. Comparison of video thoracoscopic lung biopsy to open lung biopsy in the diagnosis of interstitial lung disease. Chest. 1993;103:765–70.

31. Richeldi L, Davies HR, Ferrara G, Franco F. Corticosteroids for idiopathic pulmonary fibrosis. Cochrane Database Syst Rev. 2003;(3):CD002880.

32. Raghu G, Brown KK, Bradford WZ, et al. A Placebo-controlled trial of interferon gamma-1b in patients with idiopathic pulmonary fibrosis. N Engl J Med. 2004;350:125–33.

33. Demedts M, Behr J, Buhl R, et al. High-dose acetylcysteine in idiopathic pulmonary fibrosis. N Engl J Med. 2005;353:2229–42.

34. Azuma A, Nukiwa T, Tsuboi E, et al. Double-blind, placebo-controlled trial of pirfenidone in patients with idiopathic pulmonary fibrosis. Am J Respir Crit Care Med. 2005;171:1040–7.

35. Kubo H, Nakayama K, Yanai M, et al. Anticoagulant therapy for idiopathic pulmonary fibrosis. Chest. 2005;128:1475–82.

36. King TE, Jr., Brown KK, et al. BUILD-3: A Randomized, Controlled Trial of Bosentan in Idiopathic Pulmonary Fibrosis. Am J Respir Crit Care Med. 2011;184:92–9.

37. Raghu G, Brown KK, Costabel U, et al. Treatment of idiopathic pulmonary fibrosis with etanercept: an exploratory, placebo-controlled trial. Am J Respir Crit Care Med. 2008;178:948–55.

38. King Jr TE, Albera C, Bradford WZ, et al. Effect of interferon gamma-1b on survival in patients with idiopathic pulmonary fibrosis (INSPIRE): a multicentre, randomised, placebo-controlled trial. Lancet. 2009;374:222–8.

39. Taniguchi H, Ebina M, Kondoh Y, et al. Pirfenidone in idiopathic pulmonary fibrosis. Eur Respir J. 2010;35(4):821–9.

40. Daniels CE, Lasky JA, Limper AH, et al. Imatinib treatment for IPF: randomized placebo controlled trial results. Am J Respir Crit Care Med. 2010;181(6):604–10.

41. Zisman DA, Schwarz M, Anstrom KJ, et al. A controlled trial of sildenafil in advanced idiopathic pulmonary fibrosis. N Engl J Med. 2010;363:620–8.

42. Noble PW, Albera C, Bradford WZ, et.al. The CAPACITY Program: Pirfenidone in patients with idiopathic pulmonary fibrosis (CAPACITY): two randomised trials. Lancet. 2011; 377:1760–9.

43. Nicholson AG, Colby TV, Dubois RM, et al. The prognostic significance of the histologic pattern of interstitial pneumonia in patients presenting with the clinical entity of cryptogenic fibrosing alveolitis. Am J Respir Crit Care Med. 2000;162:2213–7.

44. Daniil ZD, Gilchrist FC, Nicholson AG, et al. A histologic pattern of nonspecific interstitial pneumonia is associated with a better prognosis than usual interstitial pneumonia in patients with cryptogenic fibrosing alveolitis. Am J Respir Crit Care Med. 1999;160:899–905.

45. Bjoraker JA, Ryu JH, Edwin MK, et al. Prognostic significance of histopathologic subsets in idiopathic pulmonary fibrosis. Am J Respir Crit Care Med. 1998;157:199–203.

46. Raghu G, Depaso WJ, Cain K, et al. Azathioprine combined with prednisone in the treatment of idiopathic pulmonary fibrosis: a prospective, double-blind randomized, placebo-controlled clinical trial. Am Rev Respir Dis. 1991;144:291–6.

47. Johnson MA, Kwan S, Snell NJC, et al. Randomized controlled trial comparing prednisolone alone with cyclophosphamide and low dose prednisolone in combination in cryptogenic fibrosing alveolitis. Thorax. 1989;44:280–8.

48. Thabut G, Mal H, Castier Y, et al. Survival benefit of lung transplantation for patients with idiopathic pulmonary fibrosis. J Thorac Cardiovasc Surg. 2003;126:469–75.

49. Raghu G, Collard HR, Egan JJ, Martinez FJ, Behr J, Brown KK, et al. An Official ATS/ERS/JRS/ALAT Statement: Idiopathic Pulmonary Fibrosis: Evidence-based Guidelines for Diagnosis and Management. Am J Respir Crit Care Med. 2011;183:788–824.

50. Hunninghake G, Zimmerman MB, Schwartz DA, et al. Utility of lung biopsy for the diagnosis of idiopathic pulmonary fibrosis. Am J Respir Crit Care Med. 2001;164:193–6.

51. Raghu G, Mageto YN, Lockhart D, et al. The accuracy of the clinical diagnosis of new-onset idiopathic pulmonary fibrosis and other interstitial lung disease: a prospective study. Chest. 1999;116:1168–74.

52. Flaherty KR, Thwaite EL, Kazerooni EA, et al. Radiological versus histological diagnosis in UIP and NSIP: survival implications. Thorax. 2003;58:143–8.

Drug Therapy for Interstitial Lung Disease

7

Robert P. Baughman, Ulrich Costabel,
and Elyse E. Lower

Abstract

This chapter summarizes the various potential medications used to treat interstitial lung diseases. The suggested administration routes and dosages are discussed. In addition, toxicity of the drugs and proposed monitoring for toxicity is presented. As newer agents become available, there is increasing information regarding the safety and efficacy of the new drugs as well as standard medications. In addition, individual drugs are used for an increasing number of interstitial lung diseases.

Keywords

Prednisone • Methotrexate • Azathioprine • Leflunomide • Mycophenolate • Infliximab • Cyclophosphamide • Rituximab

Introduction

A variety of drugs are available for the treatment of interstitial lung diseases. For many of them, the goal of therapy is to reduce inflammation and prevent subsequent fibrosis. Because of this common goal, it is not surprising that for many diseases treatment options are similar. At the same time

R.P. Baughman, MD (✉)
Department of Internal Medicine, University
of Cincinnati College of Medicine, Cincinnati, OH, USA
e-mail: bob.baughman@uc.edu

U. Costabel, MD
Department of Pneumology/Allergy, Ruhrlandklinik,
University Hospital, Essen, Germany

E.E. Lower, MD
Barnett Cancer Center, University of Cincinnati,
Cincinnati, OH, USA

some drugs may be more efficacious for one disease rather than another. Also the successful use of a drug for one disease often leads to its use for another interstitial lung disease. On the other hand, there are some drugs with a relative unique mechanism of action which makes them effective for only one or a few interstitial lung diseases.

In this chapter, we will review the various treatment options for all interstitial lung diseases. The relative benefits of one drug versus another will be discussed in the chapters regarding each specific disease.

Table 7.1 classifies the various drugs based on mechanism of action. This assignment is somewhat arbitrary since some drugs may have multiple mechanisms of action. We also list some of the diseases in which one or more reports suggest benefit. Because some drugs, such as prednisone, have been used for virtually every interstitial lung disease, the

R.P. Baughman and R.M. du Bois (eds.), *Diffuse Lung Disease: A Practical Approach*,
DOI 10.1007/978-1-4419-9771-5_7, © Springer Science+Business Media, LLC 2012

Table 7.1 Drugs used to treat interstitial lung diseases

Class	Drug	Reported as possibly useful in the following interstitial lung diseases
Glucocorticoids	Prednisone	Sarcoidosis
	Methylprednisolone	Hypersensitivity pneumonitis
		Bronchiolitis
		IPF
		NSIP
		CVD-PF
		ANCA
Cytotoxic agents	Methotrexate	Sarcoidosis
		ANCA
	Azathioprine	Sarcoidosis
		Hypersensitivity pneumonitis
		ANCA
		IPF
		CVD-PF
		NSIP
	Mycophenolate	Sarcoidosis
		ANCA
		CVD-PF
		NSIP
	Leflunomide	Sarcoidosis
	Cyclophosphamide	Sarcoidosis
		ANCA
		CVD-PF
		NSIP
		Bronchiolitis
Antimalarial agents	Chloroquine	Sarcoidosis
	Hydroxychloroquine	
Immune modulators	Thalidomide	Sarcoidosis
		IPF
Anti-TNF	Infliximab	Sarcoidosis
	Etanercept	
	Adalimumab	
B-cell depletion	Rituximab	ANCA
mTOR	Sirolimus	Lymphangioleiomyomatosis
Antifibrotic	Pirfenidone	IPF
Antioxidant	N-acetyl cysteine	IPF

IPF idiopathic pulmonary fibrosis, *NSIP* nonspecific interstitial pneumonitis, *CVD-PF* collagen vascular disease-associated pulmonary fibrosis, *ANCA* antineutrophil cytoplasmic antibody-associated vasculitis

list is not all encompassing. We have also limited the list to the main categories of interstitial lung diseases: sarcoidosis, idiopathic pulmonary fibrosis (IPF), nonspecific interstitial pneumonitis (NSIP), collagen vascular disease-associated pulmonary fibrosis (CVD-PF), hypersensitivity pneumonitis, antineutrophil cytoplasmic antibody-associated vasculitis (ANCA), and bronchiolitis. Table 7.2 lists the usual dosage, common toxicities, and some suggested monitoring for the individual drugs.

Corticosteroids

The discovery of the anti-inflammatory properties of glucocorticoids changed treatment strategies for many diseases including interstitial lung disease. During the 1950s, both the benefits of corticosteroids for multiple diseases and the significant toxicities of these drugs were discovered. As a result, corticosteroids represent the Janus of

Table 7.2 Usual dosage, common toxicities, and suggested monitoring for drugs used to treat interstitial lung diseases

Drug	Usual dosage	Common toxicity	Monitoring
Prednisone	5–40 mg a day	Weight gain, diabetes, cataracts, osteoporosis	Blood pressure, glucose, bone density
Methotrexate	2.5–15 mg once a week	Leucopenia, nausea, pneumonitis, hepatitis	CBC, renal function, hepatic function
Azathioprine	50–250 mg daily	Leucopenia, nausea, hepatitis	CBC, renal function, hepatic function
Mycophenolate	250–1,000 mg twice a day	Leucopenia, nausea	CBC, hepatic function
Leflunomide	10–20 mg daily	Leucopenia, nausea, pneumonitis, hepatitis	CBC, renal function, hepatic function
Cyclophosphamide	50–200 mg daily orally	Leucopenia, nausea, hemorrhagic cystitis	CBC, urinalysis
	100–2,000 mg intravenously every 2–4 weeks		
Chloroquine	250–500 mg daily	Ocular	Eye examination
Hydroxychloroquine	200–400 mg daily	Ocular	Eye examination
Thalidomide	50–200 mg nightly	Hypersomnolence, constipation, peripheral neuropathy, venous thrombosis, teratogenic	Monthly pregnancy testing
Adalimumab	40 mg subcutaneously every 1–2 weeks	Tuberculosis reactivation, reaction to injection, worsening congestive heart failure	Screen for latent tuberculosis, hold drug in face of active infection
Etanercept	25 mg subcutaneously twice a week	Tuberculosis reactivation, reaction to infusion, worsening congestive heart failure	Screen for latent tuberculosis, hold drug in face of active infection
Infliximab	3–10 mg/kg given initially, 2 weeks later, then every 4–8 weeks	Tuberculosis reactivation, reaction to infusion, worsening congestive heart failure	Screen for latent tuberculosis, hold drug in face of active infection
Rituximab	1,000 mg intravenously every 2 weeks for 2–4 doses and repeat every 6–12 months	Reaction to infusion, worsening of hepatitis B infection, PML	Antipyretics, antihistamines, and corticosteroids used as pretreatment
Sirolimus	1–2 mg daily	Renal dysfunction, infection	Drug levels
Pirfenidone	600–800 mg three times a day	Photosensitivity, nausea, hepatitis	Minimize direct sun exposure, sun protection cream, hepatic function
NAC	600 mg three times a day	Nausea, bloating	None

CBC complete blood count, *PML* progressive multifocal leukoencephalopathy

Table 7.3 Symptoms attributed to corticosteroids during short-term therapy

	Increased appetite (%)	Weight gain (%)	Moodiness (%)	Depression (%)	Insomnia (%)	Easy bruising (%)	GERD (%)
Always	14.2	15.9	12.5	9.1	10.8	10.8	2.8
Most of time	13.6	15,3	14.8	19.3	21.0	19.3	8.5
Some of time	21.0	19.9	13.6	11.9	26.1	26.1	17.0
Total	48.8	51.1	40.9	40.3	57.9	56.2	28.3

GERD Gastro esophageal reflux disease
Adapted from Baughman RP, Iannuzzi MC, Lower EE, et al. Use of fluticasone in acute symptomatic pulmonary sarcoidosis. Sarcoidosis Vasc Diffuse Lung Dis. 2002;19(3):198–204

therapeutic options with obvious advantages and disadvantages.

Corticosteroids have multiple effects on the inflammatory cycle. These agents directly suppress T lymphocyte number and reduce neutrophil adherence. They also modify macrophage function, including suppressing the release of tumor necrosis factor (TNF) [1]. Many cells have a glucocorticoid receptor α (GCRα) which when activated blocks a second messenger, nuclear factor-κB (NF-κB). The NF-κB normally translocates to the nucleus and leads to inflammation [2]. The proinflammatory glucocorticoid receptor β (GCRβ), which usually comprises only a small proportion of the glucocorticoid receptor numbers, is upregulated by in vivo exposure to TNF [3]. This may explain why some patients develop corticosteroid-resistant disease.

Although the dosages of corticosteroids vary, 40 mg of prednisone a day or its equivalent is a usual starting dose. Higher doses may be administered, including pulse therapy with 1,000 mg of intravenous methylprednisolone. However because of toxicity, it is desirable to establish a maintenance dose of corticosteroids using the lowest dose required to sustain a remission of symptoms. Usually that dose corresponds to 5–10 mg a day of prednisone. If that dose cannot be achieved, strategies for steroid-sparing agents have been proposed for diseases such as sarcoidosis [4]. It is often difficult for the clinician to know whether the patient is being treated with too much or too little prednisone. One guide suggests that if a patient is not responding as expected, they are receiving too little drug, but if they are doing well, they are receiving too much drug.

The toxicity for corticosteroids is dose-dependent. Patients treated with high-dose corticosteroids often express multiple drug-related complaints. Table 7.3 is a list of the common toxicities encountered by patients receiving at least 10 mg of prednisone daily during the previous 6 weeks [5]. More than half of the patients reported at least one side effect. With prednisone doses less than 10 mg daily, patients continued to experience problems but with a lower frequency. In a study of prednisone therapy for IPF, all patients had one or more side effects [6].

Diabetes and hypertension are often unmasked in susceptible patients, and weight gain is common. Although some patients may initially lose weight with prednisone therapy, this side effect is often temporary and weight gain develops with prolonged therapy [6]. In one study of 12 months of prednisone therapy for pulmonary sarcoidosis, patients gained an average of 25 lb [7].

An increased risk for infection accompanies corticosteroid usage, and this risk appears to be both dose and duration of therapy-related and influenced by the underlying disease [8]. The concomitant usage of other drugs, especially cyclophosphamide, enhances this toxicity.

Even relatively low-dose long-term corticosteroid usage can generate cumulative toxicities including cataracts and decreased bone mineral density. Although other immunosuppressive agents may lead to osteoporosis, corticosteroids are associated with the highest risk [9]. The use of calcium supplementation with vitamin D is recommended in most cases. However, sarcoidosis patients may have hypercalcemia or hypercalciuria, and therefore additional supplementation is not unwarranted but associated with toxicity. For patients with a history of hypercalcemia or nephrolithiasis, we usually do not recommend vitamin D supplementation. When oral calcium supplementation is given, we recommend monitoring serum calcium and 24 h urine calcium when clinically indicated. The bisphosphonates are effective agents in the prevention and treatment of glucocorticoid-induced osteoporosis, even in sarcoidosis patients [10].

There is no evidence to suggest that corticosteroids are carcinogenic or teratogenic. In fact, this drug class has been used for a variety of diseases such as asthma during pregnancy. However, there does appear to be an increased risk for cleft palate formation when corticosteroids are given in the first trimester of pregnancy [11].

Methotrexate

In interstitial lung diseases, the mechanism of action for methotrexate is suppression of the inflammatory response of macrophages and to lesser extent lymphocytes. Bronchoalveolar lavage studies have demonstrated that methotrexate suppresses excessive TNF and hydrogen peroxide production by alveolar macrophages in sarcoidosis patients [1]. Methotrexate is also an antiproliferative agent that inhibits the synthesis of purines and pyrimidines. However, it appears that most of the anti-inflammatory action of methotrexate is mediated by adenosine. This nucleoside is a potent endogenous anti-inflammatory mediator [12].

The dosage of methotrexate for sarcoidosis is usually 10–15 mg weekly as a single oral dose [13]. Low doses, such as 2.5 mg/week, may be safely prescribed in patients with disease-related leukopenia. In some patients, the dose may be increased to 25 mg once a week. Some clinicians prefer intramuscular rather than oral dosing [14]. Wegener's granulomatosis patients may require higher doses of methotrexate [15]. Dosage adjustments are usually performed based on toxicities,

including oral ulcers, nausea, and bone marrow suppression. Because methotrexate is cleared by the kidney, even small changes in creatinine clearance can significantly increase toxicity. Folic acid as a 1 mg oral daily supplement can reduce oral ulcers and nausea [16]. Bone marrow suppression, especially neutropenia, is usually dose-related; and holding the drug is recommended. Table 7.4 provides a general guideline for dosage adjustments in patients with hematologic impairment. In cases of significant neutropenia, the use of high-dose folinic acid may reverse the effect of methotrexate.

The long-term use of methotrexate is associated with liver toxicity in some patients. Although monitoring serum liver function is recommended by most groups who routinely prescribe methotrexate [17, 18], the role of routine liver biopsies after every 1–2 g of cumulative dosage of methotrexate is controversial. It is no longer a recommendation for rheumatoid arthritis patients [17], but is still considered an option in patients with psoriasis [18]. Because liver damage may occur without large changes in serum transaminase levels, even small increases in transaminases, which are present more than half of the time on repeated testing, may result in either drug discontinuation or a liver biopsy. For sarcoidosis patients, elevated levels of alkaline phosphatase and transaminases may occur as a result of granulomatous involvement rather than methotrexate toxicity [19]. However, many sarcoidosis centers monitor the trend of liver function tests prior to recommending a liver biopsy [20].

Pulmonary toxicity is another rare but worrisome complication of methotrexate therapy. While the drug can cause an acute hypersensitivity pneumonitis, chronic interstitial lung disease is a more common pulmonary complication [21]. The BAL findings of patients with methotrexate-associated

Table 7.4 Proposed modification of dosage of cytotoxic agents based on complete blood counts

White blood count	Platelet count	Hemoglobin	Drug dosage
>4,000	>50,0000	>10 g %	No change in dose
3–4,000	>50,000	8–10 g %	Reduce dose by 50% of usual dose
2–3,000	>25,000	8–10 g %	Reduce dose by 75% (if) of original dose
<2,000	<25,000	<8 g %	Discontinue drug and repeat blood count in 1–2 weeks[a]

[a]May continue lowered dose in cases in which count has been shown to be stable

lung disease can be similar to those seen in sarcoidosis, with increased lymphocytes and an increased CD4/CD8 ratio [22]. New or worsening cough is often the first manifestation of methotrexate toxicity. In one report of over 200 sarcoidosis patients treated with methotrexate, six developed cough attributed to the drug [23]. In that study, the discontinuation of drug led to resolution of symptoms and cough returned with methotrexate rechallenge. Only those patients with cough on rechallenge were felt to have methotrexate toxicity. Based on that observation, the recommendation for handling unexplained cough in a sarcoidosis patient on methotrexate is to withdraw the drug and consider rechallenge if one wishes to continue with that agent [23]. However, if methotrexate seems to be the cause of pulmonary toxicity, other agents, including leflunomide, may be used [24].

Methotrexate is teratogenic and should not be used during pregnancy. For both men and women, if the drug should be discontinued for at least 6 months, there seems to be no further risk. It is possible that methotrexate is carcinogenic, although large studies with long-term follow up identified a cancer risk no higher than the usual expected rate [25, 26].

Leflunomide

Leflunomide is another antimetabolite with a similar mechanism of action to methotrexate. Its toxicity profile differs from methotrexate with less gastrointestinal and pulmonary toxicity but more alopecia encountered [27]. However, gastrointestinal symptoms remain the most common indication for treatment discontinuation [28, 29]. Because of the different mechanism of action and toxicity profile, leflunomide has been successfully combined with methotrexate to treat rheumatoid arthritis [30]. The drug has also been successfully used for the treatment of sarcoidosis [24] and Wegener's granulomatosis [31].

The usual dosage of leflunomide is an oral daily dose of 10–20 mg. Dose reduction may be necessary in the setting of leukopenia. Originally, leflunomide was prescribed at 100 mg daily for three consecutive days to achieve steady-state levels. However because these high doses could lead to toxicity, this loading regimen has mostly been abandoned [28]. When given in combination with methotrexate, no dose reduction is necessary except for neutropenia [30]. Table 7.4 provides a general guideline for managing dosage in patients with reduced blood counts.

Leflunomide can also cause nausea and gastrointestinal toxicity, but usually less frequently than methotrexate. Patients who develop nausea on methotrexate can sometimes still tolerate leflunomide [24]. Liver toxicity is reported with leflunomide at rates similar to methotrexate [27].

In contrast, pulmonary toxicity is less frequent with leflunomide than with methotrexate [29]. In some cases, leflunomide was successfully prescribed for patients who manifested methotrexate pulmonary toxicity [24]. However, the drug has been associated with hypersensitivity pneumonitis, and therefore it should be discontinued in patients with new or unexpected pulmonary symptoms [32].

Peripheral neuropathy has been associated with leflunomide therapy. Risk factors for developing neuropathy include older age and underling diabetes mellitus [33]. Discontinuing the agent and using high-dose cholestyramine to assist in clearance of the drug can reduce these troublesome symptoms. Due to a high proportion of protein binding, leflunomide has a prolonged half life of over 2 weeks. Elimination of the drug can be enhanced by either cholestyramine or activated charcoal. The recommended protocol for rapid elimination of drug is 8 g of cholestyramine given three times a day for 11 days.

Because leflunomide is teratogenic, it is not recommended during pregnancy [27]. Like methotrexate, there is little indication that the drug is carcinogenic.

Azathioprine

Azathioprine is another cytotoxic drug with immunosuppressive activity. While it has been used for a variety of inflammatory conditions, most of the original data evaluated its efficacy as a steroid-sparing agent in the post solid organ transplant patient. Studies have reported it to be beneficial for several interstitial lung diseases including IPF [34], sarcoidosis [35], and ANCA-associated vasculitis [15]. The drug has a broad range of action on multiple inflammatory cells, including lymphocytes, neutrophils, and macrophages. Azathioprine has been shown to suppress the increased TNF release by alveolar macrophages of patients with active sarcoidosis [35]. This makes the drug an appealing alternative for granulomatous lung diseases.

The target dose of azathioprine is 2–3 mg/kg with the drug supplied as scored 50 mg tablets. In interstitial lung diseases, the usual initial dose is 50 mg a day with dosage increases dictated by the white blood cell count. Thiopurine S-methyltransferase (TPMT) is the rate-limiting enzymatic step in the metabolism of azathioprine. Absolute deficiency of TPMT is encountered in less than 1% of the general population [36]. However, deficient TPMT can lead to severe bone marrow suppression within weeks of initiating azathioprine [37]. Polymorphisms of this gene may lead to different levels of TPMT activity [36] and subsequent variable levels of the drug. Monitoring for both genetic and functional TPMT activity is available [38], but it remains unclear whether genetic or functional testing is better in assessing TPMT activity. Whether all patients placed on azathioprine should have TPMT screening performed is still unknown [39]. Monitoring the complete blood counts 2–4 weeks after the first dose is a relatively inexpensive method to screen for the most important toxicity of TPMT deficiency. Alternatively, drug dosage can be modified as suggested in Table 7.4.

Nausea and fatigue are common dose-dependent complaints from patients receiving azathioprine. In a case-controlled study comparing azathioprine to methotrexate in rheumatoid arthritis patients, azathioprine was associated with more gastrointestinal side effects [40]. However, in a more recent study comparing methotrexate to azathioprine for ANCA-associated vasculitis, no difference in toxicity was reported between the two drugs [15]. However, in that study methotrexate doses were higher than those prescribed for most interstitial lung diseases.

Pancreatitis and hepatotoxicity are less common but significant toxicities associated with azathioprine. Since routine blood counts are recommended for patients while receiving azathioprine, we usually monitor liver function every 2–3 months.

Azathioprine therapy is associated with an increased risk for malignancy in solid organ transplant patients [41]. Nonmelanomatous skin cancers are particularly common [42]. In the nontransplant setting, the relative risk for malignancy is unclear with some studies not able to demonstrate an increased risk [43]. Azathioprine is often prescribed concurrent with other immunomodulators which may be more important potential carcinogens. For transplant patients, this would include drugs such as cyclosporine A [41], and for inflammatory conditions, the concomitant use of anti-TNF biological agents may be associated with a higher risk factor for cancer [44, 45].

The teratogenicity of azathioprine remains unclear. Successful pregnancies have been reported in mothers treated with azathioprine with no adverse fetal outcome [46]. In one study of transplant mothers treated with azathioprine, increased rates of spontaneous abortions and low-birth-weight infants were encountered, but no congenital defects were detected [47].

N-Acetyl Cysteine

The antioxidant N-acetyl cysteine (NAC) has been reported as useful in treating pulmonary fibrosis [48]. This has been proposed as an adjunct to immunosuppressive therapy, especially in IPF where an oxidant–antioxidant imbalance may contribute to the disease process. NAC, a precursor of the major antioxidant glutathione, has been shown to restore depleted pulmonary glutathione levels [48]. A large, double-blind randomized trial demonstrated that NAC plus prednisone/azathioprine was superior to prednisone/azathioprine alone [49]. The use of NAC as a single agent for IPF is currently being studied. The toxicity of NAC is mostly gastrointestinal. It can cause nausea and bloating. Some of the preparations may have the "rotten egg" smell associated with the liquid preparation. The recommended dose is 600 mg three times a day.

Mycophenolate Mofetil

Mycophenolate mofetil (MMF) was originally approved for renal transplant recipients in the USA in 1995, and it has replaced azathioprine in many solid organ transplant programs. Recently, it has been used as another immunosuppressive agent for the treatment of interstitial lung disease [50]. MMF is rapidly hydrolyzed to its active form, mycophenolic acid, which inhibits inosine monophosphate dehydrogenase, an important enzyme in the de novo purine biosynthesis pathway. Because both T and B cells are dependent on this pathway for purine synthesis, lymphocytes are uniquely sensitive to this drug. In vitro MMF has been shown to inhibit the production of antibodies and the generation of cytotoxic T cells, and it also suppresses the expression of lymphocyte adhesion molecules.

The current recommended adult dose of MMF is 2 g a day administered in two doses. Because of potential gastrointestinal toxicity, patients often titrate up the dose by 500 mg increments. The pharmacokinetics of the drug are complex and dosage levels can be quite variable [51]. In a randomized trial of over 900 renal transplant recipients, no difference in clinical outcome or adverse reactions were noted when the drug was prescribed at a fixed dose compared to variable dosing based on MMF levels [52]. Therefore, monitoring of blood levels is generally not recommended.

MMF use is associated with diarrhea, leukopenia, and opportunistic infections. In most studies, the incidence of side effects is similar to those encountered with azathioprine [53]. In a meta-analysis of 20 clinical trials, compared with azathioprine the use of MMF was associated with slight increases in gastrointestinal adverse effects, hematologic adverse events, and CMV infections [54].

Like many solid organ transplant anti-rejection drugs, MMF has been associated with increased malignancies, particularly skin cancers [55]. Other malignancies are less frequently encountered with aggressive screening programs improving early detection [56]. Mycophenolate carries a risk for congenital abnormalities and should not be used during pregnancy [57].

Cyclophosphamide

Cyclophosphamide, an alkylating agent originally developed to treat malignancy, has a dose-dependent bimodal effect on the immune system. High doses can induce an anti-inflammatory immune reaction (i.e., suppression of T helper 1 and enhancement of T helper 2 activity), affect CD4CD25 (high) regulatory T cells, and establish a state of marked immunosuppression. It has been demonstrated efficacious for the treatment of various collagen vascular-associated lung diseases including scleroderma [58, 59] and other interstitial lung diseases [60, 61]. Additionally, it has been a standard treatment for ANCA-associated vasculitis [62].

Cyclophosphamide can be administered by either continuous oral daily dosage or intermittent intravenous pulse therapy. For several conditions, the pulse therapy appears as effective and less toxic than daily oral regimens. This includes ANCA-associated vasculitis [62, 63] as well as scleroderma-associated lung disease [58, 59]. One of the disadvantages of pulse therapy is the associated cost and need for supportive staff to administer intravenous cyclophosphamide. However, one of the advantages of pulse therapy is tailored drug dosing which can be adjusted based on the patient's individual white blood count. In one study, dosage adjustments were made in almost one-third of visits [61]. Regardless of the administration method, monitoring guidelines are similar.

Hematologic side effects are the major toxicities of cyclophosphamide. Its effect on the bone marrow, specifically the white blood cells, can create leukopenia, a dose-related complication of the drug. Although lower doses of cyclophosphamide can cause neutropenia, this complication is more common with higher dose therapy [64]. In a randomized trial of oral cyclophosphamide for scleroderma-associated pulmonary fibrosis, 19 of 79 (24%) of cyclophosphamide-treated patients developed leukopenia and 7 (9%) experienced neutropenia during the year of therapy. None of the placebo-treated patients developed leukopenia [58]. Although anemia was more common with cyclophosphamide, the difference compared to placebo was insignificant. These rates are higher than those reported for intermittent intravenous cyclophosphamide [59, 61, 62, 65]. The guidelines of Table 7.4 can be used to adjust the dose.

Hemorrhagic cystitis and bladder cancer are known toxicities of cyclophosphamide therapy. The reported complication rate is higher for continuous daily treatment compared with pulse therapy [66, 67]. Regardless of administration method, patients should be monitored for bladder toxicity. Obtaining a monthly urine analysis is the recommended assessment for bladder toxicity. A large prospective study of Wegener's granulomatosis patients treated with daily oral cyclophosphamide demonstrated that hematuria was time duration- and dose-dependent [66]. Fifty percent of patients eventually developed nonglomerular hematuria, and seven of these (5% of the total patients) developed bladder cancer. Hematuria occurred in a median of 37 months after initiating cyclophosphamide, with 15% developing hematuria within the first year of treatment. In the placebo-controlled trial of oral cyclophosphamide versus placebo for scleroderma-associated lung disease, nine of the cyclophosphamide-treated patients developed hematuria compared with three in the placebo group [58].

The hemorrhagic cystitis associated with cyclophosphamide may lead to bladder cancer [66]. While urine cytology may aid monitoring for bladder cancer in hematuria patients, cystoscopy is a more definitive test [66]. It is recommended that patients with persistent hematuria undergo further evaluation, such as cystoscopy. Some investigators have added MESNA, an uroprotectant agent against acrolein, the metabolite in part responsible for bladder toxicity from cyclophosphamide, to the treatment regimen to prevent bladder toxicity.

Despite its widespread and long-term use, there is limited information regarding the safety of cyclophosphamide during pregnancy [68]. Cyclophosphamide has been administered successfully during the second and third trimesters of pregnancy for malignancies such as lymphoma or breast cancer. Many clinicians recommend other agents, such as azathioprine, during pregnancy [69].

As an alklyating agent, cyclophosphamide can cause temporary or permanent ovarian failure. In doses used to treat malignancy, cyclophosphamide often induces early menopause [70]. Patients treated with low-dose pulse cyclophosphamide for rheumatologic diseases appear to experience lower rates of premature ovarian failure [64]. However prior to initiating treatment, women of child-bearing potential should consider oocyte or embryo cryopreservation [71].

All alkylating agents have been associated with an increased risk for cancers [72]. While cyclophosphamide is most closely associated with bladder cancer, other malignancies, including leukemia and lymphoma, may be associated with therapy.

Antimalarial Agents

Chloroquine and hydroxychloroquine were originally developed as antimicrobial agents for the treatment of malaria. However, soon after discovery these drugs were noted to possess anti-inflammatory activity leading to usage for a variety of rheumatologic diseases. Chloroquine has been reported to be superior to placebo in treating pulmonary sarcoidosis. Unfortunately, the response rates were minimal, and the drug seems most useful as a steroid-sparing agent [73]. To date, the antimalarial agents do not appear to be useful in treating other interstitial lung diseases. Although the response rates are similar between the two agents, hydroxychloroquine is less toxic and therefore preferred by some clinicians. The recommended oral dosage of hydroxychloroquine is 200–400 mg/day and chloroquine 250–500 mg/day. Toxicity for both drugs is dose-dependent [74]. To reduce ocular toxicity from hydroxychloroquine, the maximum calculated dose of 6.5 mg/kg should not be exceeded [75].

Because the antimalarial drugs are concentrated in the retina, skin, and liver, the major toxicities involve these organs. Rashes, including photosensitivity, can occur with both drugs. Gastrointestinal problems are commonly encountered with the antimalarial agents. In one retrospective analysis of various immunosuppressive agents used for sarcoidosis, the rate of toxicity, usually gastrointestinal, was double for hydroxy-chloroquine compared to either methotrexate or azathioprine [23]. For patients with drug-induced nausea, a lower dose may be tolerated. Although hepatotoxicity is rare, serum liver function should be monitored at least annually.

Ocular toxicity is the most serious adverse event with antimalarial drugs. The risk is higher for patients with impaired renal function [76]. Ocular examinations should be performed at least annually for patients receiving chloro-quine, and ocular screening has also been recommended for patients receiving hydroxy-chloroquine [77]. Ocular toxicity due to hydroxychloroquine is lower if the total drug dose remains <6.5 mg/kg [75].

There is no evidence for carcinogenicity for the antimalarial agents. However, limited data exist regarding safety during pregnancy. In one randomized trial of pregnant patients with lupus erythematosis, the use of hydroxychloroquine was associated with better clinical disease outcomes with no deleterious effect on mother or baby [78]. Hydroxychloroquine appears relatively safe when administered during pregnancy and lactation [79]. In a study using detailed neurologic testing, some infants prenatally exposed to hydroxychloroquine were found to have visual neurophysiologic disturbances [80].

Thalidomide

Thalidomide is an anti-inflammatory drug which can suppress TNF release by alveolar macrophages and inhibit production of vascular endothelial growth factor (VEGF) [81, 82]. Additionally, it can suppress lymphocyte infiltration of granulomas in successfully treated chronic cutaneous sarcoidosis patients [83].

The dosage of thalidomide varies from 50 to 200 mg orally every night. In a dose escalation study in sarcoidosis patients, 12 of 14 patients responded to 100 mg at night, while all responded to 200 mg [84]. However, toxicity was dose-dependent and 100 mg is the usual dose prescribed [83, 85].

The most common side effects of thalidomide are hypersomnolence and constipation [84]. Because they are usually dose-dependent, administering the drug prior to sleep and using agents such as fiber to minimize constipation [86] can reverse side effects. In up to 25% of patients, a dry scaly rash may occur. Although irritating, the rash is usually self-limited, successfully treated with topical corticosteroids, and not an indication for drug discontinuation. A painless peripheral neuropathy can also occur. In some cases, it will resolve with dose reduction; however, some patients may develop a permanent residual deficit.

Thalidomide can be beneficial for the treatment of intractable cough in IPF patients [87]. However, the drug rarely causes an interstitial pattern on chest roentgenogram which resolves with drug withdrawal [88, 89]. Thalidomide may also cause reversible pulmonary hypertension [90].

Pulmonary embolism is a more common cause for new onset dyspnea in a patient being treated with thalidomide. Increased rates of both arterial and venous thrombosis have been reported with thalidomide. In patients with underlying malignancy or other risk factors for hypercoagulopathy, anticoagulation prophylaxis with warfarin or aspirin can reduce rate of thrombosis [91].

Thalidomide is teratogenic. One of the great tragedies of medicine is the major skeletal malformations seen when pregnant women were exposed to thalidomide. In the USA, drug administration is carefully monitored by the System for Thalidomide Education and Prescribing Safety (STEPS) [86]. Similar programs are often used in other countries where the drug is available.

Anti-TNF Agents

Biological agents directed against TNFα have proved successful in treating various manifestations of rheumatoid arthritis. The drugs include the soluble TNF receptor–IgG fusion protein etanercept, the chimeric monoclonal anti-TNF antibody infliximab, and the humanized monoclonal antibodies adalimumab and golimumab. These agents are equally effective in treating the joint manifestations of rheumatoid arthritis [92].

Table 7.5 Monitoring guidelines for patients receiving anti-TNF therapy

Monitoring for infections
- A chest radiograph and a tuberculin skin test or similar test is recommended prior to treatment
- For patients who present with a chest roentgenogram consistent with prior tuberculosis or a positive tuberculin skin test, and/or is a high risk individual, active tuberculosis infection should be excluded prior to treatment
- For patients with latent *M. tuberculosis*, active prophylactic treatment following published guidelines before initiation of anti-TNFα therapy is recommended
- For patients with latent *M. tuberculosis* who will undergo anti-TNFα therapy, close monitoring for tuberculosis is recommended for up to 6 months after discontinuing therapy
- For patients who will undergo anti-TNFα therapy and who are at risk for viral hepatitis, serologic screening for hepatitis B is recommended prior to treatment
- For patients who have hepatitis B virus infection, anti-TNFα therapy should not be administered
- For patients who undergo anti-TNFα therapy and develop unresolved infections, discontinuation of treatment until the infection is resolved is recommended

Reactions to the medications
- For patients who undergo anti-TNFα therapy and develop local or systemic reaction to the medication (e.g., anaphylaxis), treatment should be discontinued
- For patients who undergo anti-TNFα therapy and develop symptoms of a lupus-like disorder, discontinuation of therapy is suggested

Congestive heart failure
- For patients with known grade III or IV New York Heart Association class heart failure, administration of anti-TNF therapy is not recommended
- For patients with a history of congestive heart failure (CHF) who undergo anti-TNFα therapy, close observation for CHF exacerbation is recommended

Malignancy
- Patients who develop cancer while receiving an anti-TNF therapy should be considered for discontinuing medication

Miscellaneous
- For patients with a history of demyelinating disease, alternatives to anti-TNF therapy should be considered
- For patients who undergo anti-TNF therapy and experience symptoms or display signs of a demyelinating process, discontinuation of therapy is suggested
- For patients who are pregnant, alternatives to anti-TNF therapy should be considered

However, there is evidence to suggest that only anti-TNF antibodies are useful for sarcoidosis. Infliximab has been shown to be effective in treating chronic pulmonary sarcoidosis in a double-blind randomized, placebo-controlled study [93], while etanercept was not effective in treating pulmonary sarcoidosis [94]. In a comparison of three anti-TNF agents, infliximab was more likely to induce remission than either adalimumab or etanercept [95]. Compared to placebo, etanercept has been shown more likely to stabilize the loss of lung function in IPF patients [96].

Because over the last 10 years the anti-TNF agents have proved useful for a variety of inflammatory diseases, these drugs have been administered to more than one million patients. Several guidelines for toxicity monitoring have been proposed [97–99]. Monitoring recommendations for infusion reactions, infections, worsening congestive heart failure, and malignancy are provided in Table 7.5.

An increased risk for *M. tuberculosis* is an important potential infectious complication of anti-TNF therapy. Early observations noted that patients receiving infliximab experienced a higher risk than those receiving etanercept. Most cases appeared to be latent tuberculosis rather than new infection [100, 101], hence the recommendation for intense screening for latent tuberculosis as summarized in the recommendations in Table 7.5.

This screening effort successfully reduced the rate of active tuberculosis in patients receiving anti-TNF therapy. In a registry of over 5,000 patients treated with a TNF antagonist, 15 cases of active tuberculosis were noted. Screening for latent tuberculosis was not performed in about half of the patients, and the risk for developing active tuberculosis was seven times higher for the unscreened population. Failure to perform a tuberculin skin test was the most common reason for failing to comply with the recommendations [102].

While this supports the value of a tuberculin skin test for the detection of latent tuberculosis, it is well recognized that patients receiving immunosuppressive drugs may become anergic. Recently, *M. tuberculosis* antigen-specific IFN-γ assay has been developed. In immunosuppressed patients, these tests were more specific and sensitive than routine tuberculin skin testing [103].

As noted the risk for tuberculosis differs among the various anti-TNF therapies. Etanercept is reported to have a much lower risk than infliximab therapy [100, 104]. The reported rates of active tuberculosis are similar for infliximab and adalimumab [104], which are both antibodies directed against TNF. This differential effect of tuberculosis reactivation mirrors the increased efficacy for infliximab and adalimumab for sarcoidosis treatment [95].

Because hepatitis B reactivation has occurred during anti-TNF therapy, patients should be evaluated for risk for hepatitis B and the drug should be avoided in those with known hepatitis B infection [105]. On the other hand, patients with active hepatitis C have been safely treated with anti-TNF therapy [106]. In an evidence-based analysis, Huang et al. concluded that the recommendation to screen for hepatitis C had insufficient information to support its routine use [107].

The anti-TNF agents are also associated with increased rates of fungal infections, including histoplasmosis and coccidiomycosis [108], and patients may also develop pneumonia from opportunistic organisms including *Pneumocystis jiroveci* [109] and *Legionella pneumophila* [110]. Therefore, patients who develop pneumonia while receiving anti-TNF therapy should have therapy discontinued until the pneumonia resolves.

Local and systemic reactions to anti-TNF therapy have been reported. Infliximab is associated with the highest rate of infusion reactions; and because over 10% of patients eventually develop infusion reactions [111], careful monitoring during the infusion is recommended.

A lupus-like reaction, including the development of interstitial lung disease, can occur with all the anti-TNF therapies [112]. While concurrent therapy with drugs such as methotrexate may account for some cases, severe interstitial lung disease has been reported in some patients who received only anti-TNF therapy [113]. In addition, a sarcoid-like granulomatous reaction can occur during anti-TNF therapy [114].

Shortly after the discovery of TNF, this pro-inflammatory cytokine was reported to be increased in the serum of patients with congestive heart failure. Based on these observations and studies in animal models, a potential therapeutic role for anti-TNF treatment for advanced congestive heart failure was pursued [115]. Trials of etanercept in advanced congestive heart failure demonstrated no drug benefit [116]. More worrisome was the observation that patients with advanced congestive heart failure treated with infliximab experienced a higher mortality than the placebo-controlled group [117]. Analysis of the several anti-TNF studies suggested a class effect of potentially worsening congestive heart failure in a subset of patients [118]. This led to the manufacturers' recommendations that anti-TNF therapy be avoided in patients with known grade 3 or 4 NYHA (WHO) congestive heart failure.

Randomized pulmonary disease trials have reported an increased malignancy rate in the anti-TNF-treated patients compared with the placebo-controlled group [119, 120]. Anti-TNF therapies were associated with higher rates of lymphoma in patients with Crohn's disease [121], but not in rheumatoid arthritis [122]. These variable rates could be due to sample size, underlying disease, or concurrent medications. Given the current information, it seems prudent to warn patients of the potential risk for malignancy while on therapy and to withdraw drug if cancer is detected.

Demyelinating diseases, including multiple sclerosis and optic neuritis, have been reported in patients treated with anti-TNF therapy. The risk seems greater with etanercept than with the other agents [123]. In a detailed analysis of 3,893 unique patients treated in clinical trials with etanercept, only eight cases were identified [124]. While it seems reasonable to discontinue anti-TNF therapy for patients who develop demyelinating diseases, patient outcome remains unknown. Patients may improve without stopping the drug [125], and anti-TNF agents have successfully treated optic neuritis [126, 127].

The anti-TNF agents were originally regarded as potential teratogens. With expanded clinical experience, few complications were reported during pregnancy and some have stated that these agents may be safe during pregnancy [128, 129]. However, a review from the US Food and Drug Administration database suggested an increased rate for congenital abnormalities compared to historical controls [130]. In one small study of women receiving infliximab, drug levels were easily measured in the sera but not in breast milk [131]. Although it seems prudent to seek alternatives to these drugs during pregnancy, individual risks and benefits for these drugs should be considered [128].

Rituximab

Rituximab is a chimeric anti-CD20 antibody originally developed to treat non-Hodgkin's lymphoma [132]. In the past few years, the drug has been used in a variety of nonmalignant conditions, including rheumatoid arthritis and ANCA-associated vasculitis [133]. It has also been reported to be effective in some patients with sarcoidosis [134] and relapsing polychondritis [135].

Infusion reactions associated with rituximab are attributed to the antigen–antibody interactions occurring with specific cells and tissues. Among the common reactions are flu-like symptoms such as headache, fever, sweats, skin rash, shortness of breath, hypotension, and nausea. These often occur with the first infusion. Rarely severe hypotension, bronchospasm, hypoxia, and even death have occurred [136]. Early studies of rituximab used for malignancy reported infusion reactions including mild fever, chills, and occasional skin eruptions in over half the patients after the first treatment and up to 20% of patients with subsequent infusions [137]. Because reactions

are more likely to occur in patients with high tumor burden, some side effects may be attributed to tumor lysis [138]. In trials of rheumatoid arthritis patients treated with rituximab, infusion reactions have been reported in up to 40% of patients. These are usually mild to moderate and occur with the first dose only [139].

Although pretreatment with acetaminophen, antihistamines, and corticosteroids reduces the reaction rate, severe reactions may still occur. In a retrospective analysis of 47 cases of severe reactions to rituximab, the authors found that almost all patients were pretreated. Postinfusion reactions were managed typically with corticosteroids, oxygen, and intravenous fluids, but approximately 20% of patients were hospitalized [140].

Since most reactions occur during the initial treatment [139, 141], the first dose should be infused slowly, usually over 4–6 h. For subsequent infusions, a rapid infusion over 90 min can be well tolerated in the corticosteroid pretreated patient [142]. This more rapid infusion for subsequent doses is now often employed in the rituximab-tolerant patient [143].

Like other immunosuppressive agents, rituximab is associated with an increased rate of opportunistic infections [144]. Current recommendations suggest that rituximab patients be screened for latent tuberculosis using the anti-TNF agent guidelines (see Table 7.5) [98]. However, clinical trials of rituximab have not reported a higher rate of tuberculosis [108]. In fact, a patient with rheumatoid arthritis who developed tuberculosis during anti-TNF therapy was subsequently successfully treated with rituximab [145].

Rituximab administration has also been associated with viral infection reactivation [146]. Hepatitis B reactivation was associated with a 50% mortality [146], and other viral infections were also associated with increased mortality.

Progressive multifocal leukoencephalopathy (PML) represents another case of viral infection reactivation. This is a rare demyelinating disease of the central nervous system that results from reactivation of latent Jakob Creutzfeldt virus (JCV) [147]. Cases of PML have been reported in patients with underlying malignancy as well as those with rheumatoid arthritis [147, 148].

Patients receiving rituximab who develop unexplained neurologic symptoms should discontinue the drug and be evaluated for possible PML. Unfortunately, to date there is no effective method to screen for PML since over 90% of the adult population is JCV-seropositive [149].

Sirolimus

Sirolimus, a macrolide antibiotic produced by *Streptomyces hygroscopicus*, has potent immunosuppressive and antiproliferative effects. It is structurally similar to tacrolimus as both drugs bind to intracellular FK-binding protein. However, the mechanism of action of sirolimus is different from tacrolimus. In transplant patients, sirolimus suppresses graft rejection by interfering with a cytoplasmic biochemical transducer that signals from cell membrane to the nucleus. Sirolimus binds to the mammalian target of rapamycin, mTOR, a serine/threonine kinase. The mTOR signaling system plays a key role in several transduction pathways that are necessary for cell cycle progression and cellular proliferation [150]. The drug has been found useful in treating the pulmonary manifestations of tuberous sclerosis [151] and is currently being studied for the treatment of lymphangioleiomyomatosis.

The dose of sirolimus varies based on therapy indication. Higher doses are used in transplant patients compared to nontransplant indications. In a study of tuberous sclerosis patients, the initial sirolimus dose was 0.25 mg/m^2 of body-surface area. The administered dosage was adjusted to achieve a drug blood level between 1 and 5 ng/ml [151]. Because the drug has a long half-life, dosage adjustments should be based on trough levels obtained more than 1 week after initiation of therapy or dosage change. Once the initial dose titration is complete, monitoring sirolimus trough concentrations closely is recommended for the next 2 months [152]. Although the drug can be beneficial in treating renal disease, it may also cause worsening renal function in patients with low glomerular filtration rates [153].

Pulmonary toxicity is associated with the use of the drug [154]. While an immune-mediated pneumonitis is the most common problem [154, 155], pulmonary hemorrhage can occur [156]. Withdrawal of drug and corticosteroid administration is usually sufficient to reverse the process [154, 155], but the pneumonitis can be fatal [155, 157].

Pirfenidone

Pirfenidone is a novel antifibrotic agent which has been reported to be effective in treating pulmonary fibrosis, especially IPF [158–161]. It appears to suppress known fibrotic cytokines, such as transforming growth factor $\beta1$ (TGF$\beta1$) [162], and also the proinflammatory cytokine TNFα [163].

Usual dosage ranges are 1,800–2,400 mg/day, administered in three divided doses [158–160]. Drug dosage is generally titrated up from 200 mg three times a day by increasing the dose every 2 weeks to the maximum. In one pharmacokinetic study, the administration of pirfenidone with food modestly reduced the overall drug exposure and resulted in lower peak concentrations which improved tolerability [163, 164].

The most common toxicities reported with pirfenidone are gastrointestinal symptoms and photosensitivity [158–160]. Table 7.6 combines reports from three large patient series treated with the drug, two of which included placebo-treated patients. The rate of gastrointestinal symptoms was highest in the study by Raghu et al. [159]. However, patients in that study received up to 3,600 mg/day; whereas, a maximum dose of 1,800 mg/day was prescribed in the other trials. Overall, approximately 10% of patients discontinued drug due to adverse events. Photosensitivity may be minimized by limiting exposure to sunlight and the use of sun blocks. Current recommendations suggest that liver function be monitored at least every 2 months with an elevated γ-glutamyltranspeptidase the most frequent liver function abnormality reported.

There is insufficient information regarding the use of pirfenidone during pregnancy. Given its broad effect on growth and repair, one would assume it may well be teratogenic.

Table 7.6 Reported toxicities and cause for discontinuation of pirfenidone versus placebo

	Raghu [159]	Azuma [160]		Taniguchi [158]	
	Pirfenidone	Pirfenidone	Placebo	Pirfenidone[a]	Placebo
Number of patients treated	54	73	36	163	105
Adverse reaction					
Photosensitivity	24%	43.8%[b]	0%	52.1%[b]	22.4%
Abdominal discomfort	64%	30.1%[c]	8.3%	4.3%[c]	0%
Fatigue	42%	21.9%[c]	2.8%	N.R.	N.R.
Elevated γ-GTP	N.R.	27.4%[c]	8.3%	22.7%[b]	9.3%
Photosensitivity	7%	6.8%	0%	3.1%	0%
Nausea and/or Emesis	4%	1.4%	0%	0%	0.9%
Abnormal hepatic function	0%	1.4%	0%	1.2%	0%

N.R. not reported, *g-GTP* γ-glutamyltranspeptidase
[a]Combined low and high dosage patients
[b]Significantly higher rate than placebo $p < 0.01$
[c]Significantly higher rate than placebo, $p < 0.05$

Conclusion

Treating physicians have a wide array of agents to use in the management of a variety of interstitial lung diseases that they encounter in their practices. Other drugs are being developed which may also prove useful in treating diffuse parenchymal lung disease.

References

1. Baughman RP, Lower EE. The effect of corticosteroid or methotrexate therapy on lung lymphocytes and macrophages in sarcoidosis. Am Rev Respir Dis. 1990;142:1268–71.
2. Scheinman RI, Cogswell PC, Lofquist AK, et al. Role of transcriptional activation of I kappa B alpha in mediation of immunosuppression by glucocorticoids. Science. 1995;270(5234):283–6.
3. Webster JC, Oakley RH, Jewell CM, et al. Proinflammatory cytokines regulate human glucocorticoid receptor gene expression and lead to the accumulation of the dominant negative beta isoform: a mechanism for the generation of glucocorticoid resistance. Proc Natl Acad Sci USA. 2001;98(12):6865–70.
4. Baughman RP, Costabel U, du Bois RM. Treatment of sarcoidosis. Clin Chest Med. 2008;29(3):533–48.
5. Baughman RP, Iannuzzi MC, Lower EE, et al. Use of fluticasone in acute symptomatic pulmonary sarcoidosis. Sarcoidosis Vasc Diffuse Lung Dis. 2002; 19(3):198–204.
6. Flaherty KR, Toews GB, Lynch III JP, et al. Steroids in idiopathic pulmonary fibrosis: a prospective assessment of adverse reactions, response to therapy, and survival. Am J Med. 2001;110(4):278–82.
7. Baughman RP, Winget DB, Lower EE. Methotrexate is steroid sparing in acute sarcoidosis: results of a double blind, randomized trial. Sarcoidosis Vasc Diffuse Lung Dis. 2000;17:60–6.
8. Stuck AE, Minder CE, Frey FJ. Risk of infectious complications in patients taking glucocorticosteroids. Rev Infect Dis. 1989;11(6):954–63.
9. Coulson KA, Reed G, Gilliam BE, et al. Factors influencing fracture risk, T score, and management of osteoporosis in patients with rheumatoid arthritis in the Consortium of Rheumatology Researchers of North America (CORRONA) registry. J Clin Rheumatol. 2009;15(4):155–60.
10. Gonnelli S, Rottoli P, Cepollaro C, et al. Prevention of corticosteroid-induced osteoporosis with alendronate in sarcoid patients. Calcif Tissue Int. 1997; 61(5):382–5.
11. Park-Wyllie L, Mazzotta P, Pastuszak A, et al. Birth defects after maternal exposure to corticosteroids: prospective cohort study and meta-analysis of epidemiological studies. Teratology. 2000;62(6):385–92.
12. Chan ES, Cronstein BN. Molecular action of methotrexate in inflammatory diseases. Arthritis Res. 2002; 4(4):266–73.
13. Baughman RP, Lower EE. A clinical approach to the use of methotrexate for sarcoidosis. Thorax. 1999;54: 742–6.
14. Hamilton RA, Kremer JM. Why intramuscular methotrexate may be more efficacious than oral dosing in patients with rheumatoid arthritis. Br J Rheumatol. 1997;36(1):86–90.
15. Pagnoux C, Mahr A, Hamidou MA, et al. Azathioprine or methotrexate maintenance for ANCA-associated vasculitis. N Engl J Med. 2008; 359(26):2790–803.
16. Morgan SL, Baggott JE, Vaughn WH, et al. Supplementation with folic acid during methotrexate

therapy for rheumatoid arthritis. Ann Intern Med. 1994;121:833–41.

17. Kremer JM, Alarcon GS, Lightfoot Jr RW, et al. Methotrexate for rheumatoid arthritis. Suggested guidelines for monitoring liver toxicity. American College of Rheumatology. Arthritis Rheum. 1994; 37(3):316–28.

18. Roenigk HH, Auerbach R, Mailbach HI, et al. Methotrexate guidelines revised. J Am Acad Dermatol. 1982;6:145–55.

19. Baughman RP, Koehler A, Bejarano PA, et al. Role of liver function tests in detecting methotrexate-induced liver damage in sarcoidosis. Arch Intern Med. 2003;163(5):615–20.

20. Vucinic VM. What is the future of methotrexate in sarcoidosis? A study and review. Curr Opin Pulm Med. 2002;8(5):470–6.

21. Zisman DA, McCune WJ, Tino G, et al. Drug-induced pneumonitis: the role of methotrexate. Sarcoidosis Vasc Diffuse Lung Dis. 2001;18(3): 243–52.

22. Schnabel A, Richter C, Bauerfeind S, et al. Bronchoalveolar lavage cell profile in methotrexate pneumonitis. Thorax. 1997;52:377–9.

23. Baughman RP, Lower EE. Alternatives to corticosteroids in the treatment of sarcoidosis. Sarcoidosis. 1997;14:121–30.

24. Baughman RP, Lower EE. Leflunomide for chronic sarcoidosis. Sarcoidosis Vasc Diffuse Lung Dis. 2004;21:43–8.

25. Rustin GJS, Rustin F, Dent J, et al. No increase in second tumors after cytotoxic chemotherapy for gestational trophoblastic tumors. N Engl J Med. 1982;308:473–6.

26. Balin PL, Tindall JP, Roenigk HH, et al. Is methotrexate therapy for psoriasis carcinogenic? A modified retrospective-prospective analysis. JAMA. 1975;232:359–62.

27. Alcorn N, Saunders S, Madhok R. Benefit-risk assessment of leflunomide: an appraisal of leflunomide in rheumatoid arthritis 10 years after licensing. Drug Saf. 2009;32(12):1123–34.

28. Chan V, Tett SE. How is leflunomide prescribed and used in Australia? Analysis of prescribing and adverse effect reporting. Pharmacoepidemiol Drug Saf. 2006;15(7):485–93.

29. Emery P, Breedveld FC, Lemmel EM, et al. A comparison of the efficacy and safety of leflunomide and methotrexate for the treatment of rheumatoid arthritis. Rheumatology (Oxford). 2000;39(6):655–65.

30. Kremer JM, Genovese MC, Cannon GW, et al. Concomitant leflunomide therapy in patients with active rheumatoid arthritis despite stable doses of methotrexate. A randomized, double-blind, placebo-controlled trial. Ann Intern Med. 2002;137(9): 726–33.

31. Metzler C, Miehle N, Manger K, et al. Elevated relapse rate under oral methotrexate versus leflunomide for maintenance of remission in Wegener's granulomatosis. Rheumatology (Oxford). 2007;46(7): 1087–91.

32. Savage RL, Highton J, Boyd IW, et al. Pneumonitis associated with leflunomide: a profile of New Zealand and Australian reports. Intern Med J. 2006; 36(3):162–9.

33. Martin K, Bentaberry F, Dumoulin C, et al. Peripheral neuropathy associated with leflunomide: is there a risk patient profile? Pharmacoepidemiol Drug Saf. 2007;16(1):74–8.

34. Raghu G, Depaso WJ, Cain K, et al. Azathioprine combined with prednisone in the treatment of idiopathic pulmonary fibrosis: a prospective double-blind, randomized, placebo-controlled clinical trial. Am Rev Respir Dis. 1991;144(2):291–6.

35. Muller-Quernheim J, Kienast K, Held M, et al. Treatment of chronic sarcoidosis with an azathioprine/prednisolone regimen. Eur Respir J. 1999; 14(5):1117–22.

36. Cooper SC, Ford LT, Berg JD, et al. Ethnic variation of thiopurine S-methyltransferase activity: a large, prospective population study. Pharmacogenomics. 2008;9(3):303–9.

37. Perri D, Cole DE, Friedman O, et al. Azathioprine and diffuse alveolar haemorrhage: the pharmacogenetics of thiopurine methyltransferase. Eur Respir J. 2007;30(5):1014–7.

38. Winter JW, Gaffney D, Shapiro D, et al. Assessment of thiopurine methyltransferase enzyme activity is superior to genotype in predicting myelosuppression following azathioprine therapy in patients with inflammatory bowel disease. Aliment Pharmacol Ther. 2007;25(9):1069–77.

39. Ansari A, Arenas M, Greenfield SM, et al. Prospective evaluation of the pharmacogenetics of azathioprine in the treatment of inflammatory bowel disease. Aliment Pharmacol Ther. 2008;28(8):973–83.

40. McKendry RJR, Cyr M. Toxicity of methotrexate compared with azathioprine in the treatment of rheumatoid arthritis: a case-control study of 131 patients. Arch Intern Med. 1989;149:685–9.

41. Kehinde EO, Petermann A, Morgan JD, et al. Triple therapy and incidence of de nova cancer in renal transplants. Br J Surg. 1994;81:985–6.

42. Mackenzie KA, Wells JE, Lynn KL, et al. First and subsequent nonmelanoma skin cancers: incidence and predictors in a population of New Zealand renal transplant recipients. Nephrol Dial Transplant. 2010; 25(1):300–6.

43. Lebrun C, Debouverie M, Vermersch P, et al. Cancer risk and impact of disease-modifying treatments in patients with multiple sclerosis. Mult Scler. 2008; 14(3):399–405.

44. Kempen JH, Daniel E, Dunn JP, et al. Overall and cancer related mortality among patients with ocular inflammation treated with immunosuppressive drugs: retrospective cohort study. BMJ. 2009;339:b2480. doi:10.1136/bmj.b2480.:b2480.

45. Caspersen S, Elkjaer M, Riis L, et al. Infliximab for inflammatory bowel disease in Denmark 1999–2005: clinical outcome and follow-up evaluation of malignancy and mortality. Clin Gastroenterol Hepatol. 2008;6(11):1212–7.

46. Koukoura O, Mantas N, Linardakis H, et al. Successful term pregnancy in a patient with Wegener's granulomatosis: case report and literature review. Fertil Steril. 2008;89(2):457.e1–5.

47. Miniero R, Tardivo I, Curtoni ES, et al. Pregnancy after renal transplantation in Italian patients: focus on fetal outcome. J Nephrol. 2002;15(6):626–32.

48. Behr J, Maier K, Degenkolb B, et al. Antioxidative and clinical effects of high-dose N-acetylcysteine in fibrosing alveolitis. Adjunctive therapy to maintenance immunosuppression. Am J Respir Crit Care Med. 1997;156(6):1897–901.

49. Demedts M, Behr J, Buhl R, et al. High-dose acetylcysteine in idiopathic pulmonary fibrosis. N Engl J Med. 2005;353(21):2229–42.

50. Swigris JJ, Olson AL, Fischer A, et al. Mycophenolate mofetil is safe, well tolerated, and preserves lung function in patients with connective tissue disease-related interstitial lung disease. Chest. 2006;130(1):30–6.

51. van Hest RM, Mathot RA, Pescovitz MD, et al. Explaining variability in mycophenolic acid exposure to optimize mycophenolate mofetil dosing: a population pharmacokinetic meta-analysis of mycophenolic acid in renal transplant recipients. J Am Soc Nephrol. 2006;17(3):871–80.

52. van Gelder T, Silva HT, de Fijter JW, et al. Comparing mycophenolate mofetil regimens for de novo renal transplant recipients: the fixed-dose concentration-controlled trial. Transplantation. 2008;86(8):1043–51.

53. Remuzzi G, Cravedi P, Costantini M, et al. Mycophenolate mofetil versus azathioprine for prevention of chronic allograft dysfunction in renal transplantation: the MYSS follow-up randomized, controlled clinical trial. J Am Soc Nephrol. 2007;18(6):1973–85.

54. Wang K, Zhang H, Li Y, et al. Safety of mycophenolate mofetil versus azathioprine in renal transplantation: a systematic review. Transplant Proc. 2004;36(7):2068–70.

55. Brewer JD, Colegio OR, Phillips PK, et al. Incidence of and risk factors for skin cancer after heart transplant. Arch Dermatol. 2009;145(12):1391–6.

56. Fraile P, Garcia-Cosmes P, Martin P, et al. Non-skin solid tumors as a cause of morbidity and mortality after liver transplantation. Transplant Proc. 2009;41(6):2433–4.

57. Ostensen M, Lockshin M, Doria A, et al. Update on safety during pregnancy of biological agents and some immunosuppressive anti-rheumatic drugs. Rheumatology (Oxford). 2008;47 Suppl 3:iii28–31.

58. Tashkin DP, Elashoff R, Clements PJ, et al. Cyclophosphamide versus placebo in scleroderma lung disease. N Engl J Med. 2006;354(25):2655–66.

59. Hoyles RK, Ellis RW, Wellsbury J, et al. A multicenter, prospective, randomized, double-blind, placebo-controlled trial of corticosteroids and intravenous cyclophosphamide followed by oral azathioprine for the treatment of pulmonary fibrosis in scleroderma. Arthritis Rheum. 2006;54(12):3962–70.

60. Corte TJ, Ellis R, Renzoni EA, et al. Use of intravenous cyclophosphamide in known or suspected, advanced non-specific interstitial pneumonia. Sarcoidosis Vasc Diffuse Lung Dis. 2009;26(2):132–8.

61. Baughman RP, Lower EE. Use of intermittent, intravenous cyclophosphamide for idiopathic pulmonary fibrosis. Chest. 1992;102(4):1090–4.

62. Haubitz M, Schellong S, Gobel U, et al. Intravenous pulse administration of cyclophosphamide versus daily oral treatment in patients with antineutrophil cytoplasmic antibody-associated vasculitis and renal involvement: a prospective, randomized study. Arthritis Rheum. 1998;41(10):1835–44.

63. Adu D, Pall A, Luqmani RA, et al. Controlled trial of pulse versus continuous prednisolone and cyclophosphamide in the treatment of systemic vasculitis. QJM. 1997;90(6):401–9.

64. Martin-Suarez I, D'Cruz D, Mansoor M, et al. Immunosuppressive treatment in severe connective tissue diseases: effects of low dose intravenous cyclophosphamide. Ann Rheum Dis. 1997;56(8):481–7.

65. de Groot K, Adu D, Savage CO. The value of pulse cyclophosphamide in ANCA-associated vasculitis: meta-analysis and critical review. Nephrol Dial Transplant. 2001;16(10):2018–27.

66. Talar-Williams C, Hijazi YM, Walther MM, et al. Cyclophosphamide-induced cystitis and bladder cancer in patients with Wegener granulomatosis. Ann Intern Med. 1996;124:477–84.

67. Martin F, Lauwerys B, Lefebvre C, et al. Side-effects of intravenous cyclophosphamide pulse therapy. Lupus. 1997;6(3):254–7.

68. Janssen NM, Genta MS. The effects of immunosuppressive and anti-inflammatory medications on fertility, pregnancy, and lactation. Arch Intern Med. 2000;160(5):610–9.

69. Ramsey-Goldman R, Schilling E. Immunosuppressive drug use during pregnancy. Rheum Dis Clin North Am. 1997;23(1):149–67.

70. Lower EE, Blau R, Gazder P, et al. The risk of premature menopause induced by chemotherapy for early breast cancer. J Womens Health Gend Based Med. 1999;8(7):949–54.

71. Elizur SE, Chian RC, Pineau CA, et al. Fertility preservation treatment for young women with autoimmune diseases facing treatment with gonadotoxic agents. Rheumatology (Oxford). 2008;47(10):1506–9.

72. Dorr FA, Coltman Jr CA. Second cancers following antineoplastic therapy. Curr Probl Cancer. 1985;9(2):1–43.

73. Baltzan M, Mehta S, Kirkham TH, et al. Randomized trial of prolonged chloroquine therapy in advanced pulmonary sarcoidosis. Am J Respir Crit Care Med. 1999;160(1):192–7.

74. Furst DE. Pharmacokinetics of hydroxychloroquine and chloroquine during treatment of rheumatic diseases. Lupus. 1996;5 Suppl 1:S11–5.

75. Elder M, Rahman AM, McLay J. Early paracentral visual field loss in patients taking hydroxychloroquine. Arch Ophthalmol. 2006;124(12):1729–33.

76. Leecharoen S, Wangkaew S, Louthrenoo W. Ocular side effects of chloroquine in patients with rheumatoid

arthritis, systemic lupus erythematosus and sclero-derma. J Med Assoc Thai. 2007;90(1):52–8.

77. Jones SK. Ocular toxicity and hydroxychloroquine: guidelines for screening. Br J Dermatol. 1999; 140: 3–7.

78. Levy RA, Vilela VS, Cataldo MJ, et al. Hydroxychloroquine (HCQ) in lupus pregnancy: double-blind and placebo-controlled study. Lupus. 2001;10(6):401–4.

79. Motta M, Tincani A, Faden D, et al. Follow-up of infants exposed to hydroxychloroquine given to mothers during pregnancy and lactation. J Perinatol. 2005;25(2):86–9.

80. Renault F, Flores-Guevara R, Renaud C, et al. Visual neurophysiological dysfunction in infants exposed to hydroxychloroquine in utero. Acta Paediatr. 2009;98(9):1500–3.

81. Tavares JL, Wangoo A, Dilworth P, et al. Thalidomide reduces tumour necrosis factor-alpha production by human alveolar macrophages. Respir Med. 1997;91(1):31–9.

82. Ye Q, Chen B, Tong Z, et al. Thalidomide reduces IL-18, IL-8 and TNF-alpha release from alveolar macrophages in interstitial lung disease. Eur Respir J. 2006;28(4):824–31.

83. Oliver SJ, Kikuchi T, Krueger JG, et al. Thalidomide induces granuloma differentiation in sarcoid skin lesions associated with disease improvement. Clin Immunol. 2002;102(3):225–36.

84. Baughman RP, Judson MA, Teirstein AS, et al. Thalidomide for chronic sarcoidosis. Chest. 2002;122:227–32.

85. Nguyen YT, Dupuy A, Cordoliani F, et al. Treatment of cutaneous sarcoidosis with thalidomide. J Am Acad Dermatol. 2004;50(2):235–41.

86. Ghobrial IM, Rajkumar SV. Management of thalido-mide toxicity. J Support Oncol. 2003;1(3):194–205.

87. Horton MR, Danoff SK, Lechtzin N. Thalidomide inhibits the intractable cough of idiopathic pulmonary fibrosis. Thorax. 2008;63(8):749.

88. Tilluckdharry L, Dean R, Farver C, et al. Thalidomide-related eosinophilic pneumonia: a case report and brief literature review. Cases J. 2008;1(1):143.

89. Buttin BM, Moore MJ. Thalidomide-induced reversible interstitial pneumonitis in a patient with recurrent ovarian cancer. Gynecol Oncol. 2008;111(3):546–8.

90. Younis TH, Alam A, Paplham P, et al. Reversible pulmonary hypertension and thalidomide therapy for multiple myeloma. Br J Haematol. 2003;121(1): 191–2.

91. Baz R, Li L, Kottke-Marchant K, et al. The role of aspirin in the prevention of thrombotic complications of thalidomide and anthracycline-based chemotherapy for multiple myeloma. Mayo Clin Proc. 2005;80(12):1568–74.

92. Gartlehner G, Hansen RA, Jonas BL, et al. The comparative efficacy and safety of biologics for the treatment of rheumatoid arthritis: a systematic review and metaanalysis. J Rheumatol. 2006;33(12):2398–408.

93. Baughman RP, Drent M, Kavuru M, et al. Infliximab therapy in patients with chronic sarcoidosis and pulmonary involvement. Am J Respir Crit Care Med. 2006;174(7):795–802.

94. Utz JP, Limper AH, Kalra S, et al. Etanercept for the treatment of stage II and III progressive pulmonary sarcoidosis. Chest. 2003;124(1):177–85.

95. Baughman RP. Tumor necrosis factor inhibition in treating sarcoidosis: the American experience. Revista Portuguesa de Pneumonologia. 2007;13:S47–50.

96. Raghu G, Fatenejad S, McDermott L. Efficacy and safety of etanercept in patients with idiopathic pulmonary fibrosis (IPF). Eur Respir J. 2006;28:767s.

97. Pham T, Claudepierre P, Deprez X, et al. Anti-TNF alpha therapy and safety monitoring. Clinical tool guide elaborated by the Club Rhumatismes et Inflammations (CRI), section of the French Society of Rheumatology (Societe Francaise de Rhumatologie, SFR). Joint Bone Spine. 2005;72 Suppl 1:S1–58.

98. Saag KG, Teng GG, Patkar NM, et al. American College of Rheumatology 2008 recommendations for the use of nonbiologic and biologic disease-modifying antirheumatic drugs in rheumatoid arthritis. Arthritis Rheum. 2008;59(6):762–84.

99. Smith CH, Anstey AV, Barker JN, et al. British Association of Dermatologists' guidelines for biologic interventions for psoriasis 2009. Br J Dermatol. 2009;161(5):987–1019.

100. Keane J, Gershon S, Wise RP, et al. Tuberculosis associated with infliximab, a tumor necrosis factor-alpha neutralizing agent. N Engl J Med. 2001;345:1098–104.

101. Wallis RS, Broder MS, Wong JY, et al. Granulomatous infectious diseases associated with tumor necrosis factor antagonists. Clin Infect Dis. 2004;38(9):1261–5.

102. Gomez-Reino JJ, Carmona L, Angel DM. Risk of tuberculosis in patients treated with tumor necrosis factor antagonists due to incomplete prevention of reactivation of latent infection. Arthritis Rheum. 2007;57(5):756–61.

103. Matulis G, Juni P, Villiger PM, et al. Detection of latent tuberculosis in immunosuppressed patients with autoimmune diseases performance of a mycobacterium tuberculosis antigen specific IFN-gamma assay. Ann Rheum Dis. 2008;67(1):84–90.

104. Dixon WG, Hyrich KL, Watson KD, et al. Drug-specific risk of tuberculosis in patients with rheumatoid arthritis treated with anti-TNF therapy: results from the British Society for Rheumatology Biologics Register (BSRBR). Ann Rheum Dis. 2010;69(3):522–8.

105. Nathan DM, Angus PW, Gibson PR. Hepatitis B and C virus infections and anti-tumor necrosis factor-alpha therapy: guidelines for clinical approach. J Gastroenterol Hepatol. 2006;21(9):1366–71.

106. Li S, Kaur PP, Chan V, et al. Use of tumor necrosis factor-alpha (TNF-alpha) antagonists infliximab, etanercept, and adalimumab in patients with concurrent rheumatoid arthritis and hepatitis B or hepatitis C: a retrospective record review of 11 patients. Clin Rheumatol. 2009;28(7):787–91.

107. Huang W, Cordoro KM, Taylor SL, et al. To test or not to test? An evidence-based assessment of the value of screening and monitoring tests when using systemic biologic agents to treat psoriasis. J Am Acad Dermatol. 2008;58(6):970–7.

108. Furst DE. The Risk of Infections with Biologic Therapies for Rheumatoid Arthritis. Semin Arthritis Rheum. 2010;39(5):327–46.

109. Komano Y, Harigai M, Koike R, et al. Pneumocystis jiroveci pneumonia in patients with rheumatoid arthritis treated with infliximab: a retrospective review and case-control study of 21 patients. Arthritis Rheum. 2009;61(3):305–12.

110. Tubach F, Ravaud P, Salmon-Ceron D, et al. Emergence of Legionella pneumophila pneumonia in patients receiving tumor necrosis factor-alpha antagonists. Clin Infect Dis. 2006;43(10):e95–100.

111. Kapetanovic MC, Larsson L, Truedsson L, et al. Predictors of infusion reactions during infliximab treatment in patients with arthritis. Arthritis Res Ther. 2006;8(4):R131.

112. Ramos-Casals M, Brito-Zeron P, Munoz S, et al. Autoimmune diseases induced by TNF-targeted therapies: analysis of 233 cases. Medicine (Baltimore). 2007;86(4):242–51.

113. Taki H, Kawagishi Y, Shinoda K, et al. Interstitial pneumonitis associated with infliximab therapy without methotrexate treatment. Rheumatol Int. 2009;30(2):275–6.

114. Daien CI, Monnier A, Claudepierre P, et al. Sarcoid-like granulomatosis in patients treated with tumor necrosis factor blockers: 10 cases. Rheumatology (Oxford). 2009;48(8):883–6.

115. Feldman AM, Combes A, Wagner D, et al. The role of tumor necrosis factor in the pathophysiology of heart failure. J Am Coll Cardiol. 2000;35(3):537–44.

116. Mann DL, McMurray JJ, Packer M, et al. Targeted anticytokine therapy in patients with chronic heart failure: results of the Randomized Etanercept Worldwide Evaluation (RENEWAL). Circulation. 2004;109(13):1594–602.

117. Chung ES, Packer M, Lo KH, et al. Randomized, double-blind, placebo-controlled, pilot trial of infliximab, a chimeric monoclonal antibody to tumor necrosis factor-alpha, in patients with moderate-to-severe heart failure: results of the anti-TNF Therapy Against Congestive Heart Failure (ATTACH) trial. Circulation. 2003;107(25):3133–40.

118. Anker SD, Coats AJ. How to RECOVER from RENAISSANCE? The significance of the results of RECOVER, RENAISSANCE, RENEWAL and ATTACH. Int J Cardiol. 2002;86(2–3):123–30.

119. Rennard SI, Fogarty C, Kelsen S, et al. The Safety and Efficacy of Infliximab in Moderate-To-Severe Chronic Obstructive Pulmonary Disease. Am J Respir Crit Care Med. 2007;175(9):926–34.

120. Wegener's Granulomatosis Etanercept Trial (WGET) Research Group. Etanercept plus standard therapy for Wegener's granulomatosis. N Engl J Med. 2005; 352(4):351–61.

121. Hansen RA, Gartlehner G, Powell GE, et al. Serious adverse events with infliximab: analysis of spontaneously reported adverse events. Clin Gastroenterol Hepatol. 2007;5(6):729–35.

122. Wolfe F, Michaud K. The effect of methotrexate and anti-tumor necrosis factor therapy on the risk of lymphoma in rheumatoid arthritis in 19,562 patients during 89,710 person-years of observation. Arthritis Rheum. 2007;56(5):1433–9.

123. Mohan N, Edwards ET, Cupps TR, et al. Demyelination occurring during anti-tumor necrosis factor alpha therapy for inflammatory arthritides. Arthritis Rheum. 2001;44(12):2862–9.

124. Fleischmann R, Baumgartner SW, Weisman MH, et al. Long term safety of etanercept in elderly subjects with rheumatic diseases. Ann Rheum Dis. 2006;65(3):379–84.

125. Lozeron P, Denier C, Lacroix C, et al. Long-term course of demyelinating neuropathies occurring during tumor necrosis factor-alpha-blocker therapy. Arch Neurol. 2009;66(4):490–7.

126. Katz JM, Bruno MK, Winterkorn JM, et al. The pathogenesis and treatment of optic disc swelling in neurosarcoidosis: a unique therapeutic response to infliximab. Arch Neurol. 2003;60(3):426–30.

127. Baughman RP, Bradley DA, Lower EE. Infliximab for chronic ocular inflammation. Int J Clin Pharmacol Ther. 2005;43:7–11.

128. El Mourabet M, El Hashem S, Harrison JR, et al. Anti-TNF antibody therapy for inflammatory bowel disease during pregnancy: a clinical review. Curr Drug Targets. 2010;11(2):234–41.

129. Berthelot JM, De Bandt M, Goupille P, et al. Exposition to anti-TNF drugs during pregnancy: outcome of 15 cases and review of the literature. Joint Bone Spine. 2009;76(1):28–34.

130. Carter JD, Ladhani A, Ricca LR, et al. A safety assessment of tumor necrosis factor antagonists during pregnancy: a review of the Food and Drug Administration database. J Rheumatol. 2009;36 (3): 635–41.

131. Kane S, Ford J, Cohen R, et al. Absence of infliximab in infants and breast milk from nursing mothers receiving therapy for Crohn's disease before and after delivery. J Clin Gastroenterol. 2009;43(7):613–6.

132. McLaughlin P. Rituximab: perspective on single agent experience, and future directions in combination trials. Crit Rev Oncol Hematol. 2001;40(1):3–16.

133. Keogh KA, Ytterberg SR, Fervenza FC, et al. Rituximab for refractory Wegener's granulomatosis: report of a prospective, open-label pilot trial. Am J Respir Crit Care Med. 2006;173(2):180–7.

134. Gottenberg JE, Guillevin L, Lambotte O, et al. Tolerance and short term efficacy of rituximab in 43 patients with systemic autoimmune diseases. Ann Rheum Dis. 2005;64(6):913–20.

135. Leroux G, Costedoat-Chalumeau N, Brihaye B, et al. Treatment of relapsing polychondritis with rituximab: a retrospective study of nine patients. Arthritis Rheum. 2009;61(5):577–82.

136. Dillman RO. Infusion reactions associated with the therapeutic use of monoclonal antibodies in the treatment of malignancy. Cancer Metastasis Rev. 1999;18(4):465–71.

137. Walewski J, Kraszewska E, Mioduszewska O, et al. Rituximab (Mabthera, Rituxan) in patients with recurrent indolent lymphoma: evaluation of safety and efficacy in a multicenter study. Med Oncol. 2001;18(2):141–8.

138. Byrd JC, Waselenko JK, Maneatis TJ, et al. Rituximab therapy in hematologic malignancy patients with circulating blood tumor cells: association with increased infusion-related side effects and rapid blood tumor clearance. J Clin Oncol. 1999; 17(3):791–5.

139. Fleischmann RM. Safety of biologic therapy in rheumatoid arthritis and other autoimmune diseases: focus on rituximab. Semin Arthritis Rheum. 2009;38(4):265–80.

140. Schwartzberg LS, Stepanski EJ, Fortner BV, et al. Retrospective chart review of severe infusion reactions with rituximab, cetuximab, and bevacizumab in community oncology practices: assessment of clinical consequences. Support Care Cancer. 2008;16(4):393–8.

141. Kimby E. Tolerability and safety of rituximab (MabThera). Cancer Treat Rev. 2005;31(6):456–73.

142. Sehn LH, Donaldson J, Filewich A, et al. Rapid infusion rituximab in combination with corticosteroid-containing chemotherapy or as maintenance therapy is well tolerated and can safely be delivered in the community setting. Blood. 2007;109(10): 4171–3.

143. Tuthill M, Crook T, Corbet T, et al. Rapid infusion of rituximab over 60 min. Eur J Haematol. 2009;82(4): 322–5.

144. Aksoy S, Dizdar O, Hayran M, et al. Infectious complications of rituximab in patients with lymphoma during maintenance therapy: a systematic review and meta-analysis. Leuk Lymphoma. 2009;50(3): 357–65.

145. Burr ML, Malaviya AP, Gaston JH, et al. Rituximab in rheumatoid arthritis following anti-TNF-associated tuberculosis. Rheumatology (Oxford). 2008;47(5):738–9.

146. Aksoy S, Harputluoglu H, Kilickap S, et al. Rituximab-related viral infections in lymphoma patients. Leuk Lymphoma. 2007;48(7):1307–12.

147. Carson KR, Evens AM, Richey EA, et al. Progressive multifocal leukoencephalopathy after rituximab therapy in HIV-negative patients: a report of 57 cases from the Research on Adverse Drug Events and Reports project. Blood. 2009;113(20):4834–40.

148. Fleischmann RM. Progressive multifocal leukoencephalopathy following rituximab treatment in a patient with rheumatoid arthritis. Arthritis Rheum. 2009;60(11):3225–8.

149. Major EO, Amemiya K, Tornatore CS, et al. Pathogenesis and molecular biology of progressive multifocal leukoencephalopathy, the JC virus-induced demyelinating disease of the human brain. Clin Microbiol Rev. 1992;5(1):49–73.

150. Baldo P, Cecco S, Giacomin E, et al. mTOR pathway and mTOR inhibitors as agents for cancer therapy. Curr Cancer Drug Targets. 2008;8(8):647–65.

151. Bissler JJ, McCormack FX, Young LR, et al. Sirolimus for angiomyolipoma in tuberous sclerosis complex or lymphangioleiomyomatosis. N Engl J Med. 2008;358(2):140–51.

152. Stenton SB, Partovi N, Ensom MH. Sirolimus: the evidence for clinical pharmacokinetic monitoring. Clin Pharmacokinet. 2005;44(8):769–86.

153. Rangan GK, Nguyen T, Mainra R, et al. Therapeutic role of sirolimus in non-transplant kidney disease. Pharmacol Ther. 2009;123(2):187–206.

154. Morelon E, Stern M, Israel-Biet D, et al. Characteristics of sirolimus-associated interstitial pneumonitis in renal transplant patients. Transplantation. 2001;72(5):787–90.

155. Garrean S, Massad MG, Tshibaka M, et al. Sirolimus-associated interstitial pneumonitis in solid organ transplant recipients. Clin Transplant. 2005;19(5):698–703.

156. Khalife WI, Kogoj P, Kar B. Sirolimus-induced alveolar hemorrhage. J Heart Lung Transplant. 2007;26(6):652–7.

157. Nocera A, Andorno E, Tagliamacco A, et al. Sirolimus therapy in liver transplant patients: an initial experience at a single center. Transplant Proc. 2008;40(6):1950–2.

158. Taniguchi H, Ebina M, Kondoh Y, et al. Pirfenidone in idiopathic pulmonary fibrosis. Eur Respir J. 2010;36(3):695–6.

159. Raghu G, Johnson WC, Lockhart D, et al. Treatment of idiopathic pulmonary fibrosis with a new antifibrotic agent, pirfenidone: results of a prospective, open-label Phase II study. Am J Respir Crit Care Med. 1999;159(4 Pt 1):1061–9.

160. Azuma A, Nukiwa T, Tsuboi E, et al. Double-blind, placebo-controlled trial of pirfenidone in patients with idiopathic pulmonary fibrosis. Am J Respir Crit Care Med. 2005;171(9):1040–7.

161. Noble PW, Albera C, Bradford WZ, et al. Pirfenidone in patients with idiopathic pulmonary fibrosis (CAPACITY): two randomised trials. Lancet. 2011;377(9779):1760–9.

162. Oku H, Shimizu T, Kawabata T, et al. Antifibrotic action of pirfenidone and prednisolone: different effects on pulmonary cytokines and growth factors in bleomycin-induced murine pulmonary fibrosis. Eur J Pharmacol. 2008;590(1–3):400–8.

163. Spond J, Case N, Chapman RW, et al. Inhibition of experimental acute pulmonary inflammation by pirfenidone. Pulm Pharmacol Ther. 2003;16(4): 207–14.

164. Rubino CM, Bhavnani SM, Ambrose PG, et al. Effect of food and antacids on the pharmacokinetics of pirfenidone in older healthy adults. Pulm Pharmacol Ther. 2009;22(4):279–85.

Pulmonary Hypertension in Interstitial Lung Disease

Oksana A. Shlobin and Steven D. Nathan

Abstract

Pulmonary hypertension (PH) may complicate the course of many forms of interstitial lung disease (ILD) and has been shown to portend a worse outcome. The etiology of PH is likely multifactorial and might differ among the diseases with variable contributions of many potential factors. Whether the impact of PH and thereby the course of the disease can be modified by therapy requires further study.

This chapter provides an overview of the prevalence, epidemiology, pathophysiology, diagnosis, and clinical implications of PH in ILD. The potential role of therapy is discussed and a review of current treatment trials is provided.

Keywords

Pulmonary hypertension • Interstitial lung disease • Idiopathic pulmonary fibrosis • Scleroderma • Sarcoidosis

Case 1

A 47-year-old man with sarcoidosis and moderate restrictive disease presents with worsening dyspnea on exertion (DOE) over the prior 8 weeks, associated with bilateral lower extremity swelling. He has been maintained on a stable dose of methotrexate 12.5 mg weekly and prednisone 7 mg daily. His steroids were increased for 6 weeks and subsequently tapered by his primary care physician since no improvement was noted. An echocardiogram was obtained which revealed a new finding of severe tricuspid regurgitation (TR) with an estimated elevated right ventricular systolic pressure (RVSP) of 75 mmHg.

On examination, the presence of jugular venous distention to 6 cm is noted, as is the presence of a right-sided heave, a loud pulmonic component to the second heart sound (P_2) and significant bilateral lower extremity edema. A 6-min walk test (6MWT) is performed during which the patient ambulates on room air (RA) for a distance of 290 m with desaturation to 78% from a baseline of 92%. The patient is started on oxygen and furosemide at 40 mg daily.

O.A. Shlobin, MD, FCCP (✉) • S.D. Nathan, MD, FCCP
Advanced Lung Disease and Transplant Program,
Inova Fairfax Hospital, Falls Church, VA, USA
e-mail: oksana.shlobin@inova.org

R.P. Baughman and R.M. du Bois (eds.), *Diffuse Lung Disease: A Practical Approach*,
DOI 10.1007/978-1-4419-9771-5_8, © Springer Science+Business Media, LLC 2012

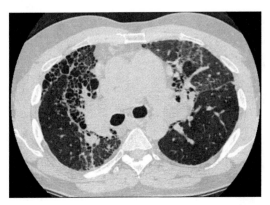

Fig. 8.1 Sarcoidosis patient with radiographic stage IV disease and moderate pulmonary hypertension (mPAP= 44 mmHg)

CAT angiography of the chest and venous Dopplers are negative for thromboembolism (Fig. 8.1). Pulmonary function tests (PFTs) show stable restrictive physiology with a stable moderate reduction in the diffusing capacity.

Right heart catheterization (RHC) demonstrates a right atrial (RA) pressure of 15 mmHg, a pulmonary artery pressure (PAP) of 69/25 mmHg with a mean pulmonary artery pressure (mPAP) of 44 mmHg, a pulmonary capillary wedge pressure (PCWP) of 8 mmHg, and a cardiac output (CO) of 3.5 L/min. Spironolactone is added to the diuretic regime and sildenafil 20 mg three times a day is started with subjective improvement. The sildenafil is titrated over a 6 months' period to 60 mg three times a day, but further dose escalation is limited by the advent of headaches. A transplant workup is initiated with repeat RHC revealing a RA pressure of 8 mmHg, a PAP of 60/21 mmHg (mPAP 37 mmHg), a PCWP of 5 mmHg, and a CO of 3.8 L/min. Bosentan is added and the patient's symptoms improve further with an increase in the 6MWT distance to 410 m with a RA saturation (SpO$_2$) nadir of 87%. A repeat RHC 1 year after bosentan is initiated reveals a RA of 6 mmHg, a PAP of 45/20 mmHg (mPAP 29), a PCWP of 5 mmHg, and an increase in the CO to 4.3 L/min. The patient is maintained on the current treatment regimen and listing for lung transplantation is deferred.

Case 2

A 59-year-old female with idiopathic pulmonary fibrosis (IPF) presents with increasing DOE. She has been on therapy with N-acetyl cysteine (NAC) since her initial diagnosis 2 years previously. Three months prior to presentation, she had a 6MWT distance of 408 m with desaturation from 97 to 92% on RA with a maximal Borg score of 2.

The patient had stable New York Heart Association (NYHA) Class II symptoms until 6 weeks prior when she noted progression in her DOE despite participation in a Pulmonary Rehabilitation program. She now gets short of breath and has to stop after walking up one flight of stairs. Physical examination is significant for bibasilar Velcro crackles, a loud P$_2$, clubbing, and trace lower extremity edema. PFTs reveal moderate restriction with a decrease in her forced vital capacity (FVC) from 65 to 58% of predicted over a 6-month period and a diffusing capacity that has decreased from 52 to 34% of predicted. A CAT scan of the chest with IV contrast shows stable interstitial disease with <10% honeycombing, no ground-glass opacities and no evidence of pulmonary emboli (Fig. 8.2). Echocardiography reveals both left ventricular (LV) size and function to be normal, but a RVSP that is estimated at 60 mmHg. A repeat 6MWT reveals a reduced

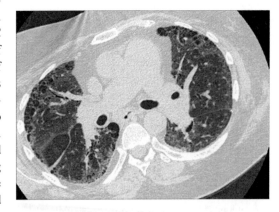

Fig. 8.2 IPF with mild pulmonary hypertension (mPAP= 32 mmHg)

distance of 320 m with her RA SpO_2 declining from 95% at rest to 85% at 6 min with a Borg score of 6. RHC demonstrates a RA pressure of 10 mmHg, a PAP of 50/14 mmHg with an mPAP of 32 mmHg, a PCWP of 13 mmHg, and a CO of 4.2 L/min. Left heart catheterization shows no coronary artery disease. Obstructive sleep apnea (OSA) is ruled out, but significant nocturnal desaturation is demonstrated with >10% of her sleep time spent with a $SpO_2 < 88\%$ and a SpO_2 nadir of 78%.

The patient is placed on furosemide 20 mg daily, sildenafil 20 mg three times a day, and oxygen with exercise and sleep. Despite these measures, over the following 6-month period, the patient demonstrated worsening in her symptoms and progressive restrictive physiology with increasing O_2 requirements. A workup for lung transplantation is completed and she is placed on the transplant list. Two months later, she undergoes a successful left single lung transplant. Noteworthy at the time of transplant, were her RHC hemodynamics which revealed a PAP 75/32 mmHg and an mPAP of 45 mmHg.

Introduction

The interstitial lung diseases (ILDs) comprise a diverse group of diseases characterized radiographically by the presence of diffuse increased interstitial lung markings. The ILDs may be idiopathic or secondary to a known cause and tend to run a variable course with an unpredictable response to therapy. They share common physiologic characteristics of restrictive physiology and impaired gas exchange. Pathological features are often similar with varying degrees of inflammation, and fibrosis and in some diseases, granuloma formation. If unresponsive to therapy, they usually progress to an advanced stage characterized by extensive scarring, which tends to be resistant to most available medical therapies [1, 2].

Since the microscopic pulmonary vessels reside within the interstitial spaces, the underlying pathologic process that characterizes most ILDs may affect the pulmonary vasculature [3].

This may manifest physiologically with elevated pulmonary pressures, and pulmonary hypertension (PH) may ensue once the mPAP exceeds the commonly accepted definition of ≥25 mmHg [4]. This may occur at various stages of the primary disease with the onset of PH often resulting in increased symptoms of shortness of breath, fatigue, and exercise limitation. As symptoms of concurrent PH tend to be similar to the primary disease presentation, the diagnosis may be missed until signs and symptoms of right-sided heart failure develop [5]. However, the onset of PH in the context of ILD does portend a worse prognosis and therefore many of these patients will succumb before they develop signs of right heart failure.

PH due to most ILDs falls into the World Health Organization (WHO) Group 3 classification of PH, last revised in 2008 [6]. The notable exceptions are sarcoidosis and pulmonary Langerhans cell histiocytosis (PLCH), which are included in the "miscellaneous" WHO Group 5 category. This categorization is based on the multiple different potential etiologic mechanisms that might be involved in these diseases. There are now seven Federal Drug Administration (FDA)-approved medications for patients with WHO Group 1 pulmonary arterial hypertension (PAH), with an ongoing growing body of data supporting their utility in this disease [6]. Whether these therapies are appropriate and safe for patients with PH due to the various ILDs remains to be answered.

This chapter provides an overview of our current state of knowledge of PH complicating the various ILDs including the prevalence, pathogenesis, diagnosis, and prognosis, specifically in IPF, sarcoidosis, PLCH, lymphangioleiomyomatosis (LAM), and connective tissue disease-related ILD. A foundation and possible rationale for therapy directed at PH in these conditions is provided, while potential drawbacks of such an approach are also underscored. The need to validate these therapies through prospective, randomized, placebo-controlled studies is therefore necessary before such therapy can be recommended routinely.

Epidemiology

Fibrotic obliteration of the normal architecture of the interstitial space and its associated vascular components may result in PH as a complication of many forms of advanced ILD. Indeed, historically the development of cor pulmonale was an expected sequela of many forms of advanced lung disease [7]. Although, this association is well documented, the prevalence of PH has not been well characterized with a wide reported range amongst the various ILDs. The reasons for this include the variability in the definition of PH associated with ILD, as well as the timing and modes of diagnosis during the course of these diseases.

The highest prevalence and severity of PH appears to be in PLCH, a smoking-related ILD characterized by proliferation and infiltration of the lungs by Langerhans cells, with the overall incidence of PH varying from 92 to 100%, and that of severe PH from 72.5 to 100% [8, 9]. Although PH seems to be more severe in advanced forms of PLCH, it can occur at any stage with a noted lack of correlation between the mPAP and spirometric indices [10, 11].

IPF is the most common of the idiopathic interstitial pneumonias. In a retrospective analysis of IPF patients awaiting transplantation, PH was evident on RHC in 31.6% of the subjects [12]. Nadrous et al. described PH in 84% of IPF patients based on echocardiographic estimates of the systolic pulmonary arterial pressures (sPAPs) [13]. Data from the United Network for Organ Sharing (UNOS) demonstrated that 45% of patients with IPF listed for transplant have RHC evidence of PH, with 9% of these patients having an mPAP above 40 mmHg [14]. Among physiologic parameters, the diffusion capacity and need for supplemental oxygen have been found to correlate inversely with the mPAP. However, there is a lack of degree of correlation with other PFT indices, including the FVC, that has been reported in several studies [12, 13, 15].

In patients with scleroderma (SSc), it can be very difficult to assess whether PH is due to the associated ILD or due to their propensity to develop a primary vasculopathy. In a registry-based cohort of patients with SSc, PAH was present in 12% of the subjects [16]. An echocardiogram-based study documented isolated PH in 19.2% and combined ILD/PH in 18.2% of patients with SSc [17]. SSc patients with both PH and ILD have worse outcomes than patients with either of these complications alone. In this regard, a recent RHC-based study reported a 3-year survival of 47% for isolated SSc-PAH, and 28% for ILD-associated SSc-PAH [18]. Similar to IPF, there is no close correlation between the severity of the restrictive ventilatory defect and the presence and severity of PH [19]. A clue to the presence of PH in the context of SSc is a low diffusion capacity for carbon monoxide ($DL_{CO}\%$), especially when this is disproportionately reduced in relation to the FVC%. Indeed, a high FVC%/$DL_{CO}\%$ ratio has been shown to be a useful predictor for the presence PH in this patient population [20].

The prevalence of PH and sarcoidosis has been evaluated in several studies. In a prospective echocardiographic study of a general sarcoidosis population, only 5.7% of 212 patients had PH based on an estimated RVSP >40 mmHg [21]. However, in a cohort of 363 patients with advanced sarcoidosis awaiting lung transplantation, 74% had PH documented on RHC [22]. This was associated with greater supplemental oxygen requirements and an increased risk of mortality while on the waiting list [23]. Spirometric indices have an uncertain relationship to the presence of PH in sarcoidosis with studies reporting both a lack of correlation and an association with lower spirometric indices and a reduced diffusing capacity [22–24].

LAM is a condition that is characterized by smooth muscle proliferation around the lymphatics, bronchioles, and blood vessels. Because of its vasculocentric propensity, a higher prevalence of PH might be anticipated. However, in this regard resting PH has been found to be relatively rare in this condition, although a rise in PAP at low exercise levels occurs frequently, in part related to exercise-induced hypoxemia [25].

Pathophysiology

PH is the physiologic consequence of a diverse group of clinicopathologic entities that affect the pulmonary vascular resistance (PVR). The WHO stratification (Table 8.1) of these disease processes categorizes PH due to the various ILDs in either group III or group V [6]. Much of what is known about PH in ILD is extrapolated from our understanding of idiopathic PAH (IPAH) and the pathologic arteriopathy found in this disease. However, while there are likely common etiologic mechanisms, the pathophysiologic processes that contribute to PH in ILD are undoubtedly more complex. There is probably a certain commonality of these factors amongst the various ILDs, while others may be unique to the specific pathologic process. Possible shared contributory factors include regional hypoxemic vasoconstriction, vascular remodeling, direct vascular involvement of the pulmonary vessels, in situ thrombosis (thrombotic angiopathy), a deranged cytokine milieu and destruction of the vascular bed by ongoing interstitial inflammation and fibrosis (Fig. 8.3) [26–29].

Other factors contributing to the development of PH may be unique to the individual ILDs, such as local compression of pulmonary arteries by hilar lymph nodes in sarcoidosis (Fig. 8.4) or pulmonary veno-occlusive disease (PVOD), which has been described in both sarcoidosis and IPF [28]. PVOD-like lesions in these conditions have emerged as a potential mechanism contributing to the development of PH and its presence may potentially contraindicate PH therapies [26, 30, 31]. Further unique mechanisms include a proliferative vasculopathy that contributes to the development of PH in PLCH and a granulomatous vasculopathy that has been described in sarcoidosis [8, 28]. Autoimmune processes, especially the presence of antiendothelial antibodies, have been implicated in the pathogenesis of PH associated with diffuse SSc and CREST syndrome [32].

Another unique aspect of the ILDs that may influence the development and severity of PH is the distribution of the primary disease, both on a macroscopic lung regional basis, as well as on a microscopic level related to the proximity and involvement of the bronchovascular bundles [2]. Fibrosis in proximity to the pulmonary arterial

Table 8.1 Current classification of pulmonary hypertension (Dana Point 2008); adapted from Simmoneau et al. [4]

World Health Organization clinical classification of pulmonary hypertension
Group I Pulmonary arterial hypertension (PAH)
Idiopathic (IPAH)
Heritable
BMPR2
ALK1, endoglin (with or without hereditary hemorrhagic telangiectasia)
Unknown
Drug and toxin induced
Associated with
Connective tissue disease
HIV infection
Portal hypertension
Congenital heart diseases
Schistosomiasis
Chronic hemolytic anemia
Persistent pulmonary hypertension of the newborn
Pulmonary veno-occlusive disease (PVOD) and/or pulmonary capillary haemangiomatosis (PCH)
Pulmonary hypertension owing to left heart diseases
Systolic dysfunction
Diastolic dysfunction
Valvular disease
Pulmonary hypertension owing to lung diseases and/or hypoxemia
Chronic obstructive pulmonary disease
Interstitial lung disease
Other pulmonary diseases with mixed restrictive and obstructive pattern
Sleep disordered breathing
Alveolar hypoventilation syndrome
Chronic exposure to high altitude
Developmental abnormalities
Chronic thromboembolic pulmonary hypertension (CTEPH)
Pulmonary hypertension with unclear multifactorial mechanisms
Hematologic disorders: myeloproliferative disorders, splenectomy
Systemic disorders: sarcoidosis, pulmonary Langerhans cell histiocytosis: lymphangioleiomyomatosis, neurofibromatosis, vasculitis
Metabolic disorders: glycogen storage disease, Gaucher disease, thyroid disorders
Others: tumoral obstruction, fibrosing mediastinitis, chronic renal failure on dialysis

ALK1 activin receptor-like kinase type 1, *BMPR2* bone morphogenetic protein receptor type 1, *HIV* human immunodeficiency virus

circulation may also adversely affect the capacitance of the vessels. It has been demonstrated in PAH that a low vascular capacitance portends a

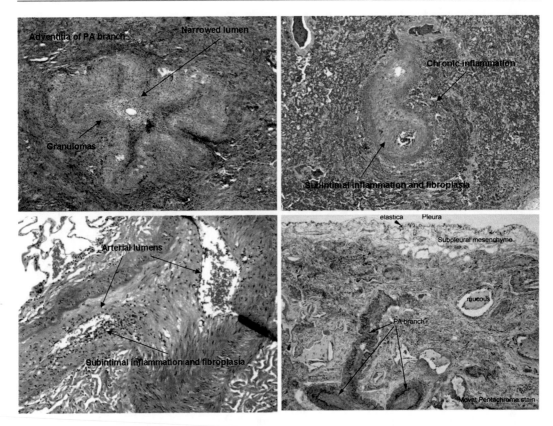

Fig. 8.3 Examples of the pathology of pulmonary hypertension in various interstitial lung diseases

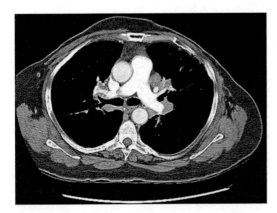

Fig. 8.4 Right pulmonary artery compression by hilar lymph nodes of sarcoidosis

worse prognosis [33]. If the same holds true for the PH of ILD, this might help explain the profound mortality implications of even mild elevations in PA pressures complicating these diseases.

On a cellular level, the role of pulmonary endothelial dysfunction has been emphasized in many studies. One mediator that may play a significant role in relation to the endothelium is endothelin-1. This is an endothelium-secreted vasoconstrictor that acts as a mitogen of pulmonary vascular smooth muscle cells and an inducer of extracellular matrix formation resulting in fibrosis. Endothelin-1 is stimulated by hypoxia and elevated circulating levels have been described in ILD patients with PH [34, 35]. Mediators that are known to be important in the genesis of PAH are also upregulated in some of the ILDs. For example, platelet-derived growth factor and transforming growth factor (TGF)-beta are upregulated in both PAH and IPF. Therefore, there might be a "spill over" effect of these mediators on the pulmonary vasculature.

An appreciation for the potential role of comorbid conditions contributing to the development of

PH in ILD is important, since most of these require further diagnostic testing and different therapeutic approaches. Diastolic dysfunction has been described in about 15–28% of patients with IPF, SSc, and sarcoidosis [36–38]. Pulmonary embolism (PE) may contribute to elevated PAPs in IPF, as a thrombotic predisposition has been described in this condition [39]. Interestingly, PE has been described as the cause of death in 3.4% of patients with IPF, and IPF lung transplant recipients are noted to be more prone to PE than other lung recipients [40, 41]. Possible mechanisms for this include elevated factor VIII levels or the presence of antiphospholipid antibodies [39]. Concomitant emphysema has been described in ~28% of IPF patients [42]. Patients with concomitant IPF and COPD exhibit a higher mortality, which is at least partially attributed to the development of severe PH. Finally, sleep disordered breathing also appears to have a greater propensity in these patients [43].

In summary, it appears that the factors contributing to the development of PH in ILD are complex and interrelated. Why some ILD patients might be more predisposed to the development of PH is unknown. Whether there are specific triggers or a genetic predisposition for PH also remains to be defined, as does the time course and progression of its development.

Diagnosis of PH in ILD

There are no current guidelines on whether, when, or how to screen for PH in patients with ILD. Therefore, this remains an individualized clinical decision based on each patient's unique circumstance. Standard physical examination findings of elevated right heart pressures might include an elevated jugular venous pressure, a parasternal heave, a pronounced P_2, and the murmur of TR [7]. However, these are usually only seen with more severe PH and may not be easy to discern in patients with mild or even moderate PH in the context of ILD. As the development of PH in patients with ILD has clear mortality implications, screening for this appears prudent.

Serum biomarkers and components of pulmonary function testing have been evaluated as predictors of PH in ILD. Brain natriuretic peptide (BNP) appears to have very good performance characteristics in predicting the presence of PH and discerning prognosis in chronic lung disease and IPF specifically [44]. However, further studies across the spectrum of ILD patients are needed to confirm the diagnostic and prognostic value of this biomarker.

PFTs have been examined in their ability to predict the development of PH in various ILDs. The single breath DL_{CO} and supplemental oxygen requirements have been found to be independent predictors of PH in IPF [12]. Exercise limitation, specifically a short 6MWT distance and a lower oxygen saturation nadir are also more common in those IPF patients with complicating PH. A reduced DL_{CO} and hypoxia have also been shown to be associated with PH in sarcoidosis [28]. Similarly, a reduced DL_{CO} appears to be the best single predictor for the development of PH in SSc. For those SSc patients with a component of pulmonary fibrosis, the $FVC\%/DL_{CO}\%$ predicted ratio has been shown to be useful in predicting the presence of PH [45]. However, this ratio has not been shown to have the same capability in patients with IPF and whether it is predictive for the presence of PH in other forms of ILD will require further study [36].

CAT scanning of the chest has not as yet proven to be a useful screening tool for PH in ILD. Neither the measurement of the main pulmonary artery (PA) segment in relation to the aorta, nor the extent of parenchymal changes in IPF patients correlates with the presence or severity of PH [46]. Whether or not measurement of the PA diameter might be useful in conditions associated with higher PA pressures, such as sarcoidosis or PLCH remains to be determined.

Echocardiography is the most commonly used tool in screening for presence of PH [47]. Measurement of the tricuspid regurgitant jet velocity with two-dimensional echocardiography allows for the estimation of the sPAP, which is synonymous with the RVSP. However, these estimates may frequently be inaccurate, especially in patients with advanced lung disease [48, 49].

In a cohort of 374 lung transplant candidates, echocardiography resulted in estimates of the RVSP in only 44% of the patients [49]. In this same cohort, 52% of patients had an estimated sPAP > 10 mmHg different than the pressure measured directly by RHC. Additionally, 48% were incorrectly estimated to have PH. The diagnostic accuracy of echocardiography may be enhanced if it is used in parallel with other indicators of PH, including the $DL_{CO}\%$, the resting SpO_2, exercise SpO_2 nadir, and BNP levels [44]. In summary, echocardiography can aid in the identification of suspected PH in ILD, but should not be solely relied upon in most circumstances for the definitive diagnosis.

Catheterization of the right heart with direct measurement of the PAPs and the PCWP remains the gold standard for the diagnosis of PH [50]. The diagnostic criteria for PH as recognized by the American College of Chest Physicians is a mPAP greater than or equal to 25 mmHg, with a PCWP less than or equal to 15 mmHg, both measured at rest by RHC [51]. Some recommend the routine practice of vasodilator testing in patients found to have PAH and in whom treatment is contemplated; however, the role of such testing in patients with ILD remains unproven and is not generally recommended outside a research setting. All current guidelines recommend the documentation of pulmonary pressures by RHC prior to the initiation of any vasoactive therapy [52].

Clinical Implications of PH in ILD

Most forms of ILD have limited effective therapeutic options. PH usually develops at a stage when the advancing parenchymal lung fibrosis is no longer responsive to therapy. Therefore, arresting or reversing the PH by treating the underlying parenchymal lung disease is usually not feasible. As the symptoms of PH are often indistinguishable from the findings of advancing ILD, the advent of PH may be subtle. Nevertheless, PH associated with ILD appears to have both significant morbidity and mortality implications. In both IPF and sarcoidosis, the presence of PH has been shown to be associated with greater

supplemental oxygen requirements, as well as a reduced functional capacity as assessed by the 6MWT.

The most ominous consequence of PH complicating ILD is its association with an increased mortality risk. In a registry of patients with limited SSc associated PAH, the 1, 2, and 3-year survival was 81%, 63%, and 56%, respectively. This registry included patients with pulmonary fibrosis on high-resolution computed tomography (HRCT) and compared these to patients with no fibrosis. There was no statistical difference in survival between those with or without fibrosis, implying that PH might be the main driver of outcomes, even in those with fibrosis [16]. In sarcoidosis patients awaiting lung transplantation, PH was demonstrated to be an independent predictor of mortality [23].

In IPF, numerous studies have consistently demonstrated the adverse prognostic implication of associated PH. In one such study, in which PH was diagnosed on RHC, the 1-year mortality was shown to be 5.5% in patients without PH as compared to 28% in those with PH [12]. Furthermore, there was a linear correlation between the mPAP and mortality. In a recent report examining the effect of severe PH (mPAP > 40 mmHg on RHC) in IPF patients listed for transplant, a 1 unit increase in the PVR was associated with a 22% greater hazard of death [53]. Although echocardiography allows only an estimate of the RVSP, it does appear to impart important prognostic information. In one study utilizing echocardiographic estimates of the RVSP, IPF patients were stratified into three groups based on the severity of their PH [13]. The median survival for those patients with a RVSP < 35 mmHg was 4.8 years, for those with a RVSP of 36–50 mmHg it was 4.1 years, while for those with a RVSP > 50 mmHg it was only 0.7 years [13]. The prognostic distinction of different levels of PH as estimated by echo has subsequently been validated in another study [44].

Since the clinical implications of PH in patients with ILD may be profound, therapy targeting the pulmonary vasculature in patients with associated PH appears attractive. However, whether PH in this setting is the primary driver of outcomes, or a surrogate for other events that drive mortality, remains uncertain. Therefore in ILD-associated PH, questions remain about the potential benefit, if any, of medications that are used to treat WHO Group 1 PAH.

Treatment

Once PH has been diagnosed, it is incumbent to rule out any comorbidities as causative or contributory, since therapies directed at these may impact and possibly reverse some or all of the PH. Entities to consider include OSA, congestive heart failure, concomitant COPD and in select case, where there is a high index of suspicion, PE [40–43, 54, 55].

Hypoxia should be actively sought and addressed. In this regard, relying on information from the resting pulse oximetry might not be sufficient. There is emerging data that this might not reflect the level of desaturation endured during the course of patients' activities of daily living or their level of nocturnal desaturation [56, 57]. Therefore, the 6MWT and nocturnal oximetry are important to detect exertional and nocturnal desaturation, respectively. In addition, postexercise recovery SpO_2 might also impart important information, as anecdotally patients can desaturate significantly after exercise has been halted. An explanation for this apparent "lag" is not readily apparent.

As the therapeutic armamentarium for WHO Group I PAH has increased, both in available agents and in the simplicity of their administration, the impetus to offer these therapies to patients with other forms of PH has also increased. In spite of this, the clear implications of treating PH beyond WHO Group 1 are not well understood. Therapies available for PH can be divided into the general treatment measures and vasoactive medications. General treatment measures include supplemental oxygen, diuretics where indicated, and therapies directed at other potential contributory comorbidities.

It makes intuitive sense that treating the underlying primary disease and reversing that process will impact on the associated PH. However, PH will have usually developed in those patients with more advanced and likely irreversible disease. Nonetheless, steroids have been reported to have potential utility in small subgroups of patients with sarcoidosis and PLCH in whom granulomatous vasculitis may be playing a role. Steroids are more likely to be of benefit in the absence of significant fibrotic changes [28, 58–61].

Digoxin is often considered for patients with PAH, but its role, if any, in other forms of PH has not been investigated and is therefore not generally recommended. Similarly, the role of anticoagulation has also not been established. In studies that support a mortality benefit for anticoagulation in IPAH, the lack of control for other variables creates difficulty in attributing the improved mortality to this therapy. There are no studies evaluating anticoagulation in ILD-related PH.

Patients with IPF, however, might be at increased risks of pulmonary emboli [40, 41]. In addition, there has been one study evaluating the role of anticoagulation in IPF demonstrating a potential mortality benefit [61]. However, the observed result might be related to a primary effect on the disease process rather than the prevention of thromboemboli [61]. At this time, the role of anticoagulant therapy for patients who have ILD and PH remains uncertain and needs to be assessed on a case-by-case basis with any potential benefit being weighed against the inherent risks.

Currently, there are seven medications FDA approved for the treatment of PAH, but none have been approved for non-WHO Group I PH (Table 8.2). Whereas there is a large body of evidence and regularly updated treatment guidelines for WHO Group I PAH, there is a paucity of data and virtually no high quality studies that have focused on other forms of PH [62].

There are a number of potential pitfalls with regards to the empiric adoption of these readily available therapies that require further consideration [52]. With any pulmonary vasodilator, there is a potential to worsen ventilation–perfusion mismatching by the reversal of regional hypoxic vasoconstriction. Moreover, PVOD lesions have been described in IPF, sarcoidosis, PLCH, and

Table 8.2 Current FDA-approved medications for the treatment of World Health Organization Group 1 pulmonary arterial hypertension

Agent	Class	Route	Recommended dose	FDA approval
Epoprostenol (Flolan)	Prostanoid	Intravenous, continuous infusion	Variable dosed in μg/kg/min	1995
Bosentan (Tracleer)	ERA	Oral	125 mg twice a day	2001
Treprostinil (Remodulin)	Prostanoid	Subcutaneous or intravenous continuous infusion; inhaled	Variable dosed in μg/kg/min	2002 (SQ) 2004 (IV) 2009 (IH)
Iloprost (Ventavis)	Prostanoid	Inhaled	5 μg 6–9 times a day	2004
Sildenafil (Revatio)	PDE5 inhibitor	Oral	20 mg three times a day	2005
Ambrisentan (Letairis)	ERA	Oral	5 or 10 mg daily	2007
Tadalafil (Adcirca)	PDE5 inhibitor	Oral	40 mg daily	2009

ERA endothelin receptor antagonist, *PDE5* inhibitor phosphodiesterase type 5 inhibitor

SSc [8, 29, 31]. As treatment with pulmonary arterial vasodilators has been reported to result in pulmonary edema in PH with concomitant PVOD [30, 31], their use in this condition is generally contraindicated.

Whether the PH itself imparts a poor prognosis, or if it is a surrogate for another upstream driver of outcomes, is unknown. It appears to make intuitive sense to abrogate a factor that has been shown to portend a worse prognosis and which impacts on patients' functional ability. However, at this point, whether therapy with medications approved for the treatment of PAH WHO Group I has any role in managing PH secondary to ILD, is a question that remains to be answered. The current literature describing outcomes of vasodilator therapy for PH in ILD is confined mostly to small series and case reports in IPF and sarcoidosis (Table 8.3).

The largest prospective study of PH in IPF was the "ACTIVE" study, which examined the effects of inhaled iloprost in a double-blind randomized trial of 51 IPF patients with presumed PH based on echocardiography [63]. Despite being preceded by a small pilot study that suggested benefit, this trial was negative and thus far has only been reported in abstract form [63, 64]. Indeed if anything, there was a trend to a greater decrement in the 6MWT distance in the active treatment arm as compared to the placebo group. These two sequential studies serve notice to the overinterpretation of small pilot series.

Sildenafil has been reported to be useful in IPF patients with PH in several small series with improvements demonstrated in the 6MWT distance [65, 66]. A recently published prospective randomized placebo-controlled trial undertaken by the National Institute of Health and sponsored IPFnetwork (STEP study) enrolled 180 IPF patients with DLCO <35% predicted and thus a high probability of concurrent PH. Although the primary endpoint based on a 20% or more increase in the 6MWT distance was not met, there were significant differences in a number of secondary endpoints including arterial oxygenation, degree of dyspnea and quality of life measurements. There was also a trend towards a mortality benefit, thus creating clinical equipoise for further research [67].

Bosentan, a dual endothelin receptor antagonist, has also been evaluated as an antifibrotic agent for IPF in the BUILD-3 study. This study also failed to meet its primary endpoint of delay in disease progression defined as either a decrease from baseline in the FVC of 10% and DLCO of 15%, acute exacerbation of IPF, or death [68]. In a small subset of patients from the ARIES-3 study of ambrisentan, a selective endothelin receptor A blocker, there did appear to be the suggestion of a salutary response in the subgroup of patients with ILD [69]. However, the subsequent prospective, randomized ARTEMIS-PH trial was stopped early based on an interim analysis of the parallel ARTEMIS-IPF study which demonstrated futility and potential harm in patients with IPF [70].

Table 8.3 Case series and treatment trials of pulmonary hypertension associated with interstitial lung disease

Type of lung disease	Investigator	Type of study	Patients	Therapy	Outcome
Sarcoid	Preston [71]	Prospective observational	8	Inhaled NO, IV epoprostenol, Ca channel blockers	Short-term decrease in PVR, mPAP; increase in 6MWT
Sarcoid	Fisher [72]	Case series	8	IV epoprostenol	Improved NYHA/WHO Class
Sarcoid	Barnett [74]	Case series	22	IV epoprostenol, inhaled iloprost, bosentan, sildenafil	Improved 6MWT, NYHA/WHO Class
Sarcoid	Millman [75]	Retrospective chart review	24	Sildenafil	Reduction in MPAP, PVR. Increase in cardiac output
Sarcoid, scleroderma, SLE, CTEPH	Sharma [76]	Case series	6	Bosentan	Improved 6MWT, decrease in NYHA Class
IPF, CTD, Sarcoid	Minai [73]	Case series	19	IV epoprostenol, bosentan	Short-term improvement in NYHA Class and 6MWT
IPF	Krowka [63]	Randomized, blinded, placebo controlled prospective trial	51	Inhaled iloprost	No improvement in 6MWT, NYHA Class
IPF	Collard [66]	Open label prospective trial	14	Sildenafil	57% had significant increase in 6MWT
Lung fibrosis	Ghofrani [65]	Randomized, controlled open label trial	16	Sildenafil, iNO, epoprostenol	Sildenafil improved pulmonary hemodynamics and gas exchange

NO nitric oxide, *PVR* pulmonary vascular resistance, *6MWT* 6-min walk test, *NYHA* New York Heart Association, *WHO* World Health Organization, *mPAP* mean pulmonary artery pressure, *CTDs* connective tissue diseases, *IPF* idiopathic pulmonary fibrosis

Inhaled and parenteral prostanoids have been reported to improve the 6MWT distance and WHO functional class in PH associated with sarcoidosis in several small restrospective reviews, but a prospective study has not as yet been published [71–74]. Sildenafil has also been reported to improve the 6MWT distance and hemodynamics in retrospective studies of sarcoidosis-associated PH, but similarly, there are no large, ongoing prospective trials to study this further [74, 75]. Bosentan has also been reported to result in functional and hemodynamic improvement in sarcoidosis-associated PH in retrospective studies [73, 74, 76, 77].

In summary, despite these small pilot series and case reports, the management of ILD-PH with PAH medications cannot routinely be recommended until the appropriate prospective double-blind placebo-controlled studies have confirmed their benefit [62].

Transplantation

The decision about transplantation for lung disease hinges on anticipated improvements in quality of life and the likelihood of mortality with and without the procedure. Patients with ILD and PH appear to have worse projected outcomes than those without PH [12, 13, 23, 53]. Thus, a prompt referral to transplant centers for appropriate candidates with ILD and PH is imperative [78]. The transplant procedure itself can be complicated by the need for cardiopulmonary bypass due to the underlying PH and the associated difficulty of maintaining these patients on single lung ventilation during the surgery. It remains controversial if these patients are better served with a single or bilateral lung transplant, but either can certainly suffice.

Patients with ILD and PH have outcomes that are similar to those without PH, although their initial postoperative course might be more challenging. There tends to be a higher incidence of primary graft dysfunction in those with PH, but the incidence of acute rejection and other posttransplant complications is no different in those ILD patients with or without PH. The PH of ILD tends to resolve

after transplantation, but can recur in the context of chronic allograft dysfunction [79].

Summary

PH frequently complicates advanced ILD and is associated with functional impairment and a worse prognosis. The pathogenesis of PH in the various ILDs is complex and multifactorial. Whether PH in the context of ILD is simply a marker of advanced parenchymal lung destruction and therefore a surrogate for poor outcomes, or if there is a primary potentially treatable vasculopathic component to these various diseases, remains to be determined. Clinical awareness of the development of PH in patients with ILD should prompt referral to a lung transplant center for an evaluation in patients in whom no transplant contraindications exist. Additionally, referral of patients with ILD-PH to specialized centers for potential enrollment in clinical studies might offer patients the most appropriate access to therapy and thereby aid in our understanding of this complex issue. Current and future trials will hopefully define the efficacy, safety, and appropriate candidates for these medications with regards to this potential expanded indication.

References

1. American Thoracic Society, European Respiratory Society. Thoracic Society/European Respiratory Society international multidisciplinary consensus classification of the idiopathic interstitial pneumonias. General principles and recommendations. Am J Respir Crit Care Med. 2002;165:277–304.
2. Thannickal VJ, Toews GB, White ES, Lynch III JP, Martinez FJ. Mechanisms of pulmonary fibrosis. Annu Rev Med. 2004;55:395–417.
3. Strange C, Highland K. Pulmonary hypertension in ILD. Curr Opin Pulm Med. 2005;11:452–5.
4. Simmoneau G, Robins IM, Beghetti M, et al. Updated clinical classification of pulmonary hypertension. J Am Coll Cardiol. 2009;54(1 Suppl):S43–S54.
5. Shapiro S. Management of pulmonary hypertension resulting from interstitial lung disease. Curr Opin Pulm Med. 2003;9:426–30.

6. McLaughlin VV, Archer SL, Badesch DB, et al. ACCF/AHA 2009 Expert Consensus Document on Pulmonary Hypertension: A Report of the American College of Cardiology Foundation Task Force on Expert Consensus Documents and the American Heart Association developed in collaboration with the American College of Chest Physicians; American Thoracic Society, Inc.; and the Pulmonary Hypertension Association. J Am Coll Cardiol. 2009;53(17): 1573–619.

7. Chronic Cor Pulmonale. Report of an expert committee. Circulation. 1963;27(4):594–615.

8. Fartoukh M, Humbert M, Capron F, et al. Severe pulmonary hypertension in histiocytosis X. Am J Respir Crit Care Med. 2000;161:216–23.

9. Dauriat G. Lung transplantation for pulmonary Langerhans' cell histiocytosis: a multicenter analysis. Transplantation. 2006;81(5):746–50.

10. Chaowalit N, Pellikka PA, Decker PA, et al. Echocardiographic and clinical characteristics of pulmonary hypertension complicating pulmonary Langerhans cell histiocytosis. Mayo Clin Proc. 2004;79(10):1269–75.

11. Harari S, Brenot F, Barberis M, Simmoneau G. Advanced pulmonary histiocytosis X is associated with severe pulmonary hypertension. Chest. 1997; 111(4):1142–4.

12. Lettieri C, Nathan SD, Barnett S, Ahmad S, Shorr AF. Prevalence and outcomes of pulmonary arterial hypertension in advanced idiopathic pulmonary fibrosis. Chest. 2006;129:746–52.

13. Nadrous HF, Pellikka PA, Krowka MJ, et al. Pulmonary hypertension in patients with idiopathic pulmonary fibrosis. Chest. 2005;128:2393–9.

14. Shorr AF, Wainright JL, Cors CS, Lettieri CJ, Nathan SD. Pulmonary hypertension in patients with pulmonary fibrosis awaiting lung transplant. Eur Respir J. 2007;30(4):715–21.

15. Nathan SD, Ahmad S, Shlobin OA, Barnett SD. Correlation of PFT with PAH in patients with IPF [abstract]. Proc Am Thorac Soc. 2006;3:A103.

16. Mukerjee D, St George D, Coleiro B, et al. Prevalence and outcome in systemic sclerosis associated pulmonary arterial hypertension: application of a registry approach. Ann Rheum Dis. 2003;62:1088–93.

17. Chang B, Wigley FM, White B, Wise RA. Scleroderma patients with combined pulmonary hypertension and interstitial lung disease. J Rheumatol. 2003;30: 2398–405.

18. Condliffe R, Kiely DG, Peacock AJ, et al. Connective tissue disease-associated pulmonary arterial hypertension in the modern treatment era. Am J Respir Crit Care Med. 2009;179:151–7.

19. Trad S, Amoura Z, Beigelman C, et al. PAH is a major mortality factor in diffuse systemic sclerosis, independent of interstitial lung disease. Arthritis Rheum. 2006;54:184–91.

20. Steen V, Medsger Jr TA. Predictors of isolated pulmonary hypertension in patients with systemic sclerosis and limited cutaneous involvement. Arthritis Rheum. 2003;48(2):516–22.

21. Handa T, Nagai S, Miki S, et al. Incidence of pulmonary hypertension and its clinical relevance in patients with sarcoidosis. Chest. 2006;129:1246–52.

22. Shorr AF, Helman DL, Davies DB, Nathan SD. Pulmonary hypertension in advanced sarcoidosis: epidemiology and clinical characteristics. Eur Respir J. 2005;25:783–8.

23. Shorr AF, Davies DB, Nathan SD. Predicting mortality in patients with sarcoidosis awaiting lung transplantation. Chest. 2003;124:922–8.

24. Sulica R, Teirstein AS, Kakarla S, Nemani N, Behnegar A, Padilla ML. Distinctive clinical, radiographic, and functional characteristics of patients with sarcoidosis-related pulmonary hypertension. Chest. 2005;128:1483–9.

25. Taveira-DaSilva AM, Hathaway OM, Sachdev V, Shizukuda Y, Birdsall CW, Moss J. Pulmonary artery pressure in lymphangioleiomyomatosis: an echocardiographic study. Chest. 2007;132(5):1573–8.

26. Portier F, Lerebours-Pigeonniere G, Thiberville L, et al. Sarcoidosis simulating pulmonary veno-occlusive disease. Rev Mal Respir. 1991;8(1):101–2.

27. Morgan JM, Griffiths M, du Bois RM, Evans TW. Hypoxic pulmonary vasoconstriction in systemic sclerosis and primary pulmonary hypertension. Chest. 1991;99:551–6.

28. Nunes H, Humbert M, Capron F, et al. Pulmonary hypertension associated with sarcoidosis: mechanisms, haemodynamics and prognosis. Thorax. 2006; 61:68–74.

29. Colombat M, Mal H, Groussard O, et al. Pulmonary vascular lesions in end-stage idiopathic pulmonary fibrosis: histopathologic study on lung explant specimens and correlations with pulmonary hemodynamics. Hum Pathol. 2007;38(1):60–5.

30. Palmer SM, Robinson LJ, Wang A, Gossage JR, Bashore T, Tapson VF. Massive pulmonary edema and death after prostacyclin infusion in a patient with pulmonary veno-occlusive disease. Chest. 1998;113: 237–40.

31. Farber HW, Graven KK, Kokolski G, Korn JH. Pulmonary edema during acute infusion of epoprostenol in a patient with pulmonary hypertension and limited scleroderma. J Rheumatol. 1999;26: 1195–6.

32. Fagan KA, Badesch DB. Pulmonary hypertension associated with connective tissue disease. Prog Cardiovasc Dis. 2002;45:225–34.

33. Mahapatra S, Nishimura RA, Sorajja P, Cha S, McGoon MD. Relationship of pulmonary arterial capacitance and mortality in idiopathic pulmonary arterial hypertension. J Am Coll Cardiol. 2006;47(4): 799–803.

34. Yamakami T, Taguchi O, Gabazza EC, et al. Arterial endothelin-1 level in pulmonary emphysema and interstitial lung disease: relation with pulmonary HTN during exercise. Eur Respir J. 1997;10:2055–60.

35. MacLean MR. Endothelin-1 and serotonin: mediators of primary and secondary pulmonary hypertension? J Lab Clin Med. 1999;134:105–14.
36. Nathan SD, Shlobin OA, Ahmad S, Urbanek S, Barnett SD. Pulmonary hypertension and pulmonary function testing in idiopathic pulmonary fibrosis. Chest. 2007;131:657–63.
37. Galie N, Manes A, Farahani KV, et al. PAH associated with CTDs. Lupus. 2005;14:713–7.
38. Fahy GJ, Marwick T, McCreery CJ, Quigley PJ, Maurer BJ. Doppler echocardiographic detection of left ventricular diastolic dysfunction in patients with pulmonary sarcoidosis. Chest. 1996;109:62–6.
39. Magro CM, Allen J, Pope-Harman A, et al. The role of microvascular injury in the evolution of idiopathic pulmonary fibrosis. Am J Clin Pathol. 2003; 119:556–67.
40. Panos R. Clinical deterioration in patients with idiopathic pulmonary fibrosis: causes and assessment. Am J Med. 1990;88(4):396–404.
41. Nathan SD, Barnett SD, Urban BA, Nowalk C, Moran BR, Burton N. Pulmonary embolism in idiopathic pulmonary fibrosis transplant recipients. Chest. 2003; 123:1758–63.
42. Mejía M, Carrillo G, Rojas-Serrano J, et al. Idiopathic pulmonary fibrosis and emphysema: decreased survival associated with severe pulmonary arterial hypertension. Chest. 2009;136(1):10–5.
43. Perez-Padilla R, West P, Lertzman M, Kryger MH. Breathing during sleep in patients with interstitial lung disease. Am Rev Respir Dis. 1985;132:224–9.
44. Song JW, Song JK, Kim DS. Echocardiography and brain natriuretic peptide as prognostic indicators in idiopathic pulmonary fibrosis. Respir Med. 2009;103: 180–6.
45. Steen V. Predictors of end stage lung disease in systemic sclerosis. Ann Rheum Dis. 2003;62:97–9.
46. Zisman DA, Karlamangla AS, Ross DJ, et al. High resolution CT findings do not predict the presence of pulmonary hypertension in advanced idiopathic pulmonary fibrosis. Chest. 2007;132:773–9.
47. Yock P. Noninvasive estimation of the right ventricular systolic pressure by Doppler ultrasound in patients with tricuspid regurgitation. Circulation. 1984;70(4): 657–62.
48. Fisher MR, Forfia PR, Chamera E, et al. Accuracy of Doppler echocardiography in the hemodynamic assessment of pulmonary hypertension. Am J Respir Crit Care Med. 2009;179(7):615–21.
49. Arcasoy S, Chrstie J, Ferrari V, et al. Echocardiographic assessment of pulmonary hypertension in patients with advanced lung disease. Am J Respir Crit Care Med. 2003;167:735–40.
50. Barst RJ, McGoon M, Torbicki A, et al. Diagnosis and differential assessment of pulmonary arterial hypertension. J Am Coll Cardiol. 2004;43:40S–7.
51. Badesch DB, Abman SH, Simonneau G, et al. Medical therapy for pulmonary arterial hypertension: updated ACCP evidence-based clinical practice guidelines. Chest. 2007;131:1917–28.
52. Hoeper MM, Barbera JA, Channick RN, et al. Diagnosis, assessment, and treatment of non-pulmonary arterial hypertension pulmonary hypertension. J Am Coll Cardiol. 2009;54:S85–96.
53. Minai OA, Santucruz JF, Thuita L, et al. Severe pulmonary hypertension in IPF: characteristics and implications (ISHLT 2009 abstract). J Heart Lung Transplant. 2009;28(2S):S109.
54. Bye PTP, Issa F, Berthon-Jones M, Sullivan CE. Studies of oxygenation during sleep in patients with interstitial lung disease. Am Rev Respir Dis. 1984;129: 27–32.
55. Papadopoulis CE, Pitsiou G, Karamitsos TD, et al. Left ventricular diastolic dysfunction in IPF: a tissue Doppler ECG study. Eur Respir J. 2008;31:701–6.
56. Corte TJ, Talbot S, Wort SJ, et al. Nocturnal desaturation is associated with pulmonary hypertension in patients with mild to moderate interstitial lung disease. Am J Respir Crit Care Med. 2009;179:A4057 (abstract).
57. Shitrit D, Rusanov V, Peled N, Amital A, Fuks L, Kramer MR. The 15-step oximetry test: a reliable tool to identify candidates for lung transplantation among patients with idiopathic pulmonary fibrosis. J Heart Lung Transplant. 2009;28:328–33.
58. Benyuones B, Crestani B, Couvelard A, Vissuzaine C, Aubter M. Steroid-responsive pulmonary hypertension in a patient with Langerhans' cell granulomatosis (histiocytosis X). Chest. 1996;110:284–6.
59. Rodman DM, Lindenfeld J. Successful treatment of sarcoidosis-associated pulmonary hypertension with corticosteroids. Chest. 1990;97:500–2.
60. Gluskowski J, Hawrylkiewicz I, Zych D, Zielinski J. Effects of corticosteroid treatment on pulmonary haemodynamics in patients with sarcoidosis. Eur Respir J. 1990;3:403–7.
61. Kubo H, Nakayama K, Yanai M, et al. Anticoagulant therapy for idiopathic pulmonary fibrosis. Chest. 2005;128:1475–82.
62. Barst RJ, Gibbs JS, Ghofrani HA, et al. Updated evidence-based treatment algorithm in pulmonary arterial hypertension. J Am Coll Cardiol. 2009;54(1):78–84. Suppl S.
63. Krowka MJ, Ahmad S, Andrade JA, et al. A randomized, double-blind, placebo-controlled study to evaluate the safety and efficacy of iloprost inhalation in adults with abnormal pulmonary arterial pressure and exercise limitation associated with idiopathic pulmonary fibrosis. Chest. 2007;132:633S (abstract).
64. Olschewski H, Ghofrani HA, Walmrath D, et al. Inhaled prostacyclin and iloprost in severe pulmonary hypertension secondary to lung fibrosis. Am J Respir Crit Care Med. 1999;160:600–7.
65. Ghofrani HA, Wiedemann R, Rose F, et al. Sildenafil for treatment of lung fibrosis and pulmonary hypertension: a randomised controlled trial. Lancet. 2002;360(9337):895–900.
66. Collard HR, Anstrom KJ, Schwarz MI, Zisman DA. Sildenafil improves walk distance in idiopathic pulmonary fibrosis. Chest. 2007;131:897–9.

67. The Idiopathic Pulmonary Fibrosis Clinical Research Network. A Controlled Trial of Sildenafil in Advanced Idiopathic Pulmonary Fibrosis. *N Engl J Med.* 2010; 363:620–628.
68. King Jr. TE, Brown KK, Raghu G, et al. BUILD-3: A Randomized, Controlled Trial of Bosentan in Idiopathic Pulmonary Fibrosis. Amer Jour Respir Crit Care Med. 2011;184:92–99.
69. Badesch DB, Feldman J, Keogh A, et al. ARIES-3: ambrisentan therapy in a diverse population of patients with pulmonary hypertension. *Am J Respir Crit Care Med.* 2009;179:A3357 (abstract).
70. http://clinicaltrials.gov/ct2/show/NCT00879229.
71. Preston IR, Klinger JR, Landzberg MJ, Houtchens J, Nelson D, Hill NS. Vasoresponsiveness of sarcoidosis-associated pulmonary hypertension. Chest. 2001;120: 866–72.
72. Fisher KA, Serlin DM, Wilson KC, Walter RE, Berman JS, Farber HW. Sarcoidosis-associated pulmonary hypertension: outcome with long-term epoprostenol treatment. Chest. 2006;130(5):1481–8.
73. Minai O, Sahoo D, Chapman J, Mehta AC. Vasoactive therapy can improve 6-min walk distance in patients with pulmonary hypertension and fibrotic interstitial lung disease. Respir Med. 2008;102(7): 1015–20.
74. Barnett CF, Bonura EJ, Nathan SD, et al. Treatment of sarcoidosis-associated pulmonary hypertension. A Two-center experience. Chest. 2009;135(6):1455–61.
75. Milman N, Burton CM, Iversen M, Videbaek R, Jensen CV, Carlsen J. Pulmonary hypertension in end-stage pulmonary sarcoidosis: therapeutic effect of sildenafil? J Heart Lung Transplant. 2008;27(3):329–34.
76. Sharma S, Kashour T, Philipp R. Secondary pulmonary arterial hypertension: treated with endothelin receptor blockade. Tex Heart Inst J. 2005;32(3):405–10.
77. Baughman RP, Engel PJ, Meyer CA, Barrett AB, Lower EE. Pulmonary hypertension in sarcoidosis. Sarcoidosis Vasc Diffuse Lung Dis. 2006;23: 108–16.
78. Behr J, Ryu JH. Pulmonary hypertension in interstitial lung disease. Eur Respir J. 2008;31:1357–67.
79. Nathan SD, Shlobin OA, Ahmad S, et al. Pulmonary hypertension in patients with bronchiolitis obliterans syndrome listed for retransplantation. Am J Transplant. 2008;8(7):1506–11.

Section II

Specific Diseases

Sarcoidosis

9

Daniel A. Culver and Marc A. Judson

Abstract

Sarcoidosis is a granulomatous syndrome with protean manifestations. Although sarcoidosis was initially described nearly 150 years ago, its etiopathogenesis remains elusive. Because sarcoidosis affects the lungs in approximately 95% of patients, pulmonologists are often called upon to manage this disease. However, since it is a systemic disease, it is essential to have an understanding of the spectrum of its extrapulmonary manifestations.

Despite many gaps in our current knowledge, there have been substantial advances in recent years regarding the diagnosis, approach to symptoms, and therapeutic options for patients with sarcoidosis. New technology such as ultrasound guided transbronchial needle aspiration has altered the approach to the diagnosis of sarcoidosis. There has been increased recognition of a spectrum of symptoms related to sarcoidosis, such as fatigue and dyspnea, which must be addressed to optimize outcomes. The development of biologic therapies and an expanded array of other steroid-sparing medications have generated new treatment options. In this chapter, we have summarized the current state of knowledge regarding the pathophysiology, diagnosis, treatment, and general clinical approach to patients with pulmonary and extrapulmonary sarcoidosis.

Keywords

Sarcoidosis • Granulomas • Extrapulmonary sarcoidosis • Endobronchial ultrasound • Steroid-sparing medications • TNF antagonists

D.A. Culver, DO (✉)
Respiratory Institute, Cleveland Clinic,
Cleveland, OH, USA
e-mail: CULVERD@ccf.org

M.A. Judson, MD
Division of Pulmonary and Critical Care,
Department of Medicine, Medical University
of South Carolina, Charleston, SC, USA

R.P. Baughman and R.M. du Bois (eds.), *Diffuse Lung Disease: A Practical Approach*,
DOI 10.1007/978-1-4419-9771-5_9, © Springer Science+Business Media, LLC 2012

Introduction

Sarcoidosis is an enigmatic disorder with protean manifestations, an undiscovered etiology, and extremely variable outcome. Since its first description by a British dermatologist, Jonathon Hutchinson, in 1869, the disease has provoked considerable interest among physicians of all specialties. However, since the lungs are involved in most cases, pulmonary physicians are often called upon to assess and manage the disease as whole.

Sarcoidosis is thought to occur when a genetically susceptible host encounters a causative antigen(s). The diagnosis of sarcoidosis depends on the identification of a constellation of clinical, radiologic, and pathologic findings, along with exclusion of similar-appearing granulomatous disorders. Since the natural history is extremely variable, decisions regarding treatment must be highly individualized.

Definition/Criteria for Diagnosis

Sarcoidosis has been defined as a multisystem granulomatous disease of unknown cause. This implies that the granulomatous inflammation must occur in more than one organ and that alternative causes of such inflammation have been excluded. Unfortunately, this definition is not air-tight. First, sarcoidosis is a diagnosis of exclusion and it is impossible to completely exclude the myriad of alternative causes of granulomatous inflammation. Second, on occasion a patient will develop a granulomatous disease where the cause is not identified but the clinical presentation is unusual for sarcoidosis. Examples of this would include granulomas that demonstrate significant necrosis on histology, or unilateral hilar adenopathy on a chest radiograph (CXR) in a patient who is a smoker, has a positive tuberculin skin test, or a history of a previous malignancy. For this reason, the American Thoracic Society/European Respiratory Society/World Association of Sarcoidosis and Other Granulomatous Disorders consensus statement on sarcoidosis requires that "the diagnosis is established when clinico-radiological findings" that

suggest sarcoidosis are present in addition to "evidence of noncaseating epithelioid cell granulomas" [1]. Third, although two or more organs involved with granulomatous inflammation are required to ensure a diagnosis of sarcoidosis, this requirement may be eliminated if the one organ is the lung. This must be done with extreme caution as isolated granulomatous diseases of the lung such as tuberculosis, fungal diseases, and hypersensitivity pneumonitis need to be reasonably excluded.

Obviously, sarcoidosis has a cause(s). A half century ago, chronic beryllium disease was diagnosed as sarcoidosis as the metal was not known to cause a granulomatous reaction. In the future, it is likely that other "sarcoidoses" of known cause will be identified that can be pared off from what is now diagnosed as sarcoidosis.

In the future, diagnosis of sarcoidosis will probably couple genetics with exposure. As more is understood about the immune response, it may be possible to identify individuals who mount a granulomatous response to specific exposures causing sarcoidosis. In this way, sarcoidosis may move from a disease of unknown cause to disease where the etiology is known.

However, at the present time the definition of sarcoidosis remains vague and its diagnosis is not absolute. Rather, the diagnosis is established when the clinical, radiographic, and histological findings are such that the statistical likelihood of an alternative cause is deemed minimal to the point that no further alternative diagnostic evaluations are warranted [2].

Immunopathogenesis and Pathology

Based on epidemiologic evidence, it is generally believed that development of sarcoidosis requires exposure to an environmental antigen(s). This hypothesis is supported by several observations, including epidemiologic studies of disease incidence, reports of case clusters in small populations, transmission by organ transplantation, and the worldwide reproducibility of intradermal granulomatous reactions only in sarcoidosis subjects

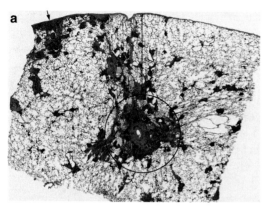

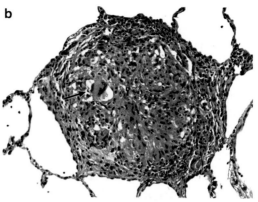

Fig. 9.1 Granulomas in sarcoidosis. The granulomas are typically distributed along the lymphatics (**a**), including the bronchovascular bundle (*circle*), the interlobular septa (*thick arrow*), and the subpleural area (*thin arrow*). This pattern accounts for the classic radiologic features as well as the excellent yield from transbronchial biopsy. The granulomas in sarcoidosis (**b**) are almost always nonnecrotizing, although some focal necrosis can occur in up to 10% of cases. *Arrow* denotes a Langerhan's-type multinucleate giant cell. Hematoxylin and eosin, ×20. Images courtesy of Carol Farver, MD

following injection of sarcoidosis lymph node homogenate (the Kveim–Siltzbach test) [1]. Molecular analyses, prolonged culture for organisms, and antimicrobial trials have all failed to reveal definite evidence for a microbial etiology, but emerging data suggest that mycobacterial proteins could be a contributor in some patients.

Genetic predisposition is assumed to play a major role in the development of sarcoidosis, based on the observations that race/ethnicity is a risk factor and that there is familial aggregation of disease risk. Much of the data suggest that the genetic effect on disease risk or severity is dependent on HLA genes governing the expression of the Type II major histocompatibility complex (MHC) on antigen-presenting cells. These observations fit well with the current concepts of disease pathogenesis, reserving a central role for activation of antigen-specific oligoclonal CD4+ T-cells by MHC Class II-restricted antigen-presenting cells, which then amplify immune mechanisms that lead to granuloma formation. A number of other genes, most commonly cytokines or chemokines, have been associated with sarcoidosis susceptibility or phenotype. However, lack of validation studies and difficulties with interpopulation genetic variability have limited progress in elucidating the genetic profiles in sarcoidosis. It is most likely that products of multiple

gene polymorphisms in combination inform susceptibility and phenotype. The responsible genes probably differ in various populations, and possibly depending on the responsible antigen as well.

Sarcoid inflammation is characterized by nonnecrotizing granulomas (Fig. 9.1), reviewed by Drs. Colby and Leslie in Chap. 4. The granuloma is a compact mass of cells that walls off foreign antigens, typically microbes. Epithelioid histiocytes, together with a few multinucleated giant cells comprise the core, surrounded by an outer margin of T-lymphocytes. The lymphocyte population is oligoclonal, with restricted T-cell receptor repertoires, consistent with an antigen-driven process. Inflammation in sarcoidosis is dependent on persistent stimulation by CD4+ T cells. A variable rim of collagen and fibroblasts surrounds the granuloma.

Most of the pathophysiologic research to present has focused on the inflammatory, or early, stages of sarcoidosis. Characterization of sarcoidosis inflammation in humans has consistently demonstrated a Th1-predominant cytokine profile, with important roles for interferon γ (IFN-γ), interleukin 12 (IL-12), IL-18, and tumor necrosis factor (TNF) [3]. IFN-γ, IL-12, and IL-18 are likely to be important in directing the development of the Th1 phenotype and may account for failure of feedback mechanisms to down-regulate immune activation. In accordance with this, IL-12 and IFN-γ knockout mice fail to develop granulomatous inflammation after challenge with granuloma-inducing agents [4]. Additionally, TNF is an essential mediator, directing monocyte proliferation and differentiation of macrophages into the epithelioid cells of granulomas. The immunology of long-standing and fibrotic sarcoidosis is less well understood.

Pulmonary Sarcoidosis

Sarcoidosis is evident in the lungs in 90–95% of patients at the time of diagnosis [1, 5]. Up to 50% of all patients with sarcoidosis exhibit pulmonary symptoms at the time of initial presentation [1]. Even when extrapulmonary manifestations dominate the clinical presentation, the lungs are usually involved. Despite the high frequency of lung involvement in sarcoidosis, presentation with pulmonary symptoms confers a delay in diagnosis, likely since the symptoms are nonspecific.

Symptoms and Signs

The most common presenting features of pulmonary sarcoidosis include dyspnea, cough, wheezing, and chest discomfort. The cough in sarcoidosis is commonly exacerbated by exposure to dusts, cold air, or other irritants, making differentiation from asthma difficult at times. The cause of the chest discomfort, which may be very severe, is unclear. It is typically described as substernal pressure or constriction in the mid-chest. Its presence does not correlate well with anatomic–radiologic features such as enlarged mediastinal lymph nodes [6]. Constitutional symptoms commonly accompany pulmonary sarcoidosis. In acute sarcoidosis, fevers, weight loss, and malaise may be prominent; later, fatigue or arthralgias are frequent complaints.

In uncomplicated pulmonary sarcoidosis, the chest exam is usually unremarkable. Clubbing or rales are distinctly unusual and should prompt consideration of alternative diagnoses. Wheezing

may indicate widespread airways involvement; however, the presence of focal wheezing should lead to consideration of large airways disease, including external constriction, focal bronchostenosis, or bronchiectasis. Flexible bronchoscopy is indicated to further evaluate the cause of focal wheezing. The examination should also include careful assessment for signs of complications, such as pulmonary hypertension, bronchiectasis, or fibrobullous disease.

Imaging Studies

The initial assessment of pulmonary sarcoidosis typically includes imaging studies and physiologic testing. The CXR is abnormal in 85–95% of patients with sarcoidosis [7]. When present, infiltrates have a predilection for the mid and upper lung zones. The most common parenchymal findings are reticulonodular infiltrates, but alveolar infiltrates, consolidation, perihilar conglomerate masses, and larger nodules may also be seen. The extent of reticulonodular infiltrates correlates most closely with the changes effected by treatment [8].

A popular CXR classification system, the Scadding scale, confers a loose sense of overall prognosis for resolution of sarcoidosis over the 5 years following the diagnosis (Fig. 9.2) [9]. The prognosis is influenced, however, by the presence of various other clinical features (see section "Prognosis," below). The Scadding stage does not describe the clinical activity of the disease. It is also important to recognize that the Scadding scale has not been validated for chest computed tomography (CT), does not describe sequential steps in the natural history of sarcoidosis, has not been validated in all populations, and is not directly correlated with the response to treatment. A recent report suggested that designation of Scadding stage by thoracic radiologists may be less straightforward than previously thought, with interobserver agreement only fair (weighted $\kappa = 0.43$) [8].

Although chest CT scanning confers advantages over CXR for diagnosis of sarcoidosis or detection of pulmonary complications, it is usually

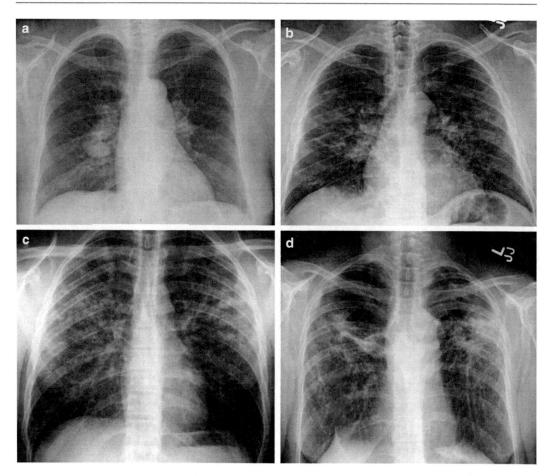

Fig. 9.2 Scadding scale. Chest radiograph (CXR) stages as proposed by Scadding [9]. Stage I disease (**a**), present in 40–67% of subjects, is characterized by bilateral hilar lymph node enlargement (*thick arrows*) with or without paratracheal adenopathy (*thin arrow*). Stage II (**b**), with parenchymal infiltrates and lymph node enlargement, occurs in 20–40% of patients. Stage III disease (**c**), defined as infiltrates without enlarged lymph nodes on the CXR, is found in 10–20% of subjects. Stage IV (**d**), which is apparent in 0–10% of patients at the time of diagnosis, implies the presence of fibrosis. Stage IV disease is most easily identified by the presence of bilateral upward hilar retraction. The prognosis for resolution of the radiologic findings after 5 years is 80–90% for stage I, 50–65% for stage II, and 20–30% for stage III

not necessary in uncomplicated cases. Characteristic features on chest CT include (Fig. 9.3): mediastinal or hilar adenopathy; micronodular infiltrates distributed along bronchovascular bundles or in a subpleural location; thickened fissures and interlobular septae, sometimes with "beading"; and bronchial wall thickening. Pulmonary fibrosis, bullae, mycetomas, bronchiectasis, and architectural distortion are seen more readily on CT than CXR. Chest CT may be indicated in the setting of atypical radiologic or clinical features (i.e., detection of mycetomas), to aid discrimination of fibrosis from reversible disease, to assist with planning diagnostic procedures (i.e., bronchoscopy), and in patients with a high degree of clinical suspicion for sarcoidosis but a normal CXR.

Pulmonary Function Tests

Baseline pulmonary function tests (PFTs) are recommended at the time of diagnosis (Table 9.1). The most reliable single test is the forced vital capacity (FVC), but the single-breath diffusing

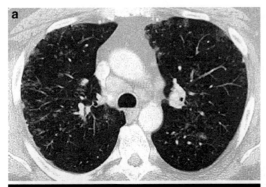

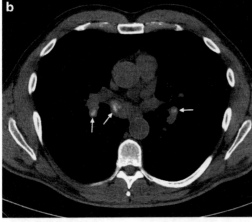

Fig. 9.3 Chest CT features in pulmonary sarcoidosis. Lung windows (**a**) demonstrating mid-lung zone predominant micronodules in a bronchovascular distribution. Much less commonly, the nodular infiltrates may predominate in a subpleural location. Mediastinal windows (**b**) usually reveal some lymph node enlargement, even when not apparent on chest radiograph. So-called frosting-type calcification in the lymph nodes is highly suggestive of sarcoidosis (*arrow*)

Table 9.1 Extent of workup for second organ involvement if a biopsy has revealed granulomatous inflammation consistent with sarcoidosis

- Chest radiograph
- Spirometry
- Liver function tests
- Complete blood count
- Ophthalmologic examination
- Electrocardiogram
- Serum calcium
- Urinalysis

capacity for carbon monoxide (DLCO) independently provides additional useful clinical information. Abnormal PFTs are found in approximately 20% of patients with Scadding stage I radiographs, whereas 40–80% of those with more advanced radiographic stages have abnormal values [7]. Although restrictive physiology is widely assumed to be typical for sarcoidosis, obstructive lung disease is seen as often. At the time of diagnosis, it is present in up to 63% of patients [10].

Along with pulmonary symptoms, serial pulmonary function testing provides the most useful information and is crucial for longitudinal management. Most investigators would consider a consistent change of at least 10% in FVC or 20% in DLCO to be clinically important [7]. It is essential, however, to recognize that PFT values correlate poorly with patient-reported outcomes such as quality of life.

Other Physiologic Tests

Other PFTs, such as cardiopulmonary exercise testing, 6-min walk tests (6MWTs), and respiratory muscle function testing are occasionally useful for the assessment of patients with unexplained dyspnea. Cardiopulmonary exercise testing may demonstrate progressively increasing dead space, dynamic hyperinflation, widening of the arterial-alveolar O_2 gradient, or evidence of excessive oxygen consumption relative to workload. The value of the information gained from addition of a 6MWT to routine clinical tests is unclear. The 6MWT does not delineate what factors are responsible for dyspnea or exercise limitation, and its routine use is probably best confined to clinical trials.

Dyspnea in Sarcoidosis

Dyspnea and impaired exercise tolerance caused by sarcoidosis are often multifactorial. Common diagnostic considerations in patients with dyspnea that is poorly explained after the initial evaluation but may be attributable to sarcoidosis include unrecognized cardiomyopathy or valvular disease, airflow obstruction (dynamic obstruction or large airways disease), anemia, respiratory muscle weakness, obesity related to corticosteroid use, depression, sarcoid involvement of joints or muscles, and sarcoidosis-associated pulmonary hypertension (SAPH). Recently data have suggested that pulmonary hypertension may be present in up to half of sarcoidosis patients with unexplained dyspnea [11]. Surface echocardiogram appears to be unreliable for diagnosing SAPH, which can be seen in any radiographic CXR stage [11].

Extrapulmonary Sarcoidosis

Although sarcoidosis most commonly affects the lung, in may involve any organ. Extrapulmonary manifestations of sarcoidosis may cause significant morbidity and have a major impact upon the patient's quality of life. In some circumstances, extrapulmonary sarcoidosis may cause potentially life-threatening complications. It is important to develop an understanding of the extrapulmonary manifestations of sarcoidosis so that they can be detected and appropriately treated. The clinical manifestations, diagnosis, and treatment of extrapulmonary sarcoidosis are beyond the scope of this text. The interested reader is referred to detailed reviews of this subject [12]. Rather, this section will focus on special nuances of sarcoidosis involvement in extrapulmonary organs in terms of the clinical presentation, diagnosis, and treatment.

Eye

Ocular sarcoidosis is very common, with frequencies of between 10 and 50% in American and European series, to as high as 89% in the Japanese [13]. Sarcoidosis may affect any part of the eye. All ocular inflammation from sarcoidosis requires treatment because it may lead to permanent visual impairment and blindness in 2–5% of cases [14].

Uveitis is the most common ocular manifestation of sarcoidosis [14]. Sarcoidosis most commonly causes an anterior uveitis that may result in symptoms of red eyes, painful eyes, or photophobia [13, 14]. However, one-third of patients with anterior uveitis from sarcoidosis present without ocular symptoms [13]. Therefore, all patients diagnosed with sarcoidosis require a slit lamp examination regardless of whether they have ocular symptoms [13].

Intermediate uveitis is defined as inflammation of the vitreous, pars plana, and peripheral retina. Patients may be asymptomatic or complain of blurred vision or floaters [13]. Posterior uveitis or inflammation of the retina is found in up to 28% of patients with ocular sarcoidosis [15]. This retinal involvement primarily affects the retinal veins. Posterior uveitis may result in significant vision impairment. Intermediate and posterior uveitis mandate a funduscopic examination for detection, and this test is therefore required in addition to a slit lamp examination for all patients diagnosed with sarcoidosis regardless of the presence of ocular symptoms.

Sarcoidosis involvement of the lacrimal gland is clinically apparent in 15–28% of sarcoidosis patients [14], and may cause a keratoconjunctivitis sicca syndrome. Optic neuritis from sarcoidosis is a rare but important manifestation because it may be vision threatening and occur suddenly. Any sarcoidosis patient who experiences sudden loss of vision or color vision requires immediate referral to an ophthalmologist and high-dose corticosteroid therapy if optic neuritis is confirmed.

The yield of granulomatous inflammation with transbronchial biopsy in patients with uveitis, suspected sarcoidosis, and a normal CXR has been shown to be greater than 60% [16]. However, a more recent study of Japanese patients with suspected sarcoid uveitis showed that the finding of parenchymal opacities on chest CT scanning was associated with a yield of 95% (19/20) on transbronchial lung biopsy (TBLB) versus 5% (1/20) when the lung parenchyma was normal [17]. The CXR and bronchoalveolar lavage (BAL) lymphocyte counts were not useful in predicting the yield of TBLB in these patients. Conjunctival biopsy has a reasonable yield (up to 67%) if conjunctival nodules are present [18]. It is controversial whether or not a blind biopsy of normal-appearing conjunctival tissue is of value with one study reporting a yield of 30% [18], while other studies suggest that such biopsies are fruitless. Lacrimal gland biopsies have a high diagnostic yield when there is uptake in the gland of ^{67}Ga on nuclear scanning or the lacrimal gland is palpable [13].

Corticosteroids are the cornerstone of treatment for ocular sarcoidosis. Topical corticosteroids (i.e., eye drops) may be used for the treatment of isolated anterior uveitis [13]. Mydriatics are instilled to suppress the inflammation and avoid synechiae (adhesion of the iris to the lens). Systemic corticosteroids are required for anterior uveitis that is refractory to eye drops and intermediate and posterior uveitis because eye drops cannot adequately penetrate deep into the eye [13].

Skin

Cutaneous sarcoidosis lesions are of two types: specific and nonspecific. Specific lesions reveal granulomatous inflammation on histology. Nonspecific skin findings are reactive inflammatory lesions that do not exhibit granulomas.

Specific sarcoid lesions may occur on any part of the skin and mucosa [19]. Almost all morphologies have been reported including macules, papules, plaques, and nodules. Despite the diversity in appearance, the most common appearance is the papular form. These lesions are firm, 2–5 mm papules that often have a yellow-brown or translucent red-brown. The yellow brown color has been likened to "apple jelly" [19].

Lupus pernio is another distinctive specific sarcoidosis skin lesion. These lesions are usually relatively symmetric, violaceous, indurated plaque-like and nodular occurring on the nose, ear lobes, and cheeks. Lupus pernio has been associated with multiorgan sarcoidosis and a poor prognosis [1]. These lesions are associated with a higher prevalence of sarcoidosis involvement of the upper respiratory tract, sometimes by direct extension into the nasal sinus.

Cutaneous sarcoidosis may occur within tattoos, scar tissue, at traumatized skin sites, and around embedded foreign material such as silica. Scar sarcoidosis usually appears as nodules within a scar. The presence of sarcoidal granulomas surrounding foreign material is not specific for the diagnosis of sarcoidosis. In this circumstance, other evidence of systemic or cutaneous involvement is required to confirm the diagnosis.

Patents with nonspecific skin lesions such as erythema nodosum do not demonstrate granulomatous inflammation on skin biopsy. Therefore, skin biopsies should be avoided in these circumstances as the procedure has no value in the diagnosis of sarcoidosis. Specific sarcoidosis skin lesions should reveal noncaseating granulomatous inflammation on biopsy.

Sarcoidosis skin lesions are never life threatening and usually do not cause significant morbidity. Therefore, the decision to treat cutaneous sarcoidosis is dependent upon their cosmetic impact to the patient. Disfiguring lesions such as lupus pernio may cause social embarrassment for the patient and adversely affect the patient's quality of life.

If lesions are of minimal cosmetic importance to the patient they may be left untreated. Patients with a few localized lesions may be treated topically with corticosteroid creams or injections. If the patient requires treatment for more generalized skin disease, some form of pharmacotherapy is required.

Corticosteroids are the drug of choice for skin sarcoidosis because of their high rate and speed of efficacy. The antimalarial drugs hydroxychloroquine and chloroquine are also often useful for patients with skin sarcoidosis. Low dose methotrexate, 10–25 mg a week, may be effective for the treatment of cutaneous sarcoidosis. Cutaneous improvement may be noted within 1 month, but the maximal therapeutic effect may require at least 6 months of treatment. Infliximab, a tumor necrosis factor α (TNF-α) antagonist, appears to be particularly useful for the treatment of lupus pernio [20].

Liver

Hepatic sarcoidosis usually causes no symptoms [21], even though the frequency with which liver biopsy shows granulomas in sarcoidosis is 50–65% [22]. The frequency of serum liver function test abnormalities in sarcoidosis is as high as 35% [21], and the frequency of signs or symptoms of hepatic involvement is lower still at approximately 5–15% [21, 23].

Pruritus and abdominal pain are two of the more common symptoms and may occur in approximately 15% of cases [23]. Jaundice, fever, and weight loss are rare [23]. Hepatomegaly is found in 5–15% of sarcoidosis patients [24]. The most common serum liver function test abnormality in hepatic sarcoidosis is an elevated serum alkaline phosphatase [21], which may occasionally exceed five to ten times the upper limits of normal. Elevations in serum transaminases are less common and usually less severe than serum alkaline phosphatase [23]. Hyperbilirubinemia, hypoalbuminemia, and hepatic encephalopathy are very rare.

Hepatomegaly is the most common liver abnormality detected on CT and is frequently associated with splenomegaly [25]. Hepatic nodules are found in less than 5% of patients in most series [25]. The nodules are typically discrete and of slightly low attenuation, usually requiring intravenous contrast to be visualized. Hepatic nodules are detectable much less frequently than splenic nodules. The differential diagnosis of low-attenuation hepatic nodules includes lymphoma, metastatic malignancy, and various infections.

Cirrhosis has been reported in 6% (6/100) of patients with hepatic sarcoidosis [23]. Most of these patients have concomitant cholestatic features with loss of bile ducts indicating a pattern of primary biliary cirrhosis. However, cirrhosis in the absence of a cholestatic pattern may also be seen [23]. Portal hypertension occurs in approximately 3% of patients with hepatic sarcoidosis [23].

Most patients with hepatic sarcoidosis do not require therapy. Although treatment with corticosteroids can improve serum liver function tests in approximately half of asymptomatic patients, without therapy serum liver function tests almost always remain stable or undergo spontaneous improvement [21]. Because of the side effect profile of corticosteroids, therapy for hepatic sarcoidosis is not indicated in asymptomatic patients with liver function test elevations. Such patients should be monitored with serial liver function tests.

Granulomatous hepatitis from sarcoidosis may require treatment if patients develop fever, pruritus, nausea, vomiting, weight loss, or right upper quadrant abdominal pain. Corticosteroids are usually effective in alleviating these symptoms. Despite the potential risk of hepatic toxicity from methotrexate, this drug has been shown to be effective, reduce liver function test abnormalities, and to be corticosteroid sparing [26].

Occasionally portal hypertension develops with hepatic sarcoidosis as a consequence of biliary fibrosis or cirrhosis. Because these fibrotic changes are permanent, sarcoidosis-induced portal hypertension is usually unresponsive to corticosteroids or other antigranulomatous therapy. However, a therapeutic trial of corticosteroids is probably warranted on the off chance that the portal hypertension is the result of granulomas in the portal areas. Otherwise, therapy for sarcoidosis-associated portal hypertension is managed in a similar fashion as portal hypertension from other causes.

Neurologic

Any part of the nervous system may be affected including the cranial nerves, meninges, parenchyma of the brain, brainstem, spinal cord, pituitary gland, hypothalamus, subependymal layer of the ventricular system, peripheral nerves, and blood vessels supplying the nervous structures [1]. Neurosarcoidosis most frequently involves the cranial nerves [1]. Peripheral seventh nerve palsy (Bell's Palsy) is the most common manifestation of neurosarcoidosis [1, 27]. It may be unilateral or bilateral, and frequently resolves before the diagnosis of sarcoidosis is considered or made. Other cranial nerves may be affected, and in many series the nerves supplying the extraocular muscles or optic nerves are not rarely involved [28].

Sarcoidosis may cause aseptic meningitis [27]. Associated symptoms include fever, stiff neck, and headache. Cerebrospinal fluid (CSF) analysis typically reveals a pleocytosis of lymphocytes, with a low CSF glucose in 20% of cases [29]. Cranial neuropathies may result from involvement of the basal meninges [27]. Sarcoid meningitis may be acute or chronic. Acute meningitis usually responds favorably to corticosteroids, whereas chronic meningitis is often recurrent and requires long-term therapy [27].

Cerebral sarcoidosis lesions may develop in any portion of the brain. These lesions are more common in supratentorial locations than the cerebellum [30]. They may cause manifestations consistent with any space occupying lesions of the brain, and therefore are potentially life threatening. The lesions have a predilection for the pituitary gland and hypothalamus [28, 30], which may result in hypogonadism, diabetes insipidus, or adrenopituitary failure.

Spinal sarcoidosis is one of the most underappreciated forms of neurosarcoidosis. Patients may present with transverse myelopathy, paresis, radicular syndrome, cauda equina syndrome, and autonomic dysfunction [27]. Other manifestations of neurosarcoidosis include peripheral neuropathy, seizures, impaired cognition, and even frank psychosis. Sarcoidosis may also cause a small fiber neuropathy that may be responsible for disabling neuropathic pain and paresthesias, and possibly cause restless leg syndrome and periodic limb movement disorder. Special testing of autonomic function or skin biopsy to assess intraepidermal nerve fiber density is often needed to secure this diagnosis.

Corticosteroids are the mainstay of treatment of neurosarcoidosis. However, the response to corticosteroids is inconsistent and high doses (a starting dose of 40–80 mg/day of prednisone equivalent) are often required [28]. Relapses are common when the dose lowered to 20–25 mg/day of prednisone equivalent [28]. If the daily corticosteroid dose cannot be tapered to 10 mg/day of prednisone equivalent over the first

several months, alternative medications should be considered. Most of these agents are not effective alone but may be corticosteroid sparing. Such agents have included hydroxychloroquine, chloroquine, methotrexate, azathioprine, mycophenolate, cyclophosphamide, and infliximab.

Heart

Sarcoidosis can affect any portion of the heart and produce a myriad of clinical conditions that may simulate other more common cardiac disorders [31]. Granulomas may infiltrate the myocardium resulting in congestive heart failure [32, 33] or deposit in papillary muscles causing mitral regurgitation. Sarcoidosis may cause a granulomatous pericarditis with or without pericardial effusion. Long-term granulomatous inflammation may result in myocardial scarring with the formation of ventricular aneurysms.

Granulomatous inflammation may involve the myocardial conducting system causing complete atrioventricular block, premature ventricular contractions, ventricular arrhythmias, or sudden death [31, 33]. The most feared complications of cardiac sarcoidosis are sudden death and progressive congestive heart failure and emphasize that patients with cardiac sarcoidosis must be diagnosed early and monitored with extreme vigilance. Therefore, all patients diagnosed with sarcoidosis are recommended to have a baseline electrocardiogram (ECG), and all unexplained electrocardiographic abnormalities should be pursued [1].

The diagnosis of cardiac sarcoidosis is often problematic. Although an endomyocardial biopsy that reveals noncaseating granulomas is highly specific for the diagnosis, it is positive in less than one-quarter of cases because of the patchy distribution of the disease [31]. Consequently, noninvasive tests are usually relied upon to establish the diagnosis of cardiac sarcoidosis. Available tests include the ECG, echocardiogram, thallium-201 perfusion scan, gallium-67 scan, gadolinium enhanced magnetic resonance (MR) scan, and positron emission tomography (PET). The accuracy of thallium and gallium scans is enhanced by using a single-photon-emission CT (SPECT) technique [33]. Thallium defects from sarcoid heart disease can often be differentiated from ischemic heart disease in that the former may decrease in size with exercise or dipyridamole (reverse distribution).

Each of these noninvasive tests has a different sensitivity and specificity. Because of the diagnostic limitations of the "gold standard," the endomyocardial biopsy, a diagnostic algorithm involving noninvasive tests is needed. Unfortunately, there are inadequate clinical data concerning these clinical tests to construct such an algorithm. In fact, when noninvasive tests are compared with each other within the same clinical trials, there is a poor concordance of the tests such that a negative result on any one test does not preclude the possibility of another test being positive [33]. Nevertheless, the Japanese Ministry of Health and Welfare and the research group that conducted A Case Control Etiology of Sarcoidosis Study (ACCESS) each developed guidelines for the application of noninvasive tests to the diagnosis of cardiac sarcoidosis [34]. Both of these guidelines involve some combination of (a) the results of diagnostic noninvasive tests for cardiac sarcoidosis; (b) histologic confirmation of noncaseating granulomatous inflammation in an extracardiac organ; and (c) evidence of conduction system abnormalities, unexplained arrhythmias, or ventricular dysfunction.

There is no consensus concerning the therapy of cardiac sarcoidosis because of the lack of controlled studies. Treatment often involves a combination of antisarcoidosis medications, antiarrhythmic drugs, ionotropes, and pacemaker/defibrillator implantation. In one large study of 95 Japanese patients with cardiac sarcoidosis, a multivariate analysis identified left ventricular end-diastolic diameter (hazard ratio = 2.6 per 10 mm increase, $p = 0.02$), New York Heart Association (NYHA) function class (hazard ratio = 7.7 per NYHA class, $p = 0.0008$), and sustained ventricular tachycardia (hazard ratio = 7.2, $p = 0.03$) as independent predictors of mortality [32]. Prognosis was excellent in patients treated with corticosteroids early before the development of left ventricular dysfunction. Although some

have advocated that high dose corticosteroids be used for cardiac sarcoidosis, this study failed to detect a difference in outcome in those receiving ≥40 of prednisone/day compared to <30 mg/day. The management of asymptomatic cardiac sarcoidosis is controversial [31], and the role of long-term treatment in patients with symptomatic or asymptomatic disease is unknown.

A recent study suggested that patients with symptomatic cardiac sarcoidosis have a poor prognosis, with a high risk of congestive heart failure, need for internal pacemaker/defibrillator placement, or sudden death [35]. This suggests that symptomatic cardiac sarcoidosis should be treated aggressively and early. Subjects should be monitored closely for the development of left ventricular dysfunction, which suggests that the corticosteroid dose be increased or an alternate agent be added; cardiac transplantation should be considered if the patient fails to respond. The value of electrophysiological examinations for estimating the probability of cardiac events, selecting antiarrhythmic therapy, and determining the need for placement of an internal defibrillator is extremely limited. Indeed, cardiac sarcoidosis patients found to be noninducible with electrophysiologic testing have experienced sudden death, probably because the granulomatous lesions are not static and can worsen over time.

There are minimal data concerning alternative medications to corticosteroids for the treatment of cardiac sarcoidosis. Medications with reported benefits include methotrexate, cyclosporine, cyclophosphamide, and infliximab. The latter drug raises concerns as infliximab has a black box warning for use in patients with congestive heart failure.

Other Organs

Calcium metabolism is dysregulated in active sarcoidosis. This primarily results from an increased 1-α hydroxylase activity in sarcoid alveolar macrophages that converts 25-hydroxyvitamin D to 1, 25-dihydroxyvitamin D, the active form of the vitamin. This may manifest as hypercalcuria, hypercalcemia, and nephrolithiasis with possible renal insufficiency. Hypercalcuria is more common than hypercalcemia in sarcoidosis. Undetected, persistent hypercalcuria and hypercalcemia can result in renal stones, nephrocalcinosis, and renal failure. Therefore, serum calcium and creatinine should be measured and a urinalysis performed in all patients diagnosed with sarcoidosis [1]. It should be noted that these screening tests will not detect hypercalcuria; therefore, renal complications may develop if these screening tests are normal. Therefore, it may be appropriate to obtain a 24-h urine for calcium and creatinine in subjects at high risk of hypercalcuria (e.g., male gender, Caucasian, diagnosis ≥ 40 years, high sunlight exposure). The treatment of sarcoidosis-related hypercalcemia includes: (a) reduction of sunlight exposure, dietary calcium, oral calcium supplements, and vitamin D; (b) maintenance of an expanded intravascular volume; (c) reduction of the inappropriate production of 1, 25-dihydroxyvitamin D by sarcoid macrophages and granulomas; and (d) reduction of 1, 25-dihydroxyvitamin D – induced intestinal calcium absorption and bone resorption. Mild hypercalcemia (serum calcium ≤ 11 mg/dl) can be treated initially with the first two approaches without pharmacotherapy. If the serum calcium is greater than 11 mg/dl, the patient has nephrolithiasis, or the serum creatinine is elevated, drug therapy is usually required. Corticosteroids are the drug of choice. Failure of the serum calcium to normalize within 2 weeks on this corticosteroid regimen should alert the clinician to an alternate or coexisting disorder such as hyperparathyroidism, lymphoma, carcinoma, and myeloma. Once the calcium disorder is brought under control, the corticosteroid dose can be lowered over 4–6 weeks. If the patient develops intolerable corticosteroid side effects or fails to respond, chloroquine, hydroxychloroquine or ketoconazole may be useful.

Patients with splenic sarcoidosis are usually asymptomatic, but left upper quadrant abdominal pain occasionally develops. Constitutional symptoms such as night sweats, fever, and malaise may occur. Massive splenomegaly is found in approximately 3% of patients with splenic involvement [12].

Splenic sarcoidosis may cause hypersplenism resulting in anemia, leukopenia, thrombocytopenia, or any combination including pancytopenia [12]. Abdominal CT may reveal splenomegaly or splenic nodules that are usually multiple and of low attenuation. Most patients with splenic sarcoidosis do not require treatment. Splenomegaly, including giant splenomegaly, may resolve spontaneously. Treatment is indicated for (1) abdominal pain from splenomegaly, (2) functional asplenia, (3) hypersplenism, or (4) splenic rupture. Corticosteroids have also been effective for hypersplenism with normalization of blood cell lines, but the corticosteroid dose is not standardized [12]. Splenectomy is rarely required. Indications for splenectomy include gross enlargement or discomfort, infarction, hypersplenism with reduction in one or several blood cell lines, and rupture. A corticosteroid trial is warranted prior to consideration of splenectomy.

Sarcoidosis of the upper respiratory tract (SURT) is probably under-recognized. The disease may affect any part of the upper airway including the sinuses, nose, larynx, tonsils, and tongue. SURT most commonly affects the nasal mucous membranes. Common symptoms of sarcoidosis nasal involvement include dryness, stuffiness, obstruction, crusting, nasal discharge, and epistaxis. A confirmatory nasal biopsy should be performed if this diagnosis is considered unless there are typical endoscopic findings and a preexisting diagnosis of sarcoidosis in other organs.

Sarcoidosis patients with lupus pernio skin lesions on the nose often have nasal sarcoidosis, and such patients should always be asked about nasal symptoms. Sinus involvement is the second most common form of SURT. Symptoms include postnasal drip, nasal obstruction, periorbital pain, and headache. Although laryngeal involvement may occur, the aryepiglottic folds, arytenoids, false cords, and suglottic areas are more commonly involved than the larynx. Common symptoms include dysphonia, hoarseness, stridor, cough, dyspnea, and a sensation of a lump in the throat. Hoarseness may also occur from cranial nerve involvement or from mediastinal adenopathy compressing the recurrent laryngeal nerve.

Tonsillar and tongue involvement with sarcoidosis are rare.

High doses of corticosteroids (20–40 mg/day of prednisone equivalent) are often required for SURT. Intralesional injections may be effective if the lesions are localized. Nasal corticosteroid inhalation may diminish nasal inflammation and obstruction. Azathioprine, chloroquine, hydroxychloroquine, methotrexate, and infliximab have all been reported to be useful in case reports and series. Chemotherapy should be attempted prior to consideration of surgical resection because lesions may recur and perforation of the nasal septum is a complication after submucosal resection. Surgery is indicated in cases of expanding mass lesions, mass lesions causing airway obstruction, acute respiratory distress, and mass lesions encroaching on the central nervous system that fail to respond to chemotherapy.

Acute sarcoid arthritis may be intermittent, migratory, and can precede other manifestations of sarcoidosis by several months. Constitutional symptoms such as fever are often present. Acute sarcoid arthritis is very common, with Lofgren's syndrome with the ankles being a common location [36]. In fact, the primary symptom of Lofgren's syndrome is often difficulty walking because of joint pain. This arthritis is usually self-limiting averaging 11 weeks in duration [36]. Chronic sarcoid arthritis is rare, affecting only 0.2% of sarcoidosis patients [37]. The arthropathy may be destructive. Synovial biopsy shows noncaseating granulomas. Sarcoidosis arthritis is usually treated with nonsteroidal anti-inflammatory agents, which are especially useful for acute sarcoid arthritis. Chronic destructive synovitis from sarcoidosis may require systemic corticosteroids or intra-articular injections. The addition of methotrexate or azathioprine may improve results and be corticosteroid sparing.

Sarcoid bone involvement is most common in patients between the ages of 30 and 50 and in African Americans [38]. The bones of the hands and feet are most commonly affected; however, the nasal bones, skull, and vertebrae may be involved [38]. The lesions are often asymptomatic and incidentally found on radiographic or MR studies. Radiological findings usually show cystic or punched-out lesions.

Four mechanisms exist by which sarcoidosis can affect the hematologic system: (1) direct involvement of the bone marrow by granulomas, (2) immunologic destruction, (3) sequestration of cells into areas of inflammation, and (4) splenic sequestration.

Sarcoidosis may cause peripheral lymphadenopathy [1]. Isolated granulomatous inflammation in a lymph node, whether it is peripheral, intrathoracic, or intra-abdominal is not diagnostic of sarcoidosis, as in this may represent a "sarcoid-like reaction" from malignancy or inflammatory disease [2].

Sarcoidosis muscle involvement is usually asymptomatic and resolves spontaneously [38]. Skeletal muscle weakness occasionally occurs. Rarely, an acute myopathy resembling polymyositis, progressive myopathy, or palpable intramuscular nodules may occur.

Sarcoidosis of the breast may occur presenting as a palpable breast mass or a lesion seen on mammography. It is important that a breast mass detected in a sarcoidosis patient is not assumed to be related to the disease, as the patient may have concomitant breast carcinoma. This is particularly pertinent as patients with breast carcinoma may have related sarcoid-like reactions in extramammary sites.

Sarcoidosis may rarely involve the male and female reproductive tracts. Sarcoidosis may affect any portion of the female genitourinary tract including the ovary, fallopian tube, uterus, and vulva. Sarcoidosis may cause testicular masses that are particularly problematic because of the concern for possible testicular malignancy. In an attempt to avoid unnecessary orchiectomy, young males with known sarcoidosis or a clinical situation compatible with sarcoidosis and normal serum alpha-fetoprotein and beta-human chorionic gonadotrophic levels could be considered for close observation and repeated ultrasound, a brief empiric trial of corticosteroids, or possibly a biopsy. It is important to recognize, however, that normal levels of these proteins do not exclude the diagnosis of cancer.

Other very unusual manifestations of extrapulmonary sarcoidosis include involvement of

Table 9.2 Manifestations and treatment of extrapulmonary sarcoidosis

Organ	Manifestations	Treatment Drug of choice	Alternatives[a]
Eye	Anterior uveitis: red eye, painful eye, photophobia	CED, CP	C, M, A, I
	Posterior uveitis: floaters, ↓ vision	C	M, A, I
	Optic neuritis: sudden loss of vision or color vision	C[e]	M, A, I
Skin	Erythema nodosum[b]: pain erythematous/ violaceous lesions on extensor surface	NSAID[c]	C
	Localized lesion(s)	CI, CC	C, M, H, CQ
	Diffuse lesions	C	M, H,CQ, I
Liver	Asymptomatic LFT ↑	Do not treat	
	Fever, nausea, vomiting	C	M, H, CQ, I
	Pruritus, cholestasis	C[d]	M, H, CQ, I
Joints	Arthritis	NSAID	C, H, CQ, M, I
	Joint destruction	C	H, CQ, M, I
Heart	Symptomatic heart block	C[e,f]	M, CYC
	Symptomatic arrhythmia	C[e,g,h]	M, CYC
	Left ventricular dysfunction	C[e,g,h]	M, CYC
Neurologic		C[e]	M, CYC, H, CQ, A, I
Hypercalcemia	Asymptomatic, serum CA++ < 11 mg/dl	∞, F	C, H, CQ
	Asymptomatic, serum CA++ ≥ 11 mg/dl	∞, F, C	H, CQ
	Nephrolithiasis, serum creatinine ↑	∞, F, C	H, CQ
Sinus	Nasal obstruction	C[i]	M
	Epistaxis, crusting	C[i]	M
	Hoarseness	C[i]	M
	Airway compromise	C[j]	M

↑, increase; ↓, decrease; ∞, restrict dietary calcium, F, high fluid intake; CED, corticosteroid eye drops; CP, cycloplegics; C, corticosteroids – usually 20–40 mg prednisone equivalent/day; M, methotrexate; A, azathioprine; I, infliximab; CC, corticosteroid creams; CI, corticosteroid injections; H, hydroxychloroquine; CQ, chloroquine; NSAID, nonsteroidal anti-inflammatory drugs; CYC, cyclophosphamide [2]
Reproduced with permission from Judson MA. The management of sarcoidosis by the primary care physician. Am J Med. 2007;120:403–7.
[a] Usually corticosteroid-sparing: require low dose corticosteroids
[b] Often presents as Lofgren's syndrome: erythema nodosum, bilateral hilar adenopathy on chest radiograph, arthritis, fever
[c] For associated arthritis
[d] Addition of ursodeoxycholate often beneficial
[e] Consider high-dose corticosteroids: 40–80 mg prednisone daily equivalent/day
[f] Consider pacemaker or internal defibrillator placement
[g] Consider internal defibrillator placement
[h] Consider heart transplantation
[i] Injection if localized
[j] Consider surgery

the renal parenchyma, peritoneum, exocrine or endocrine glands, and the gastrointestinal tract. The latter may involve any portion of the GI tract, and may be very difficult to distinguish from Crohn's disease.

The general approach to treatment of extrapulmonary sarcoidosis is outlined in Table 9.2.

Diagnosis

Sarcoidosis has been defined as a multisystem disorder of unknown cause [1]. Although it has been claimed that the method of diagnosis of sarcoidosis has been established [1], in reality the diagnosis can never be completely assured.

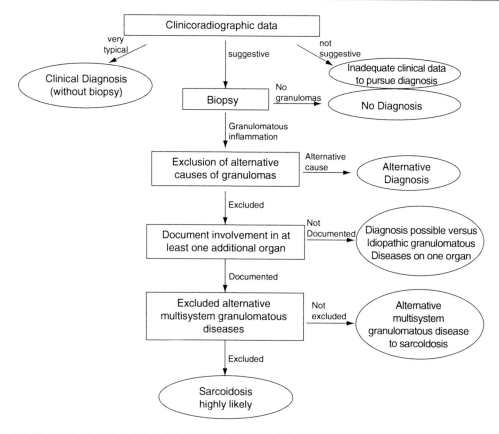

Fig. 9.4 Diagnostic algorithm. Adapted from ref. [2], with permission

There are certain clinical features that are typical of sarcoidosis but there are none that are specific for the diagnosis. The diagnostic evaluation of sarcoidosis includes gathering clinicoradiographic findings compatible with the diagnosis, histological confirmation of granulomatous inflammation, exclusion of known causes of granulomatous disease, and evidence of disease in at least two organs [2]. The end result of this diagnostic evaluation is neither a definitive diagnosis nor exclusion of the diagnosis, but rather an estimation of the statistical likelihood of the disease. This diagnostic approach is outlined in Fig. 9.4.

Clinical Findings

As with most diseases, establishing the diagnosis of sarcoidosis begins by collecting clinical data. Certain clinical findings suggest the diagnosis

of sarcoidosis although none of them is pathognomonic. The process involves judging the clinical data that support the diagnosis of sarcoidosis weighed against data that refute it. If sufficient clinical evidence accumulates to suggest the diagnosis of sarcoidosis, a tissue biopsy is normally indicated [2]. Table 9.3 outlines clinical data commonly used to gauge the pretest likelihood of the diagnosis. Although an elevated serum angiotensin-converting enzyme (SACE) level was initially thought to be diagnostic of sarcoidosis, it is neither sensitive nor specific enough to be diagnostic for the disease [2].

Because sarcoidosis is a systemic disease, evidence that a disorder is present in multiple organ systems supports the diagnosis of sarcoidosis. At presentation, 95% of patients have clinical evidence of pulmonary sarcoidosis, and more than 10% of sarcoidosis patients have evidence of involvement of the eye, skin, peripheral lymph node, or liver [5]. Therefore, sarcoidosis should

Table 9.3 Clinicoradiographic data supporting or weakening the likelihood of sarcoidosis. Adapted from ref. [2], with permission

	Supports	Weakens
Demographics	• U.S. African American • Northern European	• Age < 18 years • Age > 50 years in Male
Medical History	• Nonsmoking • No symptoms (in patients with CXR findings) • Positive family history of sarcoidosis • Symptoms involving >2 organs commonly involved with sarcoidosis (e.g., lung and eyes)	• Exposure to tuberculosis • Exposure to organic bioaerosol • Exposure to beryllium • Intravenous drug abuse
Laboratory data	• Elevated SACE	
Radiographic findings	• Bilateral hilar adenopathy (especially if without symptoms) • HRCT: Disease along the bronchovascular bundle	

CXR chest radiograph, *SACE* serum angiotensin-converting enzyme, *HRCT* high-resolution computer tomography

be considered in patients who present with pulmonary disease and concomitant disease in one of these organs.

Making a Diagnosis of Sarcoidosis Based on Clinical Findings Alone

On rare occasions, the constellation of clinical findings is so typical of sarcoidosis that the diagnosis can be assumed without a tissue biopsy (Fig. 9.4). Even in these situations the clinician often must exclude alternative diagnoses before assuming that the patient has sarcoidosis (e.g., Lofgren's syndrome, a sarcoidosis presentation consisting of bilateral hilar adenopathy on CXR and erythema nodosum skin lesions, requires the exclusion of coccidioidomycosis). Table 9.4 lists clinical presentations that may be assumed to represent sarcoidosis without tissue confirmation.

Selection of the Biopsy Site

With the exception of the rare instance where the clinical findings are highly specific for sarcoidosis, the diagnosis requires a tissue biopsy (see Fig. 9.4). Even when the patient has evidence of pulmonary or other visceral organs involved with sarcoidosis, it is in the patient's interest to select a biopsy site associated with least morbidity [2]. A skin biopsy is at lower risk of complications

Table 9.4 Clinical presentations that may be assumed to be sarcoidosis without tissue confirmation provided additional data do not suggest an alternative diagnosis. Adapted from ref. [2], with permission

• Lofgren's syndrome
  – Bilateral hilar adenopathy on chest radiograph
  – Erythema nodosum skin lesions
  – Fever (often)
  – (Ankle) arthralgias/arthritis (often)
• Heerfordt's syndrome
  – Uveitis
  – Parotitis
  – Fever (often)
• Bilateral hilar adenopathy on chest radiograph without symptoms
• Positive Panda sign (parotid and lacrimal gland uptake) and Lambda sign (bilateral hilar and right paratracheal lymph node uptake) on Gallium-67 scan

than biopsy of most other organs. Therefore, a careful skin examination should be performed in a patient with suspected sarcoidosis. The patient should be questioned about the presence of tattoos or scars because nodules that develop on these are usually granulomatous reactions. Other relatively noninvasive biopsy sites include enlarged peripheral lymph nodes and the conjunctiva if nodules are seen [18].

TBLB has a diagnostic yield for pulmonary sarcoidosis in 40 to >90% of cases [39]. Four to five lung biopsies are recommended to maximize the diagnostic yield [39]. TBLB is more likely to be diagnostic in patients with parenchymal disease evident on CXR (radiographic stage II or III) than in those with a normal lung parenchyma (radiographic stage 0 or I) [39]. Endobronchial biopsy can be performed with the TLB and has been shown to increase the diagnostic yield for sarcoidosis above that by using TLB alone. The yield of TBLB for the diagnosis of sarcoidosis is approximately 50% in patients with hilar adenopathy and no parenchymal infiltrates (radiographic stage I) [40]. Previously, the alternative diagnostic approach was mediastinoscopy, which is associated with significant cost and morbidity. Recently, the diagnostic yield from endobronchial needle aspiration has approached 90% when ultrasound guidance has been used [41].

BAL with examination of lymphocyte populations (CD4/CD8 ratio) is sometimes used as a complementary test for the diagnosis of sarcoidosis. Greater than 15% lymphocytes in BAL fluid has a sensitivity of 90% for the diagnosis of sarcoidosis, although the specificity is low [42]. In one study, a lymphocyte CD4/CD8 ratio of greater than 3.5 had a sensitivity of 53%, specificity of 94%, a positive predictive value of 76%, and a negative predictive value of 85% for the diagnosis of sarcoidosis [42].

Pathology

Although in almost all cases granulomas are required to establish a diagnosis of sarcoidosis, granulomas are nonspecific inflammatory reactions, and they are not diagnostic of sarcoidosis or any other granulomatous disease. Every biopsy should be searched for causes of granulomatous inflammation such as mycobacteria, fungi, parasites, and foreign bodies (e.g., talc).

Although there are no specific histologic features of sarcoid granulomas, there may be certain typical characteristics that suggest the diagnosis. The sarcoid granuloma usually consists of a compact (organized) collection of mononuclear phagocytes (epithelioid cells or macrophages) (see Fig. 9.1). There is typically no necrosis but occasionally there is a small to moderate amount. Usually, there is fusion of giant cells within the sarcoid granuloma to form multinucleated giant cells. These granulomas are usually surrounded

by a peripheral rim of lymphocytes. A variety of inclusions may be present such as asteroid bodies, Schaumann's bodies, birefringent crystals, and Hamazaki–Wesenberg bodies. However, these inclusions are nonspecific and not diagnostic of sarcoidosis.

Exclusion of Alternative Causes of Granulomatous Inflammation

Table 9.5 lists the differential diagnosis for granulomatous inflammation based on the organ system involved. The diagnosis of sarcoidosis requires that all of these conditions be excluded to a reasonable degree.

The exclusion of alternative causes of granulomatous inflammation requires a multifaceted approach. The histological specimen must be examined for infectious agents and foreign bodies capable of inducing a granulomatous reaction. This requires staining the specimen for mycobacteria and fungi at a minimum. Cultures for these organisms should usually be performed.

A detailed medical history is essential to exclude potential exposure to infectious agents (e.g., tuberculosis), environmental exposures (e.g., an organic bioaerosol such as significant bird or hot tub exposure causing hypersensitivity pneumonitis), and occupational exposures (e.g., beryllium). A recent study found that 40% of patients diagnosed with sarcoidosis who had a history of beryllium exposure demonstrated hypersensitivity to beryllium (6% of the total cohort) [43].

If the medical history suggests a possible alternative diagnosis, additional tests may need to be performed. Examples include antibody testing for hypersensitivity pneumonitis and a beryllium lymphocyte proliferation test for chronic beryllium disease.

Verifying Multiple Organ Involvement

The presence of noncaseating granulomata in a single organ does not conclusively establish the diagnosis of sarcoidosis because sarcoidosis, by definition, is a systemic disease that should

Table 9.5 Major pathologic differential diagnosis of sarcoidosis at biopsy. Reprinted with permission of the American Thoracic Society [1]. Copyright © American Thoracic Society

Lung	Lymph node	Skin	Liver	Bone marrow	Other biopsy sites
• Tuberculosis	• Tuberculosis	• Tuberculosis	• Tuberculosis	• Tuberculosis	• Tuberculosis
• Atypical mycobacteriosis	• Atypical mycobacteriosis	• Atypical mycobacteriosis	• Brucellosis	• Histoplasmosis	• Brucellosis
• Fungi	• Brucellosis	• Fungi	• Schistosomiasis	• Infectious mononucleosis	• Other infections
• Pneumocystis carinii	• Toxoplasmosis	• Reaction to foreign bodies: beryllium, zirconium, tattooing, paraffin, etc.	• Primary biliary cirrhosis	• Cytomegalovirus	• Crohn's disease
• Mycoplasma	• Granulomatous histiocytic necrotizing lymphadenitis (Kikuchi's disease)		• Crohn's disease	• Hodgkin's disease	• Giant cell myocarditis
• Hypersensitivity pneumonitis			• Hodgkin's disease	• Non-Hodgkin's lymphomas	• GLUS syndrome
• Pneumoconiosis: beryllium (chronic beryllium disease), titanium, aluminum	• Cat-scratch disease	• Rheumatoid nodules	• Non-Hodgkin's lymphomas	• Drugs	
	• Sarcoid reaction in regional lymph nodes to carcinoma		• GLUS syndrome	• GLUS syndrome	
• Drug reactions	• Hodgkin's disease				
• Aspiration of foreign materials	• Non-Hodgkin's lymphomas				
• Wegener's granulomatosis (sarcoid-type granulomas are rare)	• Granulomatous lesions of unknown significance (the GLUS syndrome)				
• Necrotizing sarcoid granulomatosis (NSG)					

involve multiple organs. There are idiopathic granulomatous diseases of individual organs that are distinguished from sarcoidosis. For example, idiopathic granulomatous hepatitis, where noncaseating granulomas of unknown cause are found isolated to the liver, is rarely found to be sarcoidosis (extrahepatic granulomas usually do not develop over time). Another example is idiopathic panuveitis, a granulomatous uveitis without extraocular involvement that is common in the Southeastern United States. The treatment of these single organ idiopathic granulomatous diseases is usually identical to that for sarcoidosis provided that alternative causes of granulomatous inflammation can be excluded. Therefore, it is usually unnecessary to search for involvement of a second organ to distinguish these conditions from sarcoidosis if it is not clinically obvious.

Table 9.1 lists the extent of the workup that should be performed to evaluate for a second organ involved with granulomatous inflammation.

Although the diagnosis of sarcoidosis requires proof of granulomatous involvement in a minimum of two separate organs, histologic confirmation is not necessarily required in the second organ. For example, noncaseating granulomata in the skin alone is inadequate for the diagnosis of sarcoidosis, but the concomitant presence of bilateral hilar adenopathy on CXR is thought to be sufficient evidence of second organ involvement such that a hilar lymph node or lung is not required [34]. ACCESS developed clinical criteria for when a second organ can be considered involved with sarcoidosis without biopsy (this presumes that noncaseating granulomas have been detected in the "first" organ) (Table 9.6) [34].

Table 9.6 Criteria for organ involvement in patients with preexisting sarcoidosis

Organ	Definite	Probable	Frequency[a]

Lungs	CXR with one of:
	  Bilateral hilar LAN
	  Diffuse infiltrates
	  Upper lobe fibrosis
	Restrictive PFTs
	Biopsy
		Lymphocytic alveolitis by BAL
		Any infiltrates
		Isolated reduction of DLCO
			95

Skin	Lupus pernio Annular lesion Erythema nodosum Biopsy	Maculopapular lesion New nodules	16[b]
Eyes	Lacrimal gland swelling Uveitis Optic neuritis Biopsy	Blindness	12
Liver	LFTs > 3 times normal Biopsy	Compatible CT or ultrasound Elevated ALP	12

Cardiac	Treatment-responsive
	cardiomyopathy
	IVCD or nodal block
	Positive gallium scan of the heart
	Biopsy
		No other cardiac disease and either:
		  Ventricular dysrhythmias
		  Cardiomyopathy
		Positive MRI
		Positive thallium scan
			2

Neurologic (excluding small fiber neuropathy)	Enhancement in meninges or brainstem on MRI CSF with increased lymphocytes or protein Diabetes insipidus Bell's palsy Cranial neuropathy Biopsy	Other MRI abnormalities Unexplained neuropathy Positive EMG	5
Bone marrow	Granulomas in bone marrow Unexplained anemia Marked leukopenia Thrombocytopenia		4
Spleen	Biopsy	Enlargement by exam or imaging	7
Bone/joints	Granulomas on biopsy Cystic changes in phalanges	Asymmetric, painful clubbing	<1
Lymph node	Biopsy	New palpable node above the waist Lymph node > 2 cm by imaging	15
Ear/nose/throat	Biopsy	Endoscopic examination consistent with granulomatous involvement	4
Parotid/salivary glands	Biopsy Symmetric parotitis without mumps Gallium scan (Panda sign)		4
Muscles	Biopsy Treatment-responsive elevation of CK/aldolase	Increased CK/aldolase	<1

(continued)

Table 9.6 (continued)

Organ	Definite	Probable	Frequency[a]
Calcium	Hypercalcemia without other cause	Hypercalcuria	4
		Presence of calcium-based renal stone	
Renal	Treatment responsive renal insufficiency	Treatment-responsive renal insufficiency in patients with DM/HTN	<1
	Biopsy		

These criteria are valid only in the absence of other causes for the specified abnormality
CXR chest-X-ray, *BAL* bronchoalveolar lavage, *PFT* pulmonary function test, *DLCO* diffusing capacity for carbon monoxide, *CT* computed tomogram, *LFT* liver function test, *ALP* alkaline phosphatase, *IVCD* intraventricular conduction delay, *MRI* magnetic resonance imaging, *CSF* cerebrospinal fluid, *EMG* electromyography, *CK* creatine kinase, *DM* diabetes mellitus, *HTN* hypertension
From Judson MA, Baughman RP, Teirstein AS, Terrin ML, and Yeager H, Jr. Defining organ involvement in sarcoidosis: the ACCESS proposed instrument. ACCESS Research Group. A Case Control Etiologic Study of Sarcoidosis. Sarcoidosis Vasc Diffuse Lung Dis. 1999;16(1):75–86. Reprinted with permission of the American Thoracic Society. Copyright © American Thoracic Society
[a]Incidence data at the time of diagnosis in A Case Control Study of Sarcoidosis (ACCESS)
[b]Excluding erythema nodosum

The Kveim Test

A long-standing diagnostic test for sarcoidosis is the Kveim test, where a splenic suspension from a spleen involved with sarcoidosis is inoculated intradermally. After 4–6 weeks, if a skin nodule appears at the inoculation site, is biopsied, and reveals noncaseating granulomas, this is highly specific for the diagnosis of sarcoidosis. Unfortunately, the test is not extremely sensitive, both the sensitivity and specificity vary depending upon the spleen that is used, and the suspension is not FDA approved. Therefore, the Kveim test is not a standard diagnostic test for sarcoidosis.

Other Idiopathic Systemic Granulomatous Diseases

To complicate matters further, there are other multiorgan idiopathic granulomatous syndromes that are clinically disparate from sarcoidosis such that they are thought to be separate entities. These conditions must also be excluded for a diagnosis of sarcoidosis to be established (see Fig. 9.4). Blau's Syndrome consists of iritis, granulomatous arthritis, and skin rash. It is autosomal dominant with variable penetrance, and the age of onset is usually prior to age 12 years. It is considered a separate entity from childhood sarcoidosis on the basis of a lack of pulmonary and other visceral organ involvement and the mode of inheritance.

In 1989, Brinker described a syndrome with: (a) prolonged fever; (b) epithelioid granulomata in the liver, bone marrow, spleen, and lymph nodes; (c) a benign course; and (d) a tendency for recurrence [44]. This entity has been named, "the GLUS syndrome": granulomatous lesions of unknown significance. Although it has been argued that the GLUS syndrome is a form of extrapulmonary sarcoidosis, differences include (1) elevated SACE levels have never been found with the GLUS syndrome, (2) the Kveim test has always been negative in the GLUS syndrome, (3) hypercalcemia is never found with the GLUS syndrome, (4) immunotyping of T cells in the granulomas of GLUS syndrome patients is distinctly different from that of the granulomas of sarcoidosis patients [44].

Necrotizing sarcoid granulomatosis (NSG) is a disease characterized by a granulomatous vasculitis. Because vessels are involved, necrosis is a prominent feature, unlike most cases of sarcoidosis. Although NSG may be confined to the lung, it is often a systemic disease and may involve extrapulmonary organs. It is debated whether it is a form of sarcoidosis or separate disease entity.

Treatment

Decision to Treat

Treatment of sarcoidosis requires a highly individualized approach since the pattern of organ involvement, disease duration, clinical impact, rate of progression, patient goals, and the other comorbidities all must be considered together. Most patients with sarcoidosis will remit spontaneously and there are little data to support the notion that treatment improves the chances for remission over the long term (see section "Prognosis"). Therefore, a diagnosis of sarcoidosis is not a *fait accompli* indication for treatment.

An algorithm for the treatment of pulmonary sarcoidosis is displayed in Fig. 9.5. The approach to extrapulmonary sarcoidosis is often quite similar, with specific differences outlined in the "Extrapulmonary Sarcoidosis" section.

Some authors have suggested that patients with disease duration less than 5 years can be approached differently than those with more chronic disease, since there are still reasonable prospects for spontaneous remission in this group (see section "Prognosis"). Although there are clinical features which may help predict which patients will develop bothersome long-term disease, the specificity of any individual feature is not high enough to dictate that treatment is definitely required. Thus, the decision to treat patients with sarcoidosis of less than 2–5 years' duration requires either evidence of progressive or of organ-threatening disease. There are several situations that generally warrant consideration of systemic treatment at the time of diagnosis since long-term outcomes in the affected organs are likely to be poor. The most common of these include: posterior or intermediate uveitis, or anterior uveitis refractory to topical therapy; disfiguring cutaneous disease (e.g., lupus pernio); cardiac

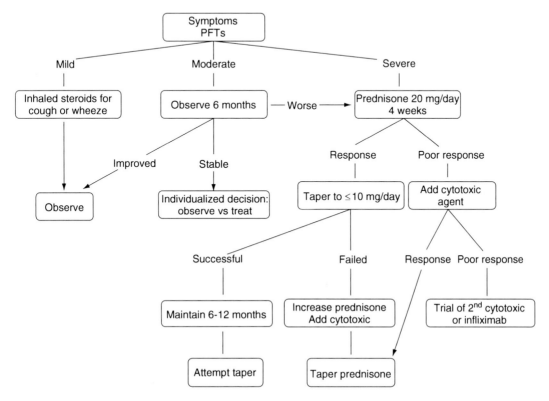

Fig. 9.5 Treatment scheme for pulmonary sarcoidosis

sarcoidosis that manifests as cardiomyopathy, dysrhythmias, or high-grade AV block; brain or spinal cord sarcoidosis, except for isolated cranial nerve 7 palsy or mild acute aseptic meningitis; symptomatic hepatosplenic sarcoidosis (i.e., pain, consumptive cytopenia, nausea); and significant hypercalcemia. Other scenarios that require case-by-case decisions include sarcoid myositis, sinonasal, gastrointestinal, exocrine gland or skin involvement, granulomatous nephritis, and bone disease.

Similarly, not all patients with long-standing sarcoidosis (more than 5 years) will require treatment, despite evidence that there is persistent granuloma formation. For example, Hunninghake et al. were able to demonstrate that the majority of patients with sarcoidosis of more than 1 years' duration who had been on prednisone were able to successfully taper off without relapse [45]. Thus, the mainstay of treatment decisions still involves an assessment of organ-specific manifestations.

Sarcoidosis Penumbra

Prior to treatment of granulomatous inflammation with immunosuppressives, it is useful to consider the range of common sarcoidosis-associated symptoms that are unlikely to respond to standard therapy. These manifestations constitute a "sarcoidosis penumbra" – features caused by the disease but which are often not the focus of the physician. Constitutional symptoms, such as fatigue and achiness, are tremendously bothersome for a large proportion of patients, and have generally been under-appreciated. However, these symptoms confer a substantial burden on quality of life for sarcoidosis patients, are often the dominant patient-identified issue, and should be explored as part of the therapeutic approach. Depression should be sought, and treated, since it occurs in up to two-thirds of patients [46]. Sleep apnea, usually obstructive, may also contribute to the symptoms. In one tertiary institution, it was present in 17% of subjects with sarcoidosis versus only 3% of other pulmonary clinic patients [47]. After other contributors to general fatigue are

identified and treated, nonspecific pharmacologic therapies such as modafinil or dexmethylphenidate may be useful.

Treatment of Pulmonary Sarcoidosis

Pulmonary disease is the most common indication for treatment of sarcoidosis, but the decision to treat pulmonary sarcoidosis is often difficult to establish at the first visit, and longitudinal follow-up is generally necessary to define the course [45]. The imperative to treat pulmonary involvement is substantially lower in patients with shorter disease duration, especially for those with mild–moderate symptoms. For cough or asthmatic symptoms, topical therapy with inhaled corticosteroids may be helpful. At times, high doses, such as 800 mcg of budesonide b.i.d. are necessary.

For patients who have severe symptoms or physiologic derangements at the time of presentation, and evidence of potentially reversible disease, treatment should be commenced immediately. Individuals with mild–moderate symptoms and/or physiologic derangements are usually observed for 6 months prior to making an individualized decision regarding whether to start treatment. A substantial proportion of this group will demonstrate either clear-cut improvement or deterioration by 6 months' time [48], avoiding steroid toxicities and better defining the clinical phenotype in this group.

In the short run, it is evident that treatment of pulmonary sarcoidosis with corticosteroids improves the chest radiographic findings, although there is less evidence for a benefit on spirometry or symptoms [49]. In the ACCESS cohort, treatment with corticosteroids was associated with a higher likelihood of either improvement or deterioration of the CXR at 2 years, likely reflecting variable responses and the presence of a subset of patients with aggressive or refractory disease [50]. Longer-term outcomes from preemptory steroid treatment are less clear, with conflicting evidence in the available literature (see section "Prognosis").

Table 9.7 Causes for apparent nonresponse to corticosteroids

Nonadherence to therapy
Irreversible (fibrotic) disease
Complications (bronchiectasis, fibrobullous disease, mycetoma)
Steroid-refractory sarcoidosis (rare)
Intercurrent infection
Masking of steroid benefit by toxicities (e.g., weight gain, myopathy)
Medication toxicities (e.g., pneumonitis)
Sarcoidosis-associated pulmonary hypertension
Nonpulmonary cause for symptoms

Responses to treatment typically are evident within 2–4 weeks [51]. Failure of pulmonary involvement to respond to therapy within 4–6 weeks should suggest several possibilities (Table 9.7). Most authors recommend starting with a dose of 20–40 mg daily of oral prednisone [1], although there are no direct controlled studies defining the optimal dose. More recent data suggest that 20 mg/day is adequate for most patients. After assessment of the initial response, tapering to the lowest effective dose is necessary to minimize steroid toxicities. The usual goal is to reduce the prednisone dose to less than 10 mg/day [1]. However, it is important to note that some patients will still develop substantial steroid toxicities at this dose, and therefore 10 mg/day is merely a general guideline. For patients with comorbidities such as poorly controlled diabetes or obesity, it may be appropriate to target lower steroid doses or steroid-free regimens. One approach to reduce steroid toxicities is alternate-day dosing, which has been shown to be effective in acute pulmonary sarcoidosis [52].

Once a decision to start systemic therapy for pulmonary sarcoidosis has been made, it is typically continued for at least 12 months, although 6 months may be adequate for patients with recent-onset disease and more moderate symptoms. Treatment for at least 12 months was associated with a lower likelihood of late relapse in one prospective observational study, although the duration of therapy was not randomized [45]. One may expect that treatment duration will more likely be prolonged in patients with long-standing (>5 years) disease, reflecting the low chance for remission in this group. Nonetheless, periodic attempts to taper steroids in these patients should still be made, since up to 30% may successfully achieve relapse-free dose reduction [53]. The rate of tapering has not been studied prospectively, but dose reductions generally should not occur more quickly than every 2 weeks.

Treatment of Extrapulmonary Sarcoidosis

Treatment of extrapulmonary sarcoidosis also requires consideration of the impact on the patient, the severity of organ derangement, and the likelihood of irreversible organ damage. Recommended treatment options are outlined in Table 9.2 and reviewed by manifestation above (see section "Extrapulmonary Sarcoidosis"). For most indications, corticosteroids are the therapy of choice – in many instances topical therapy alone is sufficient. Some of the extrapulmonary manifestations are associated with a high likelihood of refractory or bothersome long-term disease, such as lupus pernio, symptomatic myocardial involvement, severe central or peripheral nervous system disease, and severe SURT. In these situations, it is appropriate to consider alternative agents earlier in the treatment approach since the cumulative toxicities of corticosteroids will more likely be manifest. For cardiac, neurologic, and sinonasal disease, treatment may be necessary for many years.

Individual Agents

Corticosteroids

Corticosteroids are the mainstay of treatment for sarcoidosis, since they are reliable, inexpensive, easily titrated, quick-acting, and efficacious. In some situations, topical corticosteroids will provide sufficient control. Specific examples where topical therapy may be useful include limited cutaneous disease, corticosteroid eye drops for anterior uveitis, and inhaled corticosteroids for pulmonary disease manifestations referable to the airways (cough, wheeze). Some studies have also suggested a benefit for inhaled corticosteroids on pulmonary parenchymal disease, but the effect is small and the available literature is conflicting. In general, nasal steroid sprays are not very effective for SURT.

Toxicity from corticosteroids is common in sarcoidosis patients. Weight gain, worsening diabetes, and osteoporosis are most common, with the incidence of complications dependent on the dosing regimen and population. In one cohort, the median weight gain after 6 months of steroid therapy was 11 kg [54]. In contrast, the median weight gain after 12 months in the steroid-treated arm of the British Thoracic Study was only 3.6 kg [48]. Similarly, bone mineral density, which is already low in sarcoidosis in general, is adversely impacted by corticosteroids.

In patients with significant corticosteroid toxicities, it may be reasonable to attempt to use other agents to reduce the corticosteroid dose or discontinue corticosteroids. The relative value of steroid-sparing regimens will increase as the patient transitions to more chronic duration of the disease and the likelihood of remission diminishes. In practice, it is uncommon to successfully wean a corticosteroid-dependent sarcoidosis patient completely off corticosteroids using alternative medications. For most patients, the goal during prolonged corticosteroid use is to reduce the dose to less than 10 mg/day.

Antimalarials

Chloroquine and hydroxychloroquine have demonstrated effectiveness in sarcoidosis, with benefits especially apparent for cutaneous disease and hypercalcemia. In one small placebo-controlled trial, maintenance use of chloroquine 250 mg daily in patients with chronic pulmonary disease slowed the rate of lung function decline and risk of relapse [55]. These drugs may also be helpful for selected patients with neurologic sarcoidosis, although the literature for this indication is limited.

Hydroxychloroquine is generally used in practice, since retinal toxicity is lower than chloroquine. Typical dosing for hydroxychloroquine is 200 mg once or twice daily. Periodic ophthalmologic

screening is recommended for antimalarials every 6–12 months. A rare but clinically important toxicity from antimalarial medications is a reversible myopathy that may be confused with steroid or sarcoid-induced myopathy.

Methotrexate

Methotrexate is widely used as a steroid-sparing agent or for second-line treatment of sarcoidosis that is poorly responsive to steroids. Evidence from randomized, controlled trials for effectiveness is limited to demonstration of a steroid-sparing effect in symptomatic acute pulmonary disease in patients treated for 1 year [54]. Case series have also described benefits in chronic pulmonary, neurologic, ocular, and cutaneous disease; the effects may not be fully apparent for 6 months. Overall, approximately two-thirds of patients will respond [54, 56], perhaps due to variability in absorption or polymorphisms of the enzymes involved in methotrexate metabolism. Typical doses in standard use are from 10 to 25 mg once weekly. Folic acid 1–2 mg daily prevents many of the side effects and has been shown not to significantly reduce therapeutic effectiveness in rheumatoid arthritis.

Generally, methotrexate is well tolerated. The most common side effects, which are temporally related to the dose, include nausea and fatigue. Other side effects that may occur include alopecia, rash, and oral ulcers. Liver enzyme elevation is the most frequent serious toxicity that leads to discontinuation of the medication [56]. Other important toxicities include leukopenia and subacute hypersensitivity pneumonitis. Except for lung toxicity, most of the other side effects respond to dose reduction.

Periodic monitoring of liver function and blood count are recommended for the duration of methotrexate therapy. Renal function should also be assessed periodically since impaired renal clearance leads to increased toxicity. Typically, these blood tests are obtained every 6–12 weeks for chronic maintenance therapy.

Azathioprine

Azathioprine is also used frequently but has relatively less published data to support it. There are no randomized controlled trials. In a small open-label trial, a possible steroid-sparing effect was described in 11 patients with chronic sarcoidosis [57]. However, since all of the patients were also initially treated with high-dose corticosteroids, the improvement in clinical parameters may not have been due to azathioprine. In a single-center review of patients treated with azathioprine as a second-line agent, a benefit was observed in only four of the nine evaluable patients. Despite the paucity of relevant data, most sarcoidosis physicians do note benefits from the use of azathioprine to reduce steroids or in steroid-unresponsive disease.

Side effects and toxicities for azathioprine are generally similar to those for methotrexate. In patients with rheumatoid arthritis, drug discontinuation due to toxicity was similar for azathioprine and methotrexate [58]. There have been no published head-to-head comparisons of these agents for sarcoidosis. The most feared toxicity of azathioprine, severe neutropenia, can be minimized by either frequent blood counts when initiating the medication or by screening for deficiency of its major metabolic enzyme, thiopurine methyltransferase. The most common side effects are abdominal discomfort and diarrhea.

Similar to methotrexate, azathioprine requires periodic monitoring of liver function, but is probably also associated with less hepatotoxicity. Usual monitoring intervals for CBC and liver function tests are from 6 to 12 weeks, except with initiation of the medication. Typical doses range from 2 to 2.5 mg/kg/day.

Leflunomide

Leflunomide, which antagonizes lymphocyte proliferation, was reported in a single-center observational study to induce partial or complete responses in 25/32 (78%) of patients with chronic sarcoidosis unresponsive to or intolerant of methotrexate [59]. It likely has synergistic effects when used in combination with methotrexate. However, no study has evaluated what proportion of sarcoidosis patients respond to addition of leflunomide when methotrexate alone is insufficient. Typical doses are from 10 to 20 mg daily.

Side effects of leflunomide include diarrhea, abdominal cramping, fatigue, and hepatotoxicity. Liver enzymes and blood count should be monitored every 6–12 weeks with leflunomide monotherapy, and every 4–8 weeks when used in combination with methotrexate. Pulmonary toxicity, manifest as lymphocyte-predominant pneumonitis, may occasionally occur, but it appears to be less frequent than methotrexate lung toxicity. Since the half-life is approximately 14 days, mainly due to enterohepatic recirculation, leflunomide must be actively removed when severe toxicity occurs. Cholestyramine 8 g t.i.d. for 2 days is sufficient to remove 99% of the active metabolites.

Mycophenolate and Mycophenolic Acid

Anecdotal experience suggests that many clinicians have begun using mycophenolate mofetil and mycophenolic acid as a second-line agent. The mechanism of its anti-inflammatory effects is unclear, but may be due to potent suppression of de novo purine biosynthesis in lymphocytes. The largest series published described its use for ophthalmic sarcoidosis, where it appeared to have efficacy for all seven patients studied [60]. Beneficial responses have also been reported for renal and cutaneous disease as well. Theoretically, the risk for developing neutropenia may be lower than with other cytoxic agents. Liver enzyme elevations also appear to occur less frequently than with methotrexate, azathioprine, and leflunomide. Gastrointestinal side effects may limit the dose for some patients.

Cyclophosphamide

Cyclophosphamide, an alkylating agent, can be used in oral or intravenous formulations. In at least one report on neurosarcoidosis, it appears to be more efficacious than methotrexate [61]. The usefulness of cyclophosphamide for refractory brain and spinal cord sarcoidosis has been described in several series. In case reports, it has also been used to treat renal and cardiac sarcoidosis with good outcomes. Interestingly, the effect of cyclophosphamide on pulmonary sarcoidosis has not been studied. Important toxicities of this drug include neutropenia, infections, hemorrhagic cystitis, and malignancy, which may not occur until many years after its use. The side-effect profile, burdensome monitoring requirements, and availability of biologic agents have dampened enthusiasm for its use except in the most severe cases.

Biologic TNF Antagonists

Among the most recently described therapeutic options for treatment of sarcoidosis are the biologic TNF antagonists. The bulk of the evidence to date is for infusion therapy with the monoclonal antibody infliximab; the subcutaneous monoclonal agent, adalimumab has also been successful in a handful of cases. The soluble receptor antagonist, etanercept, does not appear to have efficacy for sarcoidosis.

A randomized, double-blind, placebo-controlled trial of 138 subjects demonstrated effectiveness of infliximab in chronic pulmonary disease [62]. The greatest benefits were seen in subjects with FVC < 69% predicted, disease duration >2 years, and worse dyspnea [62]. A substudy from this trial showed a benefit in the treatment of extrapulmonary sarcoidosis with infliximab [63]. Most clinical responses are apparent within 4–6 infusions, and are sometimes even dramatically evident after the first dose.

The limitations to use of these agents are primarily cost and the prospects of severe toxicities. A well-described toxicity from TNF antagonists is reactivation of tuberculosis or fungal infection. The clinical presentation of reactivation may be atypical and disseminated, leading to delayed diagnosis and mortality. It is important to screen carefully for the possibility of latent tuberculosis (TB) prior to use of these medications. Although skin testing and/or IFN-γ release assays should be checked, they may be unreliable since peripheral cellular anergy is common in sarcoidosis. Therefore, a very careful exposure history and a low threshold for presumptive treatment of latent TB prior to starting these medications are advisable.

Other potential toxicities of biologic TNF antagonists include a possible increased risk of lymphoma, de novo or worsening of cardiomyopathy, and a variety of hypersensitivity reactions. Nonetheless, in a subset of patients with refractory sarcoidosis, use of infliximab may be dramatically more effective than any other therapies [20].

Other Pharmacologic Alternatives

Thalidomide and pentoxifylline, which both inhibit TNF, are used sporadically as third- or fourth-line alternatives in patients refractory to or intolerant of other agents. Thalidomide also has antiangiogenic properties which may account for some of its effects. Dose escalation of both of these agents is commonly limited by side effects. Important toxicities of thalidomide include somnolence, peripheral neuropathy, hypercoagulability, and teratogenicity. Pentoxifylline may cause intolerable gastrointestinal symptoms at higher doses.

Minocycline, which has anti-inflammatory effects, has been reported to be useful for patients with cutaneous sarcoidosis. It most likely has a role in patients with milder forms of disease who are intolerant of or do not respond well to antimalarial agents.

Prognosis

The outcome of sarcoidosis is highly variable and difficult to predict. For most patients, the prognosis is favorable, with spontaneous remission of the disease in approximately two-thirds of affected individuals [1]. The time frame for resolution has been debated, with persistent sarcoidosis commonly defined as disease lasting more than 2 years. This definition was based, in part, on the observation that failure to improve or remit over the first 2 years portended a more difficult course, and that relapses after spontaneous regression occurred in fewer than 10% of patients [64]. Other authors have noted that continuing resolution of radiographic changes may evolve over the first 5 years [65], leading to suggestions that the term chronic be applied only to patients with disease of at least 5 years' duration. In general, patients with longer disease duration are less likely to undergo spontaneous remission; however, even after 5 years an occasional individual will remit. From a practical standpoint, the decision to define a patient as having "acute" or "chronic" sarcoidosis is less relevant than an assessment of the impact of sarcoidosis, the expected course, and the degree of reversibility.

Not all patients who fail to achieve a spontaneous remission will have clinically bothersome long-term disease. For pulmonary disease, longitudinal studies have identified several risk factors

Table 9.8 Extrapulmonary clinical prognostic factors for outcome in sarcoidosis

Favorable	Unfavorable
White race[a,d]	Black race[a]
Erythema nodosum[a,c]	Age > 40 years[b,c]
Löfgren's syndrome[b]	Organomegally[b,c]
	Lupus pernio[b]
	Cardiac disease[b]
	Nephrocalcinosis[b]
	SURT[b]
	Bone involvement[b]
	Lower family income[a]
	Extrapulmonary disease[a,b]

[a]Factors identified from ref. [50]
[b]Factors identified from ref. [73]
[c]Factors identified from ref. [72]
[d]Factors identified from ref. [74]

for deterioration or death: lower vital capacity and presence of fibrosis on CXR [66]; more prominent pulmonary symptoms at presentation regardless of radiographic stage or PFT values [67, 68]; use of corticosteroids at the time of presentation [69]; presence of pulmonary hypertension [70]; and, elevated neutrophils in the BAL [71]. There are also several extrapulmonary features that predict persistence of sarcoidosis or need for systemic immunosuppressives (Table 9.8) [50, 72–74].

It is important to consider, however, that >80% of the ACCESS cohort had stable or improved radiographs and spirometry over the 2-year follow-up period [50]. Only 6% of these patients with radiographic stages 0–II progressed to stage III or IV. Similarly, over a 5.5 year mean follow-up period, only 13% of Danish patients demonstrated radiographic deterioration [64]. The implication of these data is threefold: first, long-term longitudinal follow-up is necessary to identify patients who demonstrate progressive pulmonary deterioration that could lead to respiratory insufficiency. Second, the majority of patients with pulmonary sarcoidosis do not require treatment, and data obtained at the time of diagnosis are often insufficient to make a positive treatment decision. Third, the goals of treatment are long term, and therefore treatment strategies should be conceptualized as management regimens rather than curative.

Mortality

Assessments of mortality have been difficult, owing to the uncertain effects of treatment strategies on mortality, presence of referral bias, and the variable risk between populations. In referral centers, attributable mortality rates have been estimated to range from 4 to 7.6%, whereas they are less than 1% in community-based cohorts [65, 75]. A large epidemiologic survey of general practices in the United Kingdom conducted between 1991 and 2003 reported 7% mortality 5 years after the diagnosis, compared with 4% in age- and gender-matched controls [76]. Older age and male gender conferred increased risk. One explanation for the discrepancy between these mortality estimates may be that, for some series, a high proportion of deaths in patients are due to nonsarcoidosis causes [65]. In Europe and the United States, most of the sarcoidosis-related deaths are due to pulmonary involvement [1], whereas cardiac sarcoidosis has historically been the major cause of death in Japan.

Role of Therapy on the Natural History

There are conflicting but not compelling data to suggest that treatment of sarcoidosis influences the likelihood of remission positively or negatively. For example, Grunewald et al. found that among Swedish patients presenting with Löfgren's syndrome who were HLA-DRB1*03 negative and were treated with steroids, 80% had disease persistence at 2 years, versus only 37% of untreated patients [77]. Similarly, in a series of primarily African-American patients, those individuals who received steroids to control their disease had a 74% likelihood of relapse when therapy was tapered [74]. In the ACCESS cohort, only dyspnea and treatment within the first 6 months of diagnosis were associated with need for continued treatment at 2 years [67]. To date, there are no data to suggest that more targeted therapies, such as biologic TNF antagonists, improve the likelihood of remission.

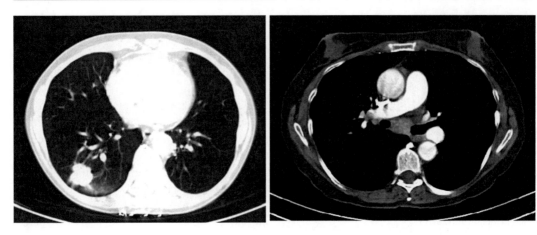

Fig. 9.6 Chest CT scan from the patient. Parenchymal window demonstrating a 3.5 cm lobulated mass in the RLL. The mediastinal window shows an enlarged subcarinal lymph node

In contradistinction, in a double-blind, randomized placebo-controlled trial of 189 Finnish patients, treatment with oral prednisolone for 3 months followed by inhaled budesonide for 15 months was associated with changes in the 5-year outcome [78]. Resolution of radiographic changes (74% for treated patients vs. 62%), rates of relapse, and (for stage II–III CXR) pulmonary function all favored a beneficial effect of treatment. A study by the British Thoracic Society examined whether individualized titrated steroid dosing for 18 months in patients with stage II–III CXRs would affect the 5-year outcome, compared to observation alone [48]. Importantly, after diagnosis, all the patients were observed for 6 months prior to randomization to select a subset without evidence of radiologic resolution or precipitous deterioration. Only 6 of 31 patients randomized to observation alone required treatment over the follow-up period. At the end of 5 years, those treated presumptively with steroids for 18 months exhibited a lower incidence of any dyspnea (15% vs. 39%) and any radiographic fibrosis (26% vs. 42%), with modest improvements in lung function. Baseline imbalances between the treated groups dilute the enthusiasm for widespread adoption of this strategy, however. At present, there are insufficient data to definitively recommend routine institution of empiric therapy for the purpose of improving the natural history for all sarcoidosis patients, even those with persistent disease.

Clinical Vignette

A 58-year-old African-American female, a never-smoker, developed fatigue and a nonproductive cough over a 3-month period. She had no history of lung disease and no other systemic symptoms. Her past medical history was notable for hypothyroidism and hyperlipidemia. A younger sister had been diagnosed with cutaneous and ocular sarcoidosis 14 years previously. She worked as a receptionist at a law office since the age of 23.

Her physical exam was entirely unremarkable. Pulmonary function testing revealed a low-normal FVC of 2.65 l (81% predicted) and forced expiratory volume in 1 s (FEV1) of 1.81 l (74% predicted). The FEV1/FVC ratio was 68%. An abnormal CXR prompted a CT scan, which showed a 3.5 cm RLL mass with subcarinal lymph node enlargement (Fig. 9.6).

A bronchoscopy was performed. The bronchoscopist noted the presence of mucosal cobblestoning in the bronchus intermedius and right lower lobe, suggesting the possibility of sarcoidosis. Endobronchial biopsy in this area revealed noncaseating granulomata; BAL cell differential showed 14% lymphocytes, with CD4/CD8 ratio of 1.7. The diagnosis of nodular sarcoidosis was made. Baseline testing revealed mild anemia (hemoglobin 11.6 g/dl); the remainder of the blood count and metabolic profile were normal. Ophthalmologic exam was likewise unremarkable.

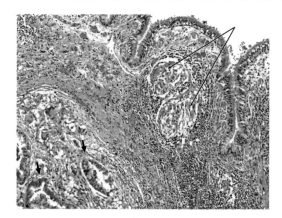

Fig. 9.7 Right lower lobe resection. There are nonnecrotizing granulomas in the submucosa (*thin arrows*). The adenocarcinoma appears as nests of malignant cells below the basement membrane (*thick arrows*), and it was not sampled by the prior endobronchial biopsy

Despite 6 weeks' treatment with inhaled budesonide/formoterol and a 2-week course of oral corticosteroids, her symptoms persisted. A repeat CXR showed no change in the size of the mass, so she underwent a diagnostic right lower lobe resection. The biopsy revealed a primary lung adenocarcinoma with a granulomatous reaction of the overlying mucosa (Fig. 9.7).

As mentioned previously, the diagnosis of sarcoidosis is never assured. The presence of noncaseating granulomas alone is insufficient to secure the diagnosis, and the clinician must carefully consider whether the clinical picture supports a diagnosis of sarcoidosis or suggests that another process could be causing a granulomatous reaction instead. Malignancies are recognized to cause granulomatous reactions. The regional mediastinal nodes are most frequently involved, with isolated granulomas present in approximately 4% of nonmalignant lymph nodes. Adjacent tissue may also exhibit granulomas, as demonstrated in this case. Adenocarcinoma and lymphoma are the most commonly associated causes of malignancy-induced granulomatous reactions in the chest.

Summary

Sarcoidosis is a multisystem granulomatous disease of unknown cause. Although the cause of sarcoidosis is unknown, evidence suggests that it results from antigen exposure eliciting a granulomatous response in genetically susceptible individuals. The disease is not definitively diagnosed. Rather, the diagnosis is established when the clinical, radiographic, and histological findings are such that the statistical likelihood of an alternate explanation is highly unlikely. Sarcoidosis may affect any organ in the body, and its major effects may be related to pulmonary or extrapulmonary involvement. Not all forms of sarcoidosis require treatment, as the disease may remain stable or remit spontaneously. When treatment is required, corticosteroids are usually the drug of choice, although alternative agents could be considered.

References

1. Hunninghake GW, Costabel U, Ando M, Baughman R, Cordier JF, du Bois R, et al. ATS/ERS/WASOG statement on sarcoidosis. American Thoracic Society/European Respiratory Society/World Association of Sarcoidosis and other Granulomatous Disorders. Sarcoidosis Vasc Diffuse Lung Dis. 1999;16(2):149–73.
2. Judson MA. The diagnosis of sarcoidosis. Clin Chest Med. 2008;29(3):415–27, viii.
3. Gerke AK, Hunninghake G. The immunology of sarcoidosis. Clin Chest Med. 2008;29(3):379–90. vii.
4. Jouanguy E, Doffinger R, Dupuis S, Pallier A, Altare F, Casanova JL. IL-12 and IFN-gamma in host defense against mycobacteria and salmonella in mice and men. Curr Opin Immunol. 1999;11(3):346–51.
5. Baughman RP, Teirstein AS, Judson MA, Rossman MD, Yeager Jr H, Bresnitz EA, et al. Clinical characteristics of patients in a case control study of sarcoidosis. Am J Respir Crit Care Med. 2001;164(10 Pt 1):1885–9.
6. Highland KB, Retalis P, Coppage L, Schabel SI, Judson MA. Is there an anatomic explanation for chest pain in patients with pulmonary sarcoidosis? South Med J. 1997;90(9):911–4.
7. Lynch 3rd JP, Ma YL, Koss MN, White ES. Pulmonary sarcoidosis. Semin Respir Crit Care Med. 2007;28(1):53–74.
8. Baughman RP, Shipley R, Desai S, Drent M, Judson MA, Costabel U, et al. Changes in chest roentgenogram of sarcoidosis patients during a clinical trial of infliximab therapy: comparison of different methods of evaluation. Chest. 2009;136(2):526–35.
9. Scadding JG. Prognosis of intrathoracic sarcoidosis in England. A review of 136 cases after five years' observation. Br Med J. 1961;5261:1165–72.
10. Sharma OP, Johnson R. Airway obstruction in sarcoidosis. A study of 123 nonsmoking black American patients with sarcoidosis. Chest. 1988;94(2):343–6.

11. Diaz-Guzman E, Farver C, Parambil J, Culver DA. Pulmonary hypertension caused by sarcoidosis. Clin Chest Med. 2008;29(3):549–63. x.

12. Judson MA. Extrapulmonary sarcoidosis. Semin Respir Crit Care Med. 2007;28(1):83–101.

13. Ohara K, Judson MA, Baughman RP. Clinical aspects of ocular sarcoidosis. Eur Respir J Monogr. 2005;10: 188–209.

14. Jabs DA, Johns CJ. Ocular involvement in chronic sarcoidosis. Am J Ophthalmol. 1986;102(3):297–301.

15. Silver MR, Messner LV. Sarcoidosis and its ocular manifestations. J Am Optom Assoc. 1994;65(5): 321–7.

16. Ohara K, Okubo A, Kamata K, Sasaki H, Kobayashi J, Kitamura S. Transbronchial lung biopsy in the diagnosis of suspected ocular sarcoidosis. Arch Ophthalmol. 1993;111(5):642–4.

17. Takahashi T, Azuma A, Abe S, Kawanami O, Ohara K, Kudoh S. Significance of lymphocytosis in bronchoalveolar lavage in suspected ocular sarcoidosis. Eur Respir J. 2001;18(3):515–21.

18. Spaide RF, Ward DL. Conjunctival biopsy in the diagnosis of sarcoidosis. Br J Ophthalmol. 1990;74(8): 469–71.

19. Marchell RM, Thiers B, Judson MA. Sarcoidosis. In: Wolff K, Goldsmith LA, Katz SI, Gilcrist BA, Paller AS, Leffell DJ, editors. Fitzpatrick's dermatology in clinical medicine. 7th ed. New York: McGraw-Hill; 2008. p. 1484–93.

20. Stagaki E, Mountford WK, Lackland DT, Judson MA. The treatment of lupus pernio: the results of 116 treatment courses in 54 patients. Chest. 2009;135(2): 468–76.

21. Vatti R, Sharma OP. Course of asymptomatic liver involvement in sarcoidosis: role of therapy in selected cases. Sarcoidosis Vasc Diffuse Lung Dis. 1997;14(1):73–6.

22. Irani SK, Dobbins 3rd WO. Hepatic granulomas: review of 73 patients from one hospital and survey of the literature. J Clin Gastroenterol. 1979;1(2): 131–43.

23. Devaney K, Goodman ZD, Epstein MS, Zimmerman HJ, Ishak KG. Hepatic sarcoidosis. Clinicopathologic features in 100 patients. Am J Surg Pathol. 1993; 17(12):1272–80.

24. Chamuleau RA, Sprangers RL, Alberts C, Schipper ME. Sarcoidosis and chronic intrahepatic cholestasis. Neth J Med. 1985;28(10):470–6.

25. Folz SJ, Johnson CD, Swensen SJ. Abdominal manifestations of sarcoidosis in CT studies. J Comput Assist Tomogr. 1995;19(4):573–9.

26. Israel HL, Margolis ML, Rose LJ. Hepatic granulomatosis and sarcoidosis. Further observations. Dig Dis Sci. 1984;29(4):353–6.

27. Hoitsma E, Shamra OP. Neurosarcoidosis. Eur Respir J Monogr. 2005;10:164–87.

28. Zajicek JP, Scolding NJ, Foster O, Rovaris M, Evanson J, Moseley IF, et al. Central nervous system sarcoidosis – diagnosis and management. Q J Med. 1999;92(2):103–17.

29. Powers WJ, Miller EM. Sarcoidosis mimicking glioma: case report and review of intracranial sarcoid mass lesions. Neurology. 1981;31(7):907–10.

30. Christoforidis GA, Spickler EM, Recio MV, Mehta BM. MR of CNS sarcoidosis: correlation of imaging features to clinical symptoms and response to treatment. AJNR Am J Neuroradiol. 1999;20(4):655–69.

31. Kim JS, Judson MA, Donnino R, Gold M, Cooper Jr LT, Prystowsky EN, et al. Cardiac sarcoidosis. Am Heart J. 2009;157(1):9–21.

32. Yazaki Y, Isobe M, Hiroe M, Morimoto S, Hiramitsu S, Nakano T, et al. Prognostic determinants of long-term survival in Japanese patients with cardiac sarcoidosis treated with prednisone. Am J Cardiol. 2001;88(9):1006–10.

33. Chapelon-Abric C, de Zuttere D, Duhaut P, Veyssier P, Wechsler B, Huong DL, et al. Cardiac sarcoidosis: a retrospective study of 41 cases. Medicine (Baltimore). 2004;83(6):315–34.

34. Judson MA, Baughman RP, Teirstein AS, Terrin ML, Yeager Jr H. Defining organ involvement in sarcoidosis: the ACCESS proposed instrument. ACCESS Research Group. A Case Control Etiologic Study of Sarcoidosis. Sarcoidosis Vasc Diffuse Lung Dis. 1999;16(1):75–86.

35. Smedema JP, Snoep G, van Kroonenburgh MP, van Geuns RJ, Dassen WR, Gorgels AP, et al. Cardiac involvement in patients with pulmonary sarcoidosis assessed at two university medical centers in the Netherlands. Chest. 2005;128(1):30–5.

36. Glennas A, Kvien TK, Melby K, Refvem OK, Andrup O, Karstensen B, et al. Acute sarcoid arthritis: occurrence, seasonal onset, clinical features and outcome. Br J Rheumatol. 1995;34(1):45–50.

37. Torralba KD, Quismorio Jr FP. Sarcoid arthritis: a review of clinical features, pathology and therapy. Sarcoidosis Vasc Diffuse Lung Dis. 2003;20(2): 95–103.

38. Jansen TLTA, Geusens PM. Sarcoidosis: joint, muscles, and bones. Eur Respir J Monogr. 2005;10:188–209.

39. Gilman MJ, Wang KP. Transbronchial lung biopsy in sarcoidosis. An approach to determine the optimal number of biopsies. Am Rev Respir Dis. 1980;122(5): 721–4.

40. Koonitz CH, Joyner LR, Nelson RA. Transbronchial lung biopsy via the fiberoptic bronchoscope in sarcoidosis. Ann Intern Med. 1976;85(1):64–6.

41. Garwood S, Judson MA, Silvestri G, Hoda R, Fraig M, Doelken P. Endobronchial ultrasound for the diagnosis of pulmonary sarcoidosis. Chest. 2007;132(4):1298–304.

42. Nagai S, Izumi T. Bronchoalveolar lavage. Still useful in diagnosing sarcoidosis? Clin Chest Med. 1997; 18(4):787–97.

43. Muller-Quernheim J, Gaede KI, Fireman E, Zissel G. Diagnoses of chronic beryllium disease within cohorts of sarcoidosis patients. Eur Respir J. 2006;27(6):1190–5.

44. Brincker H. Granulomatous lesions of unknown significance: the GLUS syndrome. In: James D, editor. Sarcoidosis and other granulomatous disorders. New York: Marcel Dekker; 1994. p. 69–76.

45. Hunninghake GW, Gilbert S, Pueringer R, Dayton C, Floerchinger C, Helmers R, et al. Outcome of the treatment for sarcoidosis. Am J Respir Crit Care Med. 1994;149(4 Pt 1):893–8.

46. Cox CE, Donohue JF, Brown CD, Kataria YP, Judson MA. Health-related quality of life of persons with sarcoidosis. Chest. 2004;125(3):997–1004.

47. Turner GA, Lower EE, Corser BC, Gunther KL, Baughman RP. Sleep apnea in sarcoidosis. Sarcoidosis Vasc Diffuse Lung Dis. 1997;14(1):61–4.

48. Gibson GJ, Prescott RJ, Muers MF, Middleton WG, Mitchell DN, Connolly CK, et al. British Thoracic Society Sarcoidosis study: effects of long term corticosteroid treatment. Thorax. 1996;51(3):238–47.

49. Paramothayan NS, Lasserson TJ, Jones PW. Corticosteroids for pulmonary sarcoidosis. Cochrane Database Syst Rev. 2005;(2):CD001114.

50. Judson MA, Baughman RP, Thompson BW, Teirstein AS, Terrin ML, Rossman MD, et al. Two year prognosis of sarcoidosis: the ACCESS experience. Sarcoidosis Vasc Diffuse Lung Dis. 2003;20(3):204–11.

51. Goldstein DS, Williams MH. Rate of improvement of pulmonary function in sarcoidosis during treatment with corticosteroids. Thorax. 1986;41(6):473–4.

52. Spratling L, Tenholder MF, Underwood GH, Feaster BL, Requa RK. Daily vs alternate day prednisone therapy for stage II sarcoidosis. Chest. 1985;88(5):687–90.

53. Johns CJ, Michele TM. The clinical management of sarcoidosis. A 50-year experience at the Johns Hopkins Hospital. Medicine (Baltimore). 1999;78(2):65–111.

54. Baughman RP, Winget DB, Lower EE. Methotrexate is steroid sparing in acute sarcoidosis: results of a double blind, randomized trial. Sarcoidosis Vasc Diffuse Lung Dis. 2000;17(1):60–6.

55. Baltzan M, Mehta S, Kirkham TH, Cosio MG. Randomized trial of prolonged chloroquine therapy in advanced pulmonary sarcoidosis. Am J Respir Crit Care Med. 1999;160(1):192–7.

56. Lower EE, Baughman RP. Prolonged use of methotrexate for sarcoidosis. Arch Intern Med. 1995;155(8):846–51.

57. Muller-Quernheim J, Kienast K, Held M, Pfeifer S, Costabel U. Treatment of chronic sarcoidosis with an azathioprine/prednisolone regimen. Eur Respir J. 1999;14(5):1117–22.

58. McKendry RJ, Cyr M. Toxicity of methotrexate compared with azathioprine in the treatment of rheumatoid arthritis. A case-control study of 131 patients. Arch Intern Med. 1989;149(3):685–9.

59. Baughman RP, Lower EE. Leflunomide for chronic sarcoidosis. Sarcoidosis Vasc Diffuse Lung Dis. 2004;21(1):43–8.

60. Bhat P, Cervantes-Castaneda RA, Doctor PP, Anzaar F, Foster CS. Mycophenolate mofetil therapy for sarcoidosis-associated uveitis. Ocul Immunol Inflamm. 2009;17(3):185–90.

61. Lower EE, Broderick JP, Brott TG, Baughman RP. Diagnosis and management of neurological sarcoidosis. Arch Intern Med. 1997;157(16):1864–8.

62. Baughman RP, Drent M, Kavuru M, Judson MA, Costabel U, du Bois R, et al. Infliximab therapy in patients with chronic sarcoidosis and pulmonary involvement. Am J Respir Crit Care Med. 2006;174(7):795–802.

63. Judson MA. Sarcoidosis: clinical presentation, diagnosis, and approach to treatment. Am J Med Sci. 2008;335(1):26–33.

64. Romer FK. Presentation of sarcoidosis and outcome of pulmonary changes. Dan Med Bull. 1982;29(1):27–32.

65. Hillerdal G, Nou E, Osterman K, Schmeke B. Sarcoidosis: epidemiology and prognosis. A 15-year European study. Am Rev Respir Dis. 1984;130(1):29–32.

66. Baughman RP, Winget DB, Bowen EH, Lower EE. Predicting respiratory failure in sarcoidosis patients. Sarcoidosis Vasc Diffuse Lung Dis. 1997;14(2):154–8.

67. Baughman RP, Judson MA, Teirstein A, Yeager H, Rossman M, Knatterud GL, et al. Presenting characteristics as predictors of duration of treatment in sarcoidosis. Q J Med. 2006;99(5):307–15.

68. Vestbo J, Viskum K. Respiratory symptoms at presentation and long-term vital prognosis in patients with pulmonary sarcoidosis. Sarcoidosis. 1994;11(2):123–5.

69. Nagai S, Shigematsu M, Hamada K, Izumi T. Clinical courses and prognoses of pulmonary sarcoidosis. Curr Opin Pulm Med. 1999;5(5):293–8.

70. Arcasoy SM, Christie JD, Pochettino A, Rosengard BR, Blumenthal NP, Bavaria JE, et al. Characteristics and outcomes of patients with sarcoidosis listed for lung transplantation. Chest. 2001;120(3):873–80.

71. Ziegenhagen MW, Rothe ME, Schlaak M, Muller-Quernheim J. Bronchoalveolar and serological parameters reflecting the severity of sarcoidosis. Eur Respir J. 2003;21(3):407–13.

72. Mana J, Salazar A, Manresa F. Clinical factors predicting persistence of activity in sarcoidosis: a multivariate analysis of 193 cases. Respiration. 1994;61(4):219–25.

73. Neville E, Walker AN, James DG. Prognostic factors predicting the outcome of sarcoidosis: an analysis of 818 patients. Q J Med. 1983;52(208):525–33.

74. Gottlieb JE, Israel HL, Steiner RM, Triolo J, Patrick H. Outcome in sarcoidosis. The relationship of relapse to corticosteroid therapy. Chest. 1997;111(3):623–31.

75. Reich JM. Mortality of intrathoracic sarcoidosis in referral vs population-based settings: influence of stage, ethnicity, and corticosteroid therapy. Chest. 2002;121(1):32–9.

76. Gribbin J, Hubbard RB, Le Jeune I, Smith CJ, West J, Tata LJ. Incidence and mortality of idiopathic pulmonary fibrosis and sarcoidosis in the UK. Thorax. 2006;61(11):980–5.

77. Grunewald J, Eklund A. Lofgren's syndrome: human leukocyte antigen strongly influence the disease course. Am J Respir Crit Care Med. 2009;179(4):307–12.

78. Pietinalho A, Tukiainen P, Haahtela T, Persson T, Selroos O. Early treatment of stage II sarcoidosis improves 5-year pulmonary function. Chest. 2002;121(1):24–31.

Idiopathic Pulmonary Fibrosis

10

Joseph P. Lynch III and John A. Belperio

Abstract

Idiopathic pulmonary fibrosis (IPF) is a specific clinicopathologic syndrome presenting in older adults with the predominant features: dyspnea, dry cough, restrictive defect on pulmonary function tests (PFTs), hypoxemia, characteristic abnormalities on high-resolution thin section computed tomographic (HRCT) scans, usual interstitial pneumonitis (UIP) pattern on lung biopsy. Surgical lung biopsy is the gold standard of diagnosis, but the diagnosis can be established in some cases by HRCT, provided the clinical features are consistent. The cause of IPF is unknown. However, IPF is more common in adults >60 years old, smokers (current or ex), and patients with specific occupational or noxious exposures. Familial IPF, associated with several distinct genetic mutations, accounts for 1.5–3% of cases. Unfortunately, the prognosis is poor, and most patients die of respiratory failure within 3–6 years of diagnosis. However, the course is highly variable. In some patients, the disease is fulminant, progressing to lethal respiratory failure within months, whereas the course may be indolent, spanning >5 years in some patients. Therapy has not been proven to alter the course of the disease or influence mortality, but recent studies with pirfenidone and tyrosine kinase inhibitors are promising. Lung transplantation is the best therapeutic option, but is limited to selected patients with severe, life-threatening disease and no contraindications to transplant.

Keywords

Idiopathic pulmonary fibrosis • Cryptogenic fibrosing alveolitis • Usual interstitial pneumonia • Idiopathic interstitial pneumonia • Honeycombing

J.P. Lynch III, MD (✉) • J.A. Belperio, MD
Division of Pulmonary and Critical Care Medicine,
David Geffen School of Medicine at UCLA,
Los Angeles, CA, USA
e-mail: jplynch@mednet.ucla.edu

R.P. Baughman and R.M. du Bois (eds.), *Diffuse Lung Disease: A Practical Approach*,
DOI 10.1007/978-1-4419-9771-5_10, © Springer Science+Business Media, LLC 2012

Idiopathic pulmonary fibrosis (IPF) is a specific clinicopathologic syndrome presenting in older adults and associated with the following features: dyspnea, dry cough, restrictive defect on pulmonary function tests (PFTs), hypoxemia (at rest or with exercise), characteristic abnormalities on thin section high-resolution computed tomographic (HRCT) scans, the presence of usual interstitial pneumonitis (UIP) pattern on lung biopsy or CT, a progressive course [1, 2]. The terms IPF and cryptogenic fibrosing alveolitis (CFA) are synonymous [1]. IPF is associated with the *histopathological pattern* of UIP [1–4], but UIP pattern can also be found in other diseases (e.g., connective tissue disease (CTD), asbestosis, diverse occupational, environmental, or drug exposures) [1, 5]. Thus, the diagnosis of IPF can be established only when these and other alternative etiologies have been excluded [1]. IPF is the most common of the idiopathic interstitial pneumonias (IIPs), constituting 47–71% of cases [2, 6]. Other IIPs (e.g., respiratory bronchiolitis interstitial lung disease (RBILD), desquamative interstitial pneumonia (DIP), acute interstitial pneumonia (AIP), lymphoid interstitial pneumonia (LIP), nonspecific interstitial pneumonia (NSIP), and cryptogenic organizing pneumonia (COP)) are distinct entities, with marked differences in prognosis and responsiveness to therapy [1, 3, 4]. These entities are discussed elsewhere in this book. In this review, we restrict our discussion to idiopathic UIP.

A *definitive* diagnosis of IPF requires the demonstration of UIP by surgical lung biopsy (SLB) unless the HRCT features are classified as "definite" according to the recently published ATS/ERS/JRS/ALAT guidelines on IPF [1a, 3]. Because of small sample size and disease heterogeneity, transbronchial lung biopsies or percutaneous needle biopsies are *not* adequate to diagnose UIP [1, 3]. However, SLB is expensive and has potential morbidity, and many clinicians are reluctant to recommend SLB for patients with suspected IPF. In clinical practice, SLB is performed in <30% of patients with IPF [2, 7]. Currently, many clinicians rely upon HRCT to corroborate the diagnosis of UIP [1, 8, 9]. SLBs are performed primarily in patients manifesting atypical or indeterminate patterns on CT [8, 10, 11].

Table 10.1 Histopathology of usual interstitial pneumonia

Cardinal features
Geographic and temporal heterogeneity
Alternating zones of normal and abnormal lung
Predilection for peripheral (subpleural) and basilar regions
Fibroblastic foci
Excessive collagen and extracellular matrix
Honeycomb change

Additional features
Smooth muscle hypertrophy
Metaplasia and hyperplasia of type II pneumocytes
Destroyed and disrupted alveolar architecture
Traction bronchiectasis and bronchioloectasis
Secondary pulmonary hypertension

What Are the Characteristic Histopathological Features of UIP?

The cardinal histopathological findings of UIP include: geographic and temporal heterogeneity, alternating zones of normal and abnormal lung, predilection for peripheral (subpleural) and basilar regions, fibroblastic foci (aggregates of proliferating fibroblasts and myofibroblasts), excessive collagen and extracellular matrix (ECM), honeycomb change (HC) [3] (Table 10.1). Additional features include: smooth muscle hypertrophy, metaplasia and hyperplasia of type II pneumocytes, destroyed and disrupted alveolar architecture, traction bronchiectasis and bronchioloectasis, secondary pulmonary hypertensive changes [3]. Histopathological features of UIP are discussed by Drs. Colby and Leslie elsewhere in this book and will not be further addressed here.

Clinical Features of UIP

Cardinal features of UIP include dry cough, exertional dyspnea, end-inspiratory velcro rales, diffuse parenchymal infiltrates on chest radiographs, honeycomb cysts on HRCT scans, a restrictive defect on PFTs, and impaired oxygenation [1, 2] (Table 10.2). Physical examination reveals crackles in >80% of patients with UIP, and clubbing in 20–50% [1, 2, 6]. IPF/UIP

Table 10.2 Clinical features of idiopathic pulmonary fibrosis

Shortness of breath, exercise limitation
Cough
Age > 50 years
Crackles on physical examination (>80%)
Clubbing on physical examination (>20–50%)
Restrictive defect (reduced lung volumes) on pulmonary function tests
Hypoxemia (at rest or with exercise)
Characteristic HRCT scan

progresses inexorably over months to years [1, 2, 6]. Extrapulmonary involvement does not occur [6] and should suggest other disorders (particularly CTD-associated pulmonary fibrosis) [12]. However, certain diseases such as ischemic cardiac disease [13, 14], deep venous thrombosis [13], diabetes mellitus [15], and gastroesophageal reflux (GER) [16] are more common in patients with IPF.

Laboratory studies are nonspecific. Elevations in the erythrocyte sedimentation rate occur in 60–90% of patients with IPF; circulating antinuclear antibodies (ANAs) or rheumatoid factor is detected in 10–26% [1, 6, 17]. Two recent retrospective studies cited circulating antineutrophil cytoplasmic antibodies (ANCAs) in a distinct minority of patients with IPF [18, 19]. None of these serological findings correlate with extent or severity of disease or predict prognosis [2, 6]. However, for new cases of *suspected* IPF, we obtain serologies for CTD [e.g., ANA and antibodies to SSA, SSB, Scl-70 (scleroderma), Sm, RNP, Jo-1, double stranded DNA] [5, 12, 20] and hypersensitivity pneumonitis (HP) to rule out those disorders as treatment and prognosis may differ from IPF.

Elevations of the glycoprotein KL-6 [21] and lung surfactant proteins (SP)-A and -D [22] have been noted in serum and bronchoalveolar lavage fluid (BALF) in patients with IPF, and may have prognostic value. These assays are available in only a few research laboratories, and additional studies are required to assess their specificity and clinical role.

Clinical Course and Prognosis

The clinical course of IPF is heterogeneous, but most patients worsen gradually (over months to years) [2]. Mean survival from the onset of symptoms is 3–5 years [2, 6, 8, 23–25]. However, the course is highly variable, and some patients remain stable for years [2, 6, 26]. In others, the course is rapid, with fatal respiratory failure evolving over a few months [27]. Additionally, some patients have gradual progression over years, followed by acute exacerbations, associated with abrupt and often fatal hypoxemic respiratory failure [26, 28]. Spontaneous remissions do not occur [2, 6]. Ten-year survival is less than 15% [2, 6, 23, 24, 29, 30].

The major cause of death is respiratory failure [31, 32]. Surveys of IPF patients in the UK and USA noted that progression of lung disease accounted for 72% [32] and 60% [33] of deaths, respectively. Other causes include pulmonary embolism [31], cardiac failure, cerebrovascular accidents (primarily in the elderly), and lung cancer [31, 34]. Lung cancer occurs in 4–13% of patients with IPF [2, 34]. The risk is higher in smokers, but the heightened risk of lung cancer is not solely due to the effects of cigarette smoking [34].

Acute Exacerbations of IPF

A subset of patients with IPF develop an accelerated course often as a terminal event, with features of diffuse alveolar damage (DAD) or organizing pneumonia on lung biopsy or autopsy [28, 35]. This syndrome, termed "acute exacerbation of IPF," is indistinguishable from idiopathic AIP [36], and is similar to acute respiratory distress syndrome (ARDS). The factors responsible for this accelerated phase of IPF are unknown, but viral infections, high concentrations of oxygen, or drug reactions are plausible etiologic factors [28, 36]. Although this syndrome is usually fatal, some patients respond dramatically to high dose corticosteroids (e.g., pulse methylprednisolone) [28, 35].

Incidence and Epidemiology of IPF

IPF is rare; depending upon criteria used to define IPF, overall rates (per 100,000) range from 14.0 to 42.7 (prevalence) and from 6.8 to 16.3 (incidence) [1, 33, 37, 38]. The incidence of IPF increased progressively in the UK between 1991 and 2003 [38]. Similarly, in the USA, deaths attributed to pulmonary fibrosis increased significantly from 1992 to 2003 (>28% increase) [33]. IPF typically affects older adults, with peak onset after the sixth decade of life; there is a slight male predominance [1, 33, 37, 38]. IPF is more common in current or former smokers [11, 39–41]. The incidence of IPF and mortality rates is markedly higher in the elderly. A retrospective study in the USA cited a prevalence (per 100,000) of 4.0 among persons aged 18–34 years and 227 among those 75 years or older [37]. In the USA, projected deaths due to IPF (per million) in 2008 were as follows: 18 (ages 45–54), 71 (age 55–64), 306 (age 65–74), 827 (age 75–84), 1,380 (age > 85) [33]. Despite its rarity, IPF accounts for more than 16,000 deaths annually in the USA [33]. Interestingly, mortality rates from IPF exhibit a seasonal variation, with the highest rates in the winter months [42]. In the USA, mortality rates from IPF are climbing more rapidly in women than men [33], possibly reflecting the impact of cigarette smoking. IPF is rare in children [except in kindreds with surfactant protein C (SFPC) mutations] [43].

Epidemiology

Environmental factors likely play a contributory role [39]. Exposure to or inhalation of minerals, dusts, organic solvents, urban pollution, or cigarette smoke has been associated with an increased risk for IPF in some studies [44]. A meta-analysis of six case–control studies found six exposures associated with IPF: ever smoking, agriculture farming, livestock, wood dust, metal dust, stone/sand [39]. Interstitial lung disease (ILD) is an occupational disease in coal miners, sandblasters, and workers exposed to asbestos, tungsten carbide,

beryllium, and other metals [44], suggesting that at least some cases of "idiopathic" UIP represent pneumoconioses. The considerable variability that exists in the development of pulmonary fibrosis among workers exposed to similar concentrations of fibrogenic/organic dusts implies that genetic factors likely modulate the lung injury [39].

Infections may trigger exacerbations of IPF [44]. Epstein–Barr virus (EBV), cytomegalovirus (CMV), human herpes virus (HHV-8), or hepatitis C have been considered as *possible* agents in the pathogenesis of IPF, but the role of these (or other infectious agents) remains conjectural [44].

Chronic aspiration secondary to GER has been suggested as a risk factor for IPF [16], but a causal relationship between acid aspiration and IPF remains controversial. Esophageal reflux has been noted in more than two-thirds of patients with IPF awaiting lung transplant (LT) [16, 45]. Aspiration of stomach contents may cause lung injury and fibrosis [44]. Among LT recipients (with or without IPF), GER can cause allograft injury [46] and appears to be a risk factor for bronchiolitis obliterans syndrome (BOS) [46, 47]. In a small series of patients with early IPF, aggressive treatment of GER was associated with stabilization or improvement of lung function [45]. Additional studies are required to assess the role of GER or aspiration in the pathogenesis or progression of IPF and therapeutic strategies to prevent or reduce GER.

Genetics

Familial IPF, which accounts for 0.5–3% of cases of IPF, is indistinguishable from nonfamilial forms, except patients tend to be younger with the familial variant [40, 41, 48, 49]. Progression of early asymptomatic ILD to symptomatic IPF may occur over a span of decades [40]. An autosomal dominant trait with variable penetrance is suspected in most, but not all, cases [41, 48, 49]. In some patients, genetic polymorphisms for interleukin-1 receptor antagonist (IL-1ra) and tumor necrosis factor-α (TNF-α) may be important in determining risk [48]. Mutations in SFPC genes have been associated with familial interstitial pneumonitis (FIP) that includes UIP, NSIP, and other histological variants [43]. Further, germ line mutations in the genes encoding telomerase reverse transcriptase (hTERT) and telomerase RNA (hTR) were implicated in dyskeratosis congenita, a rare hereditary disorder associated with pulmonary fibrosis and aplastic anemia [50]. These mutations result in telomere shortening, which has been implicated in age-related disease. Interestingly, older age and smoking also cause telomere shortening [50]. Further, short telomeres were more common in FIP and sporadic IPF compared to controls, even when mutations in hTERT and hTR were lacking [51, 52]. Pulmonary fibrosis may also complicate diverse genetic disorders such as Hermansky–Pudlak syndrome [48], familial hypocalciuric hypercalcemia [49], neurofibromatosis [49], etc. IPF occurs in Caucasians and in nonwhites; prevalence among different ethnic groups has not been studied [1]. A retrospective study of IPF in New Zealand cited a lower incidence in those of Maori or Polynesian descent than in those of European descent [53].

Differences in susceptibility to fibrogenic agents may reflect genetic polymorphisms [49]. Animal models involving different inbred strains of rodents demonstrate dramatic variability in the lung inflammatory/fibrotic response to injurious agents. We believe that IPF is a heterogeneous disorder caused by a number of environmental/occupational exposures *in combination with* genetic predispositions.

Radiographic Manifestations of IPF

Conventional Chest Radiographs

Chest radiographs in IPF typically reveal diffuse, bilateral interstitial or reticulonodular infiltrates, with a predilection for basilar and peripheral (subpleural) regions [2, 54]. The proclivity for peripheral lung zones is best demonstrated by HRCT [9] (Figs. 10.1–10.5). As the disease progresses, lung volumes shrink. Intrathoracic lymphadenopathy or pleural thickening is not evident on chest radiographs, but may be noted

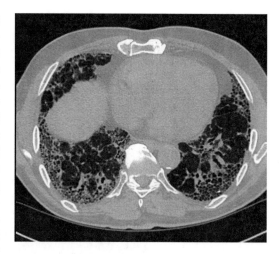

Fig. 10.1 Usual interstitial pneumonia. HRCT scan shows extensive peripheral (subpleural) honeycomb change. No significant ground-glass opacities

on CT scans [9]. Similar radiographic features are observed in asbestosis and CTD-associated pulmonary fibrosis [5, 9]. Chest radiographs have limited prognostic value, but serial radiographs (including old films) may gauge the pace and evolution of the disease.

High Resolution Thin Section CT Scan

Thin section high-resolution computed tomographic (CT) scans are invaluable to diagnose and stage IPF [8, 9, 54]. HRCT can assess the nature and extent of parenchymal abnormalities, narrow the differential diagnosis, and in some patients, substantiate a specific diagnosis, obviating the need for SLB.

How Reliable Is CT to Establish the Diagnosis of UIP?

Cardinal features of UIP on HRCT scan include: heterogeneous, "patchy" involvement; predilection for peripheral (subpleural) and basilar regions; HC; coarse reticular opacities (interlobular and intralobular septal lines); traction bronchiectasis or bronchioloectasis; minimal or no ground-glass opacities (GGOs) [8, 9, 54] (Table 10.3). The 2011 guidelines suggest that the presence of four features:

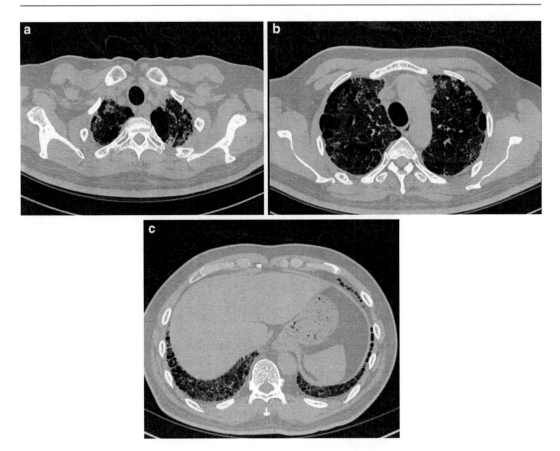

Fig. 10.2 Usual interstitial pneumonia. (**a**) HRCT scan at the level of the apices shows some focal emphysematous changes as well as a few honeycomb cysts. (**b**) HRCT from the same patient at the level of the aortic arch shows well-defined subpleural honeycomb change. Note the dilated bronchi, consistent with traction bronchiectasis. (**c**) HRCT scan from the same patient. Note classical subpleural location of the honeycomb change

subpleural, basally predominant disease; reticular abnormality; honeycombing with or without traction bronchiectasis and the absence of features listed as inconsistent with a UIP pattern allow a definitive diagnosis of a UIP pattern to be made without the need for surgical biopsy [1a]. With advanced disease, distortion, small lung volumes, and pulmonary hypertensive changes may be observed [9]. Zones of emphysema may be found in smokers [9]. Pleural involvement is not found. HC is a key feature discriminating UIP from other interstitial pneumonias [8, 9, 54]. However, CT features of UIP and NSIP overlap, and distinguishing these entities may be difficult [8, 10]. Further, classical CT features of UIP are present in only 37–67% of patients with histologically confirmed UIP [8–10]. CT scans that are "atypical" or "indeterminate" may represent UIP, NSIP, or other histological variants [8, 10].

Differential Diagnosis

Extensive GGO is *not* a feature of IPF, and suggests an alternative diagnosis such as DIP, NSIP, LIP, COP, HP, pulmonary alveolar proteinosis, etc.) [3, 4, 54]. In contrast, HC is a cardinal feature of UIP and is rare in other IIPs [8, 9]. Cystic radiolucencies may be observed in other disorders (e.g., Langerhans cell granulomatosis, sarcoidosis, lymphangioleiomyomatosis (LAM), pneumoconiosis, etc.), but the distribution of lesions and presence of concomitant abnormalities can differentiate these disorders from UIP [9, 54].

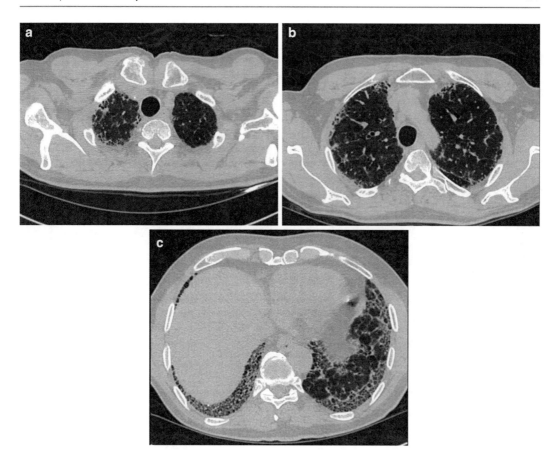

Fig. 10.3 Usual interstitial pneumonia. (**a**) HRCT at the level of the apices shows a few honeycomb cysts and thickened interlobular septa. (**b**) HRCT scan from the same patient at the level of the upper lobes. Note peripheral (subpleural) distribution of honeycomb change. (**c**) HRCT from the same patient at the level of the *lower lobes*. Subpleural (peripheral) distribution of the disease process is evident

PFTs (Including Exercise Tests) in IPF

Characteristic physiologic aberrations in UIP include: reduced lung volumes, normal or increased expiratory flow rates, increased forced expiratory volume in 1 s (FEV_1)/forced vital capacity (FVC) ratio, reduced diffusing capacity for carbon monoxide (DL_{CO}), hypoxemia or widened alveolar-arterial paO_2 gradient [$D(A-aO_2)$]) which is accentuated by exercise, reduced lung compliance, downward and rightward shift of the static expiratory pressure–volume curve, abnormalities on cardiopulmonary exercise tests (CPETs) [2] (Table 10.4). Impairments in gas exchange (i.e., DL_{CO}) and oxygenation may be evident early in the course of the disease, even when spirometry and lung volumes are normal [2].

A restrictive ventilatory defect, with reduced total lung capacity (TLC), is characteristic of IPF, but lung volumes may be normal if emphysema coexists [2]. Lung volumes (e.g., TLC, FVC) are typically higher in smokers (current or former) with IPF compared to nonsmokers [2]. When emphysema coexists, DL_{CO} and oxygenation are disproportionately reduced [2, 55]. CPET demonstrates hypoxemia, widened A-aO_2 gradient, submaximal exercise endurance, reduced oxygen consumption (VO_2), high respiratory frequency, low tidal volume (V_T) breathing pattern, increased dead space (V_D/V_T), increased minute ventilation for the level of VO_2, and a low O_2 pulse [56]. Arterial desaturation and abnormal widening of A-aO_2 gradient with exercise may be elicited with relatively simple tests, such as the 6-min

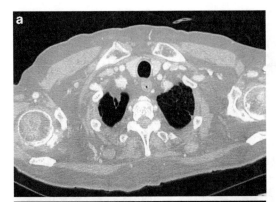

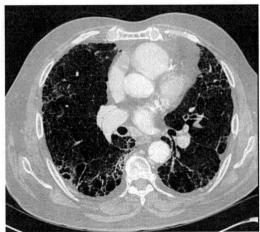

Fig. 10.5 Usual interstitial pneumonia and some areas of superimposed emphysema. HRCT scan demonstrates several emphysematous cysts as well as scattered, subpleural honeycomb cysts

Table 10.3 Usual interstitial pneumonia: HRCT features

| Heterogeneous, "patchy" involvement |
| Proclivity for peripheral (subpleural) and basilar regions |
| Reticular (linear) opacities |
| Honeycomb change |
| Minimal or no ground-glass opacities |
| Traction bronchiectasis or bronchioloectasis |
| Distortion, small lung volumes, pulmonary hypertension (advanced disease) |

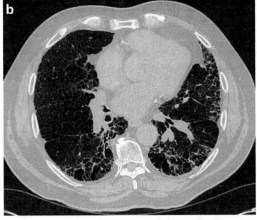

Fig. 10.4 Usual interstitial pneumonia and superimposed emphysema. (**a**) HRCT at the level of the apices shows subpleural cystic changes in the anterior segment of the *right upper lobe*, which reflects primarily paraseptal emphysema. The *upper lobes* are relatively free of interstitial changes. (**b**) HRCT from the same patient at the *lower lobes*. Extensive bilateral honeycomb change is evident. Geographic heterogeneity is present. Areas of honeycomb change are interspersed with areas of relatively normal lung. Note the peripheral (subpleural) distribution

Table 10.4 Physiologic aberrations in IPF/UIP

| Reduced lung volumes (vital capacity, total lung capacity) |
| Normal or increased expiratory flow rates |
| Increased FEV_1/FVC ratio |
| Reduced DL_{CO} |
| Widened alveolar-arterial O_2 gradient (accentuated with exercise) |
| Reduced lung compliance |
| Downward and rightward shift of the static expiratory pressure–volume curve |
| Abnormalities on cardiopulmonary exercise tests (CPET) |

walk test (6MWT) [57]. Several mechanisms are responsible for exercise-induced desaturation including: ventilation–perfusion (V/Q) mismatching, O_2 diffusing limitation, and low mixed venous pO_2 [56]. Supplemental O_2 during exercise may improve exercise performance and reduce strain to the myocardium. Dyspnea is a cardinal symptom of IPF and profoundly limits exercise performance. Other nonpulmonary factors which limit exercise performance include: deconditioning, peripheral muscle dysfunction, and nutritional status [56].

Pulmonary Arterial Hypertension

Pulmonary arterial hypertension (PAH) has been reported in 28–84% of patients with advanced IPF [58–61]. Correlations of physiological parameters with PAH are imprecise [58–60].

However, PAH is more often present when DL_{CO} is severely reduced or hypoxemia is present [59, 60]. PAH worsens as IPF progresses [62]. Transthoracic echocardiography (TTE) is a surrogate marker of PAH. Estimates of systolic pulmonary arterial pressure (sPAP) and size and functional status of the right ventricle (RV) by TTE are useful to predict PAH. In one study of 88 IPF patients, sPAP (estimated by TTE) correlated inversely with DL_{CO} and paO_2 and was an independent predictor of mortality [58]. Median survival rates according to sPAP were as follows: sPAP < 35 mmHg, 4.8 years; sPAP ≥ 36 < 50 mmHg, 4.1 years; sPAP ≥ 50 mmHg, 0.7 years [58]. In a cohort of 110 patients with IPF in Mexico, estimated sPAP ≥ 75 mmHg was an independent predictor of mortality [hazard ratio (HR) 2.25] [55]. In another study of 79 patients with IPF, PAH [defined as mean PAP (mPAP) > 25 mm by right heart catheterization (RHC)] was associated with increased 1-year mortality (28%) compared to 5.5% mortality without PAH [63]. Given the prognostic importance of PAH, we perform TTE in patients with moderate to severe IPF or those requiring supplemental oxygen. However, TTE may be unreliable in some patients, either by inability to estimate sPAP or adequately image the RV [61, 64]. In addition, specificities and negative predictive values of TTE are suboptimal [61, 64]. Given the limitations of TTE, RHC may be considered for selected IPF patients exhibiting O_2 desaturation or severe derangements in DL_{CO} (<35% predicted). However, data regarding therapy of PAH complicating IPF are limited. Anecdotal responses to prostanoids or sildenafil were cited in small nonrandomized studies [65] but survival benefit has not been examined [61].

Predictors of Survival in IPF/UIP

Median survival from the diagnosis of UIP ranges from 2 to 4 years in various studies. Advanced age [1, 17, 23, 30, 66] and male gender [1, 23, 29] were associated with a worse prognosis (higher mortality) in most studies. Interestingly, three studies cited improved survival among current or former smokers with UIP compared to never

smokers [29, 30, 67]. However, others found no such effect [68, 69]. The apparent "protective effect" of cigarette smoking may relate to inhibitory effects of cigarette smoke on lung fibroblast proliferation and chemotaxis [2]. A recent study of 249 patients with IPF noted that survival was improved in nonsmokers compared to former or current smokers after adjustment for composite physiologic index (CPI) levels [11]. In that study, current smokers had less severe disease at presentation and represented a "healthy smoker" effect. Interestingly, the concomitant presence of emphysema had no influence on survival. A recent retrospective study from Mexico cited a lower median survival time among patients with IPF and coexistent emphysema compared to IPF without emphysema (25 vs. 34 months, respectively) [55].

Prognostic Value of Histological Features

Early studies of IPF or CFA suggested that prognosis and responsiveness to therapy were improved when SLB displayed "cellularity" (as opposed to severe fibrosis) [1, 70]. In retrospect, these early studies almost certainly included IIPs other than UIP [3]. Among patients with IIPs, the finding of UIP on SLB is a robust and single most important factor influencing mortality [10, 29].

Predictive Value of PFTs (Including Exercise Tests)

Not surprisingly, severe derangements in PFTs or oxygenation predict a worse prognosis (lower survival) in patients with IPF [2, 6]. Numerous studies cited higher mortality rates when DL_{CO} or lung volumes were severely impaired [2, 24, 71]. The "cut-off" points predicting higher mortality vary considerably. Mortality increases when FVC falls below 60% of predicted values or when DL_{CO} is <30–40% predicted [2, 6, 24, 55]. Changes in TLC are less predictive of prognosis or survival [2, 6].

The relationship between any single physiologic variable and prognosis is complex and no single parameter can reliably predict prognosis in individual patients. Further, disparate results have been reported from different centers. In four studies, the following parameters correlated with mortality: % predicted FVC and widened A-aO$_2$ gradient [72], FVC < 50% predicted [55], reduced lung volumes and abnormal oxygenation during maximal exercise [30], multistage paO$_2$ on CPET (p = 0.006) [67]. British investigators examined 2-year survival among a cohort of 115 IPF patients awaiting LT [24]. The best predictors of survival (assessed at 2 years) were: DL$_{CO}$ < 39% predicted and increased fibrosis on HRCT scan [24]. In a separate study by these investigators [66], 106 nonsmokers with IPF were prospectively followed. By univariate analysis, the following parameters predicted survival: age; FEV$_1$; FVC, DL$_{CO}$, paO$_2$; O$_2$ saturation; HRCT fibrosis score; clearance of inhaled technetium ^{99}m-diethylenetriamine penta-acetic acid (^{99}mTc-DTPA) from the lungs ($t_{0.5}$) [66]. By multivariate analysis, the following parameters were independent predictors of survival: ($t_{0.5}$), percent predicted TLC, percent predicted DL$_{CO}$, age. Inclusion of other PFT or CT scores did not improve the model. Although it is intuitively obvious that severe impairment in PFTs or oxygenation predicts higher mortality, *statistical correlations* in large patient cohorts are not readily applicable to *individual* patients.

Change in pulmonary functional parameters over time may be prognostically useful. However, variability among PFTs confounds interpretation. Measurement of FVC is less variable than TLC or DL$_{CO}$ [2] and is best suited for serial measurements. Improvement or stability in VC or DL$_{CO}$ with therapy is associated with improved prognosis in patients with IPF [2, 73]. Conversely, deterioration in VC or DL$_{CO}$ at 3 or 6 months, 1 year, or later time points predicts a worse survival [2, 73–75]. In a retrospective study, serial PFTs were performed in 80 patients with IPF [73]. By multivariate analysis, >10% decrease in FVC at 6 months was an independent risk factor for mortality (HR, 2.47, p = 0.006) [73]. Collard et al. evaluated the prognostic value of serial clinical (dyspnea score) and physiologic parameters in 81 patients with IPF [75]. Not surprisingly, survival was worse among patients with deteriorating dyspnea scores or PFTs [FVC% predicted, P(A-aO$_2$)] at 6 or 12 months [75]. British investigators retrospectively reviewed the prognostic significance of histopathologic diagnosis, baseline PFTs, and serial trends in pulmonary functional indices (e.g., FVC, FEV$_1$, DL$_{CO}$) at 6 and 12 months in 104 patients with IIP (UIP, n = 63; fibrotic NSIP, n = 37) [74]. Survival was better in fibrotic NSIP compared with UIP (p = 0.001) but not in patients with severe functional impairment. Mortality during the first 2 years was linked solely to the severity of functional impairment at presentation (i.e., lower DL$_{CO}$ and FVC levels). The *CPI* score [72] was the strongest determinant of outcome (p < 0.001) [74]. At 6 months, serial PFTs and histopathologic diagnosis were prognostically equivalent [74]. However, at 12 months, serial PFT trends (DL$_{CO}$, FVC, FEV$_1$, CPI) predicted mortality better than any other covariates including histological pattern (all p < 0.0005). In this context, ΔDL$_{CO}$ provided the best prognostic information (2-year survival); histological pattern provided no additional prognostic value.

6-Min Walk Test

Hypoxemia at rest or with exertion is associated with heighted mortality in IPF [56, 76]. Further, 6-min walk distance (6MWD) correlates with DL$_{CO}$% predicted [24, 57] and has prognostic value. In one study of IPF patients awaiting LT, survival time was shorter among patients with 6MWD < 350 m [77]. In a subsequent study of 454 IPF patients awaiting LT, lower 6MWD was associated with increased mortality (assessed at 6 months) and was superior to FVC% predicted as a predictor of mortality [57]. Patients with 6MWD < 207 m had a more than fourfold greater mortality than those with 6MWD ≥ 207 m, even after adjustment for demographics, FVC% predicted, pulmonary hypertension, and medical comorbidities [57]. Flaherty et al. assessed the prognostic value of 6MWT in a cohort of 197 patients with IPF [76]. By multivariate analysis, 6MWD was not a reliable predictor of mortality, but the degree of desaturation during 6MWT had greater prognostic value. Patients with O_2 saturation $\leq 88\%$ during their initial 6MWT had a median survival of 3.2 years compared to 6.8 years for those with baseline $SaO_2 > 88\%$ ($p = 0.006$). Recently, a 6-min step test was advocated as another way of assessing exercise capacity and prognosis in patients with IPF or other ILDs [78]. Formal CPET provides additional data including measurement of maximal oxygen uptake (VO_2), an integrated measure of respiratory, cardiovascular, and neuromuscular function [56]. Fell et al. evaluated VO_2 as a predictor of survival in a cohort of 117 patients with IPF [79]. Patients with baseline $VO_2 < 8.3$ ml/kg/min had an increased risk of death after adjusting for age, smoking status, FVC, and DL_{CO}. Further, VO_2 was a stronger predictor than desaturation $< 88\%$ on 6MWT. However VO_2 did not predict survival when examined as a continuous variable. However, CPET with arterial cannulation is invasive, logistically difficult, difficult to perform for some patients, and lacks practical value.

Prognostic Value of HRCT

The extent and "pattern" of aberrations on CT have prognostic significance [8, 9, 80]. The *global extent of disease* on CT correlates roughly with severity of functional impairment in IPF [9, 72]. More importantly, the *pattern* on CT has prognostic value. Three major patterns include: GGOs, reticular or linear pattern, HC [9, 54]. GGO may reflect intra-alveolar or interstitial inflammation, fibrosis, or a combination. Reticular lines reflect fibrosis within alveolar ducts, septa, or spaces, but an inflammatory component may coexist. HC reflects irreversible destruction of alveolar walls and fibrosis [9, 54]. Reticular or "honeycomb" patterns predict a low rate of response to therapy [9, 54]. Early studies in patients with IPF (not all of whom had SLB) noted that a pattern of "predominant GGO" on CT predicted an improved prognosis and responsiveness to therapy when compared to reticular or mixed patterns [9, 54]. However, those sentinel studies may be misleading. Extensive or predominant GGO is rarely found in IPF. Patients exhibiting "predominant GGO" on CT are more likely to have NSIP than UIP [9, 54], which likely explains the more favorable prognosis in this context.

Extent of fibrosis on CT (CT-fib) correlates with functional impairment and the extent of histologic fibrosis by SLB and is an independent predictor of mortality [9, 10, 24, 29]. British investigators assessed risk factors for 2-year survival in a cohort of 115 patients with IPF awaiting LT [24]. By multivariate analysis, only CT-fib scores and DL_{CO} percent predicted were independent predictors of mortality. The risk of death increased by 106% for each unit increase in CT-fib score and 4% for every 1% decrease in DL_{CO} percent predicted [24]. Receiving operating curve (ROC) analysis gave the best fit (predictive value) using a combination of DL_{CO} and CT-fib scores. The optimal points on the ROC curves for discriminating between survivors and nonsurvivors corresponded to 39% predicted DL_{CO} and to a CT-fib score of 2.25. The curve resulting from the model yielded a sensitivity and specificity of 82% and 84%, respectively, for discriminating survivors from nonsurvivors at 2 years.

Flaherty et al. assessed the impact of CT fibrotic scores in a cohort of 168 with IIPs (UIP = 106; NSIP = 33; RBILD/DIB = 22; other = 7) [29]. A CT-fib score ≥ 2 in any lobe was highly predictive of UIP (sensitivity, 90%; specificity, 86%). The presence of an interstitial score ≥ 2 in any lobe was associated with increased mortality [relative risk (RR) of 3.35, $p = 0.02$]. The degree of fibrosis of CT is a surrogate marker for the histological pattern of UIP. CT scans that are "typical of CFA/IPF" were associated with more fibrosis and a higher mortality than "atypical" CT scans [9, 54]. In a study of 96 patients with IIP (73 had UIP and 23 had NSIP by SLB), CT scans "characteristic of UIP" (i.e., deemed as "definite" or "probable" UIP by experienced radiologists) predicted a worse survival [10]. Among patients with histologically confirmed UIP, mortality was higher when CT features were typical ("definite" or "probable") UIP compared to those with a nondiagnostic CT ($p = 0.04$) [10]. Median survival rates were 2.08 years among patients with *both* histologic *and* CT diagnosis of UIP compared to 5.76 years among patients with histologic UIP but atypical CT [10]. CT features of UIP (particularly honeycombing) likely reflect more advanced disease. A recent study retrospectively reviewed CT scans from 98 patients with a histologic diagnosis of UIP [8]. Patterns of CT scans were categorized as: (1) definite UIP, (2) probable UIP, (3) suggestive of alternative diagnosis. Mean survival rates were 45.7, 57.9, and 76.9 months, respectively, median survival rates were 34.8, 43.4, and 112 months, respectively. While these differences between groups did not achieve statistical significance, these data suggest that CT scans interpreted as definite UIP have a worse prognosis. By multivariate analysis, extent of traction bronchiectasis and fibrosis scores influenced prognosis.

Are Serial HRCT Scans Valuable?

Serial CT scans have been used to assess evolution of the disease or response to treatment in patients with IPF [2, 9, 54]. Reticular patterns or HC never regressed whereas GGO improved in 33–44% of patients [2, 9, 54]. When global extent of disease lessened on CT, it was due to reduction in the extent of GGO. Importantly, despite early regression of GGO in some patients, GGO usually progresses inexorably to a reticular pattern or HC [2, 9, 54]. Given the potential for fibrosis to evolve over months to years, the value of CT in predicting *long-term* prognosis is modest. Serial PFTs are more useful than CT scans to document the initial extent of impairment and monitor the course of the disease. Changes in CT are usually concordant with changes in FVC and DL_{CO} [2, 9, 54].

Clinical–Radiographic–Physiologic Scores

Watters et al. developed a composite score incorporating clinical (dyspnea), radiographic (chest X-rays), and physiological parameters (i.e., the clinical–radiographic–physiologic (CRP) score) as a means to more objectively monitor the course of IPF [81]. Subsequently, a modified CRP score (arbitrary total of 100 points) was

developed in a cohort of 238 patients with UIP [30]. This modified score incorporated the following variables: age (maximum 25.6 points), smoking history (maximum 13.6 points), clubbing (maximum 10.7 points), percent predicted TLC (maximum 11 points), paO_2 at maximal exercise (maximum 10.5 points), changes on chest X-rays (profusion of interstitial opacities or pulmonary hypertension) (maximum 28.6 points) [30]. In addition, an abbreviated CRP score was developed, which excluded paO_2 at maximal exercise. Importantly, the modified CRP scores predicted 5-year survival with remarkable accuracy [30]. Five-year survival rates at CRP scores of 20, 40, 60, and 80 points were 89%, 53%, 4%, and <1%, respectively. The abbreviated CRP was less accurate, but more adaptable to clinical practice. These quantitative CRP scoring systems are invaluable for research investigations, but are cumbersome for use in clinical settings.

British investigators developed a CPI incorporating CT and physiologic parameters [72]. The CPI score evaluated disease extent observed by HRCT and selected functional variables (e.g.,% predicted FVC, DL_{CO}, and FEV_1). Exercise components were not included in this index. The CPI accounts for coexisting emphysema, which may confound pulmonary functional indexes. In the CPI, both DL_{CO} and FVC were weighted positively [i.e., higher DL_{CO} or FVC resulted in lower (better) CPI scores] whereas the FEV_1 is weighted negatively [i.e., a higher FEV_1 results in a higher (i.e., worse) CPI score]. Specifically, the formula for CPI was as follows: [extent of disease on $CT = 91.0 - (0.65 \times$ percent predicted $DL_{CO}) - (0.53 \times$ percent predicted FVC) $+ (0.34 \times$ percent predicted $FEV_1)$]. CPI correlated more strongly with disease extent on CT than the individual pulmonary functional parameters. More importantly, CPI predicted mortality better than PFTs in all subgroups including 36 patients with UIP on SLB. On univariate analysis, several variables correlated with mortality including: greater extent of disease on CT ($p < 0.0005$), greater functional impairment (DL_{CO}, FVC, TLC, FEV_1, alveolar volume (VA), paO_2, A-aO_2 gradient), higher CPI scores (all had $p < 0.0005$). When compared with individual pulmonary functional components, CT disease extent was a more powerful predictor of mortality. However, the CPI index was the most powerful index and predicted survival better than the extent of disease on CT or any of the individual PFT components. Further, the CPI was compared to the original [81] or modified [30] CRP scoring systems in 30 patients with UIP who underwent CPET. The CPI was a superior predictor of outcome than the physiologic component of the original CRP score ($p = 0.02$) and the physiologic component of the modified CRP score ($p = 0.009$). Additional studies using these or similar CRP scoring systems would be of interest.

Magnetic Resonance Imaging

Dynamic magnetic resonance imaging (MRI) may discriminate inflammatory from fibrotic lesions in IIPs [82], but data are limited. The role of MRI in the diagnosis/staging of IPF needs to be further studied.

Ancillary Staging Techniques

Radionuclide scans have been used to assess prognosis in diverse ILDs. Increased intrapulmonary uptake of gallium[67] citrate (Ga[67]) may be a marker of alveolitis [83]. However, Ga[67] scans are expensive, difficult to quantitate, inconvenient (scans are performed 48 h after injection with the radioisotope), require exposure to radiation, and are nonspecific [83]. Importantly, Ga[67] scans do not predict prognosis or responsiveness to therapy and lack *practical* value in the staging or follow-up of IPF [83]. Clearance of ^{99}Tc-diethylenetriamine penta-acetate (DTPA) aerosol is accelerated in IPF and is a marker of increased lung permeability [66, 83]. Increased clearance occurs in smokers and other inflammatory lung disorders; its prognostic value is debatable [83]. Some investigators cited changes in pulmonary vascular permeability on positron emission tomographic (PET) scans in patients with IPF [83], but sensitivity, specificity, and clinical value have not been clarified. We do not employ radionuclide techniques for either the staging or follow-up of IPF.

Bronchoalveolar Lavage

Fiberoptic bronchoscopy with bronchoalveolar lavage (BAL) contributed significant insights into the pathogenesis of IPF and other ILDs but practical value is limited [1, 84]. Increases in polymorphonuclear leukocytes, eosinophils, mast cells, alveolar macrophages, and myriad cytokines are noted in BAL fluid from patients with IPF; lymphocyte numbers are usually normal [1, 84, 85]. BAL neutrophilia is present in 67–90% of patients with IPF [1, 84, 85] but does not predict prognosis or therapeutic responsiveness. By contrast, BAL lymphocytosis is rarely found in IPF and suggests an alternative diagnosis (e.g., cellular NSIP or HP) [85].

Pathogenesis of UIP

Although the etiological agent(s) in IPF has not been elucidated; two key features, that is, alveolar epithelial cell (EC) injury and dysregulation of fibroblasts (FBs) appear to be pivotal in the pathogenesis [86, 87]. Lung FBs isolated from patients with IPF demonstrate greatly enhanced proliferation and production of collagen and ECM [87]. Injury to alveolar ECs and destruction of the subepithelial basement membranes are likely early events in the pathogenesis of IPF [87]. Alveolar ECs exhibit hypertrophy/hyperplasia and ultrastructural alterations in IPF and have the potential to secrete a vast array of cytokines and growth factors [87]. Soluble mediators secreted by cells in the surrounding milieu lead to local recruitment, differentiation, and proliferation of FBs. In this context, for example, transforming growth factor-β (TGF-β), platelet-derived growth factor (PDGF), tumor necrosis factor-α (TNF-α), connective tissue growth factor (CTGF), and interleukin-8 (IL-8) likely play key roles [87]. These secreted peptides induce leukocyte influx and promote fibrosis. Historically, it was believed that inflammatory leukocytes were the source of these pro-fibrotic cytokines. However, alveolar ECs appear to be the most important source of these cytokines. Stimulation of cytokine production by injured ECs may play a critical role in initiating fibrosis in IPF; the influx of inflammatory leukocytes may be a sequela of EC activation rather than a primary event in the pathogenesis of IPF. The varying degrees of inflammation and fibrosis in the IIPs are likely dependent on, and determined by, local tissue microenvironments that are pathologically altered by a combination of host and environmental factors.

A distinctive feature of IPF/UIP is the so-called fibroblastic foci (FF), often found at the leading edge of normal and fibrotic lung [3]. It has been proposed that FF are a manifestation of ongoing lung injury [3]. Epithelial cell death is most prominent immediately adjacent to FF [3]. Further, FBs and myofibroblasts isolated from patients with IPF induce apoptosis of alveolar ECs in vitro, demonstrate increased production of collagens, increased expression of tissue inhibitors of metalloproteinases (TIMPs), and a relative decrease in collagenases [86, 87]. The combination of excessive production and deposition of ECM proteins and reduced proteolysis of ECM contributes to the fibrotic process in IPF [87]. It has been suggested that FF represent "wound healing" responses to repetitive EC injury, resulting in dysfunctional epithelial–mesenchymal cross-talk [87]. A critical aspect of this dysregulated process is the inability for alveolar ECs to regenerate, re-epithelialize, and form a normal barrier across the alveolar wall [87]. This results in a persistent "on-signal," in part mediated by chemokines, cytokines, and growth factors that activate the underlying mesenchyme. Mesenchymal cells that form FF in IPF are activated and display a contractile phenotype, commonly referred to as myofibroblasts [87]. Myofibroblast differentiation and fate is controlled by soluble growth factors such as TGF-β and matrix-derived signals [86, 87]. Under the influence of TGF-β, myofibroblasts display increased production of collagen, vimentin, β-actin, and TIMPs [86, 87]. This combination of features leads to a bias towards excessive matrix deposition and wound contraction in IFP. Greater understanding of mechanisms that mediate apoptosis of these cells, a process that has been described in the resolution of cutaneous wound healing [87], may allow development of new therapeutic targets in IPF [86].

A pro-angiogenic environment may favor fibrosis in IPF [2]. Neovascularization is a prominent feature of fibrosis in both humans and animal models [2]. Interleukin-8 (IL-8) and IFN-γ-inducible protein-10 (IP-10), members of the CXC chemokine family, affect fibrosis via angiogenic mechanisms [2]. IL-8 and its murine functional homologue macrophage inflammatory protein-2 (MIP-2) induce neutrophil and endothelial cell chemotaxis in vitro and stimulate neovascularization [2]. In contrast, IP-10 inhibits angiogenesis and endothelial cell chemotaxis [2]. In humans with IPF, IL-8 is markedly elevated in BAL fluid and serum whereas IP-10 levels in IPF lung biopsies are reduced compared to controls [2]. These findings suggest that a pro-angiogenic environment exists in IFP and may propagate fibrosis.

Several other pathophysiological processes may be critical in the abnormal lung repair process in IPF. Plausible mediators of the fibrotic process include: integrin-mediated intercellular adhesion molecules (ICAM) [86], abnormal surfactant proteins [43], imbalances in the production and/or localization of matrix metalloproteinases (MMPs) and TIMPs [87], predominance of type II cytokine profiles (particularly IL-4 and IL-13), eicosanoids, oxidative stress responses [2].

Treatment of IPF

Treatment options for IPF are still limited. Until relatively recently, randomised, double-blind, placebo-controlled (RDBPC) studies have been lacking, and optimal therapy is controversial. Historically, corticosteroids (CS) or immunosuppressive or cytotoxic agents were used, in an attempt to ablate any inflammatory component. However, inflammatory cells are *relatively* inconspicuous in IPF [88], and the degree of inflammation does not correlate with disease severity [2]. In animal models, fibrosis can occur even in the absence of neutrophils or lymphocytes [2]. Thus, it is not surprising that anti-inflammatory therapies have limited or no benefit in IPF [2, 23]. Several retrospective studies found no survival advantage with *any* form of therapy [2, 23, 24, 30]. In 2000, the ATS/ERS Consensus Statement on IPF concluded: "no data exist that adequately document any of the current treatment approaches improves survival or the quality of life for patients with IPF" [1]. More recently the 2011 ATS/ERS/JRS/ALAT guidelines stated that "the preponderance of evidence to date suggests that pharmacologic therapy for IPF is without definitive, proven benefit". Since this statement was published. three trials of therapy have been reported that suggest some treatment effect [1a, 88a, 88b, 88c]. Despite the lack of proven benefit, physicians have in the past offered treatment in an attempt to slow or prevent inexorable progression to fatal respiratory failure. In the sections that follow, we briefly discuss treatment options.

Corticosteroids

Corticosteroids were the mainstay of therapy for more than 4 decades, but are of unproven efficacy and are associated with significant toxicities [2, 23]. Early studies of patients with IPF cited response rates of 10–30% with CS (alone or combined with immunosuppressive agents), but complete or sustained remissions were rare [2, 70, 89, 90]. More importantly, many "responders" likely had IIPs other than UIP (e.g., NSIP, COP, or RBILD/DIP). In recent studies, response rates to CS among patients with histological evidence for UIP were low (0–17%) [2]. Large retrospective studies of patients with IPF showed no survival benefit with CS [2, 23, 30]. Given the potential severe toxicities associated with CS, high dose CS should *not* be used to treat IPF [1]. However, since anecdotal responses to CS are *occasionally* noted in patients with IPF, the ATS/ERS consensus statement acknowledged that *selected* patients with clinical or physiological impairment or worsening PFTs should be treated [1]. *Among patients requiring treatment*, recommended therapy was as follows: oral azathioprine (AZA) or cyclophosphamide (CP) *plus low-dose* prednisone or prednisolone [0.5 mg/kg (lean body weight per day) for 4 weeks, then 0.25 mg/kg for 8 weeks, then 0.125 mg/kg]. This represents a substantial departure from earlier regimens advocating *high-dose* prednisone (e.g., ≥1 mg/kg/day for ≥6–12 weeks)

[70, 89]. Combined therapy should be continued for 6 months in the absence of adverse effects. Treatment should be continued *beyond* 6 months only if patients improve or remain stable. These recommendations [1] reflect expert opinion, but have *not* been validated in clinical trials. We believe CS should *not* be given to patients at high risk for adverse effects (e.g., age > 70 years, osteoporosis, diabetes mellitus, extreme obesity, etc.)

Azathioprine

AZA has been used to treat IPF for more than three decades but efficacy is debatable. Only two prospective studies evaluated AZA for IPF [70, 89]. In both studies, AZA was *combined* with prednisone. In the first study, 20 patients with progressive IPF were initially treated with prednisone *alone* for 3 months [70]. At that point, AZA (3 mg/kg/day) was *added* and both agents were continued for an additional 9 months or longer. Twelve patients (60%) responded. The *independent* effect of AZA was difficult to assess since all patients received prednisone concomitantly. In a second, double-blind trial by these investigators, 27 patients with newly diagnosed, *previously untreated* IPF were randomized to receive AZA (3 mg/kg/day) *plus* high dose prednisone ($n=14$) or high dose prednisone plus placebo ($n=13$) [89]. At 1 year, PFTs (FVC, DL_{CO}, A-aO_2 gradient) were similar between groups. Vital capacity improved (>10% above baseline) in five patients receiving AZA/prednisone and in two patients receiving prednisone/placebo. DL_{CO} improved (>20% above baseline) in three patients receiving AZA/prednisone, and in two receiving prednisone/placebo. Mortality was similar at 1 year (four patients died in each group). At late follow-up (mean 9 years), 43% of AZA-treated patients had died compared to 77% in the prednisone plus placebo cohort. This survival difference was not statistically significant.

AZA has potential bone marrow, gastrointestinal toxicities, and is associated with a heightened risk for infections [91]. In contrast to cyclophosphamide, AZA does not induce bladder injury and is less oncogenic [91]. AZA (2–3 mg/kg/day) is our preferred agent for IPF patients with progressive disease. A 6-month trial is reasonable. However, in general toxicities associated with AZA outweigh benefit.

Cyclophosphamide

Cyclophosphamide (either oral or by intravenous pulse) has been used to treat IPF, but results are unimpressive [2, 30, 90]. Anecdotal responses to oral or pulse CP have been cited, but marked or sustained improvement is rarely achieved [2]. Toxicities associated with CP are substantial, and include bone marrow toxicity, opportunistic infections, infertility, bladder injury, and oncogenesis [91]. We believe that the toxicities associated with CP outweigh benefit.

Other Immunosuppressive/Cytotoxic Agents

Cyclosporin A and mycophenolate mofetil have been used to treat IPF, but data are limited to anecdotal case reports and retrospective series [2].

TNF Inhibitors

Infliximab, a chimeric anti-TNF-α antibody, has been used to treat pulmonary fibrosis complicating connective tissue disorders [92], but data affirming efficacy in IPF are lacking. Etanercept, a recombinant soluble human TNF-α receptor antagonist, has been used to treat IPF, but is of unproven benefit. A RDBPC trial in 88 patients with progressive IPF found no significant differences in predefined efficacy endpoints [i.e., $\Delta\%$ predicted FVC and DL_{CO} and $\Delta p(A-aO_2)$ gradient at rest] at 48 weeks [93]. However, a *trend* in favor of etanercept-treated patients was noted in several secondary measures. Additional trials are required before TNF-α inhibitors can be endorsed as therapy for IPF.

Colchicine

Colchicine displays antifibrotic effects in vitro and in animal models but was ineffective in IPF

in both retrospective and prospective, randomized trials [2].

N-Acetylcysteine

N-acetylcysteine (NAC) is an antioxidant that stimulates glutathione synthesis and attenuates fibrosis in animal models. A multicenter, RDBPC trial (IFIGENIA) in Europe evaluated the efficacy of oral NAC in IPF [94]. All patients received "conventional" therapy with AZA (2 mg/kg/day) plus prednisone (0.5 mg/kg/day, with taper). Patients were then randomized to oral NAC (1,800 mg/day) or placebo. At the end of 1 year, PFTs had deteriorated in both cohorts. However, the rates of decline in FVC and DL_{CO} were less in patients receiving NAC ($p<0.05$) [94]. These changes in PFTs were small (absolute difference in FVC of 4.8% and in DL_{CO} 5.1%) and of doubtful clinical significance. The benefit (if any) of NAC as therapy for IPF remains controversial. Nonetheless, NAC is inexpensive and has few side effects, making this an attractive option for IPF. A multicenter RDBPC trial sponsored by the IPFnet to address the impact of NAC in IPF is in progress.

Endothelin-1 Receptor Antagonists

Endothelin-1 (ET-1) receptor antagonists reduce collagen deposition in animal models and have a *theoretical* role to treat IPF. A multicenter RDBPC trial evaluating Bosentan Use in Interstitial Lung Disease (BUILD-1) randomized 158 IPF patients to bosentan or placebo [95]. Patients with severe pulmonary dysfunction (FVC < 50% predicted or DL_{CO} < 35% predicted) or concomitant PAH were excluded. At 12 months, 6MWD (the primary endpoint) worsened in both groups (no significant differences between groups). Mean changes from baseline in FVC at 12 months were −6.4 and −7.7% in the bosentan and placebo groups, respectively. Mean changes from baseline in DL_{CO} at 12 months were −4.3 and −5.8% in the bosentan and placebo groups, respectively. However, a *trend* in favor of bosentan was noted in the secondary endpoint [time to death or disease progression, (HR 0.64, $p = 0.12$)] [95]. In a larger study (BUILD-3), patients with mild to moderate IPF were randomized to bosentan (n=407) or placebo (n=209) for 12 months [95a]. No significant difference between groups were observed in the primary endpoint (time to IPF worsening or all-cause death).

Interferon-γ

Interferon-γ (IFN-γ) attenuates collagen synthesis by FBs in vitro and attenuates fibrosis in animal models [87]. Despite initial enthusiasm for recombinant IFN-γ-1b in humans, this agent conferred no survival benefit in two large, RDBPC trials [95b, 95c].

Indications for Therapy

Given the lack of proven efficacy of any therapeutic modality, and toxicities associated with CS or immunosuppressive agents, we reserve treatment for patients with a deteriorating course, severe or progressive symptoms, and no obvious contraindications to therapy. Empirical treatment is more attractive when surrogate markers of alveolitis are present (e.g., GGO on CT or BAL lymphocytosis). We offer treatment to *selected* patients, but only after an honest discussion with the patient and family of the low likelihood of success and the potential for significant adverse effects. For patients desiring treatment, we recommend oral AZA (2 mg/kg/day), either alone or combined with modest doses of prednisone (e.g., 0.5 mg/kg/day for 4 weeks, with gradual taper). We rarely employ CP. Prednisone is tapered to 10 mg daily (or equivalent) within 3 months. We do not recommend CS when specific contraindications or risk factors are present (e.g., obesity, diabetes mellitus, osteoporosis, age > 70 years, history of psychiatric illness, poorly controlled hypertension). Unless adverse effects necessitate early discontinuation of therapy, we treat for 6 months and reassess at that point. Treatment is continued only when improvement or stability has been demonstrated *by objective tests* (e.g., PFTs or CT). Single lung transplantation (SLT) is advised for patients with severe disease or failing medical therapy [96]. Additional novel therapies are being studied (discussed later), but therapeutic efficacy has not yet been shown.

Monitoring the Course of the Disease or Response to Therapy

The following functional measurements are essential for the initial assessment and monitoring of IPF: spirometry, DL_{CO}; 6MWT [2]. FVC is highly reproducible, and correlates better with prognosis than TLC; DL_{CO} is more variable [56]. Although authors differ regarding what constitutes "significance," the ATS/ERS defined the following changes as clinically significant: FVC or TLC ≥ 10–15%; DL_{CO} ≥ 20%; ≥4 mm increase in paO_2 saturation or >4 mm increase in paO_2 during exercise [1]. The 6MWT provides a non-invasive, simple method to assess exercise capacity and the need for supplemental O_2 [56]. We perform serial spirometry, DL_{CO}, and 6MWT at 3–4 month intervals to monitor the course of the disease. More frequent studies may be necessary in the event of clinical deterioration. More sophisticated studies (such as CPEP, measurement of compliance or elastic recoil) lack practical, clinical value [56].

Ancillary Therapies

Supplemental oxygen improves quality of life and exercise capacity in hypoxemic patients with IPF [1, 2]; impact on survival has not been studied. Pulmonary rehabilitation has been advocated to improve quality of life and exercise capacity [97], but data affirming benefit are lacking. Pulmonary hypertension may complicate advanced UIP, but the benefit of PAH-specific therapy is this context has not yet been elucidated [61]. Oral codeine or other antitussive agents may be used to control cough [1], but are of limited benefit. Opiates have been used to reduce dyspnea in patients with severe chronic lung disease, but have not been shown to be effective [2].

Lung Transplantation

SLT may be considered for patients with severe IPF [96]. Two-year survival following LT ranges from 60 to 80%; 5 year survival is 40 to 60% [98, 99]. International Society for Heart and Lung Transplant (ISHLT) Registry data for recipients with IPF cited improved survival with bilateral sequential lung transplantation (BSLT) compared to SLT ($p = 0.03$) [98]. Survival rates were similar up to 3 years, but diverged thereafter [98]. Recent data from the ISHLT cited lower survival rates at 3 months post-LT among patients with IPF (84%) or idiopathic PAH (74%) compared to cystic fibrosis (90%) and chronic obstructive pulmonary disease (COPD) (91%) [99]. Among patients surviving to 1 year, IPF and COPD had the worst long-term survival, most likely reflecting older age and comorbidities [99]. Most deaths following LT are due to chronic allograft rejection or complications of immunosuppressive therapy [99]. Due to a shortage of donor organs, waiting time for LT may be prolonged (up to 2–3 years) and many patients with IPF die while awaiting LT [96]. Unless contraindications exist, patients with severe functional impairment (e.g., FVC < 60% predicted, $DL_{CO} < 40\%$ predicted), oxygen dependency, and a deteriorating course should be listed promptly for transplantation [96].

Severe Acute Respiratory Failure Complicating IPF

Acute respiratory failure requiring mechanical ventilation (MV) may complicate IPF (either due to progression of IPF or an intercurrent illness) [100, 101]. In this context, mortality is high (>90%). Given the poor prognosis, MV is usually ill-advised in patients with severe IPF unless a potentially reversible process (e.g., pneumonia, pulmonary edema, pulmonary embolism, etc.) is diagnosed in a relatively young patient.

Novel Agents

Current therapies for IPF based upon altering the inflammatory component are only marginally effective. Major advances await the development of novel therapies that prevent fibroproliferation and/or enhance alveolar re-epithelialization [87]. Novel agents that have been tested include pirfenidone, for which there are now four reports of RDBPC, a tyrosine kinase inhibitor and anticoagulants (discussed below).

Pirfenidone

Pirfenidone (5-methyl-1-phenyl-2-[1H]-pyridone) attenuates pulmonary fibrosis in animal models, inhibits collagen synthesis in vitro, and blocks the mitogenic effect of pro-fibrotic cytokines in adult human lung FBs from IPF patients [86]. A phase II RDBPC trial compared pirfenidone to placebo (2:1 ratio) in a cohort of 107 patients with IPF [102]. The study was stopped prematurely because acute exacerbations were noted in five patients receiving placebo (14%) compared to no cases in the pirfenidone group. The primary endpoint (change in lowest O_2 saturation on 6MWT over 6 or 9 months) was not met. There were no significant differences between groups in mortality, TLC, DL_{CO}, or resting paO_2. The rate of decline in FVC at 9 months was lower in the pirfenidone group ($p = 0.037$), but differences between groups were small and of doubtful clinical significance. In a second Japanese study, 275 patients were randomised to receive either high dose (1800 mg./day), low dose (1200 mg/day) or placebo for 52 weeks. The high dose group had a lower rate of reduction in vital capacity and in the incidence of progression, defined as either death or a decrease of >10% vital capacity, compared with the placebo group [88a]. Pirfenidone has been approved for use in Japan and also in China and India. Two international placebo-controlled RDBPC evaluating pirfenidone as therapy for IPF were recently completed (InterMune, Brisbane, CA) and have been published recently. The primary end point of these

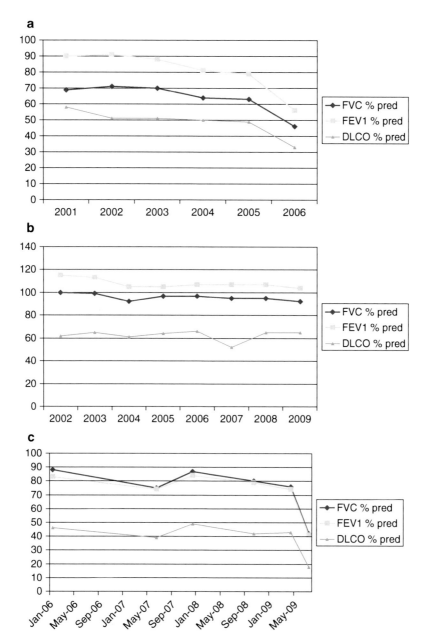

Fig. 10.6 Pulmonary function tests (PFTs) for (**a**) (case 1), (**b**) (case 2), and (**c**) (case 3). (**a**) Case 1 is a 66-year-old female who presented with cough and mild dyspnea on exertion (DOE) in March 2001. HRCT showed reticulation and honeycomb change (HC) in a peripheral and basilar distribution consistent with IPF. VATS biopsy showed temporally and spatially heterogenous pattern of interstitial fibrosis and chronic inflammation, fibroblastic foci, and focal areas of HC consistent with usual interstitial pneumonitis (UIP). Azathioprine was initiated. She developed marked hypoxemia and worsening PFTs and was listed for lung transplant (LT). Left single LT was performed in April 2007 and she has done well. (**b**) Case 2 is a 70-year-old male presented in July 2001 with mild DOE and cough. HRCT showed reticulation with a subpleural and bibasilar predominance; no ground-glass opacities or HC. PFTs revealed a mild reduction in DL_{CO} but were otherwise normal. Surgical lung biopsy (SLB) in May 2003 demonstrated temporal and spatial heterogeneity, mild chronic inflammation, frequent fibroblastic foci, and HC consistent with UIP. The patient was enrolled in the interferon-γ (IFN-γ) (Actimune) trial and remained stable. IFN-γ was discontinued in March 2007. Despite no specific therapy, he remains stable. (**c**) Case 3 is a 70-year-old male in excellent health who developed moderate DOE in October 2006. HRCT scan showed typical features of UIP. SLB in June 2007 confirmed UIP pattern. Over the next 2 years, exercise capacity worsened despite relatively stable PFTs. In May 2009, he was hospitalized with an acute exacerbation of IPF that was treated with pulse methylprednisolone. Shortly following discharge, he developed another acute exacerbation for which he was rehospitalized. In hospital, he required high flow oxygen (12 l/min) and was dyspneic at rest. He underwent single LT in July 2009

two almost identical studies that included 779 patients and that evaluated 2403 mg/day pirfenidone with placebo was change in forced vital capacity over a 72 week period. One of the studies was positive with a magnitude of effect similar to that seen in the Japanese studies. The second study did not reach its primary end point but in this and the positive study, several secondary end point indices were positive, including progression-free survival and change in distance walked in six minutes [88b]. The European Commission has recently granted marketing authorisation for Esbriet (pirfenidone) for the treatment of mild to moderate IPF in the EU.

Anticoagulants

Inflammation and vascular injury in IPF may lead to a prothrombotic state that could exacerbate lung injury [103]. Japanese investigators randomized 56 IPF patients to anticoagulants (warfarin) or placebo [104]. Three-year survival and freedom from acute exacerbations were improved in the anticoagulated group. However, dropout rate was high, and selection bias may have influenced the study. Given the risk associated with anticoagulation, additional studies involving greater numbers of patients are required before endorsing this form of therapy. Recently, a placebo-controlled study evaluating warfarin therapy for IPF conducted under the auspices of the IPFnet has been discontinued for lack of efficacy.

Tyrosine Kinase Inhibitor

A phase II RDBPC study of the effect of a tyrosine kinase inhibitor BIBF 1120 on the rate of decline of forced vital capacity has just been published [88c]. The rate of reduction of forced vital capacity was reduced by 68% with the highest dose of active drug compared with placebo and there was efficacy in a number of secondary end points including progression-free survival. In addition there was some evidence for a dose-response effect. This efficacy of the drug is now being tested in two phase III RDBPC studies.

Clinical Vignettes (See Fig. 10.6)

IPF is a heterogeneous disease, with marked differences in prognosis and disease evolution. While most patients display a gradual decline in function over months to years (case 1), some patients remain stable for years even without therapeutic intervention (case 2). Finally, a precipitous decline in lung function and marked hypoxemia may signal an acute exacerbation of IPF (case 3).

Summary

Current therapies for IPF are of limited efficacy with the exception of pirfenidone and the promise of the tyrosine kinase inhibitor BIBF 1120. In the years ahead, it will be important to identify and develop new molecular agonists or antagonists designed to interrupt or reverse the fibrotic process. Novel agents that inhibit fibrosis in vitro or in animal models and are worthy of study in future clinical trials include: angiotensin-II antagonists, platelet-activating factor receptor antagonists, inhibitors of leukocyte integrins, cytokines or proteases; agents that block IL-4, IL-12, or TGFβ; imatinib mesylate, sirolimus, keratinocyte growth factor; relaxin; lovastatin; endothelin-1 antagonists; strategies which promote matrix resorption (e.g., by enhancing the activity of MMPs) [86]. Hopefully, development of effective antifibrotic therapies may improve the outcome of what currently is a frustrating and enigmatic disease.

References

1. American Thoracic Society and the European Respiratory Society. Idiopathic pulmonary fibrosis: diagnosis and treatment. International Consensus Statement. Am J Respir Crit Care Med 2000;161: 646–64.
1a. Raghu G, Collard HR, Egan JJ, et al. ATS/ERS/JRS/ALAT Committee on Idiopathic Pulmonary Fibrosis. An official ATS/ERS/JRS/ALAT statement: idiopathic pulmonary fibrosis: evidence-based guidelines for diagnosis and management. Am J Respir Crit Care Med. 2011;183(6):788–824.

2. Lynch III J, Mahidhara RSFM, Keane MP, Zisman DA, Belperio JA. Idiopathic pulmonary fibrosis. In: Lynch III JP, editor. Interstitial pulmonary and bronchiolar disorders. New York: InformaUSA; 2008. p. 333–64. 227.

3. Katzenstein AL, Mukhopadhyay S, Myers JL. Diagnosis of usual interstitial pneumonia and distinction from other fibrosing interstitial lung diseases. Hum Pathol. 2008;39(9):1275–94.

4. American Thoracic Society/European Respiratory Society International Multidisciplinary Consensus Classification of the Idiopathic Interstitial Pneumonias. Am J Respir Crit Care Med. 2002;165:277–304.

5. Hwang JH, Misumi S, Sahin H, Brown KK, Newell JD, Lynch DA. Computed tomographic features of idiopathic fibrosing interstitial pneumonia: comparison with pulmonary fibrosis related to collagen vascular disease. J Comput Assist Tomogr. 2009;33(3):410–5.

6. Lynch 3rd JP, Saggar R, Weigt SS, Zisman DA, White ES. Usual interstitial pneumonia. Semin Respir Crit Care Med. 2006;27(6):634–51.

7. Peikert T, Daniels CE, Beebe TJ, Meyer KC, Ryu JH. Assessment of current practice in the diagnosis and therapy of idiopathic pulmonary fibrosis. Respir Med. 2008;102(9):1342–8.

8. Sumikawa H, Johkoh T, Colby TV, et al. Computed tomography findings in pathological usual interstitial pneumonia: relationship to survival. Am J Respir Crit Care Med. 2008;177(4):433–9.

9. Zisman DA, Flaherty K, Kazerooni E, Martinez F, Lynch III J. Idiopathic pulmonary fibrosis: role of high-resolution thin-section computed tomographic scanning. In: Lynch III JP, editor. Idiopathic pulmonary fibrosis. New York: Marcel Dekker; 2004. p. 237–52.

10. Flaherty KR, Thwaite E, Kazerooni EA, Gross B, et al. Radiologic vs histologic diagnosis in UIP and NSIP: survival implications. Thorax. 2003;58:143–8.

11. Antoniou KM, Hansell DM, Rubens MB, et al. Idiopathic pulmonary fibrosis: outcome in relation to smoking status. Am J Respir Crit Care Med. 2008;177(2):190–4.

12. Nunes H, Uzunhan Y, Valeyre D, Brillet PY, Kambouchner M, Wells AU. Connective tissue disease-associated interstitial lung disease. In: Lynch III JP, editor. Interstitial pulmonary and bronchiolar disorders, vol. 227. New York: InformaUSA; 2008. p. 429–86.

13. Hubbard RB, Smith C, Le Jeune I, Gribbin J, Fogarty AW. The association between idiopathic pulmonary fibrosis and vascular disease: a population-based study. Am J Respir Crit Care Med. 2008;178(12):1257–61.

14. Ponnuswamy A, Manikandan R, Sabetpour A, Keeping IM, Finnerty JP. Association between ischaemic heart disease and interstitial lung disease: a case-control study. Respir Med. 2009;103(4):503–7.

15. Gribbin J, Hubbard R, Smith C. Role of diabetes mellitus and gastro-oesophageal reflux in the aetiology of idiopathic pulmonary fibrosis. Respir Med. 2009;103(6):927–31.

16. Raghu G, Freudenberger TD, Yang S, et al. High prevalence of abnormal acid gastro-oesophageal reflux in idiopathic pulmonary fibrosis. Eur Respir J. 2006;27(1):136–42.

17. Song JW, Do KH, Kim MY, Jang SJ, Colby TV, Kim DS. Pathologic and radiologic differences between idiopathic and collagen vascular disease-related usual interstitial pneumonia. Chest. 2009;136(1):23–30.

18. Nozu T, Kondo M, Suzuki K, Tamaoki J, Nagai A. A comparison of the clinical features of ANCA-positive and ANCA-negative idiopathic pulmonary fibrosis patients. Respiration. 2009;77(4):407–15.

19. Hervier B, Pagnoux C, Agard C, et al. Pulmonary fibrosis associated with ANCA-positive vasculitides. Retrospective study of 12 cases and review of the literature. Ann Rheum Dis. 2009;68(3):404–7.

20. Kocheril SV, Appleton BE, Somers EC, et al. Comparison of disease progression and mortality of connective tissue disease-related interstitial lung disease and idiopathic interstitial pneumonia. Arthritis Rheum. 2005;53(4):549–57.

21. Yokoyama A, Kondo K, Nakajima M, et al. Prognostic value of circulating KL-6 in idiopathic pulmonary fibrosis. Respirology. 2006;11(2):164–8.

22. Takahashi H, Shiratori M, Kanai A, Chiba H, Kuroki Y, Abe S. Monitoring markers of disease activity for interstitial lung diseases with serum surfactant proteins a and D. Respirology. 2006;11(Suppl):S51–4.

23. Douglas W, Ryu J, Schroeder D. Idiopathic pulmonary fibrosis. Impact of oxygen and colchicine, prednisone, or no therapy on survival. Am J Respir Crit Care Med. 2000;161:1172–8.

24. Mogulkoc N, Brutsche MH, Bishop PW, Greaves SM, Horrocks AW, Egan JJ. Pulmonary function in idiopathic pulmonary fibrosis and referral for lung transplantation. Am J Respir Crit Care Med. 2001;164(1):103–8.

25. Flaherty KR, Colby TV, Travis WD, et al. Fibroblastic foci in usual interstitial pneumonia: idiopathic versus collagen vascular disease. Am J Respir Crit Care Med. 2003;167(10):1410–5.

26. Martinez FJ, Safrin S, Weycker D, et al. The clinical course of patients with idiopathic pulmonary fibrosis. Ann Intern Med. 2005;142(12 Pt 1):963–7.

27. Selman M, Carrillo G, Estrada A, et al. Accelerated variant of idiopathic pulmonary fibrosis: clinical behavior and gene expression pattern. PLoS One. 2007;2(5):e482.

28. Collard HR, Moore BB, Flaherty KR, et al. Acute exacerbations of idiopathic pulmonary fibrosis. Am J Respir Crit Care Med. 2007;176(7):636–43.

29. Flaherty KR, Toews GB, Travis WD, et al. Clinical significance of histological classification of idiopathic interstitial pneumonia. Eur Respir J. 2002;19(2):275–83.

30. King Jr TE, Tooze JA, Schwarz MI, Brown KR, Cherniack RM. Predicting survival in idiopathic pulmonary fibrosis: scoring system and survival model. Am J Respir Crit Care Med. 2001;164(7):1171–81.

31. Daniels CE, Yi ES, Ryu JH. Autopsy findings in 42 consecutive patients with idiopathic pulmonary fibrosis. Eur Respir J. 2008;32(1):170–4.

32. Rudd RM, Prescott RJ, Chalmers JC, Johnston ID. British Thoracic Society Study on cryptogenic fibrosing alveolitis: response to treatment and survival. Thorax. 2007;62(1):62–6.

33. Olson AL, Swigris JJ, Lezotte DC, Norris JM, Wilson CG, Brown KK. Mortality from pulmonary fibrosis increased in the United States from 1992 to 2003. Am J Respir Crit Care Med. 2007;176(3):277–84.

34. Le Jeune I, Gribbin J, West J, Smith C, Cullinan P, Hubbard R. The incidence of cancer in patients with idiopathic pulmonary fibrosis and sarcoidosis in the UK. Respir Med. 2007;101(12):2534–40.

35. Kim DS, Park JH, Park BK, Lee JS, Nicholson AG, Colby T. Acute exacerbation of idiopathic pulmonary fibrosis: frequency and clinical features. Eur Respir J. 2006;27(1):143–50.

36. Bouros D, Nicholson AC, Polychronopoulos V, et al. Acute interstitial pneumonia. Eur Respir J. 2000;15:412–8.

37. Raghu G, Weycker D, Edelsberg J, Bradford WZ, Oster G. Incidence and prevalence of idiopathic pulmonary fibrosis. Am J Respir Crit Care Med. 2006;174(7):810–6.

38. Gribbin J, Hubbard RB, Le Jeune I, Smith CJ, West J, Tata LJ. Incidence and mortality of idiopathic pulmonary fibrosis and sarcoidosis in the UK. Thorax. 2006;61(11):980–5.

39. Taskar VS, Coultas DB. Is idiopathic pulmonary fibrosis an environmental disease? Proc Am Thorac Soc. 2006;3(4):293–8.

40. Rosas IO, Ren P, Avila NA, et al. Early interstitial lung disease in familial pulmonary fibrosis. Am J Respir Crit Care Med. 2007;176(7):698–705.

41. Steele MP, Speer MC, Loyd JE, et al. Clinical and pathologic features of familial interstitial pneumonia. Am J Respir Crit Care Med. 2005;172(9):1146–52.

42. Olson AL, Swigris JJ, Raghu G, Brown KK. Seasonal variation: mortality from pulmonary fibrosis is greatest in the winter. Chest. 2009;136(1):16–22.

43. Thomas AQ, Lane K, Phillips 3rd J, et al. Heterozygosity for a surfactant protein C gene mutation associated with usual interstitial pneumonitis and cellular nonspecific interstitial pneumonitis in one kindred. Am J Respir Crit Care Med. 2002;165(9): 1322–8.

44. Garantziotis S, Schwartz DA. Host-environment interactions in pulmonary fibrosis. Semin Respir Crit Care Med. 2006;27(6):574–80.

45. Sweet MP, Patti MG, Leard LE, et al. Gastroesophageal reflux in patients with idiopathic pulmonary fibrosis referred for lung transplantation. J Thorac Cardiovasc Surg. 2007;133(4):1078–84.

46. Blondeau K, Mertens V, Vanaudenaerde BA, et al. Gastro-oesophageal reflux and gastric aspiration in lung transplant patients with or without chronic rejection. Eur Respir J. 2008;31(4):707–13.

47. Belperio JA, Weigt SS, Fishbein MC, Lynch 3rd JP. Chronic lung allograft rejection: mechanisms and therapy. Proc Am Thorac Soc. 2009;6(1):108–21.

48. Woodhead F, du Bois RM. Genetics of ILD. In: Lynch III JP, editor. Interstitial pulmonary and bronchiolar disorders. New York: InformaUSA; 2008. p. 43–91. 227.

49. du Bois RM. Genetic factors in pulmonary fibrotic disorders. Semin Respir Crit Care Med. 2006;27(6): 581–8.

50. Armanios MY, Chen JJ, Cogan JD, et al. Telomerase mutations in families with idiopathic pulmonary fibrosis. N Engl J Med. 2007;356(13):1317–26.

51. Alder JK, Chen JJ, Lancaster L, et al. Short telomeres are a risk factor for idiopathic pulmonary fibrosis. Proc Natl Acad Sci USA. 2008;105(35):13051–6.

52. Cronkhite JT, Xing C, Raghu G, et al. Telomere shortening in familial and sporadic pulmonary fibrosis. Am J Respir Crit Care Med. 2008;178(7): 729–37.

53. Young LM, Hopkins R, Wilsher ML. Lower occurrence of idiopathic pulmonary fibrosis in Maori and Pacific Islanders. Respirology. 2006;11(4):467–70.

54. Lynch III J, Weigt S, Suh R. Thoracic imaging for diffuse ILD and bronchiolar disorders. In: Lynch III JP, editor. Interstitial pulmonary and bronchiolar disorders. New York: InformaUSA; 2008. p. 13–42. 227.

55. Mejia M, Carrillo G, Rojas-Serrano J, et al. Idiopathic pulmonary fibrosis and emphysema: decreased survival associated with severe pulmonary arterial hypertension. Chest. 2009;136(1):10–5.

56. Lama VN, Martinez FJ. Resting and exercise physiology in interstitial lung diseases. Clin Chest Med. 2004;25(3):435–53. v.

57. Lederer DJ, Arcasoy SM, Wilt JS, D'Ovidio F, Sonett JR, Kawut SM. Six-minute-walk distance predicts waiting list survival in idiopathic pulmonary fibrosis. Am J Respir Crit Care Med. 2006;174(6):659–64.

58. Nadrous HF, Pellikka PA, Krowka MJ, et al. Pulmonary hypertension in patients with idiopathic pulmonary fibrosis. Chest. 2005;128(4):2393–9.

59. Nathan SD, Shlobin OA, Ahmad S, Urbanek S, Barnett SD. Pulmonary hypertension and pulmonary function testing in idiopathic pulmonary fibrosis. Chest. 2007;131(3):657–63.

60. Zisman DA, Ross DJ, Belperio JA, et al. Prediction of pulmonary hypertension in idiopathic pulmonary fibrosis. Respir Med. 2007;101(10):2153–9.

61. Zisman DA, Belperio JA, Saggar R, Saggar R, Fishbein MC, Lynch III J. Pulmonary Hypertension Complicating Interstitial Lung Disease. In: Humbert M, Lynch III JP, editors Pulmonary hypertension. New York: InformaUSA. 2009:236; pp264–291.

62. Nathan SD, Shlobin OA, Ahmad S, et al. Serial development of pulmonary hypertension in patients with idiopathic pulmonary fibrosis. Respiration. 2008;76(3):288–94.

63. Lettieri CJ, Nathan SD, Barnett SD, Ahmad S, Shorr AF. Prevalence and outcomes of pulmonary arterial hypertension in advanced idiopathic pulmonary fibrosis. Chest. 2006;129(3):746–52.

64. Arcasoy SM, Christie JD, Ferrari VA, et al. Echocardiographic assessment of pulmonary hypertension in patients with advanced lung disease. Am J Respir Crit Care Med. 2003;167(5):735–40.

65. Collard HR, Anstrom KJ, Schwarz MI, Zisman DA. Sildenafil improves walk distance in idiopathic pulmonary fibrosis. Chest. 2007;131(3):897–9.

66. Mogulkoc N, Brutsche MH, Bishop PW, et al. Pulmonary (99 m)Tc-DTPA aerosol clearance and survival in usual interstitial pneumonia (UIP). Thorax. 2001;56(12):916–23.

67. King Jr TE, Schwarz MI, Brown K, et al. Idiopathic pulmonary fibrosis: relationship between histopathologic features and mortality. Am J Respir Crit Care Med. 2001;164(6):1025–32.

68. Nicholson AG, Colby TV, du Bois RM, Hansell DM, Wells AU. The prognostic significance of the histologic pattern of interstitial pneumonia in patients presenting with the clinical entity of cryptogenic fibrosing alveolitis. Am J Respir Crit Care Med. 2000;162(6): 2213–7.

69. Hubbard R, Johnston I, Britton J. Survival in patients with cryptogenic fibrosing alveolitis: a population-based cohort study. Chest. 1998;113(2): 396–400.

70. Winterbauer R, Hammar S, Hallman K, et al. Diffuse interstitial pneumonitis. Clinicopathologic correlations in 20 patients treated with prednisone/azathioprine. Am J Med. 1978;65:661–72.

71. Nicholson AG, Fulford LG, Colby TV, du Bois RM, Hansell DM, Wells AU. The relationship between individual histologic features and disease progression in idiopathic pulmonary fibrosis. Am J Respir Crit Care Med. 2002;166(2):173–7.

72. Wells AU, Desai SR, Rubens MB, et al. Idiopathic pulmonary fibrosis: a composite physiologic index derived from disease extent observed by computed tomography. Am J Respir Crit Care Med. 2003; 167(7):962–9.

73. Flaherty KR, Mumford JA, Murray S, et al. Prognostic implications of physiologic and radiographic changes in idiopathic interstitial pneumonia. Am J Respir Crit Care Med. 2003;168(5):543–8.

74. Latsi PI, du Bois RM, Nicholson AG, et al. Fibrotic idiopathic interstitial pneumonia: the prognostic value of longitudinal functional trends. Am J Respir Crit Care Med. 2003;168(5):531–7.

75. Collard HR, King Jr TE, Bartelson BB, Vourlekis JS, Schwarz MI, Brown KK. Changes in clinical and physiologic variables predict survival in idiopathic pulmonary fibrosis. Am J Respir Crit Care Med. 2003;168(5):538–42.

76. Flaherty KR, Andrei AC, Murray S, et al. Idiopathic pulmonary fibrosis: prognostic value of changes in physiology and six-minute-walk test. Am J Respir Crit Care Med. 2006;174(7):803–9.

77. Kawut SM, O'Shea MK, Bartels MN, Wilt JS, Sonett JR, Arcasoy SM. Exercise testing determines survival in patients with diffuse parenchymal lung disease evaluated for lung transplantation. Respir Med. 2005;99(11):1431–9.

78. Dal Corso S, Duarte SR, Neder JA, et al. A step test to assess exercise-related oxygen desaturation in interstitial lung disease. Eur Respir J. 2007;29(2): 330–6.

79. Fell CD, Liu LX, Motika C, et al. The prognostic value of cardiopulmonary exercise testing in idiopathic pulmonary fibrosis. Am J Respir Crit Care Med. 2009;179(5):402–7.

80. Lynch DA, Godwin JD, Safrin S, et al. High-resolution computed tomography in idiopathic pulmonary fibrosis: diagnosis and prognosis. Am J Respir Crit Care Med. 2005;172(4):488–93.

81. Watters L, King T, Schwarz M, Waldron J, Stanford R. A clinical, radiographic, and physiologic scoring system for the longitudinal assessment of patients with idiopathic pulmonary fibrosis. Am Rev Respir Dis. 1986;133:97–103.

82. Yi CA, Lee KS, Han J, Chung MP, Chung MJ, Shin KM. 3-T MRI for differentiating inflammation- and fibrosis-predominant lesions of usual and nonspecific interstitial pneumonia: comparison study with pathologic correlation. AJR Am J Roentgenol. 2008; 190(4):878–85.

83. Singh S, Wells A, Du Bois RM. Other imaging techniques for idiopathic interstitial pneumonias. In: Lynch III JP, editor. Idiopathic pulmonary fibrosis. New York: Marcel Dekker; 2004. p. 237–52. 185.

84. Nagai S, Handa T, Ito Y, Takeuchi M, Izumi T. Bronchoalveolar lavage in idiopathic interstitial lung diseases. Semin Respir Crit Care Med. 2007;28(5): 496–503.

85. Ohshimo S, Bonella F, Cui A, et al. Significance of bronchoalveolar lavage for the diagnosis of idiopathic pulmonary fibrosis. Am J Respir Crit Care Med. 2009;179(11):1043–7.

86. Thannickal V, Flaherty K, Hyzy R, Lynch III JP. Emerging drugs for idiopathic pulmonary fibrosis. Expert Opin Emerg Drugs. 2005;10(4):707–27.

87. Selman M, Thannickal VJ, Pardo A, Zisman DA, Martinez FJ, Lynch 3rd JP. Idiopathic pulmonary fibrosis: pathogenesis and therapeutic approaches. Drugs. 2004;64(4):405–30.

88. Katzenstein A, Myers J. Idiopathic pulmonary fibrosis. Clinical relevance of pathologic classification. Am J Respir Crit Care Med. 1998;157:1301–15.

88a. Taniguchi H, Ebina M, Kondoh Y, et al. Pirfenidone Clinical Study Group in Japan. Pirfenidone in idiopathic pulmonary fibrosis. Eur Respir J. 2010;35(4):821–9. Epub 2009 Dec 8.

88b. Noble PW, Albera C, Bradford WZ, et al. Pirfenidone in patients with idiopathic pulmonary fibrosis

(CAPACITY): two randomised trials. Lancet. 2011;377(9779):1760–9. Epub 2011 May 13.

88c. Luca Richeldi, M.D., Ph.D., Ulrich Costabel, M.D., Moises Selman, M.D., Dong Soon Kim, M.D., David M. Hansell, M.D., Efficacy of a Tyrosine Kinase Inhibitor in Idiopathic Pulmonary Fibrosis N Engl J Med 2011;365:1079–87.

89. Raghu G, Depaso W, Cain K, et al. Azathioprine combined with prednisone in the treatment of idiopathic pulmonary fibrosis: a prospective double-blind, randomized, placebo-controlled clinical trial. Am Rev Respir Dis. 1991;144:291–6.

90. Johnson M, Kwan S, Snell N, Nunn A, Darbyshire J, Turner-Warwick M. Randomized controlled trial comparing prednisolone alone with cyclophosphamide and low dose prednisolone in combination in cryptogenic fibrosing alveolitis. Thorax. 1989;44: 280–8.

91. Lynch III J, McCune J. Immunosuppressive and cytotoxic pharmacotherapy for pulmonary disorders. Am J Respir Crit Care Med. 1997;155:395–420.

92. Antoniou KM, Mamoulaki M, Malagari K, et al. Infliximab therapy in pulmonary fibrosis associated with collagen vascular disease. Clin Exp Rheumatol. 2007;25(1):23–8.

93. Raghu G, Brown KK, Costabel U, et al. Treatment of idiopathic pulmonary fibrosis with etanercept: an exploratory, placebo-controlled trial. Am J Respir Crit Care Med. 2008;178(9):948–55.

94. Demedts M, Behr J, Buhl R, et al. High-dose acetylcysteine in idiopathic pulmonary fibrosis. N Engl J Med. 2005;353(21):2229–42.

95. King Jr TE, Behr J, Brown KK, et al. BUILD-1: a randomized placebo-controlled trial of bosentan in idiopathic pulmonary fibrosis. Am J Respir Crit Care Med. 2008;177(1):75–81.

95a. King Jr TE, Brown KK, Raghu G, et al. BUILD-3: a randomized, controlled trial of bosentan in idiopathic pulmonary fibrosis. Am J Respir Crit Care Med 2011:184;92–99.

95b. Raghu G, Brown KK, Bradford WZ, et al. Idiopathic Pulmonary Fibrosis Study Group. A placebo-controlled trial of interferon gamma-1b in patients with idiopathic pulmonary fibrosis. N Engl J Med. 2004;350(2):125–33.

95c. King Jr TE, Albera C, Bradford WZ, et al. Effect of interferon gamma-1b on survival in patients with idiopathic pulmonary fibrosis (INSPIRE): a multicentre, randomised, placebo-controlled trial. Lancet. 2009;374(9685):222–8.

96. Lynch 3rd JP, Saggar R, Weigt SS, Ross DJ, Belperio JA. Overview of lung transplantation and criteria for selection of candidates. Semin Respir Crit Care Med. 2006;27(5):441–69.

97. Swigris JJ, Brown KK, Make BJ, Wamboldt FS. Pulmonary rehabilitation in idiopathic pulmonary fibrosis: a call for continued investigation. Respir Med. 2008;102(12):1675–80.

98. Trulock EP, Christie JD, Edwards LB, et al. Registry of the international society for heart and lung transplantation: twenty-fourth official adult lung and heart-lung transplantation report-2007. J Heart Lung Transplant. 2007;26(8):782–95.

99. Christie JD, Edwards LB, Aurora P, et al. Registry of the international society for heart and lung transplantation: twenty-fifth official adult lung and heart/lung transplantation report-2008. J Heart Lung Transplant. 2008;27(9):957–69.

100. Saydain G, Islam A, Afessa B, Ryu JH, Scott JP, Peters SG. Outcome of patients with idiopathic pulmonary fibrosis admitted to the intensive care unit. Am J Respir Crit Care Med. 2002;166(6): 839–42.

101. Mallick S. Outcome of patients with idiopathic pulmonary fibrosis (IPF) ventilated in intensive care unit. Respir Med. 2008;102(10):1355–9.

102. Azuma A, Nukiwa T, Tsuboi E, et al. Double-blind, placebo-controlled trial of pirfenidone in patients with idiopathic pulmonary fibrosis. Am J Respir Crit Care Med. 2005;171(9):1040–7.

103. Walter N, Collard HR, King Jr TE. Current perspectives on the treatment of idiopathic pulmonary fibrosis. Proc Am Thorac Soc. 2006;3(4):330–8.

104. Kubo H, Nakayama K, Yanai M, et al. Anticoagulant therapy for idiopathic pulmonary fibrosis. Chest. 2005;128(3):1475–82.

Nonspecific Interstitial Pneumonia

11

Kevin R. Flaherty and Fernando J. Martinez

Abstract

Nonspecific interstitial pneumonia (NSIP) describes a histopathologic pattern seen on surgical lung biopsy. A careful clinical evaluation is required to determine whether the disease is idiopathic or related to systemic diseases, drug or environmental exposures. Response to therapy and prognosis for NSIP is usually better than with idiopathic pulmonary fibrosis, although some patients can progress to death or the need for lung transplantation.

Keywords

Nonspecific interstitial pneumonia • Diagnosis • Treatment

Introduction

Nonspecific interstitial pneumonia (NSIP) describes a histopathologic pattern seen on surgical lung biopsy. A careful clinical evaluation is required to determine whether the disease is idiopathic or related to systemic diseases, drug or environmental exposures. Response to therapy and prognosis for idiopathic NSIP is usually better than with idiopathic pulmonary fibrosis, although some patients can progress to death or the need for lung transplantation.

K.R. Flaherty, MD, MS (✉) • F.J. Martinez, MD, MS
Pulmonary/Critical Care Medicine,
University of Michigan, Ann Arbor, MI, USA
e-mail: flaherty@med.umich.edu

Nomenclature

The term NSIP has been used in multiple contexts. NSIP has referred to a nonspecific histopathologic lesion in immunocompromised patients [1–6], associated with connective tissue disorders [7–19], hypersensitivity pneumonitis [20], drugs [21, 22], infection, and immunosuppression including patients with HIV [1–6]. NSIP has also been recognized in "idiopathic" cases [6, 23–26]. In 2002, NSIP was included as a "provisional" type of idiopathic interstitial pneumonia (IIP) [27]. The provisional status emphasized the uncertainty surrounding the clinical manifestations and etiology of "idiopathic" NSIP. Therefore, it has been suggested that the identification of NSIP should "…prompt the clinician to redouble efforts to find potentially causative exposures" [27]. If no etiology is identified, a diagnosis of idiopathic NSIP can be made.

R.P. Baughman and R.M. du Bois (eds.), *Diffuse Lung Disease: A Practical Approach*,
DOI 10.1007/978-1-4419-9771-5_11, © Springer Science+Business Media, LLC 2012

Pathogenesis

The understanding of the pathogenesis of idiopathic NSIP is evolving. A critical question is the potential relationship between NSIP, idiopathic pulmonary fibrosis, and its histopathologic hallmark usual interstitial pneumonia (UIP) and other idiopathic or systemic disease-related interstitial pneumonias. These relationships are still under investigation. The fact that similar exposures (connective tissue disease, CTD; hypersensitivity pneumonitis), inheritance, and genetic mutations can lead to a histological pattern of NSIP or UIP suggest a potential relationship as does the finding that individual patients can harbor histopathologic lesions of both UIP and NSIP [28–30]. The varied prognosis between idiopathic NSIP and IPF/UIP [6, 23–26] and subtle variations detected between idiopathic vs. connective tissue disease-associated manifestations [31] argues for separate disease entities.

The development of fibrotic lung disease clearly involves multiple pathways. These can include injuries to the epithelial/microvascular system, varied cytokines, gene expression, and fibroblast function. An injury model with epithelial injury and dysregulated repair has been proposed as a disease model for idiopathic pulmonary fibrosis [32] and likely plays a role in the pathogenesis of NSIP [33]. Other pathways implicated in the pathobiology of NSIP include epimorphin, a cell surface-associated protein involved in epithelial morphogenesis in embryonic organs [34], matrix metalloproteinases [34, 35], heat shock protein 47 [36], surfactant protein C [37–41], the coagulation system [42, 43], intercellular adhesion molecule-1 [44], IL-4, IL-13, IL-18, interferon-γ [33, 45–47], and the pro-fibrotic chemokine, CCL7 and CCL5 [48]. Heat shock protein 47 has been reported as higher in idiopathic NSIP compared with IPF [49] and also associated negatively on prognosis [50]. While gene transcription for transforming growth factor-β (TGF-β), connective tissue growth factor, IL-13, IL-8, and interferon-γ is higher in lung tissue from patients with UIP and idiopathic NSIP compared with controls; expression between UIP and NSIP were overall similar [51]. Levels of gene transcription for TGF-B and IL-13 correlated with subsequent change in lung function. Interestingly, pirfenidone, a potential treatment for IPF was shown to decrease the expression of HSP47 in TGF-β, stimulated cultured normal human lung fibroblasts [52].

The immune system, either in response to injury or as a potential cause of injury, is also likely involved in the pathogenesis of idiopathic NSIP. Bronchoalveolar lavage fluid from patients with NSIP often shows more lymphocytes compared with patients with IPF/UIP [9, 11, 25, 53]. Dendritic cells (DC), which play a role in the immune response through antigen presentation, have been noted in greater numbers in biopsies of patients with NSIP compared with UIP and were seen in close proximity to CD4 and CD8 lymphocytes [54].

In the end, fibroblasts are believed to be a key effector cell in fibrotic lung diseases [32]. Fibroblasts from patients with IPF seem to demonstrate increased contractility compared with fibroblasts from patients with NSIP which resembled characteristics of control fibroblasts [19]. There was no difference in contractility between NSIP and control fibroblasts. Furthermore, conditioned media from IPF fibroblasts had increased levels of TGF-β and fibronectin compared with media from NSIP or controls. IPF conditioned media was able to increase the contractility of control fibroblasts, while media from NSIP fibroblasts did not. These data suggest that fibroblast phenotype as well as other factors in the fibroblast microenvironment contribute to the fibroblast function/dysfunction in idiopathic NSIP and other IIPs.

Clinical Evaluation

The assessment of patients with suspected idiopathic NSIP requires a synthesis of clinical, radiographic, and histopathologic data. Differentiating NSIP from other IIPs is difficult and a multidisciplinary approach results in more diagnostic agreement compared with clinicians, radiologists, or pathologists working in isolation [55, 56].

Clinical Characteristics

The clinical evaluation of all patients with suspected interstitial lung disease needs to focus on first confirming that interstitial lung disease is present and second, looking for clues regarding a possible etiology (drug or environmental exposure, signs of connective tissue disease). This is particularly important for NSIP. Clinical features, such as cough and dyspnea, are nonspecific and cannot differentiate NSIP from other IIPs or systemic disease-related ILDs. Exam findings are also nonspecific with crackles being present in most cases and fever present in up to 1/3 of cases. Pulmonary physiology typically manifests with restrictive pulmonary mechanics and a decreased gas transfer. Bronchoalveolar lavage is more likely to show a predominance of lymphocytes in patients with NSIP compared with UIP [55, 56], however, this is not always the case [57, 58] and BAL cell counts cannot be utilized to differentiate NSIP from other IIPs [58]. Findings on BAL may prompt the clinician that other non-IPF diseases are present leading to further historical information and changing of initial diagnostic impressions [59].

An aggressive evaluation for an associated connective tissue disease is critical as connective tissue disease-associated interstitial lung disease is often histologically manifested as NSIP [60] (see Table 11.1). The format for such an evaluation continues to evolve but should include a comprehensive clinical evaluation for extrapulmonary features. Clinical characteristics which are of particular relevance include Raynaud's phenomenon, fever, muscle symptoms, skin changes, arthralgias, and esophageal disease. These manifestations may provide clues to specific syndromes. For example, the combination of myositis, Raynaud's phenomenon, fever, mechanic's hands, and arthralgias is consistent with the antisynthetase syndrome [60]. Raynaud's phenomenon or another equivalent manifestation of peripheral vascular disease, such as digital pitting/ ulcers/gangrene or abnormal capillaries, is typically seen in scleroderma sine scleroderma [60].

The appropriate use of serological markers may be invaluable in identifying a specific causative connective tissue process or alerting the clinician that an underlying process is present. A reasonable laboratory approach to the evaluation of a patient with NISP is enumerated in Table 11.2. Table 11.3 enumerates the prevalence rate of expression of various serological markers in various connective tissue disorders. Lab values alone cannot make a specific diagnosis and must be used along with other clinical manifestations of disease. The difficulties of this diagnostic process as applied to patients with NSIP were recently highlighted by the prospective evaluation of 28 consecutive patients with interstitial pneumonia at a tertiary medical center [15]. Investigators applied diagnostic criteria proposed for undifferentiated connective tissue disease (UCTD; Table 11.4) and noted that 88% of patients previously classified as idiopathic NSIP met criteria for UCTD. Unfortunately, the significance of the criteria for UCTD remains controversial [60, 61]. It is important to note that NSIP can be the initial presentation for patients with connective tissue disease. In a large, retrospective cohort 8/83 (10%) patients initially characterized as having idiopathic disease developed a distinct connective tissue illness [62]. Interestingly, more than half the patients had an autoantibody at initial presentation.

Radiographic Characteristics

Early studies of the high resolution computed tomography features of NSIP described primarily ground glass opacification (GGO) associated with findings of fibrosis such as volume loss, reticular pattern, and/or traction bronchiectasis (Table 11.5). Honeycomb change was less common and predictive of UIP when a predominance of GGO was absent [24, 63, 64]. The HRCT features of idiopathic NSIP compared with connective tissue disease-related NSIP have been noted to be similar [8, 9, 11, 13, 20, 23, 25, 26, 53, 57, 65–75]. A recent American Thoracic Society Project provided a detailed characterization of HRCT features from 61 patients with idiopathic NSIP (Table 11.6) [76]. The majority of patients had lower lung distribution of disease that was nearly evenly split between peripheral and diffuse axial

Table 11.1 Clinical and demographic characteristics for patients with NSIP

Nonspecific interstitial pneumonia (NSIP)

Series	Number of patients	Age in years Mean ± sd or (range)	Gender	CTD n (%)	Current or previous smoking n (%)	Symptom (%)	Symptom duration in months Mean ± or (range)	Physical exam feature (%)
Collagen vascular-associated cases included								
Katzenstein and Fiorelli [8]	64	46 (9–78)	26 Male 38 Female	10 (6)	NA	Dyspnea Cough Chest pain (8) Weight loss (11)	8 (0.25–60)	Fever (22) Wheeze (6)
Cottin et al. [9]	12	53	6 Male 6 Female	3 (25)	6 (50)	Dyspnea (100) Cough (67) Fatigue (58) Weight loss (42)	31 (1–64)	Crackles (100)
Fujita et al. [11]	24	Median 60 (44–74)	7 Male 17 Female	8 (33)	NA	Cough (87) Dyspnea (71)	3 (1–8)	Crackles (100) Clubbing (0) Fever (29)
Miki et al. [19]	5	56 (42–74)	1 Male 4 Female	3 (60)	NA	Dyspnea (100)	4 (1–9)	Crackles (100)
Douglas et al. [10]	18	NA	NA	Polymyositis/ dermatomyositis in all	NA	NA	NA	NA
Bouros et al. [7]	74 (NSIP in 62)	46 (23–69)	13 Male/61 female	Scleroderma in all	25 (33)	Dyspnea (89) Cough (35)	13 (0–60)	Crackles (85) Clubbing (3)
Yamadori et al. [13]	3	60 (50–71)	1 Male/2 females	Sjogren's syndrome in all	NA	NA	NA	Crackles (100)
Kim et al. [91]	13	45	6 Males/7 females	Scleroderma in all	5 (38)	NA	6	NA
Yoshinouci et al. [14]	7	64 (52–75)	4 Male 3 Female	All rheumatoid arthritis	NA	Fever (57) Cough (86) Dyspnea (71) None (14)	NA	NA
Collagen vascular-associated cases excluded or unknown								
Park et al. [53]	7	56 (43–69)	1 Male 6 Female	NA	1 (14%)	Dyspnea (100) Cough (57) Chest pain (28)	4	Fever (29) Crackles (100)
Nagai et al. [25]	31	58 (40–72)	15 Male 16 Female	Excluded	18 (58)	Dyspnea Cough	2 (0.25–32)	Fever (32) Clubbing (10)
Bjoraker et al. [23]	14	57 (40–73)	8 Male 6 Female	Excluded	8 (57)	Dyspnea (100) Cough (85)	15 15	Crackles (79) Clubbing (21)

Study	N	Age	Sex	Association	Value	Symptoms	Duration	Findings
Daniil et al. [57]	15	43 (31–66)	7 Male / 8 Female	Excluded	9 (60)	Dyspnea (100) Cough (60)	18 (7–84)	Crackles (80) Clubbing (40)
Travis et al. [6]	22	50 (30–71)	15 Male / 7 Female	Excluded	15 (68)	Dyspnea (100) Cough (100)	NA	NA
Nicholson et al. [87]	28	53	20 Male / 8 Female	NA	19 (68)	Dyspnea	11 Median (0–180)	NA
Tekehara et al. [44]	4	52 (26–75)	2 Male / 2 Female	NA	NA	NA	15 (2–29)	NA
Flaherty et al. [24]	28 Fibrotic / 5 Cellular	56 / 50	16 Male/12 female / 3 Male/2 female	Excluded	20 (71) / 2 (40)	NA	26 / 22	NA
Riha et al. [26]	7	49 (39–67)	2 Male/5 female	Excluded	3 (43)	Dyspnea (100) Cough (57)	28 (12–36)	Crackles (71) Clubbing (57)
Vourlekis et al. [20]	6	46 (21–59)	1 Male/5 female	Hypersensitivity pneumonia in all	2 (33)	Dyspnea (100) Cough (50)	10 (1–24)	NA
Ishii et al. [33]	12	53 (28–71)	4 Males/8 females	Excluded	3 (25)	NA	NA	NA
Jegal et al. [68]	41 NSIP fibrotic / 7 NSIP cellular	54±11 / 59±10	12 Male/29 Female / 3 Male/4 Female	Excluded / Excluded	8 (19%) / 4 (57%)	NA / NA	5.5±7 / 4±4	NA / NA
Kakugawa et al. [36]	16	58 (28–75)	5 Male/11 Female	Excluded	5 (33)	NA	6 (1–74)	NA
Travis et al. [76]	56 NSIP fibrotic / 11 NSIP cellular	52 (26–73)	22 Male/45 Female	Excluded; 2 developed during follow-up	20 (31)	Dyspnea (96) Cough (87) Weight loss (22)	7 (1–120) / 6 (1–147)	Fever (22) Clubbing (8) Rash (5)
Park et al. [62]	72 NSIP fibrotic / 11 NSIP cellular	54 / 55	23 Male/49 Female / 4 Male/7 Female	Excluded; 10 developed during follow-up	21 (29) / 5 (45)	Dyspnea	5.9 / 4.9	NA

Adapted from [92, 93]

Table 11.2 Suggested laboratory evaluation of the patient with NSIP

Routine	Complete cell count
	Electrolytes
	Blood urea nitrogen/creatinine
	Liver function tests
	Urinalysis
	Creatinine phosphokinase
	Aldolase
	Sedimentation rate, C-reactive protein
Serological	ANA with pattern and titer
	Extractable nuclear antigen
	Rheumatoid factor
	Anti-CCP
	Anti-SSA/SSB
	Anti-Scl-70
	Anti-centromere
	Anti-RNP
	Myositis Panel (Jo-1, Mi-2, PL-7, PL-12, EJ, OJ, Ku, U2 snRNP)

Adapted from [60]

distribution. The most common features were reticulation, lobar volume loss, and traction bronchiectasis; ground glass was noted in only 44% of cases. A typical HRCT image from a patient with NSIP is shown in Fig. 11.1.

Numerous investigators have evaluated the ability of HRCT to predict the histopathologic pattern of IPF and NSIP, although there does not seem to be a concrete correlation between HRCT features and histopathology [76, 77]. Early series that evaluated the ability of HRCT to make a diagnosis of NSIP (as confirmed by surgical lung biopsy) had low accuracy (range 66–68%) [63, 67]. A recent retrospective series of surgical lung biopsy proven chronic hypersensitivity pneumonia ($n=18$), idiopathic pulmonary fibrosis ($n=23$), and idiopathic NSIP ($n=25$) applied statistical analysis to a detailed appraisal of HRCT features. The HRCT features most predictive of NSIP were subpleural sparing, relative absence of lobular areas with decreased attenuation, and lack of honeycombing [78]. A correct first diagnosis of NSIP was seen in 90% of NSIP cases and 94% of cases with a high level of confidence. The overall accuracy for the entire cohort was 80% with a sensitivity of 50%, specificity of 98%, and positive predictive value of 94% [78]. These data suggest

that the utility of HRCT to make a diagnosis of NSIP may improve as we develop a more thorough understanding of the HRCT features. More recent data also suggest that the accuracy of HRCT diagnosis of NSIP and UIP may be confounded by the presence of emphysema [79]. In a series of patients with UIP and NSIP, the diagnosis was correct in 136 (71%) of 192 readings, but for patients with concurrent emphysema the diagnosis was correct in only 30 (44%) of 68 readings [79].

Similar to pathology, the interpretation of HRCT is complicated and significant inter-rater variability is present [80]. In a series of HRCTs from patients with interstitial lung disease, κ for agreement of an NSIP pattern was only moderate at 0.51; NSIP was involved in 55% of the cases with disagreement [80]. More recent data showed improved κ agreement for the diagnosis of NSIP (κ=0.96) [78] which could reflect the radiologists involved, case selection, a better understanding of the HRCT features of NSIP or all. Given the prognostic and treatment implications of NSIP versus IPF these data highlight that although HRCT can suggest a diagnosis of NSIP, a surgical lung biopsy is required for confirmation until further studies can confirm the accuracy of HRCT in combination with clinical features.

Serial HRCT scans in patients with NSIP vary with some patients showing improvement and others showing evidence of disease progression (Table 11.7) [53, 66, 71, 81, 82]. A recent report of 23 patients with NSIP noted a decrease in ground glass over a mean follow-up of 66 months; in five subjects with an initial HRCT patterns suggestive of NSIP subsequent imaging was felt to be suggestive of UIP [78]. Baseline factors could not be identified to predict which patients would show progression of disease by HRCT, although the extent of consolidation, ground glass, and honeycombing has been shown to correlate with longitudinal changes in lung function [47].

Pathologic Characteristics

The histopathology of NSIP incorporates a broad spectrum of features with varied degrees of

Table 11.3 Auto-antibody prevalence by disease association

	SLE	RA	SSc	PM/DM	PSS	MCTD
ANA	90–98	40	96	25–90	70–95	83
Anti-ds DNA	50–80					
Anti-Smith	20–30					
Rheumatoid factor	15–25	65–90	10–50	10–40	30–70	
Anti-SSA/Ro	20–30				50–90	
Anti-SSB/La	10–20				50	
Anti-Scl-70			30–35[a] 10–20[b]			
Anti-centromere			40–80[b]			
Anti-Jo-1				10–50		
Anti-RNP	30–40					100
Anti-CCP		50–75				

SLE systemic lupus erythematosus, *RA* rheumatoid arthritis, *SSc* systemic sclerosis, *PM/DM* polymyositis/dermatomyositis, *PSS* primary Sjögren's syndrome, *MCTD* mixed connective tissue disease, *ANA* antinuclear antibody, *dsDNA* double-stranded DNA, *Scl* scleroderma, *Jo-1* histidyl transfer RNA synthetase, *RNP* ribonucleoprotein, *CCP* cyclic citrullinated peptide
Adapted from [60]
[a]Diffuse SSc
[b]Limited SSc

Table 11.4 Diagnostic criteria for patients with undifferentiated connective tissue disease

Diagnostic criteria	Presence of
Symptoms associated with a connective tissue process	At least one of the following: Raynaud's phenomenon Arthralgias/multiple joint swelling Photosensitivity Unintentional weight loss Morning stiffness Dry mouth or eyes Dysphagia Recurrent, unexplained fever Gastroesophageal reflux Skin changes Oral ulceration Nonandrogenic alopecia Proximal muscle weakness
Evidence of systemic inflammation in the absence of infection	At least one of the following positive: Antinuclear antigen Rheumatoid factor Anti-Scl-70 antibody SS-A or SS-B Jo-1 antibody Increased sedimentation rate of CRP

Adapted from [15]

alveolar wall inflammation or fibrosis [6, 27]. The importance of absence of heterogeneous lung architectural distortion and minimal honeycomb change and fibroblastic foci have been highlighted (Fig. 11.2). Importantly, the histopathologic features do not fit the patterns of other IIPs such as UIP, desquamative interstitial pneumonia, respiratory bronchiolitis interstitial lung disease, cryptogenic organizing pneumonia, acute interstitial pneumonia, or lymphocytic interstitial pneumonia. The recent report of the ATS NSIP project provided additional insight in describing the pathological features in 67 cases (Table 11.8) [76]. The typical findings of interstitial inflammation and varying degrees of fibrosis were noted. Interestingly, the overlapping features with other entities were noted with varying degree of organizing pneumonia and fibroblastic foci. This group has recommended revised histological criteria for a diagnosis of NSIP (Table 11.9). Others have suggested that some histological findings may be suggestive of an underlying connective tissue process including follicular bronchiolitis, lymphoid follicles, or pleural lymphoplasmacytic infiltration [83]. A separate study demonstrated a higher concentration of septal collagen and elastic fibers as well as the elastic fibers in the vascular interstitium in scleroderma-related NSIP compared with idiopathic NSIP [31].

Table 11.5 Radiologic characteristics in patients with NSIP

Series	n	CTD n (%)	CXR (%)	HRCT (%)	
				Features	Distribution
Katzenstein and Fiorelli [8]	64	10 (6)	Bilateral interstitial infiltrates (most) Diffuse alveolar or mixed alveolar/interstitial infiltrates (11) Normal (6)	NA	NA

Park et al. [75]	7	NA	Parenchymal opacification (86)	Ground glass (100)
				Irregular lines (29)
				Consolidation (71)
					Ground glass
					  Upper lobe predominant (100)
					  Lower lobe predominant (100)
					Irregular lines
					  Upper lobe predominant (100)
					  Lower lobe predominant (100)
					Consolidation
					  Upper lobe predominant (60)
					  Lower lobe predominant (100)

Park et al. [53]	7	NA	Patchy opacification (86) Normal (14)	Bilateral patchy ground glass or alveolar consolidation (71) Irregular lines (29) Honeycombing (0)	
Kim et al. [72]	23		NA	Ground glass opacity (100) Consolidation (65) Irregular lines (87) Honeycombing (0)	Subpleural (100)
Nagai et al. [25]	31	Excluded	Patchy bilateral infiltrates (77) Reticular nodular shadows (22)*	Honeycombing (26)* Ground glass (74)*	NA
Cottin et al. [9]	12	3 (25)	Diffuse infiltrate (100)	Honeycombing (8) Ground glass (82) Septal thickening (45)	Parenchymal opacities Lower lobe predominant (73) Diffuse (27) Honeycombing Subpleural (100)

			Radiographic infiltrates (93)		
Bjoraker et al. [23]	14	Excluded	NA	NA	NA
Fujita et al. [11]	24	8 (33)	NA	Interstitial, patchy parenchymal opacification[a] Honeycombing (0)	Middle/lower lobe predominance
Kim et al. [71]	13	Scleroderma 1 (8)	NA	Ground glass (100) Interstitial opacity (100) Honeycombing (8) Bronchiectasis (100)	NA
Daniil et al. [57]	15	Excluded	NA	Typical of CFA (2)* Not typical of CFA (13)*	NA
Johkoh et al. [69]	27	Excluded	NA	Ground glass (100) Interstitial opacity (93) Honeycombing (26)	Upper lobe predominant (4) Lower lobe predominant (74) Random (22) Peripheral (85)
Akira et al. [65]	9	NA	NA	Bilateral disease (100) Ground glass (100) Consolidation (78) Intralobular lines (78) Bronchiectasis (78) Honeycombing (0)	Central (100) Peripheral (100)
Nishiyama et al. [82]	15	7 (47)	Bilateral infiltrates (100) Consolidation (27) Reticular density (13) Consolidation + reticular density (60)	Ground glass (13) Interstitial thickening (37) Honeycombing (0) Traction bronchiectasis (87)	Upper lobe predominant (0) Lower lobe predominant (80) Peripheral (33) Diffuse (60)

(continued)

Table 11.5 (continued)

Series	n	CTD n (%)	CXR (%)	HRCT (%) Features	Distribution
Hartman et al. [67]	50	NA	NA	Ground glass (76) Irregular linear opacities (46) Honeycombing (30) Consolidation (16) Nodular opacities (14) Emphysema (12) Traction bronchiectasis (36)	Ground glass Upper lobe predominant (8) Lower lobe predominant (59) Random (14) Subpleural (68) Random (21) Irregular linear opacities Lower lobe predominant (87) Random (13) Subpleural (96) Honeycombing Upper lobe predominant (20) Lower lobe predominant (67) Subpleural (93)
MacDonald et al. [73]	21	Excluded	NA	Ground glass	Basal distribution (62) Subpleural distribution (60)
Riha et al. [26]	7	Excluded	Fine reticular markings (71) Vague patchy infiltrates (43) Honeycombing (14)	NA	NA
Vourlekis et al. [20]	6	Excluded	Ground glass (67) Reticular density (50) Nodular density (33) Honeycombing (17)	Centrilobular nodule (2/2) Ground glass (2/2)	Reticular opacity Upper lobe predominant (1/1)
Johkoh et al. [70]	55	Excluded	NA	Ground glass (100) Air space consolidation (98) Nodules (96) Traction bronchiectasis (95) Intralobular reticulation (87) Interlobular reticulation (71) Honeycombing (27)	Lower lobe predominance (95)

Yamadori et al. [13]	9	Sjögren's 9 (100)	NA	Ground glass (100) Honeycombing (0)	NA
Kim et al. [12]	13	Excluded	NA	Ground glass (77) Reticular opacity (54) Consolidation (23)	NA

Arakawa et al. [66]	14	DM/PM 14 (100)	NA	Reticular opacity (100)
				Ground glass (93)
				Consolidation (43)
				Traction bronchiectasis (86)
				Honeycombing (0)
					Reticular opacity
					  Peripheral (50) lower lobe (71)
					Ground glass
					  Peripheral (39) lower lobe (85)
					Consolidation
					  Peripheral (100) lower lobe (50)
					Traction bronchiectasis
					  Peripheral (60) lower lobe (100)

Jegal et al. [68]	48	Excluded	NA	Ground glass (most patients) Reticular opacity (50) Consolidation (15)	

Elliott et al. [94]	25	5 (20%)	NA		Craniocaudal distribution
					  Lower zone (90%)
					  Upper zone (2%)
					  Middle zone (2%)
					  Equal (6%)
					CT axial distribution
					  Peripheral (74%)
					  Diffuse (26%)
					Homogeneity
					  Patchy (30%)
					  Confluent (70%)

(continued)

Table 11.5 (continued)

Series	n	CTD n (%)	CXR (%)	HRCT (%) Features	Distribution
Travis et al. [76]	61	Excluded	NA	Reticular opacity (87%)	Craniocaudal distribution
				Traction bronchiectasis (82%)	Lower lobe (92%)
				Lobar volume loss (77%)	Diffuse (8%)
				Ground glass (44%)	CT axial distribution
				Subpleural sparing (21%)	Diffuse (47%)
				Emphysema/cysts (12%)	Peripheral (46%)
				Consolidation (13%)	Central (7%)
				Peribronchial thickening (7%)	
				Micronodules (3%)	
				Honeycombing (5%)	
Silva et al. [78]	23	Excluded	NA	Ground glass (100%)	Craniocaudal distribution
				Reticular opacity (91%)	Lower lobe predominance (83%)
				Traction bronchiectasis (91%)	Upper lobe fibrosis (91%)
				Traction bronchiolectasis (91%)	Basal predominance of fibrosis (83%)
				Consolidation (22%)	CT axial distribution
				Honeycombing (22%)	Regional (43%)
					Random (57%)
					Subpleural sparing (43%)
Park et al. [62]	53 Fibrotic	8 (10%)[b]	NA	Reticular opacity (95%)	NA
	11 Cellular			Ground glass (94%)	
				Consolidation (28%)	
				Honeycombing (11%)	

DM/PM dermatomyositis/polymyositis

Adapted from [92, 93]

*$p < 0.05$ UIP compared with NSIP within series

[a]Number of patients not quantified

[b]Developed connective tissue disease during course of follow-up

Table 11.6 High resolution computed tomography features in 61 cases of idiopathic nonspecific interstitial pneumonia

Radiologic feature	Number (%)	95% Confidence interval
Craniocaudal distribution		
Lower	56 (92)	82–96
Diffuse	5 (0)	4–18
Upper	0	0–6
CT axial distribution		
Diffuse	29 (47)	36–60
Peripheral	28 (46)	34–58
Central	4 (7)	3–16
Reticulation	53 (87)	76–93
Traction bronchiectasis	50 (82)	71–90
Lobar volume loss	47 (77)	65–86
Ground glass attenuation	27 (44)	33–57
Subpleural sparing	13 (21)	13–33
Emphysema/cysts	7 (12)	6–22
Consolidation	8 (13)	7–24
Peribronchial thickening	4 (7)	3–16
Substantial micronodules	2 (3)	1–11
Honeycombing	3 (5)	2–13

Adapted from [6]

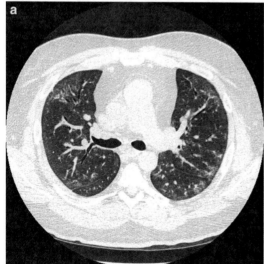 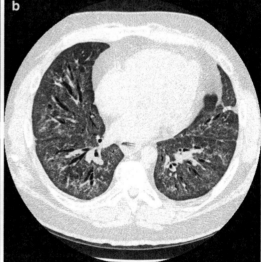

Fig. 11.1 Images from a patient with surgical lung biopsy proven nonspecific interstitial pneumonia (NSIP). High resolution computed tomography images from the mid- and lower lung zones of a patient with NSIP. The images demonstrate a peripheral and lower lobe predominance of ground glass, septal thickening, and bronchiectasis. Honeycombing is not present

Table 11.7 Results of serial radiographic studies in patients with NSIP

Series	N	Follow-up	Results
Park et al. [75]	6	13 Months	3 Complete resolution 3 Improvement
Kim et al. [71]	13	11 Months	Improved ground glass opacity > irregular linear opacity
Nishiyama et al. [74]	15	15.6 Months	3 Complete resolution 9 Improvement 1 Persistent 1 Worsened
Akira et al. [65]	9	3.1 Years	4 Complete resolution 1 Improvement 2 Persistent 2 Worsened
Arakawa et al. [66]	14	3–61 Months, mean 28 months	Reticular opacity – improved 11, worse 3 Ground glass – improved 12, progressed 2 Consolidation – improved 5, progressed 1 Traction bronchiectasis – improved 4, progressed 2 Honeycombing – no patient developed honeycombing
Silva et al. [78]	23	66 Months (median)	5/18 Patients with initial NSIP pattern developed UIP-like pattern

Adapted from [92, 93]

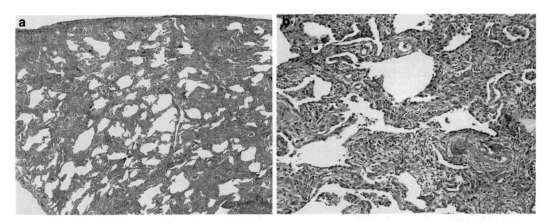

Fig. 11.2 Surgical lung biopsies. Low- and high power fields from a surgical lung biopsy of a patient with nonspecific interstitial pneumonia

Although the histopathologic features of NSIP can be defined as noted earlier, the separation of NSIP from other IIPs, particularly UIP, remains difficult. The level of agreement (κ) for the diagnosis of various interstitial lung diseases between ten experts thoracic pathologists in the UK was only 0.32 (fair) and NSIP was involved in the majority of divergent cases [84]. In a subsequent studies, significant discordance between general and specialty pathologists has been reported, especially in the diagnosis of NSIP and other non-IPF IIPs [55, 85].

The classification of NSIP is further complicated by the fact that areas of both NSIP and UIP can be located in the same patient when biopsies are taken from multiple locations. Studies evaluating patients with multiple lobe biopsies found a pattern of UIP in one lobe and NSIP in another lobe in 13–26% of patients [28, 29]. These discordant IPF cases had a similar prognosis to patients with IPF in all lobes arguing that patients should have multiple lobes biopsied and if UIP is found in any lobe the patient should be treated as such.

Table 11.8 Pathological features in 67 cases of idiopathic NSIP

Pathological feature	Number (%)
NSIP pattern	
Cellular	11 (16)
Fibrosing	56 (84)
Bronchiolocentricity (minor finding)	9 (13%)
Lymphoid follicles	38 (57%)
Interstitial fibrosis with enlarged airspaces	
Absent	9 (13)
<10%	23 (34)
10–50%	24 (36)
>50%	11 (17)
Interstitial cellular inflammation	
Mild	31 (46%)
Moderate	36 (54%)
Organizing pneumonia	
Absent	32 (48%)
0–9%	33 (49%)
10–19%	2 (3)
Smooth muscle hyperplasia	14 (36)
Fibroblastic foci	14 (21)
Bronchiolar metaplasia	13 (19)

Adapted from [76]

Table 11.9 Proposed revised histological features of NSIP

Key features
Cellular pattern
  Mild to moderate interstitial chronic inflammation
  Type II pneumocyte hyperplasia in areas of inflammation
Fibrosing pattern
  Dense or loose interstitial fibrosis with uniform appearance
  Lung architecture is frequently preserved
    Interstitial chronic inflammation-mild or moderate
Pertinent negative findings
  Cellular pattern
    Dense interstitial fibrosis is absent
    Organizing pneumonia is note prominent feature (>20% biopsy specimen)
    Lack of diffuse severe alveolar septal inflammation
  Fibrosing pattern
    Temporal heterogeneity pattern – fibroblastic foci with dense fibrosis are inconspicuous or absent
    Honeycombing inconspicuous or absent
    (Enlarged fibrotic airspaces may be present)
  Both patterns
    Acute lung injury pattern is absent
    Eosinophils are inconspicuous or absent
    Granulomas absent
    Lack of viral inclusions and organisms on special stains
    Dominant airway disease such as extensive peribronchiolar metaplasia

Adapted from [76]
Italicized text reflects modifications from the 2002 ATS/ERS statement [27]

Management and Treatment

Data regarding response to treatment for patients with idiopathic NSIP comes from patients initially treated as IPF/UIP and then reclassified as NSIP. Most patients were treated with corticosteroids with or without the addition of cytotoxic agents such as azathioprine or cyclophosphamide (Table 11.10). Treatment regimens and duration of treatment were variable [6–12, 20, 23–26, 57, 86, 87]. Following an initial response to treatment some patients will relapse following the cessation of immunosuppressive treatment, suggesting that long-term treatment may be required [9, 62]. Adverse reactions to corticosteroid treatment can be substantial [88] and a careful assessment of risks and benefits needs to be discussed prior and during the course of treatment.

The optimal dose and duration of corticosteroid therapy is not known. We typically begin with 1 mg/kd/day up to a dose of 60 mg for 1 month followed by 40 mg/day for an additional 2 months. Patients responding or stabilizing with treatment are gradually tapered to complete at least 1 year of therapy. Patients with progressive disease, relapsing disease, or intolerance to treatment with corticosteroids should be considered for treatment with cytotoxic agents such as azathioprine or cyclophosphamide. Patients with progressive disease should also be considered for lung transplant.

Prognosis

There are no prospective studies of untreated patients with NSIP. Data regarding the outcome of patients with NSIP has been gleaned from retrospective analyses of patients previously classified as IPF/CFA (see Table 11.9). The vast

Table 11.10 Survival and response to treatment in patients with NSIP

Series	N	Survival	Treatment	Follow-up time	Follow-up response
Katzenstein and Fiorelli [8]	Group I – 31	NA	NA	61 Months	Alive and Well (13/22)
				60 Months	Alive with disease (9/22)
					Dead (0/22)
	Group II – 24			40 Months	Alive and Well (7/20)
				7 Months	Alive with disease (7/20)
				18 Months	Dead of disease (3/20)
				3 Months	Dead of other (3/20)
	Group III – 9			8 Months	Alive and Well (1/6)
				36 Months	Alive with disease (2/6)
				15 Months	Dead of disease (2/6)
				17Months	Dead of other (1/6)
Nagai et al. [25]	Cellular NSIP – 16	NA	None (8/16)	NA	Improved (10/16)
			CS (6/16)		Remission (4/16)
			CS+IS (2/16)		No change (2/16)
					Worse (0/16)
					Dead (0/16)
	Fibrotic NSIP – 15		None (4/15)		Improved (8/15)
			CS (5/15)		Remission (1/15)
			CS+IS (6/15)		No change (1/156)
					Worse (3/156)
					Dead (2/15)
Cottin et al. [9]	12	NA	CS (5/12)	50 Months	Improved (10/12)
			CS+IS (7/12)		Worse (2/12)
					Dead (0/12)
Bjoraker et al. [23]	14	Median>13 years	NA	NA	
Douglas et al. [10]	70	Median>7 years	CS (67/70)	NA	
Daniil et al. [57]	15	Median>7 years	None (2/14)	NA	Improved (2/12)
			CS (1/14)		Stable (4/12)
			CS+IS (11/14)		Worse (3/12)
					Dead (1/12)

Nicholson et al. [87]	28	Median 52 months	CS (12/28) CS+IS (9/28)	NA	NA
Bouros et al. [7]	62	Median > 10 years 5 Years – 91%	NA	NA	Dead (16/62)
Fujita et al. [11]	24	NA	CS (21/24) CS+IS (3/24)	NA	Improved (17/24) Worse (1/24) Dead of disease (4/24) Dead of other (2/24)
Travis et al. [6]	Cellular NSIP – 7 Fibrotic NSIP – 22	10 Years – 100% 10 Years – 35%	NA	NA	NA
Flaherty et al. [24]	33	Median > 9 years	None (2/33) CS (18/33) CS+IS (4/33) Other (9/33)	NA	Improved (4/10)[a] Stable (4/10) Worse (1/10)
Riha et al. [26]	7	Median 178 months	None (2/7) CS (2/7) CS+IS (2/7) Other (1/7)	NA	NA
Vourlekis et al. [20]	6 with hypersensitivity pneumonitis	NA	CS (3/6) CS+IS (3/6)	5.5 Years	NA
Shimizu et al. [54]	Cellular NSIP – 13 Fibrotic NSIP – 2	NA	NA	NA	Improved (9/15) Stable (5/15) Died (1/15)
Kim et al. [12]	13	NA	CS (1/12) CS+IS (11/12)	34.5 Months	Improved (5/8) Stable (3/8) Died (1/8)
Kondoh et al. [86]	12	Median > 12 years	CS+IS	Mean 92 months range (60–148)	Improved (5/12) Stable (4/12) Worse (3/12)

(continued)

Table 11.10 (continued)

Series	N	Survival	Treatment	Follow-up time	Follow-up response
Park et al. [95]	Idiopathic – 66	3 Years – 77.6% 5 Years – 67.4% Mean – 91.5 months	NA	NA	NA
	CTD – 57	3 Years – 88.9% 5 Years – 81.5% Mean – 132.2 months			
Travis et al. [76]	Cellular NSIP – 11 Fibrotic NSIP – 56	5 Years – 82.3% 10 Years – 73.2%	NA	NA	NA
Park et al. [62]	Cellular NSIP – 11 Fibrotic NSIP – 72	NA 2 Years – 85%[b] 5 Years – 74%[b]	CS±IS (11) CS±IS (68)		NA Improved/stable – 81% Recurrence – 36% Worsening – 19%

CS corticosteroids, IS immunosuppressive therapy, CTD connective tissue disease
Adapted from [92, 93]
[a]After 3-month trial of high-dose steroids in subset of NSIP patients
[b]Disease-related death

majority of these patients were treated with immunosuppressive agents. At baseline, compared with IPF, the overall prognosis and response to therapy for NSIP is favorable [6, 23–26]. In series of patients with IPF/UIP and NSIP changes in FVC, FEV_1, DL_{CO}, and/or a composite physiologic index have been shown to correlate with subsequent survival and over time. Furthermore, an individual's physiologic course may become as important or more important that the baseline histopathology [68, 89, 90]. In a Korean study, the baseline decrement in DL_{CO}, older age, and histopathology (UIP vs. NSIP) were risk factors for subsequent mortality, while gender, FVC, and PaO_2 were not [68]. After 6 months of follow-up, initial DL_{CO}, change in FVC, and gender were predictors of mortality, while age, histopathology, baseline FVC, and PaO_2 were not [68]. A more recent study showed that HRCT findings of ground glass or consolidation correlated with subsequent improvement in lung function, while findings of honeycombing were associated with increased risk of subsequent mortality [62]. Overall these data suggests that histopathology is a good baseline predictor of subsequent mortality, while changes in physiology become more important than histopathology over time. Patients with NSIP that show signs of progression despite treatment should be considered for lung transplantation, similar to patients with IPF.

Acknowledgments Supported in part by National Institutes of Health Grants 5P50HL56402, 2 K24 HL04212, 1 K23 HL68713, R01 HL 091743-01AI, and U10HL080371.

References

1. Bojko T, Notterman DA, Greenwald BM, De Bruin WJ, Magid MS, Godwin T. Acute hypoxemic respiratory failure in children following bone marrow transplantation: an outcome and pathologic study. Crit Care Med. 1995;23(4):755–9.
2. Griffiths MH, Miller RF, Semple SJ. Interstitial pneumonitis in patients infected with the human immunodeficiency virus. Thorax. 1995;50(11):1141–6.
3. Sattler F, Nichols L, Hirano L, Hiti A, Hofman F, Hughlett C, et al. Nonspecific interstitial pneumonitis mimicking Pneumocystis carinii pneumonia. Am J Respir Crit Care Med. 1997;156(3 Pt 1):912–7.
4. Simmons JT, Suffredini AF, Lack EE, Brenner M, Ognibene FP, Shelhamer JH, et al. Nonspecific interstitial pneumonitis in patients with AIDS: radiologic features. AJR Am J Roentgenol. 1987;149(2):265–8.
5. Suffredini AF, Ognibene FP, Lack EE, Simmons JT, Brenner M, Gill VJ, et al. Nonspecific interstitial pneumonitis: a common cause of pulmonary disease in the acquired immunodeficiency syndrome. Ann Intern Med. 1987;107(1):7–13.
6. Travis W, Matsui K, Moss J, Ferrans V. Idiopathic nonspecific interstitial pneumonia: prognostic significance of cellular and fibrosing patterns. Am J Surg Path. 2000;24(1):19–33.
7. Bouros D, Wells A, Nicholson A, Colby T, Polychronopoulos V, Pantelidis P, et al. Histopathologic subsets of fibrosing alveolitis in patients with systemic sclerosis and their relationship to outcome. Am J Respir Crit Care Med. 2002;165(12):1581–6.
8. Katzenstein A, Fiorelli R. Nonspecific interstitial pneumonia/fibrosis. Histologic features and clinical significance. Am J Surg Pathol. 1994;18(2):136–47.
9. Cottin V, Donsbeck A-V, Revel D, Loire R, Cordier J-F. Nonspecific interstitial pneumonia: individualization of a clinicopathologic entity in a series of 12 patients. Am J Respir Crit Care Med. 1998;158:1286–93.
10. Douglas WW, Tazelaar HD, Hartman TE, Hartman RP, Decker PA, Schroeder DR, et al. Polymyositis-dermatomyositis-associated interstitial lung disease. Am J Respir Crit Care Med. 2001;164(7):1182–5.
11. Fujita J, Yamadori I, Suemitsu I, Yoshinouchi T, Ohtsuki Y, Yamaji Y, et al. Clinical features of nonspecific interstitial pneumonia. Respir Med. 1999;93:113–8.
12. Kim EA, Lee KS, Johkoh T, Kim TS, Suh GY, Kwon OJ, et al. Interstitial lung diseases associated with collagen vascular diseases: radiologic and histopathologic findings. Radiographics. 2002;22:S151–65.
13. Yamadori I, Fujita J, Bandoh S, Tokuda M, Tanimoto Y, Kataoka M, et al. Nonspecific interstitial pneumonia as pulmonary involvement of primary Sjogren's syndrome. Rheumatol Int. 2002;22(3):89–92.
14. Yoshinouchi T, Ohtsuki Y, Fujita J, Yamadori I, Bandoh S, Ishida T, et al. Nonspecific interstitial pneumonia pattern as pulmonary involvement of rheumatoid arthritis. Rheumatol Int. 2005;26(2):121–5.
15. Kinder BW, Collard HR, Koth L, Daikh DI, Wolters PJ, Elicker B, et al. Idiopathic nonspecific interstitial pneumonia: lung manifestation of undifferentiated connective tissue disease? Am J Respir Crit Care Med. 2007;176(7):691–7.
16. Hwang JH, Misumi S, Sahin H, Brown KK, Newell JD, Lynch DA. Computed tomographic features of idiopathic fibrosing interstitial pneumonia: comparison with pulmonary fibrosis related to collagen vascular disease. J Comput Assist Tomogr. 2009;33(3):410–5.
17. Okayasu K, Ohtani Y, Takemura T, Uchibori K, Tamaoka M, Furuiye M, et al. Nonspecific interstitial pneumonia (NSIP) associated with anti-KS antibody: differentiation from idiopathic NSIP. Intern Med. 2009;48(15):1301–6.

18. Richards TJ, Eggebeen A, Gibson K, Yousem S, Fuhrman C, Gochuico BR, et al. Characterization and peripheral blood biomarker assessment of anti-Jo-1 antibody-positive interstitial lung disease. Arthritis Rheum. 2009;60(7):2183–92.

19. Miki H, Mio T, Nagai S, Hoshino Y, Nagao T, Kitaichi M, et al. Fibroblast contractility. Usual interstitial pneumonia and nonspecific interstitial pneumonia. Am J Respir Crit Care Med. 2000;162:2259–64.

20. Vourlekis JS, Schwarz MI, Cool CD, Tuder RM, King TE, Brown KK. Nonspecific interstitial pneumonitis as the sole histologic expression of hypersensitivity pneumonitis. Am J Med. 2002;112(6):490–3.

21. Lantuejoul S, Brambilla E, Brambilla C, Devouassoux G. Statin-induced fibrotic nonspecific interstitial pneumonia. Eur Respir J. 2002;19(3):577–80.

22. Pesenti S, Lauque D, Daste G, Boulay V, Pujazon MC, Carles P. Diffuse infiltrative lung disease associated with flecainide. Report of two cases. Respiration. 2002;69(2):182–5.

23. Bjoraker J, Ryu J, Edwin M, Myers J, Tazelaar H, Schoreder D, et al. Prognostic significance of histopathologic subsets in idiopathic pulmonary fibrosis. Am J Respir Crit Care Med. 1998;157:199–203.

24. Flaherty K, Toews G, Travis W, Colby T, Kazerooni E, Gross B, et al. Clinical significance of histological classification of idiopathic interstitial pneumonia. Eur Respir J. 2002;19:275–83.

25. Nagai S, Kitaichi M, Itoh H, Nishimura K, Izumi T, Colby TV. Idiopathic nonspecific interstitial pneumonia/fibrosis: comparison with idiopathic pulmonary fibrosis and BOOP. Eur Respir J. 1998;12:1010–9.

26. Riha R, Duhig E, Clarke B, Steele R, Slaughter R, Zimmerman P. Survival of patients with biopsy-proven usual interstitial pneumonia and nonspecific interstitial pneumonia. Eur Respir J. 2002;19(6):1114–8.

27. Society AT, Society ER. American Thoracic Society/European Respiratory Society international multidisciplinary consensus classification of the Idiopathic Interstitial Pneumonias. Am J Respir Crit Care Med. 2002;165:277–304.

28. Flaherty K, Travis W, Colby T, Toews G, Kazerooni E, Gross B, et al. Histologic variability in usual and nonspecific Interstitial pneumonias. Am J Resp Crit Care Med. 2001;164:1722–7.

29. Monaghan H, Wells AU, Colby TV, du Bois RM, Hansell DM, Nicholson AG. Prognostic implications of histologic patterns in multiple surgical lung biopsies from patients with idiopathic interstitial pneumonias. Chest. 2004;125(2):522–6.

30. Maher TM, Wells AU, Laurent GJ. Idiopathic pulmonary fibrosis: multiple causes and multiple mechanisms? Eur Respir J. 2007;30(5):835–9.

31. de Carvalho EF, Parra ER, de Souza R, A'B Saber AM, Machado Jde C, Capelozzi VL. Arterial and interstitial remodelling processes in non-specific interstitial pneumonia: systemic sclerosis versus idiopathic. Histopathology. 2008;53(2):195–204.

32. Selman M, King Jr T, Pardo A. Idiopathic pulmonary fibrosis: prevailing and evolving hypotheses about its pathogenesis and implications for therapy. Ann Intern Med. 2001;134:136–51.

33. Ishii H, Mukae H, Kadota J, Fujii T, Abe K, Ashitani J, et al. Increased levels of interleukin-18 in bronchoalveolar lavage fluid of patients with idiopathic nonspecific interstitial pneumonia. Respiration. 2005; 72(1):39–45.

34. Terasaki Y, Fukuda Y, Suga M, Ikeguchi N, Takeya M. Epimorphin expression in interstitial pneumonia. Respir Res. 2005;6(1):6.

35. Suga M, Iyonaga K, Okamoto T, Gushima Y, Miyakawa H, Akaike T, et al. Characteristic elevation of matrix metalloprotinase activity in idiopathic interstitial pneumonias. Am J Respir Crit Care Med. 2000;162:1949–56.

36. Kakugawa T, Mukae H, Hayashi T, Ishii H, Nakayama S, Sakamoto N, et al. Expression of HSP47 in usual interstitial pneumonia and nonspecific interstitial pneumonia. Respir Res. 2005;6(1):57.

37. Brasch F, Griese M, Tredano M, Johnen G, Ochs M, Rieger C, et al. Interstitial lung disease in a baby with a de novo mutation in the SFTPC gene. Eur Respir J. 2004;24(1):30–9.

38. Chibbar R, Shih F, Baga M, Torlakovic E, Ramlall K, Skomro R, et al. Nonspecific interstitial pneumonia and usual interstitial pneumonia with mutation in surfactant protein C in familial pulmonary fibrosis. Mod Pathol. 2004;17(8):973–80.

39. Nogee LM, Dunbar 3rd AE, Wert SE, Askin F, Hamvas A, Whitsett JA. A mutation in the surfactant protein C gene associated with familial interstitial lung disease. N Engl J Med. 2001;344(8):573–9.

40. Stevens PA, Pettenazzo A, Brasch F, Mulugeta S, Baritussio A, Ochs M, et al. Nonspecific interstitial pneumonia, alveolar proteinosis, and abnormal proprotein trafficking resulting from a spontaneous mutation in the surfactant protein C gene. Pediatr Res. 2005;57(1):89–98.

41. Thomas AQ, Lane K, Phillips 3rd J, Prince M, Markin C, Speer M, et al. Heterozygosity for a surfactant protein C gene mutation associated with usual interstitial pneumonitis and cellular nonspecific interstitial pneumonitis in one kindred. Am J Respir Crit Care Med. 2002;165(9):1322–8.

42. Eitzman DT, McCoy RD, Zheng X, Fay WP, Shen T, Ginsburg D, et al. Bleomycin-induced pulmonary fibrosis in transgenic mice that either lack or overexpress the murine plasminogen activator inhibitor-1 gene. J Clin Invest. 1996;97(1):232–7.

43. Kim KK, Flaherty KR, Long Q, Hattori N, Sisson TH, Colby TV, et al. A plasminogen activator inhibitor-1 promoter polymorphism and idiopathic interstitial pneumonia. Mol Med. 2003;9(1–2):52–6.

44. Takehara H, Tada S, Kataoka M, Matsuo K, Ueno Y, Ozaki S, et al. Intercellular adhesion molecule-1 in patients with idiopathic interstitial pneumonia. Acta Med Okayama. 2001;55(4):205–11.

45. Jakubzick C, Choi ES, Kunkel SL, Evanoff H, Martinez FJ, Puri RK, et al. Augmented pulmonary

IL-4 and IL-13 receptor subunit expression in idiopathic interstitial pneumonia. J Clin Pathol. 2004; 57(5):477–86.

46. Keogh KA, Limper AH. Characterization of lymphocyte populations in nonspecific interstitial pneumonia. Respir Res. 2005;6:137.

47. Park SW, Ahn MH, Jang HK, Jang AS, Kim DJ, Koh ES, et al. Interleukin-13 and its receptors in idiopathic interstitial pneumonia: clinical implications for lung function. J Korean Med Sci. 2009;24(4):614–20.

48. Choi ES, Jakubzick C, Carpenter KJ, Kunkel SL, Evanoff H, Martinez FJ, et al. Enhanced monocyte chemoattractant protein-3/CC chemokine ligand-7 in usual interstitial pneumonia. Am J Respir Crit Care Med. 2004;170(5):508–15.

49. Kakugawa T, Yokota S, Mukae H, Kubota H, Sakamoto N, Mizunoe S, et al. High serum concentrations of autoantibodies to HSP47 in nonspecific interstitial pneumonia compared with idiopathic pulmonary fibrosis. BMC Pulm Med. 2008;8:23.

50. Amenomori M, Mukae H, Sakamoto N, Kakugawa T, Hayashi T, Hara A, et al. HSP47 in lung fibroblasts is a predictor of survival in fibrotic nonspecific interstitial pneumonia. Respir Med. 2010;104:895–901.

51. Golec M, Lambers C, Hofbauer E, Geleff S, Bankier A, Czerny M, et al. Assessment of gene transcription demonstrates connection with the clinical course of idiopathic interstitial pneumonia. Respiration. 2008; 76(3):261–9.

52. Nakayama S, Mukae H, Sakamoto N, Kakugawa T, Yoshioka S, Soda H, et al. Pirfenidone inhibits the expression of HSP47 in TGF-beta1-stimulated human lung fibroblasts. Life Sci. 2008;82(3–4):210–7.

53. Park C, Jeon J, Park S, Lim G, Jeong S, Uh S, et al. Nonspecific interstitial pneumonia/fibrosis: clinical manifestations, histologic and radiologic features. Korean J Intern Med. 1996;11:122–32.

54. Shimizu S, Yoshinouchi T, Ohtsuki Y, Fujita J, Sugiura Y, Banno S, et al. The appearance of S-100 protein-positive dendritic cells and the distribution of lymphocyte subsets in idiopathic nonspecific interstitial pneumonia. Respir Med. 2002;96(10):770–6.

55. Flaherty KR, Andrei AC, King Jr TE, Raghu G, Colby TV, Wells A, et al. Idiopathic interstitial pneumonia: do community and academic physicians agree on diagnosis? Am J Respir Crit Care Med. 2007;175: 1054–60.

56. Flaherty KR, King Jr TE, Raghu G, Lynch 3rd JP, Colby TV, Travis WD, et al. Idiopathic interstitial pneumonia: what is the effect of a multidisciplinary approach to diagnosis? Am J Respir Crit Care Med. 2004;170(8):904–10.

57. Daniil Z, Gilchrist F, Nicholson A, Hansell D, Harris J, Colby T, et al. A histologic pattern of nonspecific interstitial pneumonia is associated with a better prognosis than usual interstitial pneumonia in patients with cryptogenic fibrosing alveolitis. Am J Respir Crit Care Med. 1999;160:899–905.

58. Veeraraghavan S, Latsi P, Wells A, Pantelidis P, Nicholson A, Colby T, et al. BAL findings in idiopathic nonspecific interstitial pneumonia and usual interstitial pneumonia. Eur Respir J. 2003;22(2):239–44.

59. Ohshimo S, Bonella F, Cui A, Beume M, Kohno N, Guzman J, et al. Significance of bronchoalveolar lavage for the diagnosis of idiopathic pulmonary fibrosis. Am J Respir Crit Care Med. 2009;179(11):1043–7.

60. Tzelepis GE, Toya SP, Moutsopoulos HM. Occult connective tissue diseases mimicking idiopathic interstitial pneumonias. Eur Respir J. 2008;31(1):11–20.

61. Kim DS, Nagai S. Idiopathic nonspecific interstitial pneumonia: an unrecognized autoimmune disease? Am J Respir Crit Care Med. 2007;176(7):632–3.

62. Park IN, Jegal Y, Kim DS, Do KH, Yoo B, Shim TS, et al. Clinical course and lung function change of idiopathic nonspecific interstitial pneumonia. Eur Respir J. 2009;33(1):68–76.

63. Flaherty K, Thwaite E, Kazerooni E, Gross B, Toews G, Colby T, et al. Radiological versus histological diagnosis in UIP and NSIP: survival implications. Thorax. 2003;58(2):143–8.

64. Hunninghake G, Lynch D, Galvin J, Muller N, Schwartz D, King Jr T, et al. Radiologic findings are strongly associated with a pathologic diagnosis of usual interstitial pneumonia. Chest. 2003;124: 1215–23.

65. Akira M, Inoue G, Yamamoto S, Sakatani M. Nonspecific interstitial pneumonia: findings on sequential CT scans of nine patients. Thorax. 2000;55:854–9.

66. Arakawa H, Yamada H, Kurihara Y, Nakajima Y, Takeda A, Fukushima Y, et al. Nonspecific interstitial pneumonia associated with polymyositis and dermatomyositis: serial high-resolution CT findings and functional correlation. Chest. 2003;123(4): 1096–103.

67. Hartman T, Swensen S, Hansell D, Colby T, Myers J, Tazelaar H, et al. Nonspecific interstitial pneumonia: variable appearance at high-resolution chest CT. Radiology. 2000;217:701–5.

68. Jegal Y, Kim DS, Shim TS, Lim CM, Do Lee S, Koh Y, et al. Physiology is a stronger predictor of survival than pathology in fibrotic interstitial pneumonia. Am J Respir Crit Care Med. 2005;171(6):639–44.

69. Johkoh T, Muller N, Cartier Y, Kavanagh P, Hartman T, Akira M, et al. Idiopathic interstitial pneumonias: diagnostic accuracy of thin-section CT in 129 patients. Radiology. 1999;211:555–60.

70. Johkoh T, Muller N, Colby T, Ichikado K, Taniguchi H, Kondoh Y, et al. Nonspecific interstitial pneumonia: correlation between thin-section CT findings and pathologic subgroups in 55 patients. Radiology. 2002;225:199–204.

71. Kim E, Lee K, Chung M, Kwon O, Kim T, Hwang J. Nonspecific interstitial pneumonia with fibrosis: serial high-resolution CT findings with functional correlation. AJR Am J Roentgenol. 1999;173:1734–9.

72. Kim T, Lee K, Chung M, Han J, Park J, Hwang J, et al. Nonspecific interstitial pneumonia with fibrosis: high-resolution CT and pathologic findings. AJR Am J Roentgenol. 1998;171:1645–50.

73. MacDonald S, Rubens M, Hansell D, Copley S, Desai S, DuBois R, et al. Nonspecific interstitial pneumonia and usual interstitial pneumonia: comparative appearances at and diagnostic accuracy of thin-section CT. Radiology. 2001;221:600–5.

74. Nishiyama O, Kondoh Y, Taniguchi H, Yamaki K, Suzuki R, Yokoi T, et al. Serial high resolution CT findings in nonspecific interstitial pneumonia/fibrosis. J Comput Assist Tomogr. 2000;24(41–6).

75. Park J, Lee K, Kim J, Park C, Suh Y, Choi D, et al. Nonspecific interstitial pneumonia with fibrosis: radiographic and CT findings in seven patients. Radiology. 1995;195:645–8.

76. Travis WD, Hunninghake G, King Jr TE, Lynch DA, Colby TV, Galvin JR, et al. Idiopathic nonspecific interstitial pneumonia: report of an American Thoracic Society Project. Am J Respir Crit Care Med. 2008;177(12):1338–47.

77. Sumikawa H, Johkoh T, Ichikado K, Taniguchi H, Kondoh Y, Fujimoto K, et al. Nonspecific interstitial pneumonia: histologic correlation with high-resolution CT in 29 patients. Eur J Radiol. 2009;70(1): 35–40.

78. Silva CI, Muller NL, Hansell DM, Lee KS, Nicholson AG, Wells AU. Nonspecific interstitial pneumonia and idiopathic pulmonary fibrosis: changes in pattern and distribution of disease over time. Radiology. 2008;247(1):251–9.

79. Akira M, Inoue Y, Kitaichi M, Yamamoto S, Arai T, Toyokawa K. Usual interstitial pneumonia and nonspecific interstitial pneumonia with and without concurrent emphysema: thin-section CT findings. Radiology. 2009;251(1):271–9.

80. Aziz ZA, Wells AU, Hansell DM, Bain GA, Copley SJ, Desai SR, et al. HRCT diagnosis of diffuse parenchymal lung disease: inter-observer variation. Thorax. 2004;59(6):506–11.

81. Akira M, Yamamoto S, Hara H, Sakatani M, Ueda E. Serial computed tomographic evaluation in desquamative interstitial pneumonia. Thorax. 1997;52: 333–7.

82. Nishiyama O, Kondoh Y, Taniguchi H, Yamaki K, Suzuki R, Yokoi T, et al. Serial high resolution CT findings in nonspecific interstitial pneumonia/fibrosis. J Comput Assist Tomogr. 2000;24(1):41–6.

83. Tansey D, Wells AU, Colby TV, Ip S, Nikolakoupolou A, du Bois RM, et al. Variations in histological patterns of interstitial pneumonia between connective tissue disorders and their relationship to prognosis. Histopathology. 2004;44(6):585–96.

84. Nicholson AG, Addis BJ, Bharucha H, Clelland CA, Corrin B, Gibbs AR, et al. Inter-observer variation between pathologists in diffuse parenchymal lung disease. Thorax. 2004;59(6):500–5.

85. Lettieri CJ, Veerappan GR, Parker JM, Franks TJ, Hayden D, Travis WD, et al. Discordance between general and pulmonary pathologists in the diagnosis of interstitial lung disease. Respir Med. 2005;99(11): 1425–30.

86. Kondoh Y, Taniguchi H, Yokoi T, Nishiyama O, Ohishi T, Kato T, et al. Cyclophosphamide and low-dose prednisone in idiopathic pulmonary fibrosis and fibrosing nonspecific interstitial pneumonia. Eur Resir J. 2005;25:528–33.

87. Nicholson A, Colby T, DuBois R, Hansell D, Wells A. The prognostic significance of the histologic pattern of interstitial pneumonia in patients presenting with the clinical entity of cryptogenic fibrosing alveolitis. Am J Respir Crit Care Med. 2000;162: 2213–7.

88. Flaherty K, Toews G, Lynch III J, Kazerooni E, Gross B, Strawderman R, et al. Steroids in idiopathic pulmonary fibrosis: prospective assessment of adverse reactions, response to therapy, and survival. Am J Med. 2001;110:278–82.

89. Flaherty K, Mumford J, Murray S, Kazerooni E, Gross B, Colby T, et al. Prognostic implications of physiologic and radiographic changes in idiopathic interstitial pneumonia. Am J Respir Crit Care Med. 2003;168(5):543–8.

90. Latsi PI, du Bois RM, Nicholson AG, Colby TV, Bisirtzoglou D, Nikolakopoulou A, et al. Fibrotic idiopathic interstitial pneumonia: the prognostic value of longitudinal functional trends. Am J Respir Crit Care Med. 2003;168(5):531–7.

91. Kim DS, Yoo B, Lee JS, Kim EK, Lim CM, Lee SD, et al. The major histopathologic pattern of pulmonary fibrosis in scleroderma is nonspecific interstitial pneumonia. Sarcoidosis Vasc Diffuse Lung Dis. 2002;19(2): 121–7.

92. Martinez F, Flaherty K, Travis W, Lynch III J. Nonspecific interstitial pneumonia. In: Lynch III J, editor. Idiopathic pulmonary fibrosis. New York: Marcel Dekker; 2004. p. 101–36.

93. Flaherty K, Martinez F, Travis W, Lynch III J. Nonspecific interstitial pneumonia (NSIP). Semin Respir Crit Care Med. 2001;22:423–33.

94. Elliot TL, Lynch DA, Newell Jr JD, Cool C, Tuder R, Markopoulou K, et al. High-resolution computed tomography features of nonspecific interstitial pneumonia and usual interstitial pneumonia. J Comput Assist Tomogr. 2005;29(3):339–45.

95. Park IN, Kim DS, Shim TS, Lim CM, Lee SD, Koh Y, et al. Acute exacerbation of interstitial pneumonia other than idiopathic pulmonary fibrosis. Chest. 2007;132(1):214–20.

A Practical Approach to Connective Tissue Disease-Associated Lung Disease

12

Aryeh Fischer and Roland M. du Bois

Abstract

The goal of this chapter is to provide a practical approach to connective tissue disease (CTD)-associated lung disease by focusing on commonly encountered problems in the management of this complex and heterogeneous patient population. Several illustrative cases are incorporated into the text and interstitial lung disease is a major focus because it occurs across the spectrum of the CTDs, is potentially the most devastating of pulmonary manifestations, and often poses the most significant challenges to the practicing clinician.

Keywords

Connective tissue disease • Collagen vascular disease • Interstitial lung disease • Lung disease • Lung-dominant connective tissue disease

Introduction

The designations "connective tissue disease" (CTD) or "collagen vascular disease" are used interchangeably and refer to the spectrum of systemic rheumatologic diseases that are characterized by autoimmune phenomena (i.e., autoantibodies) and organ dysfunction. Although these disorders are grouped together, there is significant heterogeneity with respect to the clinical features associated with each specific CTD. The CTDs are rheumatoid arthritis, systemic lupus erythematosus (SLE), systemic sclerosis (SSc), polymyositis/dermatomyositis (including antisynthetase syndrome), primary Sjögren's syndrome, mixed CTD (MCTD), and undifferentiated CTD (UCTD) (Table 12.1). Other rheumatologic disorders that are characterized by inflammatory features – but not necessarily autoimmunity – are traditionally excluded from the grouping of CTD and these disorders include the family of spondyloarthropathy, Behçet's disease, and relapsing polychondritis. The systemic vasculitides are typically considered as a distinct group and not considered within the spectrum of CTD.

The goal of this chapter is to provide a practical approach to CTD-associated lung disease by

A. Fischer, MD (✉)
Department of Medicine, National Jewish Health,
Denver, CO, USA
e-mail: fischera@njhealth.org

R.M. du Bois, MA, MD, FRCP
National Heart & Lung Institute, Imperial College,
London, UK

R.P. Baughman and R.M. du Bois (eds.), *Diffuse Lung Disease: A Practical Approach*,
DOI 10.1007/978-1-4419-9771-5_12, © Springer Science+Business Media, LLC 2012

Table 12.1 Rheumatologic diseases associated with lung disease

CTD	Non-CTD
• Rheumatoid arthritis	• Ankylosing spondylitis
• Systemic lupus erythematosus	• Relapsing polychondritis
	• Behçet's disease
• Systemic sclerosis	• Systemic vasculitis
• Sjögren's syndrome	– Granulomatosis with polyangiitis (Wegener's)
• Polymyositis/ dermatomyositis	
– Antisynthetase syndrome	– Microscopic polyangiitis
• Mixed CTD	– Churg–Strauss vasculitis
• Undifferentiated CTD	

CTD connective tissue disease

Table 12.2 Pulmonary manifestations of rheumatologic diseases

• Pleural disease	• Parenchymal
– Pleurisy	– Interstitial lung disease
– Effusion/thickening	(a) NSIP, UIP, OP, LIP, DAD, DIP
• Airways	
– Upper	– Diffuse alveolar hemorrhage
(a) Cricoarytenoid disease	– Acute pneumonitis
(b) Tracheal disease	• Rheumatoid nodules
– Lower	• Infections
(a) Bronchiectasis	• Drug toxicity
(b) Bronchiolitis	• Lung cancer
• Vascular	

NSIP nonspecific interstitial pneumonia, *UIP* usual interstitial pneumonia, *LIP* lymphocytic interstitial pneumonia, *OP* organizing pneumonia, *DAD* diffuse alveolar damage, *DIP* desquamative interstitial pneumonia

focusing on commonly encountered problems in the management of lung disease in CTD rather than structuring the chapter in the more traditional anatomic compartment-based descriptions.

By definition, the CTDs manifest with autoimmune-mediated organ dysfunction and the lungs are a frequent target. Certain CTDs are more likely to include lung involvement – such as SSc, poly-/dermatomyositis (PM/DM), and rheumatoid arthritis (RA) – but all patients with CTD are at risk for developing associated lung disease.

There is a myriad of pulmonary manifestations – with varied incidence and prevalence – associated with the CTDs; essentially every component of the respiratory tract is at risk of injury in these patients (Table 12.2). In addition to the heterogeneous nature of the CTDs, there is also a wide spectrum of lung involvement among the specific CTDs and certain of these diseases are associated with specific types of lung involvement (Table 12.3). As examples, in patients with SSc, pulmonary involvement is the leading cause of mortality, and is typically manifest by interstitial lung disease (ILD) and/or pulmonary hypertension (PH). In contrast, in SLE, ILD and PH occur much less frequently – yet, pleural disease occurs quite commonly. Patients with RA and Sjogren's syndrome often develop airways disease (bronchiolitis and bronchiectasis) and ILD, whereas patients with PM/DM frequently develop ILD and yet rarely ever develop airway complications.

Table 12.3 Most common CTD-associated pulmonary manifestations

	SSc	RA	Primary Sjögren's	MCTD	PM/DM	SLE
Airways	–	++	++	+	–	+
ILD	+++	++	++	++	+++	+
Pleural	–	++	+	+	–	+++
Vascular	+++	–	–	++	+	+
DAH	–	–	–	–	–	++

SSc systemic sclerosis, *RA* rheumatoid arthritis, *MCTD* mixed connective tissue disease, *PM/DM* polymyositis/dermatomyositis, *SLE* systemic lupus erythematosus, *ILD* interstitial lung disease, *DAH* diffuse alveolar hemorrhage. The number of + signs indicates relative prevalence of each manifestation

It is not known why specific CTDs are more likely to be associated with certain types of lung involvement, and there is much to learn about the natural history of lung involvement among CTD.

Because there already are a number of excellent comprehensive reviews describing in detail the pulmonary manifestations that are associated with CTD [1–4], we chose to focus this chapter on common dilemmas that clinicians encounter in the care of patients with CTD-associated lung disease with an aim to provide a "practical approach" to this complex intersect of diseases.

Several illustrative cases are incorporated into the text and we will largely focus on ILD because it occurs across the spectrum of CTD, is potentially the most devastating of pulmonary manifestations, and often poses the most significant challenges to the practicing clinician.

Case 1

A 55-year-old man, former smoker, has a 10-year history of rheumatoid factor (RF) and anticyclic citrullinated peptide (anti-CCP) positive erosive RA and develops progressive exertional dyspnea and cough. The articular manifestations of his disease are well controlled with combined adalimumab, methotrexate, and ibuprofen. On examination, he appears well, there is no tachypnea or tachycardia, his resting pulse oximetry is 91% but with walking drops to 87%. On respiratory examination he has audible crackles at the bases of both lungs. He has chronic rheumatoid deformities of his hands and feet, but no active synovitis. His forced vital capacity (FVC) is 2.3 L (74% predicted), forced expiratory volume (FEV-1) is 2.1 L (73%), and his DLCO is 64% predicted. A chest X-ray shows bilateral pulmonary infiltrates, and high-resolution computed tomography (HRCT) has a pattern most suggestive of fibrotic lung disease (Fig. 12.1).

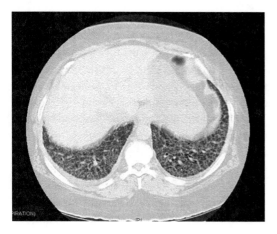

Fig. 12.1 Case 1 – 55-year-old man with well-characterized rheumatoid arthritis and high-resolution computed tomography evidence of fibrotic lung disease

This case serves to illustrate a common scenario whereby ILD has developed in a patient with well-characterized CTD and further evaluation is needed to determine whether the ILD is a manifestation of the underlying CTD or reflects an alternative process.

ILD Within Preexisting CTD

It is not uncommon to detect ILD in patients with preexisting CTD. Of the CTDs, ILD is particularly common in patients who have SSc, PM/DM, RA, primary Sjögren's syndrome, and MCTD [1–4]. When ILD is identified in patients with well-characterized CTD – such as the patient in Case 1 who has erosive, RF-positive, anti-CCP positive, well-characterized and long-standing RA – a variety of questions need to be considered by the clinician.

ILD Within Preexisting CTD: True–True and Unrelated?

Just because ILD is identified in a patient with a CTD does not mean the two are interrelated. In other words, the presence of preexisting RA does not preclude the development of ILD due to other causes (e.g., hypersensitivity pneumonitis). Given that patients with preexisting CTD are often being treated with immunosuppressive therapies, the findings of new pulmonary infiltrates in an immunocompromised host should raise strong suspicions for respiratory infection – with either typical or atypical pathogens. Furthermore, there should be consideration for drug-induced lung toxicity because some of the anti-inflammatory and immunomodulatory therapies including aspirin, non-steroidal anti-inflammatory drugs (NSAIDs), sulfasalazine, methotrexate, leflunomide, and the antitumor necrosis factor (anti-TNF) agents are all associated with drug-induced pneumonitis (discussed further in the next section) [4–23]. In this regard, just as with patients who present with de novo ILD, a thorough evaluation is needed to explore potential etiologies for the development of ILD. This evaluation should be comprehensive in scope in order to consider infection, drug toxicity, environmental and occupational exposures, familial disease, smoking-related lung disease, malignancy, and even idiopathic disease. As these other entities are being considered, the possibility of CTD-associated ILD (CTD-ILD) needs to be considered given that the patient presented with a preexisting CTD, but determining whether the ILD is associated with the preexisting CTD is often decided through a process of elimination.

Thoracic HRCT imaging plays a central role in the evaluation of ILD by providing detailed information on the pattern, distribution, and extent of the ILD; assessment of disease severity; and the presence of extraparenchymal abnormalities including pleural disease and lymphadenopathy [24–26]. Recent data show that certain extrapulmonary findings on HRCT are suggestive of underlying CTD – and these include the presence of a dilated esophagus or pericardial thickening/effusion [27]. ILD occurring with CTD is almost always bilateral, bibasilar, and peripheral-predominant [24, 26, 27]. The most common patterns are those that reflect the underlying pathologies of nonspecific interstitial pneumonia (NSIP), usual interstitial pneumonia (UIP), organizing pneumonia (OP), diffuse alveolar damage (DAD), and lymphocytic interstitial pneumonia (LIP) [24–27]. Although there is a high degree of concordance between HRCT and lung biopsy for UIP pattern lung disease, HRCT is not as reliable when it comes to distinguishing cellular NSIP from fibrotic NSIP; identifying LIP, OP, or DAD; or evaluating for infection or malignancy.

ILD Within Preexisting CTD: Drug-Induced Lung Disease

In patients who are being treated for their CTD, consideration for drug-induced lung toxicity is indicated if respiratory symptoms develop because a broad array of medication commonly used for patients with CTD – and particularly RA – are associated with drug-induced lung adverse events [18]. In particular, of the disease-modifying antirheumatic drugs (DMARDs), methotrexate is most commonly associated with drug-induced pneumonitis as this drug is the most frequently used DMARD and is considered the gold standard of therapy for RA. Methotrexate-induced pneumonitis occurs in as many as 3% [18, 22, 23, 28] of those on the drug, and does not appear to be dose dependent or related to duration of treatment. Patients with methotrexate-induced pneumonitis typically present with a relatively insidious onset of progressive breathlessness and are found to have peripheral-predominant pulmonary infiltrates on chest imaging. A mild peripheral eosinophilia is noted in 40% of patients and bronchoalveolar lavage (BAL) often produces a lymphocytic return [18]. Transbronchial or surgical lung biopsy may reveal a hypersensitivity pattern of poorly formed nonnecrotizing granulomata and eosinophilia and occasionally there are components of organizing pneumonia in addition. In many instances, the diagnosis of methotrexate-induced pneumonitis is not definitive and is made on the basis of excluding other etiologies and associations for pneumonitis, particularly infection. When methotrexate-induced pneumonitis is suspected, treatment includes withdrawal of the offending drug and high-dose corticosteroids (CS) [18]. In some instances, drug withdrawal is sufficient provided there is no significant lung function impairment that requires corticosteroids. Most patients respond favorably although there is potential for progression and for the development of an acute respiratory distress syndrome [18]. Re-challenge of patients is not acceptable as it usually leads to recurrence of pneumonitis that can be more intense [18, 23].

Other immunosuppressive agents commonly used in CTD including sulfasalazine, leflunomide, etanercept, infliximab, adalimumab, and rituximab have also been associated with lung toxicity but these situations occur far less commonly or convincingly than with methotrexate [5–9, 15, 18, 29, 30]. There are far fewer data to confirm a direct causal effect of lung toxicity with these agents but scattered case reports continue to suggest a possible association.

ILD Within Preexisting CTD: Is Bronchoscopic Evaluation Needed?

BAL is an integral part of the evaluation of CTD-associated lung disease to exclude respiratory infection or alveolar hemorrhage in the immuno-compromised CTD patient with new onset pulmonary infiltrates and in the evaluation of drug-induced disease. In this regard, BAL eosino-philia, with or without an associated lymphocy-tosis, may suggest drug-induced pneumonitis – but this is neither a sensitive nor specific finding. Silver and colleagues have suggested that BAL neutrophilia or eosinophilia in patients with SSc-ILD is useful as a predictor of progressive ILD [31]. However, two recent well-designed large prospective studies [32, 33] failed to demonstrate any prognostic significance of either an eosino-philia or neutrophilia obtained from BAL in patients with SSc-ILD, and hence the routine use of BAL to solely predict the likelihood of disease progression in CTD-ILD cannot be recom-mended. Transbronchial biopsy is of limited value in the evaluation of parenchymal lung dis-ease in CTD, but may be diagnostic in more air-way-centric complications such as bronchiolitis.

ILD Within Preexisting CTD: Is a Surgical Lung Biopsy Needed?

Because data have yet to show that determining a specific type of IP impacts on prognosis in CTD-ILD, the role of surgical lung biopsy in patients with preexisting CTD remains controversial [34]. The distinction between the specific ILD types (e.g., UIP vs. NSIP) is known to have prognostic significance among patients with idiopathic inter-stitial pneumonia (IIP) [35–37] – but does not appear to be as prognostically significant in patients with CTD. In the largest series of biopsied SSc-ILD subjects ($n = 80$), Bouros and colleagues showed that changes in diffusing capacity over time – but not histopathologic distinction between NSIP and UIP – predicted prognosis [38]. Similarly, in their cohort of 93 patients with a variety of CTD-ILD, Park and colleagues demonstrated that

age, pulmonary function, and degree of dyspnea were of prognostic importance – but differences in IP type did not impact survival [39]. In contrast, although among a much smaller cohort of patients with SSc-ILD, Fischer and colleagues have shown that those patients with SSc-NSIP ($n = 14$) have a median survival of 15.3 years compared with 3 years for those with SSc-UIP ($n = 8$) [40]. The rela-tively small cohort sizes of existing studies and the impact of selection and referral bias cannot be dis-counted and therefore the predictive power of dif-ferent patterns of lung histopathology remains uncertain in CTD-ILD. Furthermore, CTD-ILD patients tend to be treated with immunosuppres-sive therapies – targeting both progressive ILD and the extrathoracic inflammatory features – irre-spective of specific ILD pattern. In this context, because the biopsy finding may not impact on treatment decisions, including immunosuppres-sion, clinicians often elect not to proceed with a surgical biopsy [34].

In general, we believe that it is important to the patient with CTD-ILD to discuss obtaining a surgical lung biopsy unless the HRCT is strongly suggestive of UIP pattern lung disease – with pat-terns of consolidation, because of the wide dif-ferential diagnosis; with patterns suggestive of LIP because this will heighten awareness for pos-sible subsequent development of lymphoma; and in patterns suggestive of NSIP because the radio-logical "diagnosis" is often not correct. In patients with SSc, and perhaps other well-characterized CTD, however, a "convincing" pattern of NSIP on HRCT may obviate the need for a surgical biopsy. HRCT pattern has high concordance with histopathology for cases of UIP, but is much less reliable in its ability to distinguish the other pat-terns encountered in patients with CTD. In addi-tion, biopsy is helpful to exclude malignancy or infection, particularly when the HRCT shows areas of consolidation. In practice, we incorpo-rate knowledge of the underlying histopathology into our discussions with the patient, and have found that it can impact on treatment plans, par-ticularly the use of corticosteroids as discussed below. In general, therefore, we find it useful for management to confirm a definitive pattern of ILD in our patients with chronic ILD.

We also believe that a surgical lung biopsy is indicated in patients with preexisting CTD in cases when there are concerns for a co-existent and alternative etiology (e.g., hypersensitivity pneumonitis), when the ILD pattern on HRCT is atypical for underlying CTD (e.g., upper lobe disease prominence), when the HRCT features suggest malignancy or infection (e.g., progressive nodules, cavitation, consolidation, pleural thickening or effusion), or as discussed above – when a specific pattern cannot be identified by HRCT (i.e., all patterns other than typical UIP). In addition, when the preexisting CTD is not as well defined – such as with sero-negative (RF and anti-CCP negative) RA – or not fully confirmed – such as with patients who have weakly positive antinuclear antibodies and "soft" features of any definable CTD – a surgical lung biopsy should be performed. In these circumstances, the histopathology of the ILD may have some of the features that have come to be considered as characteristic features of autoimmune lung histopathology including dense perivascular collagen, plasmacytic infiltration, pleuritis, or lymphoid aggregates with germinal center formation – and thus may actually help confirm CTD when the extrathoracic manifestations and serologies cannot! Ultimately, the decision of whether to proceed with surgical lung biopsy is individualized to each patient, but our approach is to have a low threshold to proceed with biopsy in CTD patients when the presence of the "preexisting" CTD is

not convincing, when there are any atypical HRCT features that would suggest an alternative diagnosis, or when the imaging does not provide ample support for a definitive diagnosis.

Case 2

A 60-year-old woman, never smoker, presents with the insidious onset of dyspnea and a cough that is worse at night. Her past medical history is notable only for hypothyroidism. On symptom review she describes blanching, tingling, and pain in both hands on exposure to cold. On physical examination, she is noted to have puffy hands with some tethering of the skin distal to the proximal interphalangeal joints, and a few scattered palmar telangiectasia. Nail fold capillary microscopy of the fourth and fifth nail beds is abnormal and shows dilated and tortuous capillaries with scattered areas of capillary loop dropout (Fig. 12.2a). She has audible crackles on respiratory examination limited to the bases of both lungs and HRCT evidence of ILD (Fig. 12.2b). Laboratory testing is notable for a positive antinuclear antibody (ANA) at moderate titer (1:320) with a nucleolar staining pattern.

This case serves to illustrate a scenario whereby ILD has developed in a patient without any prior history of CTD, yet features obtained in the history (Raynaud's phenomenon), physical examination (digital edema, telangiectasia, abnormal

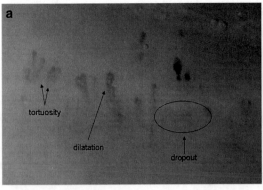
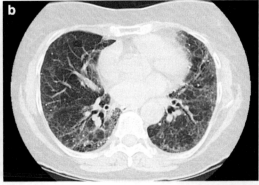

Fig. 12.2 (a) Nailfold capillaroscopy demonstrating capillary dropout, dilatation, and tortuosity (digital photograph at ×40 magnification). (b) Case 2 – high-resolution computed tomography evidence of interstitial lung disease in a 60-year-old woman without prior history of connective tissue disease

nail fold capillaroscopy), and laboratory testing (nucleolar-ANA positive) raise strong suspicions that this patient has a SSc spectrum of disease with ILD as the presenting manifestation.

ILD as the Presenting Manifestation of CTD

Identifying CTD

The detection of "occult" CTD in patients presenting with ILD is optimized by rheumatologic evaluation and multidisciplinary collaboration [41]. Identifying underlying CTD is challenging [42–44] but finding CTD is not uncommon: it has been estimated that among those presenting with an apparently idiopathic IP, roughly 15% are found to have underlying CTD after more thorough evaluation [2]. Rheumatologic expertise can be particularly helpful in the identification and assessment of subtle extrathoracic features of CTD – such as the symptomatic keratoconjunctivitis sicca (KCS) of primary Sjögren's syndrome, or the puffy hands/digital edema associated with SSc – and with autoantibody interpretation. As an example of the challenges of CTD detection, Homma and colleagues evaluated whether IP as the sole presentation of CTD can be differentiated from IIP [45]. They described 68 patients who had presented with IIP and were followed prospectively over 11 years. Thirteen (19%) patients eventually developed classifiable CTD. The prevalence of the presence of ANA or RF was no different in the group who developed CTD compared with those who did not. The authors concluded that patients who are defined as having an IIP cannot be distinguished from those with CTD-ILD before the systemic manifestations appear [45]. While we support their findings that detecting occult CTD is challenging and that ANA and RF positivity alone are not very useful in this endeavor, we offer an alternative set of conclusions: engaging rheumatologists to help evaluate for subtle extrathoracic features of underlying CTD, assessing more specific autoantibodies, and incorporating ANA titer and pattern of immunofluorescence are all important

components of an ILD evaluation and make it more likely that occult CTD will be detected.

Autoantibodies and ILD

Despite the knowledge that detecting CTD in patients presenting with ILD is not only important but common, there are no protocols or guidelines to aid the clinician. The current standard practice in most units is to draw an ANA and RF (and occasionally other autoantibodies) in patients presenting with ILD, and if any are positive, a rheumatologic evaluation is requested. In our opinion, this approach is less than ideal for a number of reasons. Foremost, ANA and RF are poor screening tests: they have low specificity – particularly when present at low titer – and can be seen in healthy individuals. Furthermore, given that a negative ANA and RF are likely to dissuade the pulmonologist from requesting a rheumatologic evaluation, cases of occult CTD that may be ANA and RF negative (e.g., antisynthetase syndrome) are missed. We recently described a cohort of antisynthetase patients who presented with ILD and were characteristically ANA negative [46]. All patients had subtle features of the antisynthetase syndrome (e.g., mechanic's hands) which were detected only after referral for rheumatologic evaluation, and all patients were antisynthetase antibody (PL-7 and PL-12) positive. Prior to evaluation at our center, none had undergone rheumatologic evaluation – and we suspect this was due to the negative ANA, RF, and ANA profile that had been performed elsewhere as screening tests. In addition, further highlighting the importance of engaging rheumatologists in the evaluation of undefined forms of ILD, we recently described a cohort of "idiopathic" IP patients identified to have occult Sjögren's syndrome as confirmed by the presence of chronic sialadenitis on minor labial salivary gland biopsy [47].

More specific antibodies do serve as integral components in the assessment for CTD-ILD. Practitioners evaluating what appears to be idiopathic disease should consider ordering more than an ANA and RF if they wish to screen for CTD more effectively (for the full list of antibodies for

Table 12.4 Proposed provisional criteria for "*lung-dominant CTD*"

1. NSIP, UIP, LIP, OP, DAD (or DIP if no smoking history) as determined by surgical lung biopsy or suggested by HRCT

2. Insufficient extrathoracic features of a definite CTD to allow a specific CTD designation

3. No identifiable alternative etiology for IP

4. Any *one* of these autoantibodies or *at least two* of these histopathology features:

(a) High-titer ANA (>1:320) or RF (>60 IU/mL)	(a) Lymphoid aggregates with germinal centers
(b) Nucleolar-ANA	
(c) Anti-CCP	(b) Extensive pleuritis
(d) Anti-Scl-70	(c) Prominent plasmacytic infiltration
(e) Anti-Ro	(d) Dense perivascular collagen
(f) Anti-La	
(g) Anti-dsDNA	
(h) Anti-Smith	
(i) Anti-RNP	
(j) Anti-tRNA synthetase	
(k) Anti-PM-Scl	
(l) Anticentromere	

NSIP nonspecific interstitial pneumonia, *UIP* usual interstitial pneumonia, *LIP* lymphocytic interstitial pneumonia, *OP* organizing pneumonia, *DAD* diffuse alveolar damage, *DIP* desquamative interstitial pneumonia, *HRCT* high-resolution computed tomography, *CTD* connective tissue disease, *MCPs* metacarpal-phalangeal joints, *KCS* keratoconjunctivitis sicca, *IP* interstitial pneumonia, *ANA* antinuclear antibody, *CCP* cyclic citrullinated peptide, *Scl-70* anti DNA topoisomerase I, *Ro* anti-Sjögren's syndrome A (anti-SS-A), *La* anti-Sjögren's syndrome B (anti-SS-B), *RNP* ribonucleic protein

Adapted from Fischer A, West SG, Swigris JJ, Brown KK, du Bois RM. Connective tissue disease-associated interstitial lung disease: a call for clarification. Chest. 2010;138(2):251–6

which we suggest screening, see Table 12.4). Furthermore, we believe it is important to take note of the pattern of immunofluorescence when the ANA is positive, as the nucleolar-staining ANA pattern in patients with ILD suggests SSc spectrum of disease [48]. Particularly helpful antibodies to request in patients with ILD as part of a CTD evaluation include anti-Scl-70, antisynthetase antibodies (e.g., Jo-1, PL-7, PL-12, and others), anti-Ro (SS-A), antiribonucleoprotein (RNP), and anti-CCP. Anti-Scl-70 is highly specific for SSc, anti-Ro is present in a broad array of CTDs characteristically associated with ILD (such as Sjögren's syndrome, antisynthetase syndrome, and SSc), anti-RNP is specific for MCTD, anti-tRNA synthetase antibodies confirm the antisynthetase syndrome, and anti-CCP antibodies are highly specific for RA.

Histopathological Considerations

Careful review of the histopathology from surgical lung biopsy specimens may provide clues that the ILD is a manifestation of an underlying CTD.

There are a number of "suggestive" patterns and features observed on histopathology with known associations with CTD [49–52]. A higher index of suspicion for possible occult CTD is warranted in any case of NSIP or LIP as these are two of the more commonly recognized patterns in patients with CTD. In addition, secondary histopathologic features that should raise strong suspicions for underlying CTD include: dense perivascular collagen, extensive pleuritis, lymphoid aggregates with germinal center formation, and prominent plasmacytic infiltration [49–52]. These histologic features alert the pathologist that the injury pattern is likely due to an underlying CTD. In such cases, the pulmonologist may conclude that the biopsy is consistent with CTD-ILD – and choose to manage the patient as such.

There are recent data to suggest that the presence of circulating autoantibodies is associated with histopathology findings – even in the absence of characterizable CTD. Song et al. [52] compared and contrasted secondary histopathologic features among three groups of patients with UIP pattern lung injury: Group 1 (*n*=39) was comprised of subjects with CTD-UIP; Group

2 ($n=27$) with subjects who had idiopathic UIP with ANA or RF positivity; and Group 3 ($n=34$) subjects had idiopathic UIP and were antibody negative [52]. Among those with CTD-UIP there were more germinal centers, plasma cells, and fewer fibroblastic foci when compared with all subjects who had idiopathic UIP. Interestingly, however, histopathologic features differed between the subgroups (Groups 2 and 3) of idiopathic UIP based on autoantibody status: although none of the antibody-positive idiopathic-UIP subjects (Group 2) had extrathoracic features of CTD, they had higher germinal center scores and more plasma cells than antibody-negative idiopathic-UIP subjects (Group 3). Moreover, no histopathologic features distinguished CTD-UIP (Group 1) from antibody-positive idiopathic-UIP (Group 2). Among those with idiopathic UIP, antibody status did not impact survival – although as the authors point out, this might have been due to the small sample sizes in each group, but those with idiopathic UIP had a worse prognosis than those with CTD-UIP [52]. The significance of these findings is not known, but we believe they merit further investigation.

An Interdisciplinary Roadblock

Paradoxically, the detection of autoantibodies often raises more questions and may not clarify classification. This is in part due to what we consider to be shortcomings of existing rheumatologic classification criteria. In the absence of extrathoracic manifestations attributable to CTD (such as inflammatory arthritis or sclerodactyly), rheumatologists are reluctant to diagnose CTD, even when highly specific autoantibodies and a fitting ILD pattern are present. To illustrate this point, consider a 35-year-old man with a positive anti-Ro antibody, fibrotic NSIP, and no extrathoracic features of CTD: based on currently available criteria, this patient would not be classified as having CTD. Similarly, a 40-year-old woman with LIP, a high-titer speckled ANA, and esophageal hypomotility as her only extrathoracic abnormality would not be defined as having CTD.

Neither case meets diagnostic criteria for CTD, nor would either be considered as "idiopathic" by pulmonologists.

UCTD and NSIP

The concept has been proposed that all patients with idiopathic NSIP – even those without extrathoracic features or serum autoantibodies – actually have UCTD [53, 54]. In our opinion, although this is an interesting hypothesis, the revised application of this CTD diagnosis to encompass all NSIP cases raises problems. Redefining the UCTD diagnosis in this way requires input from rheumatologists who are generally skeptical about accepting ILD as a diagnostic criterion for CTD. As an example, rheumatologists would classify a 55-year-old woman with inflammatory arthritis and a positive ANA as UCTD, but not a 55-year-old woman with NSIP and a positive ANA. Patients with isolated NSIP are not considered to have CTD by rheumatologists unless there are extrathoracic features present. Rheumatologists will only classify patients with NSIP as having a CTD if there are extrathoracic features (e.g., Raynaud's phenomenon or inflammatory arthritis) and specific autoantibodies to lend more certainty to the CTD label. Another difficulty with the use of the term UCTD is that UCTD is considered by rheumatologists to be indicative of mild disease [55, 56]. To attempt to redefine UCTD to include isolated, and often life-threatening, ILD is unlikely to succeed, because we strongly suspect it would not be adopted by rheumatologists.

A Novel Term to Consider: "Lung-Dominant" CTD (Table 12.4)

We have recently proposed the use of the term "*lung-dominant CTD*" for cases where the ILD has a "rheumatologic flavor" as supported by specific autoantibodies or histopathologic features and yet does not meet criteria for a defined CTD based on the lack of adequate extrathoracic features to confer a diagnosis of definite CTD [57]. Implicit in the use of the proposed term "lung-dominant CTD" is the recognition that specific autoantibodies and histopathologic features alone can be enough to characterize and classify a patient as having a CTD-ILD. The presence of extrathoracic features highly suggestive of CTD (e.g., Raynaud's phenomenon, esophageal hypomotility, inflammatory arthritis of the metacarpal phalangeal joints [MCPs] or wrists, digital edema, or symptomatic KCS) is important and will lend further support for an underlying CTD, but their absence should not preclude a diagnosis of lung-dominant CTD. Based on limitations of the current classification schemes, such cases are presently classified (we would actually say misclassified) as idiopathic or, worse, left unclassified.

The following two cases are examples of patients with lung-dominant CTD: (1) a 60-year-old woman with biopsy-proven UIP with the secondary histopathologic features of extensive pleuritis and lymphoid aggregates with germinal center formation, a positive anti-Ro antibody, along with esophageal hypomotility; (2) a 45-year-old man with biopsy-proven NSIP and a positive ANA of 1:640 with a speckled pattern, without any extrathoracic features of CTD.

The diagnostic criteria for lung-dominant CTD listed in Table 12.4 have been recently proposed, should be viewed as provisional, and we hope they will serve as a platform for further investigation, including validation via prospective study [57].

Multidisciplinary Approach to Evaluation

Given the challenges of detecting CTD and the limited utility of nonspecific autoantibodies – such as RF or ANA – a multidisciplinary approach to evaluation is indicated and we suggest that the best way to assess for occult CTD is by having a rheumatologist evaluate patients with undefined forms of ILD. However, given the international shortage of rheumatologists available to evaluate even "traditional" rheumatology patients, suggesting that rheumatologists should also evaluate all cases of ILD is unrealistic and impractical. Instead, we advise that a rheumatologic consult is needed as part of an ILD evaluation for the following groups of patients because they are more likely to have CTD (Table 12.5): (1) women, particularly those younger than 50, (2) any patient with extrathoracic manifestations highly suggestive of CTD (e.g., Raynaud's phenomenon, esophageal hypomotility, inflammatory arthritis of the MCPs or wrists, digital edema, or symptomatic KCS), (3) all cases of NSIP, LIP, or any ILD pattern with secondary histopathology features that might suggest CTD (i.e., extensive pleuritis, dense perivascular collagen, lymphoid aggregates with germinal center formation, prominent plasmacytic infiltration), and (4) patients with a positive ANA or RF in high titer (generally considered to be ANA > 1:320 or RF > 60 IU/mL), a nucleolar-staining ANA at any titer, or any positive autoantibody specific as to a particular CTD

Table 12.5 Suggested categories of ILD patients who require further rheumatologic evaluation

1. Women, particularly those younger than 50
2. Any patient with extrathoracic manifestations highly suggestive of CTD
(a) i.e., Raynaud's phenomenon, esophageal hypomotility, inflammatory arthritis of the metacarpal-phalangeal joints or wrists, digital edema, or symptomatic keratoconjunctivitis sicca
3. All cases of NSIP, LIP, or any ILD pattern with secondary histopathology features that might suggest CTD
(a) i.e., Extensive pleuritis, dense perivascular collagen, lymphoid aggregates with germinal center formation, or prominent plasmacytic infiltration
4. Patients with a positive ANA or RF in high titer (generally considered to be ANA > 1:320 or RF > 60 IU/mL), a nucleolar-staining ANA at any titer, or any positive autoantibody specific to a particular CTD
(a) i.e., Anti-CCP, anti-Scl-70, anti-Ro, anti-La, anti-dsDNA, anti-Smith, anti-RNP, anti-tRNA synthetase

(see list of autoantibodies in Table 12.4a–j). Collaborative assessments and ongoing dialogue between pulmonologists and rheumatologists will only lead to bridging some of the current deficiencies and limitations of CTD-ILD detection and classification terminology.

Management Considerations for CTD-ILD

CTD-ILD: Is Treatment Indicated?

Not all patients with CTD-ILD require pharmacologic treatment. Although radiographic findings of ILD on HRCT are common in patients with CTD, only a subset of patients will show clinically significant, progressive disease. For example, SSc patients with anticentromere antibody positivity often have mild bibasilar ILD that is nonprogressive [58]. Furthermore, because CTD patients are at increased risk for a myriad of pulmonary manifestations as well as cardiovascular disease, the assessment of respiratory impairment in a patient with CTD should be comprehensive in scope. This is particularly relevant when evaluating dyspneic/hypoxic SSc patients as they have such a high prevalence of PH – occurring either in isolation or concomitant with ILD. The decision to treat CTD-ILD often rests upon whether the patient has respiratory impairment, whether the ILD is progressive, and in consideration of any mitigating factors. Therapy for CTD-ILD is generally reserved for those patients with clinically significant, progressive disease, and this determination is based upon a constellation of clinical assessment tools that include both subjective and objective measures of respiratory impairment [59].

When considering immunomodulatory therapy options for CTD-ILD, both intrathoracic and extrathoracic disease manifestations and degrees of activity need to be considered. The extrathoracic manifestations of a specific CTD often require immunosuppressive therapy yet the drug selected for the treatment of extrathoracic CTD manifestations (such as inflammatory arthritis)

may be one not typically employed for managing ILD (such as anti-TNF agents) or may be an agent with significant potential for lung toxicity (e.g., methotrexate). In some cases, the extrathoracic manifestations of the underlying CTD determine the choice of the initial immunomodulatory regimen, and in others it is the ILD that predominates clinically and determines the choice of immunosuppression and the intensity of therapy.

In all cases of CTD-ILD, disease monitoring, choice of therapy, and on-going longitudinal assessment and re-assessment of treatment response are complex – and are optimized by effective cross-specialty collaboration [59]. Efforts should be made to tailor any treatment recommendation to the individual, fully considering the myriad of factors besides the CTD-ILD itself including the specific underlying CTD, medical comorbidities, patient preferences and compliance, insurance coverage, and access to care. In reality, we are left with few data to guide choice specific therapeutic agents, and in many cases, the disease progresses despite therapeutic intervention.

CTD-ILD: Therapeutic Agents to be Considered

Corticosteroids

Because they have a rapid onset of action and anti-inflammatory properties, CS have served as an initial and mainstay of therapy for CTD-ILD. There are some small case series supporting the use of CS for CTD-ILD [60–62] but no controlled studies. We incorporate knowledge of underlying histopathology when making treatment decisions, particularly as it relates to the use of corticosteroids. In general, in our experience, the more fibrotic forms of CTD-ILD (UIP and fibrotic NSIP) tend to be less corticosteroid responsive when compared with more cellular forms of ILD (cellular NSIP, OP, LIP). Therefore, in cases of UIP or fibrotic NSIP, we do not use high doses of CS (>40 mg/day) for prolonged periods of time. In contrast, in more cellular forms – particularly

OP – we often implement high-dose CS (~60 mg/day) for 4–6 weeks followed by slow taper along with titration of CS-sparing agents described below.

The toxicity and adverse side effects associated with long-term use of CS are numerous and frequently limit their use. CS are commonly introduced early in the treatment course at a moderate to high dose (e.g., between 20 and 60 mg PO daily of prednisone or equivalent, or 0.25–0.75 mg/kg/day) in order to obtain early improvement in symptoms and induce a response. As steroid-sparing agents are added and dose-escalated (see below) CS are slowly tapered towards a lower maintenance dose to minimize the cumulative toxicity of the CS (e.g., 10 mg PO daily or every other day of prednisone or equivalent). In many cases, CS may be tapered to complete discontinuation. One caveat to this strategy, based on data suggesting that SSc patients treated with moderate-high dose CS may be at increased risk of scleroderma renal crisis [63], is that one should consider limiting the daily prednisone dose to less than 15 mg/day for patients with SSc-ILD though this is determined on a case-by-case basis.

Cyclophosphamide

Cyclophosphamide (CYC) is one of the most potent steroid-sparing immunosuppressive medications employed for organ-threatening damage caused by CTD. The efficacy of CYC in the treatment of rheumatic diseases is based on controlled trials of patients with systemic vasculitis, lupus nephritis, and SSc-ILD [64–67]. Retrospective studies have shown that in patients with progressive SSc-ILD, treatment with CYC is associated with improved pulmonary function and better survival [68–70]. Data from two recently completed controlled trials show that SSc-ILD patients treated with CYC for 12 months have improved quality of life, stabilization or modest improvement of pulmonary function, and less radiographic progression of fibrosis [65–67, 71]. Interestingly, it appears that unless CYC therapy is continued beyond 12 months, or is followed by another effective immunosuppressive agent, the

gains in pulmonary function attributed to the CYC treatment are lost once therapy has been discontinued [67].

CYC is administered in either oral or intravenous form. Both forms have been studied with apparent equal efficacy and there is less bladder toxicity with the intravenous route. With intravenous therapy, a typical starting dose is 500 mg/m^2 for the first infusion and subsequent infusions are then dose escalated based upon the tolerability of the previous dose(s) and the white blood cell count nadir. Peak dosing is often in the 750–1,000 mg/m^2 range (to a maximum absolute dose of ~2,000 mg per infusion). Hydration with intravenous fluids and administration of MESNA pre- and post-CYC infusion, and encouraging oral intake of liquids over the 24-h postinfusion period can minimize the potential for bladder toxicity. Because intravenous dosing of CYC is emetogenic, antiemetics are given prior to the infusion and on as needed basis for the 1 or 2 days post the infusion. To optimize use of the drug, it is often useful to engage health care providers (usually rheumatologists or oncologists) with experience in administration of intravenous CYC. When CYC is given orally, the initial dose is 50 mg/day and the medication is dose escalated as tolerated towards a recommended goal maintenance dose of ~2 mg/kg/day. Ongoing periodic assessment of the complete blood count, hepatic function, and urinalysis is important to assess its safe administration [72].

Mycophenolate Mofetil

There are no controlled trials evaluating the efficacy of mycophenolate mofetil (MMF) for CTD-ILD, though data from controlled trials have supported the use of MMF in subsets of patients with lupus nephritis [73]. In 2006, our group published our experience with MMF for the treatment of 28 patients with CTD-ILD [74]. Over the course of therapy, we found that the daily prednisone dose decreased from 15 to 10 mg/day and that the percent predicted FVC increased by 2.3% and the percent predicted of DLCO increased by 2.6%. Moreover, the drug was well tolerated with a paucity of side effects [74]. Similarly, Liossis and colleagues reported their experience with SSc-ILD in six patients and found improvement in five of six patients both clinically and with objective testing [75]. More recently, two additional centers published case series of 17 patients and 13 patients, respectively, both demonstrating that patients with SSc-ILD who were treated with MMF had stable or improved lung function, and that the drug was again well tolerated [76, 77]. Collectively, these data support the rationale of the ongoing Scleroderma Lung Study II, a large, randomized, multicenter trial of MMF vs. CYC in the treatment of SSc-ILD.

As with other cytotoxic agents, MMF is initiated at a low starting dosage (250–500 mg twice daily) and dose escalated with close drug-specific monitoring towards a target dose of 1.0–1.5 g twice daily as tolerated. Periodic serologic monitoring for myelosuppression, hepatotoxicity, and other potential adverse effects of the drug is emphasized [72]. In patients with gastrointestinal intolerance to MMF, a dose reduction of the MMF or a switch to mycophenolic acid (Myfortic©) may be considered.

Azathioprine

Controlled trials in rheumatoid arthritis, SLE, and other CTDs suggest that azathioprine (AZA) is an effective steroid-sparing agent [78–80]. In a recent placebo-controlled trial, Hoyles and colleagues demonstrated that in patients with SSc, administration of intravenous CYC for 6 monthly infusions followed by AZA appears to stabilize ILD [65]. In addition, isolated case reports, small case series, and anecdotal experience suggest that AZA has some degree of efficacy for CTD-ILD [81–83]. In one large trial of IPF patients, AZA plus CS plus the antioxidant N-acetylcysteine has been shown to preserve lung function as measured by FVC and DLCO compared with CS plus AZA alone [83]. It is not known whether similar efficacy can be extrapolated for CTD-related UIP.

Prior to initiating AZA, testing should be undertaken to assess thiopurine methyltransferase (TPMT) enzyme activity. Patients with normal or high levels of enzyme activity have a lower frequency of toxicity [84] and for these patients therapy may be initiated at an initial dose of 50 mg PO daily followed by dose escalation towards a target dose of ~2 mg/kg/day. Because patients with absent or very low levels of TPMT activity are at high risk for severe myelosuppression, AZA should ideally be avoided in these patients, but if used, dose reduced by ~50% for a target dose closer to ~1 mg/kg/day [85]. Actual dosing regimens must be tailored to the individual patient's tolerance of the agent, disease severity and disease responsiveness, and based on safety demonstrated by periodic serologic monitoring for myelosuppression and hepatotoxicity [72].

Cyclosporine and Tacrolimus

There are no controlled trials evaluating the efficacy of either agent in CTD-ILD. Controlled trials have demonstrated its effectiveness in the management of RA [86, 87]. Anecdotal experience suggests that these agents are effective in other rheumatic diseases [88, 89]. Interestingly, small case series suggest that these agents may be particularly effective in treating refractory PM/DM-related ILD [90, 91].

Anti-TNF Drugs

Over the past decade, the management of the rheumatic diseases has been revolutionized by the advent of targeted biologic therapy. In particular, anti-TNF agents (etanercept, infliximab, adalimumab) have been shown to have a high degree of efficacy for RA [92, 93]. The effect of these agents on ILD is not known. There have been isolated case reports describing the development of ILD in patients being treated with each of these agents [5–7, 94] and at least one report demonstrating efficacy of anti-TNF therapy for RA-associated ILD [94]. Though they have little role in managing the ILD component of the CTD, the anti-TNF class of drugs is commonly needed to effectively control the extrathoracic CTD manifestations (e.g., rheumatoid synovitis) and in our experience can be used safely in patients with CTD-ILD.

CTD-ILD: Is Lung Transplantation an Option?

Lung transplantation is a reasonable consideration for any patient with severe ILD that is refractory to conventional therapies [95]. Historically, patients with CTD have been considered to be less than ideal candidates based on the systemic nature of their illness. In particular, the frequent finding of esophageal dilation, reflux, and hypomotility (such as in patients with SSc and PM/DM) has had a negative impact on the potential for lung transplantation – although recent data suggest that laparoscopic fundoplication favorably impacts on transplantation outcomes in CTD patients [96]. Furthermore, severe extrathoracic disease activity or comorbidity may dissuade lung transplantation consideration. That being said, for selective CTD-ILD patients, lung transplantation is a viable option and for these carefully selected cases, posttransplant outcomes appear to be similar to other transplanted cohorts [97–100].

CTD-ILD: Assessment and Management of ILD Exacerbation

Little is known about the natural history of CTD-ILD. Some patients with CTD-ILD are asymptomatic and do not progress, others present with an insidious onset characterized by chronic disease progression, and yet others present with an acute and fulminant course associated with rapid deterioration and death. In addition to the heterogeneity in presentation and clinical course, similar to other ILDs, patients with CTD-ILD can also have disease exacerbations – and these are not well characterized or described, but in our experience are typically associated with a poor outcome. When a patient with CTD-ILD develops worsening breathlessness or cough, ILD exacerbation is a concern, but comprehensive evaluation is indicated to exclude more common entities such as respiratory infection, thromboembolism, or acute cardiovascular events. Such evaluation usually requires a multidisciplinary

approach and includes pulmonary physiologic re-assessment, HRCT imaging, and bronchoscopic evaluation. Certain scenarios require CT-angiography or ventilation/perfusion scanning, echocardiography, or other cardiac testing. Drug-induced pneumonitis associated with immunosuppressive agents (such as CYC-associated pneumonitis) [18, 101–103] cannot be ignored as a possibility – but tends to be quite rare and is difficult to prove with any degree of certainty. When HRCT imaging shows progression of the ILD, and infectious causes have been excluded, alteration and intensification of the immunosuppressive regimen is often indicated. Our approach is to use high-dose CS as a first-line approach to treating acute exacerbations, followed by consideration of switching steroid-sparing therapies. There are no formal guidelines to follow, decisions are individualized to each patient, and we emphasize the importance of a thorough evaluation (including BAL) to exclude infection in these immunocompromised patients.

CTD-ILD: Screening for and Treatment of Concomitant Pulmonary Hypertension

Patients with ILD are at an increased risk of developing secondary PH at least in part related to chronic hypoxia [104]. In addition, patients with SSc, SLE, and MCTD are at risk for a primary vasculopathy resulting in pulmonary arterial hypertension (PAH). As exertional dyspnea is seen with ILD and PH, it is often difficult to dissect the relative contributions of these pulmonary manifestations in a given patient. Periodic screening with echocardiography is recommended for all CTD-ILD patients; a study by Arcasoy and colleagues, however, that assessed the sensitivity (85%), specificity (55%), and positive predictive value (52%) of a finding of PH in patients with advanced lung disease found that the estimated systolic pulmonary artery pressure is frequently inaccurate [105]. In patients with SSc-ILD, Steen has shown that a disproportionate reduction in the DLCO relative to the FVC (ratio of FVC%/DLCO% > 1.6) suggests concomitant PAH. In patients with SSc, elevations in the serum brain-natriuretic peptide level also suggest the presence of PH. In patients with CTD-ILD suspected to have PH based on noninvasive assessment, definitive evaluation with right-heart catheterization is warranted. Although the decision to proceed with right-heart catheterization is individualized to each patient, factors that should prompt strong consideration for right-heart catheterization include echocardiographic estimates of significant right ventricular systolic pressure elevation (>45 mmHg) or a tricuspid regurgitation velocity jet of >2.8 m/s, pulmonary function tests that show a declining DLCO relative to the FVC (i.e., FVC%/DLCO% > 1.6), examination findings that suggest PH (such as an accentuated pulmonic component of the second heart sound, increased lower extremity edema, right ventricular heave), or unexplained worsening dyspnea or exertional hypoxemia in the absence of other explanations [106–110].

Because SSc patients have the highest prevalence of ILD and PAH, most if not all of the controlled data from trials for CTD-ILD or CTD-PAH are based on studying CTD patients with an SSc spectrum of disease. The controlled trials that have demonstrated efficacy for SSc-ILD therapies excluded patients with SSc-PAH, and trials that have demonstrated efficacy for novel vasodilatory therapies for SSc-PAH have excluded patients with SSc-ILD patients. As a result, there are no controlled data to inform evidence-based decisions for cohorts of CTD-ILD patients with co-existent PAH/PH. In practice, it is not uncommon to combine immunosuppressive regimens for ILD with PAH-specific therapies (e.g., prostanoids, phosphodiesterase-inhibitor therapy, or endothelin-antagonist therapy) but these strategies are only based on anecdotal evidence [111, 112].

Case 3

A 40-year-old woman, current smoker, presents with cough, and exertional dyspnea. She was recently diagnosed with asthma but feels her respiratory symptoms have worsened despite inhaled corticosteroid and bronchodilator therapy. Her CTD symptom review is notable for

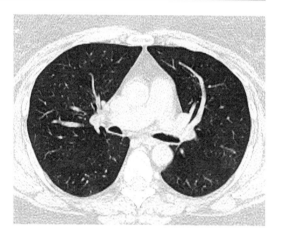

Fig. 12.3 Case 3 – High-resolution computed tomography expiratory image demonstrating mosaicism consistent with the presence of severe obstructive lung disease. *Arrows* show areas of air trapping

fatigue and symptoms of keratoconjuctivits sicca (KCS). She has end-expiratory wheeze on respiratory examination. A Schirmer's tear test is performed to objectify her symptoms of KCS, and profound ocular dryness is confirmed with <5 mm of tear wetting after 5 min of tear filter paper application. Her FEV-1 is 2.0 L (60% predicted) and improves by 8% with inhaled bronchodilator. Her FVC is proportionally reduced. Her CXR is normal but expiratory HRCT images show evidence of mosaic attenuation (Fig. 12.3) in the absence of any significant parenchymal abnormality. Laboratory assessment is notable for an elevated IgG level, a polyclonal hypergammaglobulinemia, positive ANA of 1:320 speckled, high-titer RF, anti-Ro and anti-La antibodies.

This case serves to illustrate a scenario in which obstructive lung disease has developed in a patient without any prior history of CTD, yet features obtained in the history (KCS), examination (positive Schirmer's tear test), and laboratory assessments (positive ANA, anti-Ro, anti-La, RF, polyclonal hypergammaglobulinemia, elevated IgG) confirm that this patient has primary Sjögren's syndrome. The presence of this CTD, the irreversible obstructive defect, the presence of mosaicism, and anatomical confirmation of severe airways obstruction on HRCT, all raise suspicions that this is Sjögren's associated bronchiolitis.

Bronchiolitis in CTD

Bronchiolar disease occurs less commonly than parenchymal disease in patients with CTD. Little is known about the incidence or prevalence of bronchiolitis in CTD, and it appears to occur most commonly in patients with RA or primary Sjögren's syndrome. The spectrum encountered with CTD includes obliterative bronchiolitis, lymphocytic bronchiolitis, and follicular bronchiolitis. Clinically, patients present with an insidious onset of dyspnea and cough, and are found to have obstructive defects by spirometric testing. It is not uncommon for there to be a component of reactivity with bronchodilator therapy, but classically, in bronchiolitis, the airways are not responsive to bronchodilator therapy and the FEV-1 does not improve as it does with reactive airways diseases. Chest radiography is usually normal or demonstrates hyperinflated lungs. Although the definitive diagnosis requires lung histopathology obtained by surgical biopsy, the airways-centric process may be diagnosed by transbronchial biopsy, and expiratory HRCT imaging is becoming increasingly sensitive in detecting bronchiolitis and distinguishing among the various subtypes [113]. Ultimately – and similar to the process of evaluation for an interstitial pneumonia – the diagnosis of bronchiolitis needs to be made by the clinician, incorporating a synthesis of the available clinical, radiologic, and pathologic data. As the data for CTD-associated bronchiolitis are based only on small case series or case reports, little is known about its natural history, and decisions on therapy are not evidence based. In our experience, bronchiolitis may be the first manifestation of an underlying CTD but more commonly is seen in those with existing CTD – and particularly RA. The clinical course appears to be variable but potentially quite devastating – particularly in those with obliterative bronchiolitis. It is not known whether treatment with macrolides, inhaled therapies, or immunosuppression alter the clinical course of the disease. At our center, most patients with CTD bronchiolitis are treated with a combination of therapies including various combinations of inhaled corticosteroids, macrolides, and immunosuppressive drugs including corticosteroids, methotrexate, MMF, AZA, anti-TNF agents, and rituximab. We refer patients for lung transplantation if the disease is progressive and refractory to medical interventions.

Screening CTD Patients for Lung Disease

An area of continued debate relates to whether screening for lung disease is indicated for CTD patients. Most authorities agree that screening for lung disease in patients with SSc is indicated [107]. In this regard, although no exact screening protocols exist, clinicians are advised to screen SSc patients for both ILD and PH [107]. This recommendation is based on the fact that pulmonary disease is the leading cause of morbidity and mortality for SSc and the belief that earlier detection of SSc-associated ILD or SSc-associated PAH may lead to improved survival. Recent data show that therapeutic interventions for SSc-associated ILD and SSc-associated PAH lead to subjective and objective improvement in quality of life and pulmonary disease status [66, 67, 114]. Although not yet proven by clinical trials, it is likely that these novel therapies (particularly those for SSc-associated PAH) also will lead to improved survival. Given the prevalence of lung disease in SSc, and the potentially favorable impact of therapeutic intervention, the concept of screening for the presence of lung disease in SSc is justified.

It is of much more significant debate when the discussion of screening for lung disease is extended to the other CTDs in which the prevalence of lung disease is lower and where there are no convincing data to suggest that specific intervention leads to improved outcomes. In our practice, we in fact do "screen" for lung disease among all of our CTD patients (including those with RA) by carefully assessing for respiratory symptoms or physical examination signs of impairment at each clinical encounter. Any abnormality detected – even if only mild or subtle – will prompt further investigation with office spirometry, ambulatory oximetry, and chest radiography that may lead to

Fig. 12.4 Algorithm for investigation of lung disease in connective tissue disease patients. *CxR* chest radiograph, *HRCT* high-resolution computed tomography, *BAL* bronchoalveolar lavage, *PFT* pulmonary function testing

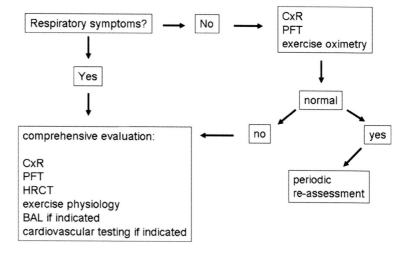

pulmonary consultation (Fig. 12.4). In other words, although we cannot yet advocate for wide-scale screening HRCT imaging to assess for lung disease in all CTD patients, we do highlight the importance of clinical vigilance in this situation while maintaining a low threshold to proceed with full pulmonary evaluation given the potentially devastating manifestations of lung disease that can occur in all CTD.

Summary

Lung disease occurs commonly in patients with CTD and varies in severity from nonprogressive, clinically insignificant disease to that of life-threatening respiratory impairment. Collaborative evaluations by pulmonologists, rheumatologists, and other health care providers are indicated when CTD patients develop respiratory symptoms to assess whether the abnormalities represent CTD-associated lung disease or an alternative etiology. Lung disease – and particularly ILD – may be the presenting manifestation of CTD, and in these scenarios, the lung may be the dominant manifestation of CTD (i.e., "lung-dominant CTD") with the CTD component being either incomplete or in partial form that is not classifiable using the traditional rheumatological defining criteria. Recent studies support the use of immunosuppressive therapies for progressive CTD-ILD but further controlled studies are needed to better inform medical decision-making for these groups of patients. There remain many unanswered questions about the natural history of the spectrum of CTD-associated lung disease and how best to treat them; more research is needed to better understand the complex intersect of lung disease with systemic autoimmunity.

References

1. Lamblin C, Bergoin C, Saelens T, Wallaert B. Interstitial lung diseases in collagen vascular diseases. Eur Respir J Suppl. 2001;32:69s–80.
2. Strange C, Highland KB. Interstitial lung disease in the patient who has connective tissue disease. Clin Chest Med. 2004;25(3):549–59, vii.
3. Wiedemann HP, Matthay RA. Pulmonary manifestations of the collagen vascular diseases. Clin Chest Med. 1989;10(4):677–722.
4. Frankel SK, Brown KK. Collagen vascular diseases of the lung. Clin Pulm Med. 2006;13(1):25–36.
5. Huggett MT, Armstrong R. Adalimumab-associated pulmonary fibrosis. Rheumatology (Oxford). 2006; 45(10):1312–3.
6. Peno-Green L, Lluberas G, Kingsley T, Brantley S. Lung injury linked to etanercept therapy. Chest. 2002; 122(5):1858–60.
7. Villeneuve E, St-Pierre A, Haraoui B. Interstitial pneumonitis associated with infliximab therapy. J Rheumatol. 2006;33(6):1189–93.
8. Ognenovski VM, Ojo TC, Fox DA. Etanercept-associated pulmonary granulomatous inflammation in patients with rheumatoid arthritis. J Rheumatol. 2008; 35(11):2279–82.

9. Zimmer C, Beiderlinden M, Peters J. Lethal acute respiratory distress syndrome during anti-TNF-alpha therapy for rheumatoid arthritis. Clin Rheumatol. 2006;25(3):430–2.

10. Hirabayashi Y, Shimizu H, Kobayashi N, Kudo K. Leflunomide-induced pneumonitis in a patient with rheumatoid arthritis. Intern Med. 2006;45(10):689–91.

11. Jenks KA, Stamp LK, O'Donnell JL, Savage RL, Chapman PT. Leflunomide-associated infections in rheumatoid arthritis. J Rheumatol. 2007;34(11):2201–3.

12. Martin N, Innes JA, Lambert CM, Turnbull CM, Wallace WA. Hypersensitivity pneumonitis associated with leflunomide therapy. J Rheumatol. 2007; 34(9):1934–7.

13. Ochi S, Harigai M, Mizoguchi F, Iwai H, Hagiyama H, Oka T, et al. Leflunomide-related acute interstitial pneumonia in two patients with rheumatoid arthritis: autopsy findings with a mosaic pattern of acute and organizing diffuse alveolar damage. Mod Rheumatol. 2006;16(5):316–20.

14. Sakai F, Noma S, Kurihara Y, Yamada H, Azuma A, Kudoh S, et al. Leflunomide-related lung injury in patients with rheumatoid arthritis: imaging features. Mod Rheumatol. 2005;15(3):173–9.

15. Sato T, Inokuma S, Sagawa A, Matsuda T, Takemura T, Otsuka T, et al. Factors associated with fatal outcome of leflunomide-induced lung injury in Japanese patients with rheumatoid arthritis. Rheumatology (Oxford). 2009;48(10):1265–8.

16. Takeishi M, Akiyama Y, Akiba H, Adachi D, Hirano M, Mimura T. Leflunomide induced acute interstitial pneumonia. J Rheumatol. 2005;32(6):1160–3.

17. Wong SP, Chu CM, Kan CH, Tsui HS, Ng WL. Successful treatment of leflunomide-induced acute pneumonitis with cholestyramine wash-out therapy. J Clin Rheumatol. 2009;15(8):389–92.

18. Camus P. Drug induced infiltrative lung diseases. 4th ed. Hamilton: BC Decker; 2003.

19. Imokawa S, Colby TV, Leslie KO, Helmers RA. Methotrexate pneumonitis: review of the literature and histopathological findings in nine patients. Eur Respir J. 2000;15(2):373–81.

20. Suda T, Sato A, Toyoshima M, Imokawa S, Yoshitomi A, Tamura R, et al. Weekly low-dose methotrexate therapy for sarcoidosis. Intern Med. 1994;33(7): 437–40.

21. Heffner JE, Sahn SA. Salicylate-induced pulmonary edema. Clinical features and prognosis. Ann Intern Med. 1981;95(4):405–9.

22. Alarcon GS, Kremer JM, Macaluso M, Weinblatt ME, Cannon GW, Palmer WR, et al. Risk factors for methotrexate-induced lung injury in patients with rheumatoid arthritis. A multicenter, case-control study. Methotrexate-Lung Study Group. Ann Intern Med. 1997;127(5):356–64.

23. Kremer JM, Alarcon GS, Weinblatt ME, Kaymakcian MV, Macaluso M, Cannon GW, et al. Clinical, laboratory, radiographic, and histopathologic features of methotrexate-associated lung injury in patients with rheumatoid arthritis: a multicenter study with literature review. Arthritis Rheum. 1997;40(10):1829–37.

24. Lynch DA, Quantitative CT. of fibrotic interstitial lung disease. Chest. 2007;131(3):643–4.

25. Lynch DA, Travis WD, Muller NL, Galvin JR, Hansell DM, Grenier PA, et al. Idiopathic interstitial pneumonias: CT features. Radiology. 2005;236(1): 10–21.

26. Tanaka N, Newell JD, Brown KK, Cool CD, Lynch DA. Collagen vascular disease-related lung disease: high-resolution computed tomography findings based on the pathologic classification. J Comput Assist Tomogr. 2004;28(3):351–60.

27. Hwang JH, Misumi S, Sahin H, Brown KK, Newell JD, Lynch DA. Computed tomographic features of idiopathic fibrosing interstitial pneumonia: comparison with pulmonary fibrosis related to collagen vascular disease. J Comput Assist Tomogr. 2009;33(3): 410–5.

28. Cottin V, Tebib J, Massonnet B, Souquet PJ, Bernard JP. Pulmonary function in patients receiving long-term low-dose methotrexate. Chest. 1996;109(4): 933–8.

29. Burton C, Kaczmarski R, Jan-Mohamed R. Interstitial pneumonitis related to rituximab therapy. N Engl J Med. 2003;348(26):2690–1. discussion 2690-1.

30. Hagiwara K, Sato T, Takagi-Kobayashi S, Hasegawa S, Shigihara N, Akiyama O. Acute exacerbation of preexisting interstitial lung disease after administration of etanercept for rheumatoid arthritis. J Rheumatol. 2007;34(5):1151–4.

31. Silver RM, Miller KS, Kinsella MB, Smith EA, Schabel SI. Evaluation and management of scleroderma lung disease using bronchoalveolar lavage. Am J Med. 1990;88(5):470–6.

32. Strange C, Bolster MB, Roth MD, Silver RM, Theodore A, Goldin J, et al. Bronchoalveolar lavage and response to cyclophosphamide in scleroderma interstitial lung disease. Am J Respir Crit Care Med. 2008;177(1):91–8.

33. Goh NS, Veeraraghavan S, Desai SR, Cramer D, Hansell DM, Denton CP, et al. Bronchoalveolar lavage cellular profiles in patients with systemic sclerosis-associated interstitial lung disease are not predictive of disease progression. Arthritis Rheum. 2007;56(6):2005–12.

34. Antoniou KM, Margaritopoulos G, Economidou F, Siafakas NM. Pivotal clinical dilemmas in collagen vascular diseases associated with interstitial lung involvement. Eur Respir J. 2009;33(4):882–96.

35. Bjoraker JA, Ryu JH, Edwin MK, Myers JL, Tazelaar HD, Schroeder DR, et al. Prognostic significance of histopathologic subsets in idiopathic pulmonary fibrosis. Am J Respir Crit Care Med. 1998;157(1): 199–203.

36. Daniil ZD, Gilchrist FC, Nicholson AG, Hansell DM, Harris J, Colby TV, et al. A histologic pattern of nonspecific interstitial pneumonia is associated with a better prognosis than usual interstitial pneumonia in patients with cryptogenic fibrosing alveolitis. Am J Respir Crit Care Med. 1999;160(3):899–905.

37. Nicholson AG, Colby TV, du Bois RM, Hansell DM, Wells AU. The prognostic significance of the histologic pattern of interstitial pneumonia in patients presenting with the clinical entity of cryptogenic fibrosing alveolitis. Am J Respir Crit Care Med. 2000;162(6):2213–7.

38. Bouros D, Wells AU, Nicholson AG, Colby TV, Polychronopoulos V, Pantelidis P, et al. Histopathologic subsets of fibrosing alveolitis in patients with systemic sclerosis and their relationship to outcome. Am J Respir Crit Care Med. 2002; 165(12):1581–6.

39. Park JH, Kim DS, Park IN, Jang SJ, Kitaichi M, Nicholson AG, et al. Prognosis of fibrotic interstitial pneumonia: idiopathic versus collagen vascular disease-related subtypes. Am J Respir Crit Care Med. 2007;175(7):705–11.

40. Fischer A, Swigris JJ, Groshong SD, Cool CD, Sahin H, Lynch DA, et al. Clinically significant interstitial lung disease in limited scleroderma: histopathology, clinical features, and survival. Chest. 2008;134(3): 601–5.

41. Fischer A. Interstitial lung disease: a rheumatologist's perspective. J Clin Rheumatol. 2009;15(2): 95–9.

42. Cottin V. Interstitial lung disease: are we missing formes frustes of connective tissue disease? Eur Respir J. 2006;28(5):893–6.

43. Mittoo S, Gelber AC, Christopher-Stine L, Horton MR, Lechtzin N, Danoff SK. Ascertainment of collagen vascular disease in patients presenting with interstitial lung disease. Respir Med. 2009;103(8): 1152–8.

44. Tzelepis GE, Toya SP, Moutsopoulos HM. Occult connective tissue diseases mimicking idiopathic interstitial pneumonias. Eur Respir J. 2008;31(1): 11–20.

45. Homma Y, Ohtsuka Y, Tanimura K, Kusaka H, Munakata M, Kawakami Y, et al. Can interstitial pneumonia as the sole presentation of collagen vascular diseases be differentiated from idiopathic interstitial pneumonia? Respiration. 1995;62(5):248–51.

46. Fischer A, Swigris JJ, du Bois RM, Lynch DA, Downey GP, Cosgrove GP, et al. Anti-synthetase syndrome in ANA and anti-Jo-1 negative patients presenting with idiopathic interstitial pneumonia. Respir Med. 2009;103(11):1719–24.

47. Fischer A, Swigris JJ, du Bois RM, Groshong SD, Cool CD, Sahin H, et al. Minor salivary gland biopsy to detect primary Sjogren syndrome in patients with interstitial lung disease. Chest. 2009;136(4):1072–8.

48. Fischer A, Meehan RT, Feghali-Bostwick CA, West SG, Brown KK. Unique characteristics of systemic sclerosis sine scleroderma-associated interstitial lung disease. Chest. 2006;130(4):976–81.

49. Fukuoka J, Lesile KO. Practical pulmonary pathology. A diagnostic approach. 1st ed. Philadelphia, PA: Churchill-Livingstone; 2005.

50. Travis WD, Colby TV, Koss MN, Rosado-de-Christenson ML, Muller NL, King Jr TE. Nonneoplastic disorders of the lower respiratory tract.

1st ed. Washington, DC: American Registry of Pathology and the Armed Forces Institute of Pathology; 2002.

51. Leslie KO, Trahan S, Gruden J. Pulmonary pathology of the rheumatic diseases. Semin Respir Crit Care Med. 2007;28(4):369–78.

52. Song JW, Do KH, Kim MY, Jang SJ, Colby TV, Kim DS. Pathologic and radiologic differences between idiopathic and collagen vascular disease-related usual interstitial pneumonia. Chest. 2009;136(1): 23–30.

53. Fujita J, Ohtsuki Y, Yoshinouchi T, Yamadori I, Bandoh S, Tokuda M, et al. Idiopathic non-specific interstitial pneumonia: as an "autoimmune interstitial pneumonia". Respir Med. 2005;99(2):234–40.

54. Kinder BW, Collard HR, Koth L, Daikh DI, Wolters PJ, Elicker B, et al. Idiopathic nonspecific interstitial pneumonia: lung manifestation of undifferentiated connective tissue disease? Am J Respir Crit Care Med. 2007;176(7):691–7.

55. Mosca M, Neri R, Bombardieri S. Undifferentiated connective tissue diseases (UCTD): a review of the literature and a proposal for preliminary classification criteria. Clin Exp Rheumatol. 1999;17(5):615–20.

56. Vaz CC, Couto M, Medeiros D, Miranda L, Costa J, Nero P, et al. Undifferentiated connective tissue disease: a seven-center cross-sectional study of 184 patients. Clin Rheumatol. 2009;28(8):915–21.

57. Fischer A, West SG, Swigris JJ, Brown KK, du Bois RM. Connective tissue disease-associated interstitial lung disease: a call for clarification. Chest. 2010;138(2):251–6.

58. Steen VD. Autoantibodies in systemic sclerosis. Semin Arthritis Rheum. 2005;35(1):35–42.

59. Fischer A, Brown KK, Frankel SK. Treatment of connective tissue disease related interstitial lung disease. Clin Pulm Med. 2009;16(2):74–80.

60. Walker WC, Wright V. Diffuse interstitial pulmonary fibrosis and rheumatoid arthritis. Ann Rheum Dis. 1969;28(3):252–9.

61. Holgate ST, Glass DN, Haslam P, Maini RN, Turner-Warwick M. Respiratory involvement in systemic lupus erythematosus. A clinical and immunological study. Clin Exp Immunol. 1976;24(3):385–95.

62. Sullivan WD, Hurst DJ, Harmon CE, Esther JH, Agia GA, Maltby JD, et al. A prospective evaluation emphasizing pulmonary involvement in patients with mixed connective tissue disease. Medicine (Baltimore). 1984;63(2):92–107.

63. Steen VD, Medsger Jr TA. Case-control study of corticosteroids and other drugs that either precipitate or protect from the development of scleroderma renal crisis. Arthritis Rheum. 1998;41(9):1613–9.

64. Reinhold-Keller E, Kekow J, Schnabel A, Schmitt WH, Heller M, Beigel A, et al. Influence of disease manifestation and antineutrophil cytoplasmic antibody titer on the response to pulse cyclophosphamide therapy in patients with Wegener's granulomatosis. Arthritis Rheum. 1994;37(6):919–24.

65. Hoyles RK, Ellis RW, Wellsbury J, Lees B, Newlands P, Goh NS, et al. A multicenter, prospective, randomized,

double-blind, placebo-controlled trial of corticosteroids and intravenous cyclophosphamide followed by oral azathioprine for the treatment of pulmonary fibrosis in scleroderma. Arthritis Rheum. 2006;54(12):3962–70.

66. Tashkin DP, Elashoff R, Clements PJ, Goldin J, Roth MD, Furst DE, et al. Cyclophosphamide versus placebo in scleroderma lung disease. N Engl J Med. 2006;354(25):2655–66.

67. Tashkin DP, Elashoff R, Clements PJ, Roth MD, Furst DE, Silver RM, et al. Effects of 1-year treatment with cyclophosphamide on outcomes at 2 years in scleroderma lung disease. Am J Respir Crit Care Med. 2007;176(10):1026–34.

68. Silver RM, Warrick JH, Kinsella MB, Staudt LS, Baumann MH, Strange C. Cyclophosphamide and low-dose prednisone therapy in patients with systemic sclerosis (scleroderma) with interstitial lung disease. J Rheumatol. 1993;20(5):838–44.

69. Steen VD, Lanz Jr JK, Conte C, Owens GR, Medsger Jr TA. Therapy for severe interstitial lung disease in systemic sclerosis. A retrospective study. Arthritis Rheum. 1994;37(9):1290–6.

70. White B, Moore WC, Wigley FM, Xiao HQ, Wise RA. Cyclophosphamide is associated with pulmonary function and survival benefit in patients with scleroderma and alveolitis. Ann Intern Med. 2000; 132(12):947–54.

71. Goldin J, Elashoff R, Kim HJ, Yan X, Lynch D, Strollo D, et al. Treatment of scleroderma-interstitial lung disease with cyclophosphamide is associated with less progressive fibrosis on serial thoracic high-resolution CT scan than placebo: findings from the scleroderma lung study. Chest. 2009;136(5):1333–40.

72. Furst DE, Clements, PJ. Immunosuppressives. In: Hochberg MC SA, Smolen JS, Weinblatt ME, Weisman MH, editors. Rheumatology. 3rd ed. Spain: Mosby; 2003. p. 439–48.

73. Chan TM, Li FK, Tang CS, Wong RW, Fang GX, Ji YL, et al. Efficacy of mycophenolate mofetil in patients with diffuse proliferative lupus nephritis. Hong Kong-Guangzhou Nephrology Study Group. N Engl J Med. 2000;343(16):1156–62.

74. Swigris JJ, Olson AL, Fischer A, Lynch DA, Cosgrove GP, Frankel SK, et al. Mycophenolate mofetil is safe, well tolerated, and preserves lung function in patients with connective tissue disease-related interstitial lung disease. Chest. 2006;130(1): 30–6.

75. Liossis SN, Bounas A, Andonopoulos AP. Mycophenolate mofetil as first-line treatment improves clinically evident early scleroderma lung disease. Rheumatology (Oxford). 2006;45(8):1005–8.

76. Zamora AC, Wolters PJ, Collard HR, Connolly MK, Elicker BM, Webb WR, et al. Use of mycophenolate mofetil to treat scleroderma-associated interstitial lung disease. Respir Med. 2008;102(1):150–5.

77. Gerbino AJ, Goss CH, Molitor JA. Effect of mycophenolate mofetil on pulmonary function in scleroderma-associated interstitial lung disease. Chest. 2008;133(2):455–60.

78. Felson DT, Anderson J. Evidence for the superiority of immunosuppressive drugs and prednisone over prednisone alone in lupus nephritis. Results of a pooled analysis. N Engl J Med. 1984;311(24): 1528–33.

79. Nicholls A, Snaith ML, Maini RN, Scott JT. Proceedings: controlled trial of azathioprine in rheumatoid vasculitis. Ann Rheum Dis. 1973;32(6): 589–91.

80. Yazici H, Pazarli H, Barnes CG, Tuzun Y, Ozyazgan Y, Silman A, et al. A controlled trial of azathioprine in Behcet's syndrome. N Engl J Med. 1990;322(5): 281–5.

81. Nadashkevich O, Davis P, Fritzler M, Kovalenko W. A randomized unblinded trial of cyclophosphamide versus azathioprine in the treatment of systemic sclerosis. Clin Rheumatol. 2006;25(2):205–12.

82. Dheda K, Lalloo UG, Cassim B, Mody GM. Experience with azathioprine in systemic sclerosis associated with interstitial lung disease. Clin Rheumatol. 2004;23(4):306–9.

83. Demedts M, Behr J, Buhl R, Costabel U, Dekhuijzen R, Jansen HM, et al. High-dose acetylcysteine in idiopathic pulmonary fibrosis. N Engl J Med. 2005;353(21):2229–42.

84. Stolk JN, Boerbooms AM, de Abreu RA, de Koning DG, van Beusekom HJ, Muller WH, et al. Reduced thiopurine methyltransferase activity and development of side effects of azathioprine treatment in patients with rheumatoid arthritis. Arthritis Rheum. 1998;41(10):1858–66.

85. Clunie GP, Lennard L. Relevance of thiopurine methyltransferase status in rheumatology patients receiving azathioprine. Rheumatology (Oxford). 2004;43(1):13–8.

86. Tugwell P, Pincus T, Yocum D, Stein M, Gluck O, Kraag G, et al. Combination therapy with cyclosporine and methotrexate in severe rheumatoid arthritis. The Methotrexate-Cyclosporine Combination Study Group. N Engl J Med. 1995;333(3): 137–41.

87. Wells G, Tugwell P. Cyclosporin A in rheumatoid arthritis: overview of efficacy. Br J Rheumatol. 1993;32 Suppl 1:51–6.

88. Clements PJ, Lachenbruch PA, Sterz M, Danovitch G, Hawkins R, Ippoliti A, et al. Cyclosporine in systemic sclerosis. Results of a forty-eight-week open safety study in ten patients. Arthritis Rheum. 1993;36(1):75–83.

89. BenEzra D, Cohen E, Chajek T, Friedman G, Pizanti S, de Courten C, et al. Evaluation of conventional therapy versus cyclosporine A in Behcet's syndrome. Transplant Proc. 1988;20(3 Suppl 4):136–43.

90. Oddis CV, Sciurba FC, Elmagd KA, Starzl TE. Tacrolimus in refractory polymyositis with interstitial lung disease. Lancet. 1999;353(9166):1762–3.

91. Wilkes MR, Sereika SM, Fertig N, Lucas MR, Oddis CV. Treatment of antisynthetase-associated interstitial lung disease with tacrolimus. Arthritis Rheum. 2005;52(8):2439–46.

92. Koopman WJ. Dawn of the era of biologics in the treatment of the rheumatic diseases. Arthritis Rheum. 2008;58(2 Suppl):S75–8.

93. Toussirot E, Wendling D. The use of TNF-alpha blocking agents in rheumatoid arthritis: an overview. Expert Opin Pharmacother. 2004;5(3):581–94.

94. Vassallo R, Matteson E, Thomas Jr CF. Clinical response of rheumatoid arthritis-associated pulmonary fibrosis to tumor necrosis factor-alpha inhibition. Chest. 2002;122(3):1093–6.

95. Alalawi R, Whelan T, Bajwa RS, Hodges TN. Lung transplantation and interstitial lung disease. Curr Opin Pulm Med. 2005;11(5):461–6.

96. Gasper WJ, Sweet MP, Golden JA, Hoopes C, Leard LE, Kleinhenz ME, et al. Lung transplantation in patients with connective tissue disorders and esophageal dysmotility. Dis Esophagus. 2008;21(7):650–5.

97. Rosas V, Conte JV, Yang SC, Gaine SP, Borja M, Wigley FM, et al. Lung transplantation and systemic sclerosis. Ann Transplant. 2000;5(3):38–43.

98. Shitrit D, Amital A, Peled N, Raviv Y, Medalion B, Saute M, et al. Lung transplantation in patients with scleroderma: case series, review of the literature, and criteria for transplantation. Clin Transplant. 2009; 23(2):178–83.

99. Massad MG, Powell CR, Kpodonu J, Tshibaka C, Hanhan Z, Snow NJ, et al. Outcomes of lung transplantation in patients with scleroderma. World J Surg. 2005;29(11):1510–5.

100. Schachna L, Medsger Jr TA, Dauber JH, Wigley FM, Braunstein NA, White B, et al. Lung transplantation in scleroderma compared with idiopathic pulmonary fibrosis and idiopathic pulmonary arterial hypertension. Arthritis Rheum. 2006;54(12):3954–61.

101. Brieva J. Cyclophosphamide-induced acute respiratory distress syndrome. Respirology. 2007;12(5):769–73.

102. Spector JI, Zimbler H. Cyclophosphamide pneumonitis. N Engl J Med. 1982;307(4):251.

103. Malik SW, Myers JL, DeRemee RA, Specks U. Lung toxicity associated with cyclophosphamide use. Two distinct patterns. Am J Respir Crit Care Med. 1996;154(6 Pt 1):1851–6.

104. Ryu JH, Krowka MJ, Pellikka PA, Swanson KL, McGoon MD. Pulmonary hypertension in patients with interstitial lung diseases. Mayo Clin Proc. 2007;82(3):342–50.

105. Arcasoy SM, Christie JD, Ferrari VA, Sutton MS, Zisman DA, Blumenthal NP, et al. Echocardiographic assessment of pulmonary hypertension in patients with advanced lung disease. Am J Respir Crit Care Med. 2003;167(5):735–40.

106. Steen V, Medsger Jr TA. Predictors of isolated pulmonary hypertension in patients with systemic sclerosis and limited cutaneous involvement. Arthritis Rheum. 2003;48(2):516–22.

107. Steen VD. The lung in systemic sclerosis. J Clin Rheumatol. 2005;11(1):40–6.

108. Hachulla E, de Groote P, Gressin V, Sibilia J, Diot E, Carpentier P, et al. The three-year incidence of pulmonary arterial hypertension associated with systemic sclerosis in a multicenter nationwide longitudinal study in France. Arthritis Rheum. 2009;60(6):1831–9.

109. Hachulla E, Launay D, Mouthon L, Sitbon O, Berezne A, Guillevin L, et al. Is pulmonary arterial hypertension really a late complication of systemic sclerosis? Chest. 2009;136(5):1211–9.

110. Bull TM. Screening and therapy of pulmonary hypertension in systemic sclerosis. Curr Opin Rheumatol. 2007;19(6):598–603.

111. Olschewski H, Ghofrani HA, Walmrath D, Schermuly R, Temmesfeld-Wollbruck B, Grimminger F, et al. Inhaled prostacyclin and iloprost in severe pulmonary hypertension secondary to lung fibrosis. Am J Respir Crit Care Med. 1999;160(2):600–7.

112. Shapiro S. Management of pulmonary hypertension resulting from interstitial lung disease. Curr Opin Pulm Med. 2003;9(5):426–30.

113. Pipavath SJ, Lynch DA, Cool C, Brown KK, Newell JD. Radiologic and pathologic features of bronchiolitis. AJR Am J Roentgenol. 2005;185(2):354–63.

114. Denton CP, Pope JE, Peter HH, Gabrielli A, Boonstra A, van den Hoogen FH, et al. Long-term effects of bosentan on quality of life, survival, safety and tolerability in pulmonary arterial hypertension related to connective tissue diseases. Ann Rheum Dis. 2008; 67(9):1222–8.

Hypersensitivity Pneumonitis: A Clinical Perspective

13

Moisés Selman, Mayra Mejía, Héctor Ortega, and Carmen Navarro

Abstract

Hypersensitivity pneumonitis (HP) is a complex interstitial lung disease provoked by the inhalation of a wide variety of organic particles and characterized by a diffuse immune-mediated inflammatory reaction of the lung parenchyma. Importantly, the list of environments and antigens that can cause this disease is always increasing. According to the antigen exposure and genetic characteristics, patients may present an acute, subacute, or chronic form of the disease, the later usually evolving to lung fibrosis with the consequent poor prognosis. HP represents a diagnostic challenge not only in the context of other interstitial lung diseases, but also with other clinical syndromes that may occur as a result of inhalation of organic agents. Treatment includes avoiding further exposure and, in a number of cases, the use of corticosteroids, although preventive measures are always desirable.

Keywords

Hypersensitivity pneumonitis • Allergic alveolitis • Farmer's lung • Pigeon breeder's disease • Bronchoalveolar lavage • T-lymphocytes • Lung fibrosis

Hypersensitivity pneumonitis (HP), also known as extrinsic allergic alveolitis, is a complex syndrome of varying intensity, clinical presentation, and natural history [1]. Numerous provocative agents have been identified around the world, including, but not limited to, agricultural dusts, fungi and bacteria, mammalian and insect proteins, and low molecular weight chemicals (Table 13.1). The disease is the result of an immunologically induced inflammation of the lung parenchyma provoked by repeated inhalation of antigen(s).

M. Selman, MD (✉) • M. Mejía, MD • C. Navarro, MD
Instituto Nacional de Enfermedades Respiratorias "Ismael Cosio Villegas", Mexico D.F., Mexico
e-mail: mselmanl@yahoo.com.mx

H. Ortega, MD
Medicine Development Center, Glaxosmithkline, Research Triangle Park, NC, USA

Epidemiology and Risk Factors

The prevalence and incidence of HP vary considerably around the world, depending upon disease definitions and diagnosis, intensity of exposure to

R.P. Baughman and R.M. du Bois (eds.), *Diffuse Lung Disease: A Practical Approach*, DOI 10.1007/978-1-4419-9771-5_13, © Springer Science+Business Media, LLC 2012

Table 13.1 Some etiologic agents related to hypersensitivity pneumonitis

Disease	Antigen	Source
Fungal and bacterial		
Farmer's lung	*Faeni rectivirgula*	Moldy hay, grain, silage
Air conditioner/humidifier lung	*Thermoactinomyces vulgaris, Thermoactinomyces sacchari*	Contaminated forced-air systems, water reservoirs
Mushroom worker's lung	*T. sacchari*	Moldy mushroom compost
Suberosis	*Thermoactinomyces viridis, Aspergillus fumigatus, Penicillium frequentans*	Moldy cork
Detergent lung	*Bacillus subtilis enzymes*	Detergents
Malt worker's lung	*Aspergillus fumigatus, Aspergillus clavatus*	Moldy barley
Sequoiosis	*Graphium, Pullularia, Aureobasidium pullulans*	Moldy wood dust
Maple bark stripper's lung	*Cryptostroma corticale*	Moldy maple bark
Cheese washer's lung	*Penicillium casei, A. clavatus*	Moldy cheese
Woodworker's lung	*Alternaria* spp., *wood dust*	Oak, cedar, mahogany dust, pine and spruce pulp
Paprika slicer's lung	*Mucor stolonifer*	Moldy paprika pods
Sauna taker's lung	*Aureobasidium* spp., other sources	Contaminated sauna water
Composter's lung	*T. vulgaris, Aspergillus*	Compost
Hot tub lung	*Mycobacterium avium complex*	Hot tub mists; mold on ceiling
Wine maker's lung	*Botrytis cincrea*	Mold on grapes
Thatched roof lung	*Saccharomonospora viridis*	Dead grasses and leaves
Tobacco grower's lung	*Aspergillus* spp.	Tobacco plants
Summer-type pneumonitis	*Trichosporon cutaneum*	Contaminated old houses
Dry rot lung	*Merulius lacrymans*	Rotten wood
Machine operator's lung	*Mycobacterium immunogenum; Pseudomona fluorescens*	Aerosolized metalworking fluid
Animal proteins		
Pigeon breeder's disease	Avian droppings, feathers, serum	Parakeets, budgerigars, pigeons,
Pituitary snuff taker's lung	Pituitary snuff	Bovine and porcine pituitary proteins
Fish meal worker's lung	Fish meal	Fish meal dust
Bat lung	Bat serum protein	Bat droppings
Furrier's lung	Animal fur dust	Animal pelts
Animal handler's lung	Rats, gerbils	Urine, serum, pelts, proteins
Insect proteins		
Miller's lung	*Sitophilus granarius* (i.e., *wheat weevil*)	Dust-contaminated grain
Lycoperdonosis	Puffball spores	Lycoperdon puffballs
Chemical		
Pauli's reagent alveolitis	Sodium diazobenzene sulfate	Laboratory reagent
Chemical worker's lung	Isocyanates, trimellitic anhydride	Polyurethane foams, spray paints

offensive antigens, geographical and local conditions, cultural practices, proximity to a variety of industries, and host risk factors. Overall, the prevalence and incidence of HP are low, perhaps because a large number of individuals with mild or subclinical HP are not detected or are misdiagnosed as suffering from viral illnesses, asthma, or other interstitial lung diseases that may mimic HP.

Since not all exposed individuals develop clinically significant HP, genetic factors appear to influence an individual's risk of disease. However, studies regarding genetic susceptibility are scanty. Polymorphisms of MHC class II alleles have been associated with a higher risk to develop the disease, and more recently, it was reported that transporters associated with antigen processing (TAP) genes which play an important role transporting peptides across the endoplasmic reticulum membrane for MHC class I molecules assembly may be involved in the HP genetic susceptibility [2–4]. In addition, exposure to a second offending agent such as respiratory viral infections or use of organochlorine and carbamate pesticides has been associated with increased risk for developing the disease [5, 6].

By contrast, cigarette smoking appears to have a protective role. Thus, HP occurs more frequently in nonsmokers than in smokers under similar risk exposure and also nonsmokers exhibit a significantly higher IgG response against the offending antigen [1]. In an extensive study of almost 6,000 dairy farmers conducted in France, it was noticed that the risk of developing farmer's lung was significantly higher to nonsmokers [7]. Recent findings indicate that nicotine may affect the expression of key inflammatory cytokines in vivo and in vitro, suggesting that the reduction of the inflammatory response could be, at least in part, responsible for the observed protection of disease in smokers [8]. However, it is important to emphasize that even though smoking seems to protect from development of HP, when the disease does occur in smokers, it has a more chronic clinical course [1].

Farmer's lung disease is one of the most common forms of HP, affecting 0.4–7% of the farming population. Prevalence of the disease varies by country, climate, and farming practices, from approximately 9% in farmers in humid zones to 2% in drier zones [9, 10]. However, the replacement of old farming methods by more modern techniques of haymaking, hay drying, hay storage, and by silage making has decreased the incidence of farmer's lung [11].

Another frequent form of HP is pigeon (or more appropriate bird) breeder's disease (PBD). Old data indicate that the prevalence of HP among bird fanciers ranges from 20 to 20,000 per 100,000 persons at risk [1]. New studies among this at high-risk population are necessary to better define the prevalence and risk factors associated with PBD. The prevalence of PBD among people with only a few birds at home, which usually provokes a more chronic lung disease, is largely unknown. Importantly, exposure to feather pillows and down comforters can also be a source of HP [12]. The disease seems to be less common in childhood in which PBD appears as the most common form. Clinical presentation is similar to adult disease [13].

HP also seems to occur sporadically in some individuals. For example, lifeguards exposed to public swimming pools, workers at plants manufacturing polyurethane foam parts for automobiles, workers exposed to metalworking fluids, and office workers [14–16]. A wide range of other occupations result in contact with airborne antigens that increase the risk of developing HP. More than 300 of such agents have been reported. For example, in the last 10 years, a large body of evidence has demonstrated that individuals exposed to aerosolized environmental nontuberculous mycobacteria (NTM) can develop HP-like granulomatous lung. Exposure to NTM may occur in unexpected places such as home saunas, indoor swimming pools, and enclosed hot tubs where *Mycobacterium avium complex* has been usually identified [17]. Likewise, outbreaks of HP have been reported in workplaces with metalworking fluids containing NTM, most frequently *Mycobacterium immunogenum* [15, 18].

Clinical Features

Patients with HP have several characteristic features that help to suspect the diagnosis in most of the cases. The clinical presentation of HP has been categorized as acute, subacute, or chronic depending upon the frequency, length, and intensity of exposure and the duration of symptoms.

Acute

This form of HP usually follows a heavy exposure to a provoking agent. Without a history of exposure to an identifiable agent, acute HP can be overlooked because symptoms may be indistinguishable from an acute viral or bacterial respiratory infection. The course is characterized by the abrupt onset (4–8 h following exposure) of fever, chills, malaise, nausea, cough, chest tightness, and shortness of breath without wheezing. On physical examination, subjects present with tachypnea and diffuse fine rales. Removal from exposure to the provoking antigen results in improvement of symptoms within 12 h to several days and complete resolution of clinical and radiographic findings within several weeks. The disease may recur with re-exposure to the same antigen. Actually, recurrent acute episodes should prompt consideration of HP and a careful search for relevant historical exposures is mandatory.

Acute HP in farmers must be distinguished from febrile, toxic reactions to inhaled mold dusts (organic dust toxic syndrome [ODTS]), which is a nonimmunologic reaction that occurs nearly 50 times more often than HP. ODTS is an influenza-like illness characterized by fever, chills, shivering, malaise, fatigue, muscle and joint aches, headache, nasal irritation, throat burning, mild dyspnea, chest tightness with or without dry cough, and wheezing [19]. Bacterial endotoxins and fungal toxins of moldy hay have been proposed as causative agents of ODTS. In contrast to patients with acute HP, ODTS patients generally have no precipitins to antigens of molds, and usually present with normal clinical findings upon respiratory examination and chest radiographs.

Laboratory tests are of limited utility. Some nonspecific markers of inflammation such as erythrocyte sedimentation rate, rheumatoid factor, and C-reactive protein may be increased. Serum LDH may be increased in acute phases of the disease and may decline as clinical symptoms improve. Immunoglobulins, precipitating IgG antibodies, and circulating immune complexes are also elevated in some patients. Increase of neutrophils and lymphocytes are observed in bronchoalveolar lavage (BAL). Pulmonary function tests usually reveal a restrictive defect during symptomatic episodes. In some cases, however, an obstructive pattern may be found.

Chest X-rays may be normal. However, when positive findings are present a micronodular pattern and/or ground-glass attenuation in the lower and middle lung zones may be identified. Consolidation is rarely seen [20] (Fig.13.1). The use of high-resolution computed tomography (HRCT) is often required to confirm the presence

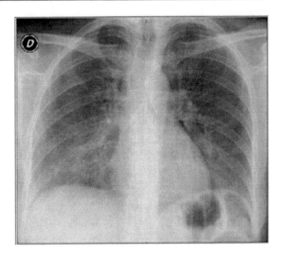

Fig. 13.1 Chest radiograph exhibiting moderate diffuse ground-glass opacities in an acute episode of HP

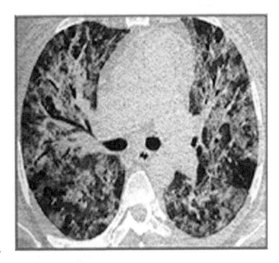

Fig. 13.2 High-resolution computed tomography showing ground-glass attenuation and consolidation in a severe acute form of HP

of pneumonitis [21]. Main changes include patchy ground-glass opacities and occasionally images of consolidation (Fig. 13.2). However, the sensitivity of HRCT is not absolute and must be interpreted in the context of the clinical symptoms.

Subacute

This is characterized by gradual development of productive cough, dyspnea, fatigue, anorexia, and weight loss. Some patients present fever during

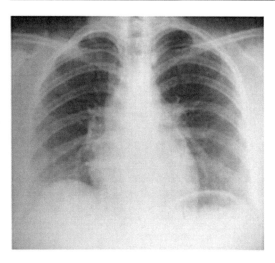

Fig. 13.3 Chest radiograph showing ground-glass attenuation with shortening of the lung fields in a subacute HP patient

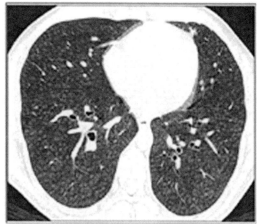

Fig. 13.4 High-resolution computed tomography scan illustrating poorly defined bronchiolocentric micronodules diffusely distributed throughout both lungs and some ground-glass attenuation in subacute HP

the first weeks. Similar findings may occur in patients who suffer repeated, infrequent acute attacks of HP characterized by cough and malaise. Physical examination usually reveals tachypnea and diffuse rales. Improvement of symptoms takes longer than with the acute form of the disease (weeks to months), and usually pharmacological treatment is necessary. Chest X-rays may occasionally be normal but usually show ground-glass attenuation, micronodular or fine reticular opacities (as in the case of acute HP) (Fig. 13.3). The abnormalities are sometimes more prominent in the middle to upper lung zones. HRCT shows diffuse micronodules, ground-glass attenuation, and mild fibrotic changes (Fig. 13.4) [20, 21]. A mosaic pattern caused by a combination of patchy areas of ground glass and focal air trapping is usually noticed. Air trapping is best seen as a failure of an area to increase in attenuation on an expiratory CT scan (Fig. 13.5) [21]. These findings often undergo dramatic improvement when patients with subacute disease are removed from the offending exposure and treated with corticosteroids. Pulmonary function testing usually presents a predominantly restrictive pattern with associated moderate hypoxemia. Occasionally, a mixed pattern of both obstructive and restrictive ventilatory abnormalities can be observed. The DL_{CO} is reduced in most cases. However, the primary use

of pulmonary function tests is to determine the degree of the associated impairment but they have no discriminative properties in differentiating HP from other interstitial lung diseases.

Histopathological findings are characterized by bronchiolocentric lymphocytic pneumonitis, and poorly formed, noncaseating granulomas in the interstitium (Fig. 13.6). A major laboratory abnormality in subacute HP is a striking increase of lymphocytes in the BAL (Fig. 13.7). The differential diagnosis for subacute HP includes infectious and noninfectious diffuse interstitial lung diseases such as sarcoidosis, organizing pneumonia, and cellular nonspecific interstitial pneumonia (NSIP). Lymphocytic interstitial pneumonitis in HIV-infected individuals as well as some drug-induced lung disease should also be included in the differential diagnosis. Infections resulting from mycobacteria, fungi, HIV, and respiratory viruses should always be ruled out by PCR, cultures, special stains, and clinical correlation.

Chronic

Unrecognized and untreated acute/subacute episodes of HP may progress to chronic disease (recurrent HP) while other patients have no history of acute episodes but has slowly progressive

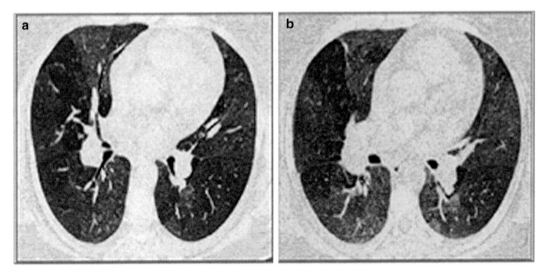

Fig. 13.5 (**a**) High-resolution computed tomography exhibiting diffuse bronchiolocentric micronodules, ground-glass opacities, and a mosaic pattern gives by the presence of areas of air trapping. (**b**) The mosaic pattern is better defined on expiration

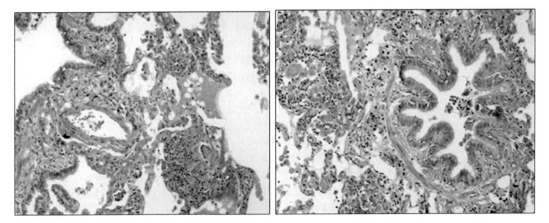

Fig. 13.6 Peribronchiolar inflammation of mononuclear predominance and poorly formed noncaseating granulomas in two patients with subacute HP (hematoxylin and eosin, ×40)

(insidious) chronic respiratory disease [22]. The patient with chronic HP usually presents with progressive dyspnea on exertion. Associated symptoms include cough, fatigue, malaise, and weight loss. Digital clubbing may be seen in advanced disease and may help to predict clinical deterioration [1]. Disabling and irreversible respiratory findings due to pulmonary fibrosis are characteristic. At this stage clinical and radiological features may be similar to idiopathic pulmonary fibrosis (IPF), making it difficult to differentiate the disease [1]. Chronic HP is more

frequently seen in patients who have been exposed to low levels of antigen for prolonged period. Some patients with HP, primarily those with recurrent farmer's lung attacks, develop an obstructive lung disease with emphysematous changes instead of a fibrotic response [23].

Laboratory findings are of minimal utility in this stage, and even the specific antibodies against the offending antigen may be negative. Lymphocytosis may still be present in BAL, but other abnormalities, neutrophilia or eosinophilia, may also be seen. A moderate to severe restrictive

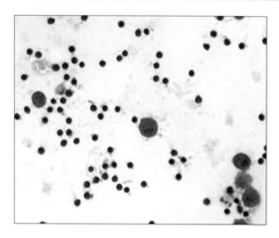

Fig. 13.7 Light micrograph of bronchoalveolar lavage (BAL) cell population from a subacute patient of hypersensitivity pneumonitis. Most of the inflammatory cells recovered from BAL are lymphocytes (hematoxylin and eosin; ×40)

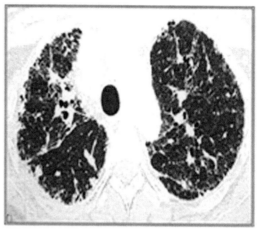

Fig. 13.9 High-resolution computed tomography from a chronic HP patient. It can be observed mild patchy ground-glass attenuation and numerous reticular opacities with architectural distortion

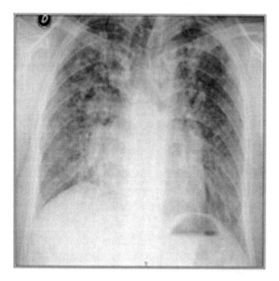

Fig. 13.8 Chest X-ray showing fibrotic changes in a chronic HP patient. There is diffuse coarse reticulonodular opacities and pulmonary hypertension

defect is common; however, since bronchiolitis is a prominent feature, mixed obstructive and restrictive physiology may be present. The DL_{CO} is reduced, and hypoxemia at rest worsening with exercise is commonly present. Chest radiographs typically show progressive fibrotic changes with loss of lung volume that may affect the upper or the lower lobes (Fig. 13.8). Nodular or ground-glass densities are less commonly seen. HRCT

shows typically ground-glass attenuation and parenchymal micronodules, accompanied by fibrotic changes and honeycombing (Fig. 13.9). In chronic farmer lung, emphysematous alterations may be prominent.

The diagnosis of the chronic form of HP usually requires lung biopsy. In addition to bronchiolocentric or diffuse interstitial pneumonitis and some multinucleated giant cells, biopsy specimens reveal distal destruction of alveoli (honeycombing) in association with dense fibrotic zones. However, advanced chronic HP may closely mimic UIP or fibrotic NSIP.

Diagnostic Assessment

HP represents a diagnostic challenge not only in the context of other interstitial lung diseases, but also with other clinical syndromes that may occur as a result of inhalation of organic agents. Some of these conditions include inhalation fever, ODTS, chronic bronchitis, asthma, and chronic airflow limitation. History of exposure to birds, ventilation systems or agricultural products, wood dust, water-based aerosols, etc., provides a powerful clue to identify potential exposures associated with HP.

In general, the criteria for HP diagnosis should include a high index of suspicion by the clinician

Table 13.2 Diagnostic criteria for hypersensitivity pneumonitis

Clinical form	Time of symptoms	Symptoms	HRCT	BAL	Pathology
Acute	Few hours after heavy exposure	Flu-like syndrome	Patchy or diffuse ground-glass attenuation	Lymphocytes > 30% Neutrophils > 20%	Acute inflammatory infiltrate
Subacute	Weeks, few months	Progressive dyspnea, cough and malaise Often fever	Ground-glass opacities, poorly defined centrilobular nodules, mosaic attenuation	Lymphocytes > 40%. Usually higher than 50%	Bronchiolocentric lymphoplasmacytic interstitial pneumonitis, poorly formed nonnecrotizing granulomas, isolated giant cells. Occasional areas of organizing pneumonia
Chronic	Several months, few years	Progressive dyspnea, cough, fatigue, malaise, weight loss. Digital clubbing	Reticulation, and traction bronchiectasis superimposed on findings of subacute HP In some cases, emphysematous changes	Lymphocytes > 30%	Fibrotic pattern superimposed to subacute changes

that face a patient with a flu-like syndrome or an ILD of obscure origin. Unfortunately, there is no diagnostic test that by itself allows the diagnosis. Instead, diagnosis is based on a constellation of findings, including a suggestive environmental history and positive antibodies against the offending antigen, symptoms, physical findings, radiographic abnormalities (mainly HRCT), pulmonary function and immunologic tests, and BAL results. Precipitating IgG antibodies against antigens, such as fungi, bacteria, or animal secretions can be identified in the patient's serum. However, a large percent (30–40% farmers) of individuals with a high degree of exposure have positive serum precipitins in the absence of clinical disease. The incidence of serum precipitins in asymptomatic bird breeders is even higher, probably due to intense and prolonged exposure to provoking antigens. On the other hand, in many patients with chronic insidious disease-specific antibodies are not found. In this context, it is important to emphasize that the absence of serum precipitins does not rule out HP. Ideally, it will be better to obtain a sample of the suspected causative agent from the original source and test it against the patient's blood.

Recently, a prospective multicentre cohort study aimed to develop a clinical prediction rule

for the diagnosis of HP to help clinicians to decide whether further investigation is needed to either rule in or rule out HP was published [24]. Consecutive adult patients presenting with an interstitial lung disease for which HP was considered in the differential diagnosis were included in this study. Regression analyses identified six significant predictors of active HP: exposure to a known offending antigen, positive precipitating antibodies, recurrent episodes of symptoms, symptoms 4–8 h after exposure, inspiratory crackles, and weight loss. These results indicate that a simple clinical prediction rule may guide clinical practice by providing estimates of the probability of acute, subacute, or chronic progressive HP from noninvasive testing.

In the acute form, a notorious improvement after removing the patient from the suspected environment, and worsening after re-exposure is a key feature in the assessment of these patients. In the case of subacute or chronic forms, these usually behave as most interstitial lung diseases, and the diagnostic criteria should include: history of exposure with cause–effect relationship; antibodies against the offending antigen; BAL lymphocytosis, and some characteristic changes on HRCT (Table 13.2). An algorithm for diagnosis is shown in Fig. 13.10.

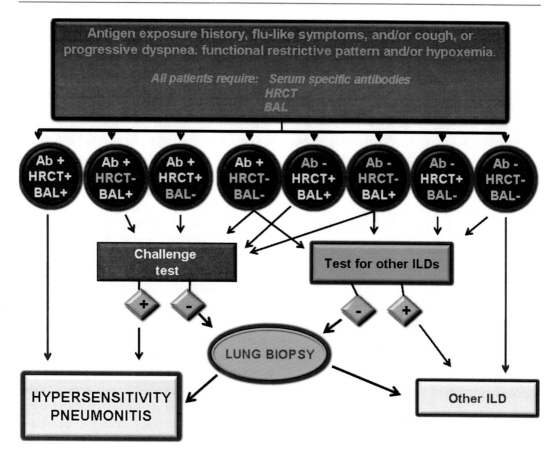

Fig. 13.10 Diagnostic algorithm for hypersensitivity pneumonitis. In a patient suspected of having hypersensitivity pneumonitis, three tests should be performed initially: a panel of specific antibodies, high-resolution computed tomography, and bronchoalveolar lavage. If the three tests are positive (see Table 13.2), diagnosis of HP can be done. If the three tests are negative diagnosis of HP can be ruled out. In presence of two positive results, the patient can be challenged either naturally in the suspected environment or, if the antigen is known and available, in a controlled in-hospital test. In the case that the patient have only one positive test it is necessary to explore for other ILDs. If the challenge test is negative or unavailable, or there is any evidence indicative for other ILD, surgical lung biopsy is required

Invasive Tools for Diagnosis

Bronchoalveolar Lavage

BAL may be helpful in supporting the diagnosis of HP. It is a highly sensitive tool to detect an alveolitis in patients suspected of having HP [25]. It is important to recognize, however, that BAL abnormalities may be also found in asymptomatic individuals with antigen exposure [26]. A marked BAL lymphocytosis (greater than 30% and often exceeding 50% of the inflammatory cells recovered) is a nonspecific but helpful finding in HP patients primarily with the subacute form of the disease. This level of BAL lymphocytosis is uncommon in other diseases generally considered in the differential diagnosis such as IPF. However, BAL lymphocytosis can also be found in infectious and noninfectious granulomatous diseases such as sarcoidosis, berylliosis, or miliary tuberculosis.

The CD4/CD8 ratio varies significantly according to a number of situations including the causative agent, the intensity of exposure, the smoking habit, and the stage of the disease when the BAL is performed. In general, CD4/CD8 ratio is within a normal range or lower in acute/subacute cases and is increased in chronic patients [27]. BAL neutrophils are significantly elevated in acute cases and after recent antigen exposure. Patients with advanced disease may also show a modest but significant increase of neutrophils. The finding of substantial numbers of mast cells (>1%), especially if associated with a marked BAL lymphocytosis, is very useful for diagnosing HP in the appropriate clinical setting.

Increased levels of immunoglobulins may be found in patients with HP. The presence of plasma cells, higher immunoglobulin and IgG to albumin ratios in BAL may be a sign of active alveolitis [28].

If it is not possible to confirm the diagnosis, two additional tools can be used: challenge test and lung biopsy.

Inhalation Challenge

Inhalation challenge can be performed by re-exposure of the patient to the environment of the suspected agent or testing the patient in the hospital under standardized conditions. It can demonstrate a relationship between symptoms and a particular environment and thus support the diagnosis of HP. Two patterns of response are observed, in the first one and most common, patients present fever, malaise, headache, crackles on chest exam, peripheral neutrophilia, and decrease of the forced vital capacity (FVC) 8–12 h after exposure. Consequently, the patient should be monitored closely or have ready access to medical care for at least 24 h. The second pattern is a less common one where a two-stage reaction can occur with immediate, transient wheezing and a decrease in the FEV_1 but preservation of the diffusing capacity. This is followed in 4–6 h by decreased FEV_1 and FVC, fever, and leukocytosis.

Inhalation challenge of a suspected antigen in the hospital is not generally performed because of lack of standardized antigens and limited access to a specialized setting to conduct the study [29–31]. As a result, aerosols prepared in medical laboratories may contain an imprecise mixture of the antigen or may be contaminated with nonspecific irritants. If the test must be done, this should always be conducted carefully to elicit a controlled, mild-to-moderate clinical and functional reaction. Certain workers under even heavy exposure will, for unknown reasons, report less frequent symptoms as compared to those who are less heavily exposed to a particular respiratory irritant.

We have determined the diagnostic usefulness of a provocation test with pigeon serum in patients with subacute/chronic PBD [32]. Patients with other interstitial lung diseases, and exposed but asymptomatic individuals were challenged as controls. After the inhalation challenge, an increase in body temperature and a significant decrease in FVC, PaO_2, and SO_2 were observed in all HP patients. An increase of 0.5°C in temperature (point a) was the best cut point displaying a sensitivity (S) of 100%, a specificity (SP) of 82%, a positive predictive value of (PPV) of 100%, and a negative predictive value (NPV) of 86%. There were no challenge test complications reported during the study. False negative results were obtained in approximately 15% of patients with other ILD but not in avian antigen exposed subjects, suggesting that provocation test can identify patients with HP in the majority of the cases.

Histopathology

Histopathological confirmation of the diagnosis is required in some subacute or chronic cases that may mimic any ILD. Subacute disease is characterized by the presence of small, poorly formed noncaseating granulomas located near respiratory or terminal bronchioles. Other findings include patchy mononuclear cell infiltration (predominantly lymphocytes and plasma cells) of the alveolar walls, typically in a bronchiolocentric distribution [33, 34]. Patients with chronic HP exhibit variable degrees of fibrosis which can be prominent in advanced cases of HP, particularly in those with chronic progressive disease. In these cases, it may be extremely difficult to pathologically distinguish HP from other fibrotic lung disorders including usual interstitial pneumonia. When fibrosis is severe the presence of mild or moderate infiltration with lymphocytes, some giant cells, and the occasional poorly formed granulomas suggests that the pulmonary fibrosis may be secondary to HP.

Additionally, it is important to emphasize that around 10–20% of the patients with documented subacute or chronic HP will show a NSIP either cellular (subacute HP) or fibrotic, (chronic HP) [35, 36]. Because of the diagnostic difficulties in the morphological assessment, it is critical that the pathologist is informed when HP is being considered; the typical HP findings may be subtle and must be interpreted with knowledge of the clinical presentation.

Treatment and Outcome

Because both environmental and host factors are involved in the development of the disease, management should entail modification of the environment or of the host immune response. However, the pathogenesis of HP is incompletely understood, and emphasis on environmental control remains the central part of the treatment. Therefore, decreasing exposure to provocative antigens can reduce the incidence of HP. This may be accomplished by minimizing contact with potential antigens, reducing microbial contamination of the work or home environment, or using protective equipment. Improvement in farming practices and conditions has helped to decrease the incidence of farmer's lung. Likewise, elimination of the yeast from the domestic environment decreased the frequency of summer-type HP provoked by *T. cutaneum* in Japan [37]. Wetting compost prior to handling decreases dispersion of actinomycetes spores, and use of antimicrobial solutions in sugar cane processing diminishes fungal growth and the development of bagassosis.

A reasonable likelihood of causation should lead to preventive actions. In the case of detection of a sentinel case in the workplace, an epidemiological approach is desirable including the careful evaluation of the suspected association.

Indoor microbial contamination is usually related to problems with moisture control. Appropriate design of facilities may reduce stagnant water that promotes microbial overgrowth. Humidity in occupied buildings should be maintained below 50%, and carpeting should be avoided in areas where persistent moisture is likely to be present. Preventive maintenance should be performed routinely to ensure that all heating, ventilation, and air conditioning equipment is properly maintained and that the indoor environment is clean. Buildings with water incursions should be immediately repaired because microbial colonization occurs quickly and can be very difficult to eradicate. Newly wetted areas can be prevented from becoming moldy if they can get dry within 24 h. However, water-damaged furnishings, drywall, and carpeting should be removed because most of the times cannot be adequately dried. Mold colonies are remarkably persistent, and may continue to thrive without the original source. In the case of PBD, birds should be eliminated from homes. However, high levels of antigens may persist for prolonged periods of time in the patient's home, regardless the removal of the birds and a complete environmental cleanup [38].

Corticosteroids are recommended in acute, severe disease. However, long-term efficacy of these agents has yet to be determined. In progressive subacute/chronic cases, the empiric scheme consists of 0.5 mg/kg/day of prednisone for a month followed by a gradual reduction until a maintenance dose of 10–15 mg/day is reached. Prednisone is discontinued when the patient is considered to be healed or when there is no clinical and/or functional response. If the patient worsens after prednisone taper, the maintenance regimen should be prolonged indefinitely. Patients with NTM-related HP have been treated with corticosteroids alone or with antimycobacterial agents or even both, with significant improvement at the time of follow-up [17]. There is no antifibrotic treatment for chronic advanced HP patients. For these cases, lung transplantation should be considered.

The outcome is usually good in acute or subacute cases if the preventive and therapeutic procedures are done quickly and appropriately. By contrast, the prognosis in chronic patients that develop fibrosis and destruction of the lung architecture is poor. Different studies have demonstrated that the presence and degree of fibrosis is associated with higher mortality [39–41].

Conclusions

The diagnosis of HP requires a high index of suspicion by the clinicians. Unfortunately, many cases go unrecognized both in the workplace and in other settings. The physician should determine whether a workplace or home exposure is related with the disease in question. When establishing associations between environmental exposures and clinical symptoms it is important to consider the potential for mixed exposures.

The presence of a normal chest X-ray should not be used to dismiss HP, a normal X-ray can be observed in a number of patients with HP, mainly with an acute attack. Studies have shown significant decline in the sensitivity of chest X-rays for the diagnosis of HP. In one study, chest X-rays were less likely to be abnormal when a population-based approach to the diagnosis of disease was assumed [42]. The presence of negative serum precipitins should not be used to rule out the possibility of HP, but the opposite also is true. The presence of serum precipitins is not a confirmatory test and must be evaluated in the context of clinical symptoms. Other possible problems related with the diagnosis of HP are the presence of abnormal pulmonary function test (obstructive pattern), the presence of a "negative" or "inadequate" lung biopsy accepted to rule out HP, an incorrect pathological interpretation of the lung biopsy (because subtle findings are assumed to be unimportant). These problems are particularly common in mild disease or early stages of the disease. Because most of the test previously discussed are not very specific or are too invasive, a development of new biomarkers, preferable non-invasive will provide new opportunities to better assess patients with HP.

References

1. Selman M. Hypersensitivity pneumonitis: a multifaceted deceiving disorder. Clin Chest Med. 2004;25: 531–47.
2. Ando M, Hirayama K, Soda K, Okubo R, Araki S, Sasazuki T. HLA-DQw3 in Japanese summer-type hypersensitivity pneumonitis induced by Trichosporon cutaneum. Am Rev Respir Dis. 1989; 140:948–50.
3. Camarena A, Juarez A, Mejia M, et al. Major histocompatibility complex and tumor necrosis factor-alpha polymorphisms in pigeon breeder's disease. Am J Respir Crit Care Med. 2001;163:1528–33.
4. Aquino-Galvez A, Camarena A, Montaño M, et al. Transporter associated with antigen processing (TAP) 1 gene polymorphisms in patients with hypersensitivity pneumonitis. Exp Mol Pathol. 2008;84:173–7.
5. Dakhama A, Hegele RG, Laflamme G, Israël-Assayag E, Cormier Y. Common respiratory viruses in lower airways in patients with acute hypersensitivity pneumonitis. Am J Resp Crit Care Med. 1999;159: 1316–22.
6. Hoppin JA, Umbach DM, Kullman GJ, et al. Pesticides and other agricultural factors associated with self-reported farmer's lung among farm residents in the Agricultural Health Study. Occup Environ Med. 2007;64:334–41.
7. Dalphin JC, Debieuvre D, Pernet D, et al. Prevalence and risk factors for chronic bronchitis and farmer's lung in French dairy farmers. Br J Ind Med. 1993;50: 941–4.
8. Blanchet M-R, Israel-Assayag E, Cormier Y. Inhibitory effect of nicotine on experimental hypersensitivity pneumonitis in vivo and in vitro. Am J Respir Crit Care Med. 2004;169:903–9.
9. Madsen D, Klock LE, Wenzel FJ, Robbins JL, Schmidt CD. The prevalence of farmer's lung in an agricultural population. Am Rev Respir Dis. 1976;113: 171–4.
10. Depierre A, Dalphin JC, Pernet D, Dubiez A, Faucompré C, Breton JL. Epidemiological study of farmer's lung in five districts of the French Doubs province. Thorax. 1988;43:429–35.
11. Arya A, Roychoudhury K, Bredin CP. Farmer's lung is now in decline. Ir Med J. 2006;99:203–5.
12. Inase N, Ohtani Y, Sumi Y, Umino T, Usui Y, Miyake S, et al. A clinical study of hypersensitivity pneumonitis presumably caused by feather duvets. Ann Allergy Asthma Immunol. 2006;96:98–104.
13. Stauffer-Ettlin M, Pache JC, Renevey F, Hanquinet-Ginter S, Guinand S, Barazzone-Argiroffo C. Bird breeder's disease: a rare diagnosis in young children. Eur J Pediatr. 2006;165:55–61.
14. Moreno-Ancillo A, Vicente J, Gomez L, et al. Hypersensitivity pneumonitis related to a covered and heated swimming pool environment. Int Arch Allergy Immunol. 1997;114:205–6.
15. Gupta A, Rosenman KD. Hypersensitivity pneumonitis due to metal working fluids: sporadic or under reported? Am J Ind Med. 2006;49:423–33.
16. Hodgson MJ, Morey PR, Simon JS, Waters TD, Fink JN. An outbreak of recurrent acute and chronic hypersensitivity pneumonitis in office workers. Am J Epidemiol. 1987;125(4):631–8.
17. Hanak V, Kalra S, Aksamit TR, Hartman TE, Tazelaar HD, Ryu JH. Hot tub lung: presenting features and clinical course of 21 patients. Respir Med. 2006;100: 610–5.
18. Rosenman KD. Asthma, hypersensitivity pneumonitis and other respiratory diseases caused by metalworking

fluids. Curr Opin Allergy Clin Immunol. 2009;9: 97–102.

19. Seifert SA, Von Essen S, Jacobitz K, Crouch R, Lintner CP. Organic dust toxic syndrome: a review. J Toxicol Clin Toxicol. 2003;41:185–93.

20. Glazer CS, Rose CS, Lynch DA. Clinical and radiologic manifestations of hypersensitivity pneumonitis. J Thorac Imaging. 2002;17:261–72.

21. Silva CI, Churg A, Müller NL. Hypersensitivity pneumonitis: spectrum of high-resolution CT and pathologic findings. AJR Am J Roentgenol. 2007;188: 334–44.

22. Ohtani Y, Saiki S, Sumi Y, et al. Clinical features of recurrent and insidious chronic bird fancier's lung. Ann Allergy Asthma Immunol. 2003;90: 604–10.

23. Malinen AP, Erkinjuntti-Pekkanen RA, Partanen PL, Rytkönen HT, Vanninen RL. Long-term sequelae of Farmer's lung disease in HRCT: a 14-year follow-up study of 88 patients and 83 matched control farmers. Eur Radiol. 2003;13:2212–21.

24. Lacasse Y, Selman M, Costabel U, et al. Clinical diagnosis of hypersensitivity pneumonitis. Am J Respir Crit Care Med. 2003;168:952–8.

25. Semenzato G, Bjermer L, Costabel U, Haslam PL, Olivieri D. Clinical guidelines and indications for bronchoalveolar lavage (BAL): extrinsic allergic alveolitis. Eur Respir J. 1990;3:945–9.

26. Cormier Y, Belanger J, Laviolette M. Persistent bronchoalveolar lymphocytosis in asymptomatic farmers. Am Rev Respir Dis. 1986;133:843–7.

27. Barrera L, Mendoza F, Zuñiga J, et al. Functional diversity of T-cell subpopulations in subacute and chronic hypersensitivity pneumonitis. Am J Respir Crit Care Med. 2008;177:44–55.

28. Drent M, Wagenaar SS, Van Velzen Blad H, et al. Relationship between plasma cell levels and profile of bronchoalveolar lavage fluid in patients with subacute extrinsic allergic alveolitis. Thorax. 1993;48: 835–9.

29. Reynolds SP, Jones KP, Edwards JH, Davies BH. Inhalation challenge in pigeon breeder's disease: BAL fluid changes after 6 hours. Eur Respir J. 1993;6: 467–76.

30. Ohtani Y, Kojima K, Sumi Y, et al. Inhalation provocation tests in chronic bird Fancier's lung. Chest. 2000;118:1382–9.

31. Ortega H, Weissman D, Carter D, Banks D. Use of specific inhalation challenge in the evaluation of workers at risk for occupational asthma: a survey of pulmonary, allergy and occupational medicine residency training programs in the United States and Canada. Chest. 2002;121:1323–8.

32. Ramirez-Venegas A, Sansores RH, Pérez-Padilla R, Carrillo G, Selman M. Utility of a provocation test for diagnosis of chronic pigeon breeder's disease. Am J Respir Crit Care Med. 1998;158:862–9.

33. Coleman A, Colby TV. Histologic diagnosis of extrinsic allergic alveolitis. Am J Surg Pathol. 1988;12: 514–8.

34. Cheung OY, Muhm JR, Helmers RA, et al. Surgical pathology of granulomatous interstitial pneumonia. Ann Diagn Pathol. 2003;7:127–38.

35. Vourlekis JS, Schwarz MI, Cool CD, Tuder RM, King TE, Brown KK. Nonspecific interstitial pneumonitis as the sole histologic expression of hypersensitivity pneumonitis. Am J Med. 2002;112:490–3.

36. Churg A, Muller NL, Flint J, Wright JL. Chronic hypersensitivity pneumonitis. Am J Surg Pathol. 2006;30:201–8.

37. Yoshida K, Ando M, Sakata T, Araki S. Prevention of summer-type hypersensitivity pneumonitis: effect of elimination of Trichosporon cutaneum from the patient's homes. Arch Environ Health. 1989;44: 317–22.

38. Craig TJ, Hershey J, Engler RJM, Davis W, Carpenter GB, Salata K. Bird antigen persistence in the home environment after removal of the bird. Ann Allergy. 1992;69:510–2.

39. Pérez-Padilla R, Salas J, Chapela R, et al. Mortality in Mexican patients with chronic pigeon breeders lung compared to those with usual interstitial pneumonia. Am Rev Respir Dis. 1993;148:49–53.

40. Vourlekis JS, Schwarz MI, Cherniack RM, et al. The effect of pulmonary fibrosis on survival in patients with hypersensitivity pneumonitis. Am J Med. 2004;116:662–8.

41. Churg A, Sin DD, Everett D, Brown K, Cool C. Pathologic patterns and survival in chronic hypersensitivity pneumonitis. Am J Surg Pathol. 2009;33(12): 1765–70.

42. Hodgson MJ, Parkinson DK, Karpf M. Chest X-rays in hypersensitivity pneumonitis: a meta-analysis of secular trend. Am J Ind Med. 1989;16:45–52.

Smoking and Interstitial Lung Disease

14

Joshua J. Solomon and Kevin K. Brown

Abstract

Cigarette smoke contains over 4,000 compounds, contributes to over 400,000 deaths annually and causes or exacerbates a large number of diseases. Recently, a variety of less common interstitial lung diseases have been associated with tobacco exposure. Respiratory bronchiolitis (RB) is a clinically silent histologic finding in the lungs of smokers consisting of pigmented macrophages in the bronchiolar duct and alveolar space. Respiratory bronchiolitis interstitial lung disease (RB-ILD) is the pathologic finding of RB in the presence of clinicoradiographic evidence of interstitial lung disease. Computed tomography (CT) shows bronchial wall thickening with centrilobular nodularity and smoking cessation leads to resolution in most patients with a good prognosis. Desquamative interstitial pneumonia (DIP) is associated with tobacco exposure in 80–90% of patients, is characterized by computed tomography evidence of ground glass opacities in the mid and lower lung zones and has the major histologic feature of a uniform cellular infiltrate of pigmented macrophages within the alveolar spaces. Corticosteroids and tobacco cessation lead to improvement in most patients and relapse is common. Pulmonary Langerhans' cell histiocytosis (PLCH) is associated with tobacco smoke in 90–100% of cases. It has the CT findings of diffuse nodules and cysts with upper lone zone predominance and histopathology shows nodules with Langerhans' cells, pigmented macrophages and occasional necrosis and cavitation. Pneumothorax is common during the course of illness and prognosis is variable with mortality rates greater than 30% at 10 years. Idiopathic pulmonary fibrosis (IPF) is a progressive fibrotic lung disease seen more commonly in smokers. When IPF is seen concomitantly with emphysema, the syndrome is called combined pulmonary fibrosis and emphysema (CPFE). Acute eosinophilic pneumonia (AEP), a syndrome

J.J. Solomon, MD (✉) • K.K. Brown, MD
Department of Medicine, National Jewish Health,
University of Colorado, Denver, CO, USA
e-mail: solomonj@njhealth.org

R.P. Baughman and R.M. du Bois (eds.), *Diffuse Lung Disease: A Practical Approach*,
DOI 10.1007/978-1-4419-9771-5_14, © Springer Science+Business Media, LLC 2012

of diffuse pulmonary infiltrates and pulmonary eosinophilia, is strongly associated with smoking and a significant number of cases are seen in new-onset smokers. Finally, anti-glomerular basement disease (anti-GBM) is a pulmonary renal disease that shows an increased risk of alveolar hemorrhage in active smokers.

Keywords

Smoking-related interstitial lung disease • Respiratory bronchiolitis interstitial lung disease • Desquamative interstitial pneumonia • Eosinophilic granuloma • Pulmonary Langerhans' cell histiocytosis • Combined pulmonary fibrosis and emphysema • Acute eosinophilic pneumonia • Anti-glomerular basement membrane disease

---

Background

The first documented reports of tobacco use date to the Mayans in Pre-Columbian times. Subsequently brought to Spain by Columbus, it gained popularity in Western Europe during the sixteenth and seventeenth centuries as something to be chewed or smoked in a pipe. The cigarette was not introduced until the 1840s, but by the early decades of the 1900s it had gained wide acceptance in the Western world [1]. Cigarette smoking in the USA likely peaked sometime between 1955 and 1965 at over 40% of the adult population, but has since declined in all sociodemographic subpopulations to approximately 19.8% of U.S. adults and 21.9% of high-school students [2, 3]. Unfortunately, worldwide consumption of tobacco has continued to grow, now with over 1.2 billion active users.

Cigarette smoke is a known toxin. It contains over 4,000 compounds [4], approximately 10^{17} oxidant molecules per puff [5] and over 60 tumor initiators, promoters, and carcinogens. Long suspected to cause illness, it was not until the 1950s that research directly linked tobacco use to disease [6], with diseases of the lung the first to be recognized [6, 7]. In 1964, the U.S. Surgeon General concluded that smoking was the primary cause of lung cancer [8] and currently an estimated 90% of current lung cancer deaths worldwide are linked to tobacco use [9]. The link between cigarettes and chronic obstructive pulmonary disease (COPD)

was established in the 1970s [10]. Tobacco use is now a recognized risk factor in six of the eight leading worldwide causes of death, including respiratory cancers, COPD, heart disease, stroke, pneumonia, and TB [11]. It is estimated that tobacco use leads to 443,000 premature deaths and $193 billion in health-care expenditures and productivity loss yearly [12].

It has recently been recognized that less common lung diseases may be caused or exacerbated by tobacco smoke. This chapter reviews the impact of cigarette use on a variety of these interstitial lung diseases (ILDs) (Table 14.1).

Respiratory Bronchiolitis Interstitial Lung Disease

History

In 1974, Niewoehner et al. described pathologic changes in the small airways of young smokers [13]. All had abnormalities of the respiratory bronchioles consisting of "clusters of brown macrophages in the first-order and second-order respiratory bronchiole distal to the terminal membranous bronchiole… frequently associated with edema, fibrosis and epithelial hyperplasia in the adjacent bronchiolar and alveolar walls." The authors concluded that these changes were a possible precursor to centriacinar emphysema, responsible for physiologic abnormalities seen in

Table 14.1 Smoking-related interstitial lung diseases

	RB-ILD	DIP	PLCH	CPFE
Age of onset	40s–50s	30s–40s	30s–40s	50s–70s
M:F ratio	3:2	1:1	1:1	2:1
% current or former smokers	>98%	80–90%	90–100%	100%
HRCT findings	Bronchial wall thickening, upper centrilobular nodules, GG	GG opacities mid lower lung zones. reticulation	Diffuse nodules and cysts with upper and mid lung predominance	Upper lobe emphysema with lower lobe fibrosis
Physiology	Reduced DLCO, restriction	Restriction, reduced VC, reduced DLCO	Variable, normal or reduced DLCO	Volumes normal, severely reduced DLCO
Pathology	Peribronchiolar pigmented macrophages	Uniform macrophage infiltration of alveolar spaces	LCs accumulate in and around bronchioles, patchy and focal	Upper lobe centrilobular emphysema, lower lobe UIP
Treatment	Smoking cessation	Corticosteroids	Smoking cessation, +/– immunosuppression	Smoking cessation with therapy similar to IPF
Outcome	Excellent	Excellent, rare progressive fibrosis	Median survival 12–13 years	5-Year survival 25–75% (with or without pHTN)

RB-ILD respiratory bronchiolitis interstitial lung disease, *DIP* desquamative interstitial pneumonia, *PLCH* pulmonary Langerhans' cell histiocytosis, *CPFE* combined pulmonary fibrosis and emphysema, *GG* ground glass, *DLCO* diffusion capacity for carbon monoxide, *VC* vital capacity, *UIP* usual interstitial pneumonia, *IPF* idiopathic pulmonary fibrosis, *pHTN* pulmonary hypertension, *LCs* Langerhans' cells, *M* male, *F* female, *HRCT* high-resolution computer tomography asymptomatic smokers, and likely reversible with smoking cessation. This was the first description of the pathologic pattern of respiratory bronchiolitis (RB), a clinically silent histologic finding in the lungs of smokers. A follow-up study in 1980, looking at smokers over the age of 40, found similar bronchiolar abnormalities with coexistent emphysema [14]. In 1983, Wright et al. found significant differences in the small airways between lifelong nonsmokers and both current and former smokers [15]. These changes were the same in current and former smokers despite an improvement in physiology after tobacco cessation. These findings were the first to suggest that smoking-induced small airway changes might persist well after smoking cessation.

In 1987, Myers et al. described a series of active smokers with clinicoradiographic evidence of ILD who were found to have RB as the sole pathologic pattern on surgical lung biopsy [16]. They speculated that this RB-associated ILD might be on a clinical spectrum with desquamative interstitial pneumonia (DIP), a more diffuse and symptomatic smoking-related lung disease. Eighteen additional cases were subsequently reported by Yousem and the term respiratory bronchiolitis-interstitial lung disease (RB-ILD) was proposed to distinguish the clinical disease from the histologic finding seen in asymptomatic smokers [17].

Relationship to Smoking

The best evidence for a relationship with smoking was reported by Fraig in 2002. In 156 cases, RB was found in all 83 of the current smokers and 24 of 49 ex-smokers. Only two subjects with RB had no discernable tobacco history [18]. These findings have been supported by a number of other studies [17–24]. The histologic changes appear to resolve in some patients, although this likely takes years [the increased numbers of macrophages with smoking-related inclusions seen on bronchoalveolar (BAL) in active smokers takes 3 years to fall to nonsmoker levels] [25]. While smoking appears to be the dominant cause of histologic RB, similar findings have been described in asbestos and nonasbestos mineral dust exposures, as well as rheumatoid arthritis [18, 20].

Clinical Features

Based on clinical data from 245 patients, the average age is 49 with a large range (21–83) [16–24, 26]. Males constitute 59% of subjects. Symptoms have an insidious onset. The most common, progressive dyspnea, is seen in 67–100% of patients. Cough is seen 30–80% of the time, and is most often productive of sputum. Infrequently, chest pain and wheeze are present [16, 17, 19, 20, 22–24, 26].

Chest Imaging

A variety of abnormal plain chest radiographic findings can be seen. The most common include airway wall thickening in central and peripheral airways, diffuse ground glass opacities, and emphysema [22]. Additional findings include low lung volumes, bibasilar bands and atelectasis, and reticulonodular densities [16, 17, 20, 24, 26]. Up to 15% of patients may have normal plain chest radiographs [22]. In contrast, high-resolution computerized tomographic (HRCT) scanning is universally abnormal (Fig. 14.1). The most common findings are bronchial wall thickening in central and peripheral airways in 90% of patients, mid and upper lung zone centrilobular nodules in 70%, and upper zone ground glass opacities in 67%. About half the patients will have centrilobular emphysema [21, 22, 27]. More rarely, reticular changes and increased intralobular septa have been reported [20, 24, 26]. The HRCT changes correlate with pathologic findings. Centrilobular nodularity equates to macrophage accumulation and chronic inflammation of the respiratory bronchioles and the ground glass opacification equates to macrophage accumulation in the alveolar ducts and spaces [21, 22].

Physiology

The physiologic abnormalities are variable and generally mild. The most common is a mild to moderate reduction in diffusion capacity for carbon monoxide (DLCO%) [16, 17, 20, 22–24]. The severity of the DLCO% reduction appears to

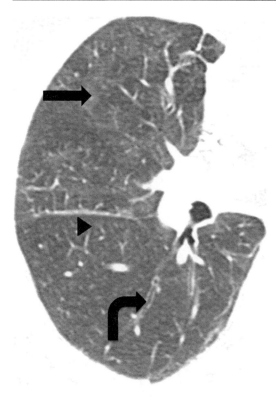

Fig. 14.1 CT in respiratory bronchiolitis. CT scans in respiratory bronchiolitis are universally abnormal and show upper zone ground glass abnormalities (*arrow*), mid and upper zone centrilobular nodularity (*arrowhead*) and bronchial wall thickening in central and peripheral airways (*curved arrow*)

correlate with the extent of centrilobular nodularity and ground glass abnormality on HRCT [21]. Both restrictive and obstructive physiologic abnormalities occur with restriction (31–66%) being more common than obstruction (24–47%).

Pathology

Histopathologic findings are patchy and airway-centered, predominately around the bronchiole [18, 28]. The lung tissue distal to the involved airways is normal unless there is superimposed emphysema. The defining characteristic is the presence of pigmented macrophages in the bronchiolar duct, alveolar space, and peribronchiolar space (Fig. 14.2). The macrophages have a finely granular golden-brown cytoplasm with inclusions that stain with both periodic acid-Schiff (PAS) and

Prussian blue [28]. These inclusions are thought to be components of cigarette smoke. Variable numbers of lymphocytes and histiocytes are seen in the peribronchiolar and submucosal spaces with occasional mild peribronchiolar fibrosis. This inflammation and fibrosis can involve contiguous alveolar septa and is often accompanied by hyperplasia of type II pneumocytes, goblet cell hyperplasia, and metaplastic cuboidal epithelium [16, 29]. If fibroblast foci, granulomas or Langerhans' cells are present, one should consider an alternative diagnosis. Though early studies sought to separate the simple finding of pathologic RB from the clinical syndrome of RB-ILD by the extent of the histologic findings [17, 20, 27, 30], later studies have confirmed that the histologic pattern is indistinguishable between the two.

Diagnosis

The definitive diagnosis of RB-ILD requires a clinical syndrome of ILD, i.e., the presence of respiratory symptoms with clinically significant pulmonary physiologic and chest imaging abnormalities in combination with the histologic pattern of RB on surgical lung biopsy [31]. In the absence of any clinical signs or symptoms, the histologic pattern of RB simply suggests that the patient is or was a smoker. Given that the symptoms, clinical signs and physiologic abnormalities are nonspecific, the HRCT pattern helps to support the diagnosis when pathology is not available. The HRCT findings can overlap with findings in DIP and hypersensitivity pneumonitis, but the extent and distribution of ground glass abnormalities seen in DIP (see below) and the general lack of smoking history for hypersensitivity pneumonitis aid in these distinctions [32].

Treatment and Outcome

There are only limited data on therapy. Smoking cessation appears to be the most important intervention [15, 18, 23, 24]. A significant reduction in symptoms, decreased ground glass opacity and centrilobular nodularity, as well as improvements in DLCO and PaO_2 have all been described in

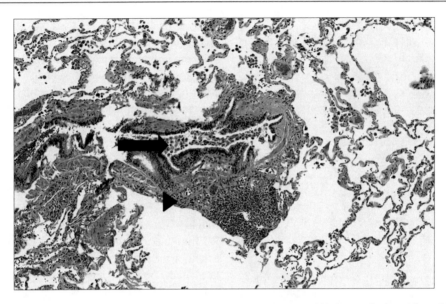

Fig. 14.2 Pathology in respiratory bronchiolitis. Respiratory bronchiolitis is characterized by pigmented macrophages in the bronchiolar duct, alveolar space, and peribronchiolar space (*arrow*). There are variable numbers of lymphocytes and histiocytes in the peribronchiolar and submucosal spaces (*arrowhead*) with occasional mild peribronchiolar fibrosis

response to smoking cessation, although this is clearly not seen in all patients [21–23]. The use of corticosteroids with or without other agents has been reported to be effective in improving symptoms, physiology, and radiologic findings in some patients [16, 17, 19–21, 24, 29]. However, these results are not universal, and lack of clinical improvement or even worsening in the face of smoking cessation with or without corticosteroids is routinely seen [20, 23, 24]. Death from progressive RB-ILD appears extremely rare. In a study looking at long-term outcome, the median survival could not be calculated due to the prolonged survival. Seventy-five percent of patients are expected to survive ≥7 years [23].

Desquamative Interstitial Pneumonia

History

In 1965, Liebow described the clinical, radiographic and surgical lung biopsy findings in 18 patients with a clinical syndrome of ILD and a histologic pattern on surgical lung biopsy characterized by "massive proliferation and desquamation of large alveolar cells, by slight thickening of the walls of distal airspaces, by the absence of necrosis and by minimal loss of tissue" [33]. Termed desquamative interstitial pneumonia (DIP) because the accumulated "large alveolar cells" were thought to be desquamated pneumocytes, it was felt that the distinctive pathologic features and response to therapy warranted a separation between it and the other interstitial pneumonias. In a follow-up study, Gaensler and colleagues described an additional 12 cases with long-term follow up [34]. They noted a more benign course when compared to the other fibrosing interstitial pneumonias and documented a brief remission with steroid treatment. Subsequent studies determined that the "large alveolar cells" were in fact macrophages [35, 36], and were thought to be a nonspecific response to injury and the precursor lesion to the usual interstitial pneumonia (UIP) pathologic pattern. It is now widely accepted that UIP and DIP are separate entities [24, 28, 37–39].

Relationship to Smoking

Early studies focused on a potential virologic etiology due to the rare intranuclear inclusion bodies seen histologically [33, 34]. Subsequent investigation revealed that 80–90% of patients are current or former smokers [17, 24, 27, 40], though numerous case reports describe CMV and hepatitis C infection, exposures to aluminum, mycotoxins, nitrofurantoin, and inorganic particulates, as well as monomyelocytic leukemia to be associated with DIP [41–47].

Clinical Features

Patients are generally young with an average age at presentation between the late 30s to mid 40s. Women and men are equally represented. Most complain of the insidious onset of dyspnea with half describing a dry cough. A minority describe a systemic illness with weight loss and lethargy. Physical examination ranges from normal to auscultatory findings of crackles. Finger clubbing is seen in less than half. Pneumothorax at some point during the course of illness has been reported in up to 25% [17, 24, 33, 34].

Chest Imaging

Plain chest radiographs commonly show bibasilar ground glass and/or interstitial infiltrates, but are normal in up to a quarter of patients [17, 24, 33, 34]. The predominate HRCT findings are ground glass opacities in the mid and lower lung zones with a peripheral distribution (Fig. 14.3). Fibrotic features, represented by reticular lines with or without architectural distortion, are seen in just over half of the patients. These also have a peripheral and basilar location. Other findings such as nodules, emphysema, and foci of consolidation are rare [27, 48].

Physiology

Pulmonary physiology is variable. Most have a restrictive defect with a low normal total lung

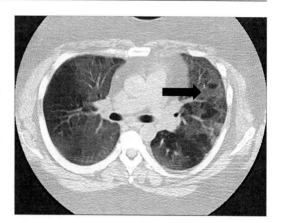

Fig. 14.3 CT in desquamative interstitial pneumonia. CT findings in desquamative interstitial pneumonia consist of ground glass opacities in the mid and lower lung zones with a peripheral distribution (*arrow*). Fibrotic features are seen in just over half of the patients and nodules, emphysema and foci of consolidation are rare

capacity (TLC%) and mildly reduced forced vital capacity (FVC%). Diffusing capacity is impaired in almost all and exercise-induced desaturation is common. Airflow obstruction is rare [17, 24, 33, 34, 40].

Pathology

The distinguishing histologic feature is a uniform cellular infiltrate of pigmented macrophages within the alveolar spaces (Fig. 14.4) [28, 48, 49]. These macrophages have golden-brown cytoplasms, fine black particles, and stain with PAS and Prussian blue in a manner similar to macrophages in RB. This infiltrate is evenly distributed throughout the involved area, leading to an early description of "monotonous uniformity" [33]. It is this uniformity of findings that helps distinguish DIP from RB and its patchy bronchiolocentric distribution [28]. The alveolar space findings are accompanied by diffuse and uniform septal thickening consisting predominately of mononuclear cells with occasional eosinophils. The septal thickening is accompanied by comparatively minor collagen deposition and hyperplasia of type 2 pneumocytes. The alveolar architecture is maintained and significant fibrosis or honeycombing is rare.

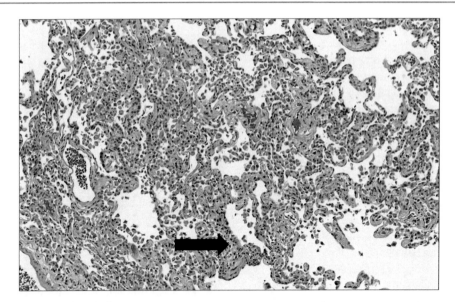

Fig. 14.4 Pathology in desquamative interstitial pneumonia. Desquamative interstitial pneumonia has a uniform and evenly distributed cellular infiltrate of pigmented macrophages within the alveolar spaces (*arrow*). This is accompanied by diffuse and uniform septal thickening consisting predominately of mononuclear cells with occasional eosinophils. Alveolar architecture is maintained and significant fibrosis or honeycombing is rare

A focal DIP-like reaction can occasionally be seen in the surgical lung biopsies of smoking patients with other ILDs such as IPF, RB-ILD or nonspecific interstitial pneumonia (NSIP), eosinophilic pneumonia, chronic pulmonary hemorrhage, veno-occlusive disease, rheumatoid nodules, hamartomas, and eosinophilic granulomas [50, 51].

Diagnosis

Similar to RB-ILD, the definitive diagnosis of DIP requires a clinical syndrome of ILD in the setting of a DIP pattern on surgical pathology. As a DIP-like reaction may be seen in other diffuse lung diseases, the possibility of a sampling error must be considered. When pathology is not available, a confident diagnosis rests on a suggestive clinical syndrome in younger persons with characteristic HRCT findings. Active smoking supports the diagnosis, but up to 20% of cases are seen in nonsmokers.

Treatment and Outcome

In the initial descriptions of DIP, the majority of patients showed stabilization or improvement with corticosteroid treatment [33]. In Gaensler's subsequent study, corticosteroids resulted in marked improvement in the majority of patients, responses that were "striking and immediate." However, when the steroid dose was reduced or discontinued, all patients relapsed [34]. Current expert opinion favors a 2-month trial of moderate doses (up to 40 to 60 milligrams daily) of prednisone followed by a slow taper over another 2 months. A steroid-sparing agent should be considered if the clinical response is inadequate or in the face of unacceptable corticosteroid side effects [52]. Prognosis is good. A 10-year survival of up to 100% has been reported with a mean survival from the date of diagnosis of 12 years [40, 53, 54]. A subset may develop progressive fibrosis with honeycombing and an associated shorter lifespan [34].

Pulmonary Langerhans' Cell Histiocytosis

History

In 1950, Lichtenstein coined the term "Histiocytosis X" to describe a group of disorders of varying clinical features and prognoses whose common feature was tissue infiltration with histiocytes [55]. He described three specific diseases: Hand–Schüller–Christian, Letterer–Siwe, and eosinophilic granuloma of bone. In 1978, the infiltrating histiocytes were found to be pathologically similar to the Langerhans' cells (LCs) normally present in skin and other epithelia [56] and the new term "Langerhans'-cell histiocytosis" (LCH) was offered as an alternative. In 1985, the Histiocyte Society was formed to study these diseases and to clarify a confusing nomenclature [57]. The Society divided the clinical syndromes into subgroups based on the site of involvement and extent of disease [58]. Acute disseminated LCH (Letterer–Siwe) is a multifocal multisystem disease with a poor prognosis seen mainly in children under the age of 2. Multifocal unisystem LCH (Hand–Schüller–Christian syndrome) is usually seen in children, carries a better prognosis and is often characterized by fever, lytic bone lesions and skin eruptions. Unifocal LCH (eosinophilic granuloma) involves either the bones, skin, lungs or stomach. Though the lung can be involved in multisystem disease, the localized pulmonary form of the disease (pulmonary Langerhans' cell histiocytosis [PLCH]) is the one most commonly encountered by pulmonologists. Its unique clinical picture warrants its consideration as a variant of LCH and separation from pulmonary involvement seen in childhood multisystem disease [58].

Relationship to Smoking

The consistent risk factor associated with the development of PLCH is tobacco smoke. Ninety to 100% of patients are current or previous smokers [59–65]. There is an association with the amount of tobacco consumption. Smokers who develop PLCH have a higher average daily tobacco consumption than smokers without PLCH [59]. Clinical and radiographic resolution has also been seen with tobacco cessation alone [66].

Langerhans' cells (dendritic or antigen-presenting cells produced in the marrow and found in most tissues of the body) are normally present in the healthy lung and are sparsely distributed in the tracheobronchial epithelia [67]. Their numbers

significantly increase in the presence of tobacco smoke, cancer, and chronic pulmonary inflammation [68, 69]. Though multiorgan LCH seems to display a clonal proliferation of LCs, PLCH appears to be generally a nonclonal reactive proliferation to tobacco smoke in which nonmalignant clonal proliferations may arise [70]. Though described associations other than smoking are rare, PLCH has been described in the setting of malignancy including Hodgkin's lymphoma and lung carcinoma [71].

Clinical Features

Early studies suggested a male predominance, likely reflecting differences in tobacco use [59, 61, 63], As tobacco use by women has increased, the ratio appears closer to 1:1 [62, 64]. While described cases have been predominately in Caucasians, the racial distribution is not known [72]. A clinico-epidemiologic study conducted in Japan described a similar age of onset, smoking relationship, and male predominance [65].

Isolated pulmonary LCH has a younger age of onset than other ILDs, usually presenting in the third or fourth decade. Two-thirds of the patients present with cough or dyspnea. Extrapulmonary symptoms are common and include malaise, fevers and weight loss, while 15–30% of patients will have extrapulmonary manifestations with bone, skin and pituitary being the most common [60–65]. Pneumothorax is seen in up to 25% of patients either at diagnosis or during the course of their illness, and can be recurrent [73].

Chest Imaging

The characteristic plain chest radiograph finding is multiple small- to medium-sized nodules with either an upper or mid-zone predominance that spare the costophrenic angles [62, 74]. Micronodules up to 2 mm in size are seen in over 90% of patients with larger nodules and cysts seen in half of the patients [74]. HRCT findings have been well described and consist of diffuse nodules and cysts with an upper and mid-lung zone predominance (Fig. 14.5) [75, 76]. The nodules tend

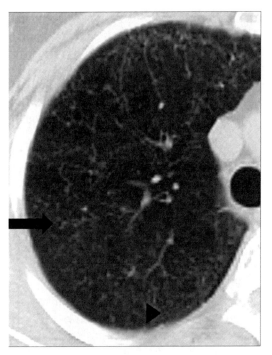

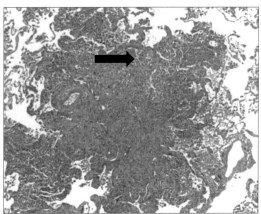

Fig. 14.6 Pathology in pulmonary Langerhans' cell histiocytosis. In pulmonary Langerhans' cell histiocytosis, Langerhans' cells accumulate in and around the bronchioles in a patchy and focal fashion. This forms a nodule, usually with a stellate pattern, that consists of Langerhans' cells, eosinophils, neutrophils, lymphocytes, fibroblasts, and macrophages (*arrow*). These can have cavitation or necrosis

Fig. 14.5 CT in pulmonary Langerhans' cell histiocytosis. In pulmonary Langerhans' cell histiocytosis, CT findings consist of diffuse cysts (*arrow*) and nodules (*arrowhead*) with upper and mid-lung zone predominance. The nodules and cysts also tend to be small, usually less than 10 mm. Linear and ground glass opacities are rare

volume in 1 second (FEV1)/FVC ratio is rare in early and mild disease [60, 61, 63, 64]. Progression to late-stage disease can be heralded by reductions in TLC%, FVC%, FEV1%, FEV1/FVC and variable changes in residual volume (RV) [60, 63].

Pathology

In normal healthy lungs, LCs are sparse while in PLCH these cells accumulate in and around the bronchioles in a patchy and focal fashion (Fig. 14.6). They are different from other histiocytes in that they stain positive for CD1a and have pentalaminar Birbeck granules visible by electron microscopy [77]. Macroscopic findings in surgically exposed lungs consist of palpable small subpleural nodules occasionally associated with cysts [78]. The predominant microscopic finding is bronchiolocentric nodules most commonly in a stellate pattern [28]. The nodules consist of a varying number of LCs, eosinophils, neutrophils, lymphocytes, fibroblasts and macrophages (often containing smoker's pigment), and can display necrosis or cavitation. The eosinophils vary in number, are occasionally the dominant cell type and are situated at the periphery of the nodule [78].

to be small, the majority less than 10 mm in size. Cysts also tend to be small (<10 mm) and thin walled, with larger cysts, confluent cysts, and thick-walled cysts being less common. Linear and ground glass opacities tend to be rare. Studies looking at evolution of CT findings with disease progression suggest that active disease is represented by the presence of nodular lesions, which regress or progress and transform into cysts.

Physiology

The severity of physiologic impairment is variable. Normal physiology has been reported in up to 35% of patients, likely representing early diagnosis [61, 62, 64]. The most common abnormality is a reduction in DLCO%, seen in up to 90%. TLC% and FVC% can be mildly reduced and obstruction with a reduced forced expiratory

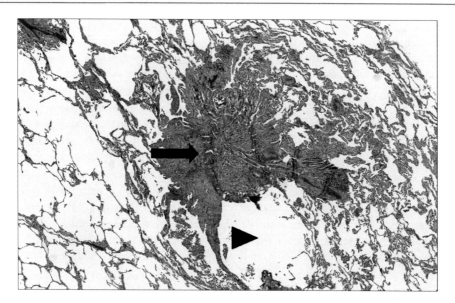

Fig. 14.7 The stellate scar in pulmonary Langerhans' cell histiocytosis. The stellate scar is the final fibrotic stage of pulmonary Langerhans' cell histiocytosis. They are seen around the bronchioles and are usually void of Langerhans' cells (*arrow*). Cystic spaces are formed by traction of the surrounding normal airspaces by contraction of the scar (*arrowhead*)

A "DIP-like" reaction with macrophages filling the airways can often be seen [62]. Histologic progression is associated with fibroblast proliferation in the center with collagen deposition and scarring. Stellate scars are seen around the bronchioles (bronchiolocentric), are void of LCs, and presumed to be the final fibrotic stage (Fig. 14.7) [28].

Diagnosis

In the absence of alternative explanations, a young smoker with characteristic HRCT findings has a diagnosis of PLCH with a high degree of confidence. In the correct clinical setting, BAL findings of >5% LCs that stain for CD1a makes a diagnosis of PLCH likely [79]. When the clinical and radiographic data are less clear, tissue biopsy may be required. As the lesions are focal in nature, the yield of transbronchial biopsy is low (in the range of 10–40%) and a definitive diagnosis often requires a surgical lung biopsy [80]. Tissue should be stained with antibodies for S-100 and CD1a [28, 72].

Treatment and Outcome

Smoking cessation should be encouraged as there has been documented near-complete symptomatic and radiographic improvement with tobacco cessation alone [66]. In asymptomatic patients, additional therapy does not appear warranted. Patients with symptoms or significant physiologic derangement are often treated with corticosteroids alone or, in the case of multisystem disease, corticosteroids with another immunosuppressive agent [64]. Many immunosuppressive agents have been used, including cyclophosphamide, vinblastine, chlorambucil, methotrexate, etoposide, and cladribine [64, 78]. No strong data exist on the efficacy of these regimens. For subjects with pneumothoraces, surgical pleurodesis should be considered [73].

Prognosis is variable. Fifty to 60% of patients will show a decline in symptoms with or without steroid therapy. The mortality rate has been estimated to be as high as 36% at 10 years [64], with a median survival of 12–13 years [61, 64]. Death usually results from respiratory failure, but patients appear to be at increased risk of neoplasm, usually pulmonary or hematologic [61, 64]. Factors associated with a worsened survival include age, reduced FEV1/FVC ratio, increased RV/TLC, and in DLCO% [61, 64].

Idiopathic Pulmonary Fibrosis and Combined Pulmonary Fibrosis and Emphysema

Ever-smoking is a known risk factor for the development of IPF. Studies looking at environmental and occupational exposures in patients with IPF have found that when compared to never-smokers, ever-smokers have an increased risk of disease development (odds ratio ranging from 1.57 to 2.9) [81–83]. A meta-analysis has provided additional support for a relationship [84] as have studies of subjects genetically at risk for the development of fibrosis [85]. More recently, patients with IPF, severe breathlessness, and a marked reduction in DLCO% in spite of normal or near normal lung volumes on pulmonary function testing have been described [86]. HRCT scanning revealed upper-lobe emphysema and lower lobe UIP patterns. All patients were former or current smokers. This was an early description of a proposed distinct entity, the combination of pulmonary fibrosis and emphysema (CPFE) [87–92], a syndrome reported almost exclusively in smokers [92]. It has been estimated that it may account for 5–10% of diffuse ILDs [87].

At least two-thirds of described patients are men with a primary complaint of breathlessness. Cough is less frequent. Clubbing is seen in up to half of patients [86, 87, 89–92]. HRCT scans show predominately upper lobe centrilobular emphysema and lower lobe UIP pattern fibrosis [87, 93]. The prevalence of ground glass abnormalities and the distribution of fibrotic lesion are similar to that seen in IPF [91]. In contrast to typical emphysema, near normal lung volumes, 80–90% of predicted, are seen and air trapping is rare. Decreases in FEV1/FVC ratio are mild with a mean ratio of 0.70 [87, 90]. DLCO% is markedly reduced, usually 30–40% of predicted. The physiologic findings represent the additive effects of emphysema and IPF on gas transfer

and the opposing effects on total lung volume and airflows [86]. Pathology obtained from surgical lung biopsy or explants reveals upper lung zone centrilobular emphysema and lower lung zone UIP pattern fibrosis [87]. There are variable amounts of intra-alveolar pigmented macrophage deposition representing a smoker's "DIP-like" reaction. Histologic patterns other than UIP have been reported including DIP, organizing pneumonia and unclassifiable interstitial pneumonia [87]. Therapy is similar to that for IPF [87]. The risk of pulmonary hypertension (PH) is high (50–90%) and the presence of echocardiographically proven PH decreases 5-year survival from 75 to 25% [92].

Acute Eosinophilic Pneumonia

Acute eosinophilic pneumonia (AEP) is a rare syndrome characterized by fever, diffuse pulmonary infiltrates, and pulmonary eosinophilia. Patients often develop fever, dyspnea, and cough 3–4 days before diagnosis [94]. Chest x-ray and HRCT scans show diffuse airspace opacities with effusions present in up to 70% [95]. Peripheral blood eosinophilia is not seen. While diagnostic criteria are debated, other common causes of pulmonary eosinophilia must be excluded, including helminthic, fungal and bacterial infections, drugs, toxins, radiation exposure, Churg–Strauss vasculitis and Hodgkin's disease [96]. BAL eosinophilia in the range of 36–54% is seen [94]. Reported treatment regimens consist of varying doses of IV methylprednisolone, ranging from 240 to 1,000 mg daily with an expected response with rapid clearing of chest radiographs and resolution of respiratory failure. Prednisone tapers last from days to months and reoccurrences have not been reported. While AEP has been associated with various inhaled exposures including World Trade Center dust [97], cocaine [98] and Scotchguard inhalation [99], the strongest association has been with smoking. Up to 97% of patients are active smokers, with new-onset smokers being over-represented [95, 100, 101]. In a study of military personnel deployed in or near Iraq, all 18 cases of AEP identified were in current smokers, with 78% of cases noted in new-onset smokers (within the last 2 months prior to diagnosis) [102].

Anti-glomerular Basement Membrane Disease

Anti-glomerular basement membrane (anti-GBM) disease is a rare autoimmune disease characterized by circulating antibodies against type IV collagen. While classically considered a pulmonary renal syndrome, it presents with either isolated renal disease, renal disease with diffuse alveolar hemorrhage (DAH), or rarely with alveolar hemorrhage alone [103]. There is a correlation between active cigarette smoking and both the development and relapse of DAH, with active smokers making up from 50 to 89% of patients [104–108]. There is also speculation that smoking may play a more general role in precipitating hemoptysis in patients with a predisposition to hemorrhage, as heavy smoking appears associated with an increased risk of DAH in immunocompromised patients and in idiopathic pulmonary hemosiderosis [109–112].

Conclusion

Tobacco smoke is associated with a wide range of effects in the human lung. Beyond its known association with the development of lung cancer and emphysema, it is associated with the development of both incidental bronchiolar changes as well as a number of specific ILDs. For example, RB as an incidental histologic finding in ever smokers may persist without clinical impact for years, while RB-ILD is a clinically significant ILD disease with identical pathologic changes. Its impact is not limited to its known associations with RB-ILD/DIP and PLCH as it also appears to be associated with the development of lung fibrosis, eosinophilic pneumonia, and alveolar hemorrhage in susceptible individuals. Overall, the impact of tobacco smoke is wide and almost universally detrimental.

References

1. Kumra V, Markoff BA. Who's smoking now? The epidemiology of tobacco use in the United States and abroad. Clin Chest Med. 2000;21(1):1–9, vii.
2. Centers for Disease Control and Prevention (CDC). Cigarette smoking among adults – United States, 2007. MMWR Morb Mortal Wkly Rep. 2008;57(45): 1221–6.
3. Centers for Disease Control and Prevention (CDC). Cigarette use among high school students – United States, 1991–2007. MMWR Morb Mortal Wkly Rep. 2008;57(25):686–8.
4. Smith CJ, Hansch C. The relative toxicity of compounds in mainstream cigarette smoke condensate. Food Chem Toxicol. 2000;38(7):637–46.
5. Pryor WA, Stone K. Oxidants in cigarette smoke. Radicals, hydrogen peroxide, peroxynitrite, and peroxynitrite. Ann N Y Acad Sci. 1993;686:12–27. discussion 27–18.
6. Wynder EL, Graham EA. Tobacco smoking as a possible etiologic factor in bronchiogenic carcinoma; a study of 684 proved cases. J Am Med Assoc. 1950; 143(4):329–36.
7. Doll R, Hill AB. Smoking and carcinoma of the lung; preliminary report. Br Med J. 1950;2(4682): 739–48.
8. Service USPH. Smoking and health: a report of the Surgeon General. Washington, DC: US Government Printing Office; 1964.
9. Bilello KS, Murin S, Matthay RA. Epidemiology, etiology, and prevention of lung cancer. Clin Chest Med. 2002;23(1):1–25.
10. Petty TL. The history of COPD. Int J Chron Obstruct Pulmon Dis. 2006;1(1):3–14.
11. World Health Organization. WHO report on the global tobacco epidemic. Geneva: World Health Organization; 2008.
12. Centers for Disease Control and Prevention (CDC). State-specific smoking-attributable mortality and years of potential life lost – United States, 2000–2004. MMWR Morb Mortal Wkly Rep. 2009;58(2): 29–33.
13. Niewoehner DE, Kleinerman J, Rice DB. Pathologic changes in the peripheral airways of young cigarette smokers. N Engl J Med. 1974;291(15):755–8.
14. Cosio MG, Hale KA, Niewoehner DE. Morphologic and morphometric effects of prolonged cigarette smoking on the small airways. Am Rev Respir Dis. 1980;122(2):265–71.
15. Wright JL, Lawson LM, Pare PD, Wiggs BJ, Kennedy S, Hogg JC. Morphology of peripheral airways in current smokers and ex-smokers. Am Rev Respir Dis. 1983;127(4):474–7.
16. Myers JL, Veal Jr CF, Shin MS, Katzenstein AL. Respiratory bronchiolitis causing interstitial lung disease. A clinicopathologic study of six cases. Am Rev Respir Dis. 1987;135(4):880–4.

17. Yousem SA, Colby TV, Gaensler EA. Respiratory bronchiolitis-associated interstitial lung disease and its relationship to desquamative interstitial pneumonia. Mayo Clin Proc. 1989;64(11):1373–80.

18. Fraig M, Shreesha U, Savici D, Katzenstein AL. Respiratory bronchiolitis: a clinicopathologic study in current smokers, ex-smokers, and never-smokers. Am J Surg Pathol. 2002;26(5):647–53.

19. Craig PJ, Wells AU, Doffman S, et al. Desquamative interstitial pneumonia, respiratory bronchiolitis and their relationship to smoking. Histopathology. 2004; 45(3):275–82.

20. Moon J, du Bois RM, Colby TV, Hansell DM, Nicholson AG. Clinical significance of respiratory bronchiolitis on open lung biopsy and its relationship to smoking related interstitial lung disease. Thorax. 1999;54(11):1009–14.

21. Nakanishi M, Demura Y, Mizuno S, et al. Changes in HRCT findings in patients with respiratory bronchiolitis-associated interstitial lung disease after smoking cessation. Eur Respir J. 2007;29(3):453–61.

22. Park JS, Brown KK, Tuder RM, Hale VA, King Jr TE, Lynch DA. Respiratory bronchiolitis-associated interstitial lung disease: radiologic features with clinical and pathologic correlation. J Comput Assist Tomogr. 2002;26(1):13–20.

23. Portnoy J, Veraldi KL, Schwarz MI, et al. Respiratory bronchiolitis-interstitial lung disease: long-term outcome. Chest. 2007;131(3):664–71.

24. Ryu JH, Myers JL, Capizzi SA, Douglas WW, Vassallo R, Decker PA. Desquamative interstitial pneumonia and respiratory bronchiolitis-associated interstitial lung disease. Chest. 2005;127(1):178–84.

25. Agius RM, Rutman A, Knight RK, Cole PJ. Human pulmonary alveolar macrophages with smokers' inclusions: their relation to the cessation of cigarette smoking. Br J Exp Pathol. 1986;67(3):407–13.

26. Holt RM, Schmidt RA, Godwin JD, Raghu G. High resolution CT in respiratory bronchiolitis-associated interstitial lung disease. J Comput Assist Tomogr. 1993;17(1):46–50.

27. Heyneman LE, Ward S, Lynch DA, Remy-Jardin M, Johkoh T, Muller NL. Respiratory bronchiolitis, respiratory bronchiolitis-associated interstitial lung disease, and desquamative interstitial pneumonia: different entities or part of the spectrum of the same disease process? AJR Am J Roentgenol. 1999;173(6):1617–22.

28. Aubry MC, Wright JL, Myers JL. The pathology of smoking-related lung diseases. Clin Chest Med. 2000;21(1):11–35, vii.

29. King Jr TE. Respiratory bronchiolitis-associated interstitial lung disease. Clin Chest Med. 1993;14(4): 693–8.

30. Cottin V, Streichenberger N, Gamondes JP, Thevenet F, Loire R, Cordier JF. Respiratory bronchiolitis in smokers with spontaneous pneumothorax. Eur Respir J. 1998;12(3):702–4.

31. Davies G, Wells AU, du Bois RM. Respiratory bronchiolitis associated with interstitial lung disease and desquamative interstitial pneumonia. Clin Chest Med. 2004;25(4):717–26.

32. Wells AU, Nicholson AG, Hansell DM, du Bois RM. Respiratory bronchiolitis-associated interstitial lung disease. Semin Respir Crit Care Med. 2003;24(5): 585–94.

33. Liebow AA, Steer A, Billingsley JG. Desquamative interstitial pneumonia. Am J Med. 1965;39: 369–404.

34. Gaensler EA, Goff AM, Prowse CM. Desquamative interstitial pneumonia. N Engl J Med. 1966;274(3): 113–28.

35. Farr GH, Harley RA, Hennigar GR. Desquamative interstitial pneumonia. An electron microscopic study. Am J Pathol. 1970;60(3):347–70.

36. Valdivia E, Hensley G, Leory EP, Wu J, Jaeschke W. Morphology and pathogenesis of desquamative interstitial pneumonitis. Thorax. 1977;32(1):7–18.

37. Scadding JG, Hinson KF. Diffuse fibrosing alveolitis (diffuse interstitial fibrosis of the lungs). Correlation of histology at biopsy with prognosis. Thorax. 1967; 22(4):291–304.

38. Nagai S, Kitaichi M, Izumi T. Classification and recent advances in idiopathic interstitial pneumonia. Curr Opin Pulm Med. 1998;4(5):256–60.

39. Akira M, Yamamoto S, Hara H, Sakatani M, Ueda E. Serial computed tomographic evaluation in desquamative interstitial pneumonia. Thorax. 1997;52(4): 333–7.

40. Carrington CB, Gaensler EA, Coutu RE, FitzGerald MX, Gupta RG. Natural history and treated course of usual and desquamative interstitial pneumonia. N Engl J Med. 1978;298(15):801–9.

41. Iskandar SB, McKinney LA, Shah L, Roy TM, Byrd Jr RP. Desquamative interstitial pneumonia and hepatitis C virus infection: a rare association. South Med J. 2004;97(9):890–3.

42. Schroten H, Manz S, Kohler H, Wolf U, Brockmann M, Riedel F. Fatal desquamative interstitial pneumonia associated with proven CMV infection in an 8-month-old boy. Pediatr Pulmonol. 1998;25(5): 345–7.

43. Lougheed MD, Roos JO, Waddell WR, Munt PW. Desquamative interstitial pneumonitis and diffuse alveolar damage in textile workers. Potential role of mycotoxins. Chest. 1995;108(5):1196–200.

44. Herbert A, Sterling G, Abraham J, Corrin B. Desquamative interstitial pneumonia in an aluminum welder. Hum Pathol. 1982;13(8):694–9.

45. Goldstein JD, Godleski JJ, Herman PG. Desquamative interstitial pneumonitis associated with monomyelocytic leukemia. Chest. 1982;81(3):321–5.

46. Abraham JL, Hertzberg MA. Inorganic particulates associated with desquamative interstitial pneumonia. Chest. 1981;80(1 Suppl):67–70.

47. Bone RC, Wolfe J, Sobonya RE, et al. Desquamative interstitial pneumonia following long-term nitrofurantoin therapy. Am J Med. 1976; 60(5):697–701.

48. Singh G, Katyal SL, Whiteside TL, Stachura I. Desquamative interstitial pneumonitis. The intra-alveolar cells are macrophages. Chest. 1981;79(1): 128.

49. Fromm GB, Dunn LJ, Harris JO. Desquamative interstitial pneumonitis. Characterization of free intraalveolar cells. Chest. 1980;77(4):552–4.

50. Bedrossian CW, Kuhn 3rd C, Luna MA, Conklin RH, Byrd RB, Kaplan PD. Desquamative interstitial pneumonia-like reaction accompanying pulmonary lesions. Chest. 1977;72(2):166–9.

51. American Thoracic Society/European Respiratory Society International Multidisciplinary Consensus Classification of the Idiopathic Interstitial Pneumonias. This joint statement of the American Thoracic Society (ATS), and the European Respiratory Society (ERS) was adopted by the ATS board of directors, June 2001 and by the ERS Executive Committee, June 2001. Am J Respir Crit Care Med. 2002;165(2):277–304.

52. Elkin SL, Nicholson AG, du Bois RM. Desquamative interstitial pneumonia and respiratory bronchiolitis-associated interstitial lung disease. Semin Respir Crit Care Med. 2001;22(4):387–98.

53. Nicholson AG, Colby TV, du Bois RM, Hansell DM, Wells AU. The prognostic significance of the histologic pattern of interstitial pneumonia in patients presenting with the clinical entity of cryptogenic fibrosing alveolitis. Am J Respir Crit Care Med. 2000;162(6): 2213–7.

54. Travis WD, Matsui K, Moss J, Ferrans VJ. Idiopathic nonspecific interstitial pneumonia: prognostic significance of cellular and fibrosing patterns: survival comparison with usual interstitial pneumonia and desquamative interstitial pneumonia. Am J Surg Pathol. 2000;24(1):19–33.

55. Lichtenstein L, Histiocytosis X. Integration of eosinophilic granuloma of bone, Letterer-Siwe disease, and Schuller-Christian disease as related manifestations of a single nosologic entity. AMA Arch Pathol. 1953; 56(1):84–102.

56. Nezelof C, Basset F, Rousseau MF. Histiocytosis X histogenetic arguments for a Langerhans cell origin. Biomedicine. 1973;18(5):365–71.

57. Histiocytosis syndromes in children. Writing Group of the Histiocyte Society. Lancet. 1987;1(8526): 208–9.

58. Favara BE, Feller AC, Pauli M, et al. Contemporary classification of histiocytic disorders. The WHO Committee on Histiocytic/Reticulum Cell Proliferations. Reclassification Working Group of the Histiocyte Society. Med Pediatr Oncol. 1997;29(3): 157–66.

59. Hance AJ, Basset F, Saumon G, et al. Smoking and interstitial lung disease. The effect of cigarette smoking on the incidence of pulmonary histiocytosis X and sarcoidosis. Ann N Y Acad Sci. 1986;465:643–56.

60. Crausman RS, Jennings CA, Tuder RM, Ackerson LM, Irvin CG, King Jr TE. Pulmonary histiocytosis X: pulmonary function and exercise pathophysiology. Am J Respir Crit Care Med. 1996;153(1):426–35.

61. Delobbe A, Durieu J, Duhamel A, Wallaert B. Determinants of survival in pulmonary Langerhans' cell granulomatosis (histiocytosis X). Groupe d'Etude en Pathologie Interstitielle de la Societe de Pathologie Thoracique du Nord. Eur Respir J. 1996; 9(10):2002–6.

62. Friedman PJ, Liebow AA, Sokoloff J. Eosinophilic granuloma of lung. Clinical aspects of primary histiocytosis in the adult. Medicine (Baltimore). 1981;60(6): 385–96.

63. Schonfeld N, Frank W, Wenig S, et al. Clinical and radiologic features, lung function and therapeutic results in pulmonary histiocytosis X. Respiration. 1993;60(1):38–44.

64. Vassallo R, Ryu JH, Schroeder DR, Decker PA, Limper AH. Clinical outcomes of pulmonary Langerhans'-cell histiocytosis in adults. N Engl J Med. 2002;346(7):484–90.

65. Watanabe R, Tatsumi K, Hashimoto S, Tamakoshi A, Kuriyama T. Clinico-epidemiological features of pulmonary histiocytosis X. Intern Med. 2001;40(10): 998–1003.

66. Mogulkoc N, Veral A, Bishop PW, Bayindir U, Pickering CA, Egan JJ. Pulmonary Langerhans' cell histiocytosis: radiologic resolution following smoking cessation. Chest. 1999;115(5):1452–5.

67. Mellman I, Steinman RM. Dendritic cells: specialized and regulated antigen processing machines. Cell. 2001;106(3):255–8.

68. Soler P, Moreau A, Basset F, Hance AJ. Cigarette smoking-induced changes in the number and differentiated state of pulmonary dendritic cells/Langerhans cells. Am Rev Respir Dis. 1989;139(5): 1112–7.

69. Tazi A, Bouchonnet F, Grandsaigne M, Boumsell L, Hance AJ, Soler P. Evidence that granulocyte macrophage-colony-stimulating factor regulates the distribution and differentiated state of dendritic cells/Langerhans cells in human lung and lung cancers. J Clin Invest. 1993;91(2):566–76.

70. Yousem SA, Colby TV, Chen YY, Chen WG, Weiss LM. Pulmonary Langerhans' cell histiocytosis: molecular analysis of clonality. Am J Surg Pathol. 2001;25(5):630–6.

71. Egeler RM, Neglia JP, Puccetti DM, Brennan CA, Nesbit ME. Association of Langerhans cell histiocytosis with malignant neoplasms. Cancer. 1993;71(3): 865–73.

72. Tazi A. Adult pulmonary Langerhans' cell histiocytosis. Eur Respir J. 2006;27(6):1272–85.

73. Mendez JL, Nadrous HF, Vassallo R, Decker PA, Ryu JH. Pneumothorax in pulmonary Langerhans cell histiocytosis. Chest. 2004;125(3):1028–32.

74. Lacronique J, Roth C, Battesti JP, Basset F, Chretien J. Chest radiological features of pulmonary histiocytosis X: a report based on 50 adult cases. Thorax. 1982;37(2):104–9.

75. Brauner MW, Grenier P, Mouelhi MM, Mompoint D, Lenoir S. Pulmonary histiocytosis X: evaluation with high-resolution CT. Radiology. 1989;172(1): 255–8.

76. Brauner MW, Grenier P, Tijani K, Battesti JP, Valeyre D. Pulmonary Langerhans cell histiocytosis: evolution of lesions on CT scans. Radiology. 1997;204(2): 497–502.

77. Gasent Blesa JM, Alberola Candel V, Solano Vercet C, et al. Langerhans cell histiocytosis. Clin Transl Oncol. 2008;10(11):688–96.

78. Basset F, Corrin B, Spencer H, et al. Pulmonary histiocytosis X. Am Rev Respir Dis. 1978;118(5): 811–20.

79. Auerswald U, Barth J, Magnussen H. Value of CD-1-positive cells in bronchoalveolar lavage fluid for the diagnosis of pulmonary histiocytosis X. Lung. 1991;169(6):305–9.

80. Vassallo R, Ryu JH, Colby TV, Hartman T, Limper AH. Pulmonary Langerhans'-cell histiocytosis. N Engl J Med. 2000;342(26):1969–78.

81. Iwai K, Mori T, Yamada N, Yamaguchi M, Hosoda Y. Idiopathic pulmonary fibrosis. Epidemiologic approaches to occupational exposure. Am J Respir Crit Care Med. 1994;150(3):670–5.

82. Hubbard R, Lewis S, Richards K, Johnston I, Britton J. Occupational exposure to metal or wood dust and aetiology of cryptogenic fibrosing alveolitis. Lancet. 1996;347(8997):284–9.

83. Baumgartner KB, Samet JM, Stidley CA, Colby TV, Waldron JA. Cigarette smoking: a risk factor for idiopathic pulmonary fibrosis. Am J Respir Crit Care Med. 1997;155(1):242–8.

84. Taskar VS, Coultas DB. Is idiopathic pulmonary fibrosis an environmental disease? Proc Am Thorac Soc. 2006;3(4):293–8.

85. Steele MP, Speer MC, Loyd JE, et al. Clinical and pathologic features of familial interstitial pneumonia. Am J Respir Crit Care Med. 2005;172(9):1146–52.

86. Wiggins J, Strickland B, Turner-Warwick M. Combined cryptogenic fibrosing alveolitis and emphysema: the value of high resolution computed tomography in assessment. Respir Med. 1990;84(5): 365–9.

87. Cottin V, Nunes H, Brillet PY, et al. Combined pulmonary fibrosis and emphysema: a distinct underrecognised entity. Eur Respir J. 2005;26(4):586–93.

88. Cottin V, Cordier JF. The syndrome of combined pulmonary fibrosis and emphysema. Chest. 2009;136(1): 1–2.

89. Grubstein A, Bendayan D, Schactman I, Cohen M, Shitrit D, Kramer MR. Concomitant upper-lobe bullous emphysema, lower-lobe interstitial fibrosis and pulmonary hypertension in heavy smokers: report of eight cases and review of the literature. Respir Med. 2005;99(8):948–54.

90. Jankowich MD, Polsky M, Klein M, Rounds S. Heterogeneity in combined pulmonary fibrosis and emphysema. Respiration. 2008;75(4):411–7.

91. Rogliani P, Mura M, Mattia P, et al. HRCT and histopathological evaluation of fibrosis and tissue destruction in IPF associated with pulmonary emphysema. Respir Med. 2008;102(12):1753–61.

92. Mejia M, Carrillo G, Rojas-Serrano J, et al. Idiopathic pulmonary fibrosis and emphysema: decreased survival associated with severe pulmonary arterial hypertension. Chest. 2009;136(1):10–5.

93. American Thoracic Society. Idiopathic pulmonary fibrosis: diagnosis and treatment. International consensus statement. American Thoracic Society (ATS), and the European Respiratory Society (ERS). Am J Respir Crit Care Med. 2000;161(2 Pt 1):646–64.

94. Janz DR, O'Neal Jr HR, Ely EW. Acute eosinophilic pneumonia: a case report and review of the literature. Crit Care Med. 2009;37(4):1470–4.

95. Philit F, Etienne-Mastroianni B, Parrot A, Guerin C, Robert D, Cordier JF. Idiopathic acute eosinophilic pneumonia: a study of 22 patients. Am J Respir Crit Care Med. 2002;166(9):1235–9.

96. Hayakawa H, Sato A, Toyoshima M, Imokawa S, Taniguchi M. A clinical study of idiopathic eosinophilic pneumonia. Chest. 1994;105(5):1462–6.

97. Rom WN, Weiden M, Garcia R, et al. Acute eosinophilic pneumonia in a New York City firefighter exposed to World Trade Center dust. Am J Respir Crit Care Med. 2002;166(6):797–800.

98. Oh PI, Balter MS. Cocaine induced eosinophilic lung disease. Thorax. 1992;47(6):478–9.

99. Kelly KJ, Ruffing R. Acute eosinophilic pneumonia following intentional inhalation of Scotchguard. Ann Allergy. 1993;71(4):358–61.

100. Pope-Harman AL, Davis WB, Allen ED, Christoforidis AJ, Allen JN. Acute eosinophilic pneumonia. A summary of 15 cases and review of the literature. Medicine (Baltimore). 1996;75(6): 334–42.

101. Uchiyama H, Suda T, Nakamura Y, et al. Alterations in smoking habits are associated with acute eosinophilic pneumonia. Chest. 2008;133(5):1174–80.

102. Shorr AF, Scoville SL, Cersovsky SB, et al. Acute eosinophilic pneumonia among US Military personnel deployed in or near Iraq. JAMA. 2004;292(24): 2997–3005.

103. Pusey CD. Anti-glomerular basement membrane disease. Kidney Int. 2003;64(4):1535–50.

104. Donaghy M, Rees AJ. Cigarette smoking and lung haemorrhage in glomerulonephritis caused by autoantibodies to glomerular basement membrane. Lancet. 1983;2(8364):1390–3.

105. Lazor R, Bigay-Game L, Cottin V, et al. Alveolar hemorrhage in anti-basement membrane antibody disease: a series of 28 cases. Medicine (Baltimore). 2007;86(3):181–93.

106. Herody M, Bobrie G, Gouarin C, Grunfeld JP, Noel LH. Anti-GBM disease: predictive value of clinical,

histological and serological data. Clin Nephrol. 1993;40(5):249–55.

107. Levy JB, Lachmann RH, Pusey CD. Recurrent Goodpasture's disease. Am J Kidney Dis. 1996;27(4): 573–8.

108. Klasa RJ, Abboud RT, Ballon HS, Grossman L. Goodpasture's syndrome: recurrence after a five-year remission. Case report and review of the literature. Am J Med. 1988;84(4):751–5.

109. Leaker B, Walker RG, Becker GJ, Kincaid-Smith P. Cigarette smoking and lung haemorrhage in anti-glomerular-basement-membrane nephritis. Lancet. 1984;2(8410):1039.

110. De Lassence A, Fleury-Feith J, Escudier E, Beaune J, Bernaudin JF, Cordonnier C. Alveolar hemorrhage. Diagnostic criteria and results in 194 immunocom-promised hosts. Am J Respir Crit Care Med. 1995;151(1):157–63.

111. Lowry R, Buick B, Riley M. Idiopathic pulmonary haemosiderosis and smoking. Ulster Med J. 1993; 62(1):116–8.

112. Montana E, Etzel RA, Allan T, Horgan TE, Dearborn DG. Environmental risk factors associated with pediatric idiopathic pulmonary hemorrhage and hemosiderosis in a Cleveland community. Pediatrics. 1997;99(1):E5.

Childhood Interstitial Lung Disease

15

Lisa R. Young

Abstract

Childhood interstitial lung diseases (ILDs) are a heterogeneous group of disorders characterized by common clinical features and diffuse radiographic abnormalities. There are important differences between the types and prognosis of ILD in children than in adults. Additionally, several unique disease entities occur only in infants and young children, including pulmonary interstitial glycogenosis, neuroendocrine cell hyperplasia of infancy, and some disorders affecting lung development. The approach to diagnosis depends on the age of presentation and clinical severity, and may include laboratory investigations, genetic testing, pulmonary function testing, chest HRCT scanning, bronchoscopy, and surgical lung biopsy. Establishing a specific etiology of ILD can have profound management and prognostic implications.

Keywords

Children • Pediatric • NEHI • Surfactant • Interstitial lung disease • Pulmonary alveolar proteinosis • Lung biopsy • Chest computerized tomography scan

L.R. Young, MD (✉)
Division of Allergy, Immunology, and Pulmonary Medicine,
Department of Pediatrics, Vanderbilt University School
of Medicine, Nashville, TN, USA

Division of Allergy, Pulmonary, and Critical Care Medicine,
Department of Medicine, Vanderbilt University School
of Medicine, Nashville, TN, USA
e-mail: lisa.young@vanderbilt.edu

R.P. Baughman and R.M. du Bois (eds.), *Diffuse Lung Disease: A Practical Approach*,
DOI 10.1007/978-1-4419-9771-5_15, © Springer Science+Business Media, LLC 2012

Case 1

A 7-month-old female infant presents with rhinorrhea, tachypnea, and cough. The infant was the full-term product of an uncomplicated pregnancy, and there were no neonatal respiratory concerns. Family history is significant for mother with asthma and a great-grandfather who died of pulmonary fibrosis. Physical examination is notable for clear rhinorrhea, tachypnea, mild intercostal retractions, and scattered crackles. Oxygen saturation on room air is 93% when awake but 86–89% with feeding and sleep. A nasal washing is positive for RSV antigen. Chest radiograph shows hyperinflation and diffuse interstitial markings. The infant is hospitalized and treated with supplemental oxygen and supportive care.

Over the subsequent weeks, the infant's cough and tachypnea persist, and she develops progressive hypoxemia with need for continuous supplemental oxygen. Her weight declines from the 25th percentile to the 10th percentile for age, with length at the 50th percentile. An echocardiogram, sweat chloride testing, a complete blood count, and serum immunoglobulins are all normal. A flexible bronchoscopy shows normal anatomy and no infectious pathogens are identified on bronchoalveolar lavage (BAL). The BAL cytology shows a mild inflammatory profile with 15% neutrophils and increased numbers of lipid-laden macrophages. A barium swallow and pH/impedance probe demonstrates mild gastroesophageal reflux. Acid suppression therapy is initiated yet the infant fails to improve.

A controlled ventilation chest high-resolution computed tomography (HRCT) scan is performed and shows lower lobe predominant ground-glass opacities with increased interstitial markings and a few subpleural cysts. Genetic testing identifies the I73T mutation in the surfactant protein C gene (*SFTPC*).

Case 2

A 4-month-old term male infant is seen for a well-child appointment. He is smiling and playful, but has a respiratory rate of 70 breaths per minute and prominent intercostal and subglottic retraction. His weight is at the 5th percentile. His parents do not think he is acutely ill, and his grandmother emphasizes that she has always thought the infant breathed a bit fast. Chest examination reveals hyperinflation and diffuse crackles, most prominent in the mid-lung zones. A chest radiograph shows mild hyperinflation but is otherwise normal.

The child is referred to a pulmonologist. Room air oxygen saturations are 88% and the child is started on continuous supplemental oxygen via nasal cannula. Testing for respiratory viruses, cystic fibrosis, and general laboratory studies are normal. An echocardiogram is normal. Flexible bronchoscopy reveals normal airway anatomy, no evidence of infectious pathogens, and normal cytology without evidence of inflammation. Controlled ventilation chest HRCT (see Fig. 15.1a) shows apparent geographic ground-glass opacities in the right middle lobe and lingula, and marked air-trapping is demonstrated with the expiratory images. Video-assisted thoracoscopic surgery (VATS) lung biopsy is performed. The histology is near-normal on hematoxylin and eosin staining, with only very mild increase in airway smooth muscle and mild peri-bronchiolar lymphoid aggregates, without other histologic abnormalities (see Fig. 15.1b). Bombesin staining demonstrates prominent increase in the numbers of neuroendocrine cells and neuroendocrine bodies (see Fig. 15.1c), confirming the diagnosis of neuroendocrine cell hyperplasia of infancy (NEHI).

Case 3

A 9-year-old girl with common variable immunodeficiency presents with chronic cough and recurrent pneumonia. She has been maintained on intravenous immunoglobulin infusions and amoxicillin prophylaxis. Previous sputum cultures have been positive for *Moraxella catarrhalis* and *Haemophilus influenzae*. Despite frequent courses of oral and intravenous antibiotics, she has chronic cough and exercise intolerance. She has not responded to bronchodilator therapy and airway clearance with a Vest and DNase. Pulmonary function testing reveals a moderate

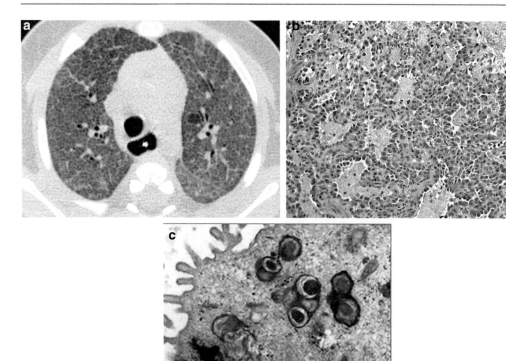

Fig. 15.1 Neuroendocrine cell hyperplasia of infancy. (**a**) Chest high-resolution computed tomography (at total lung capacity) in a 24 month old with tachypnea and hypoxemia who was being treated for recurrent pneumonia and refractory asthma. Sharply defined areas of apparent ground-glass opacity are seen most prominent in the *right middle lobe* and *lingula*, but also in the medial portions of the *upper lobes* (not shown). Diffuse air-trapping was seen on expiratory images (not shown). No additional abnormalities were identified. (**b**) H&E staining of the lung biopsy reveals near-normal lung architecture with only a mild increase in bronchiolar smooth muscle. (**c**) Bombesin immunostaining reveals an increased number of neuroendocrine cells (images provided by Gail H. Deutsch, MD)

obstructive defect without bronchodilator response, and lung volumes demonstrate air-trapping. DLco is normal. Exercise oximetry shows desaturation to 87%. Chest HRCT shows mild bronchiectasis in the right middle lobe and diffuse ground-glass opacities and mosaic attenuation. Extensive axillary, supraclavicular, hilar, and mediastinal adenopathy is present. Flexible bronchoscopy reveals a diffuse nodularity of the bronchial mucosa with only scant thin secretions. Microbiologic studies are negative. VATS lung biopsy is performed. There is severe airway-centric lymphocytic inflammation with reactive follicles, which infiltrate and obscure some bronchioles. Interstitial inflammation and fibrosis are absent. Treatment with Rituxan and corticosteroids are initiated, and the patient later undergoes bone marrow transplantation.

Introduction

Childhood interstitial lung diseases (ILDs) are a heterogeneous group of disorders characterized by common clinical features and diffuse radiographic abnormalities. ILD has remained the preferred clinical term despite the fact that the primary pathology occurs outside the interstitial compartment in some entities, making diffuse lung disease is a more accurate description. Some types of childhood ILD share considerable overlap with adult forms of ILD (such as those associated with connective tissue disease), yet in many areas there are significant differences, and efforts to establish clinical descriptions and therapeutic strategies have been limited by the relative rarity in children. Historically the approach to ILD in children has been patterned after nomenclature and prognosis in adults, and such practice has unfortunately created a great deal of confusion.

Recent experience increasingly demonstrates that there are important areas of departure between disease etiology and natural history in the pediatric age group. Specifically, idiopathic pulmonary fibrosis (IPF) does not occur in children, and there are forms of ILD which are either unique to young children or have differing manifestations. Further, in the last decade, several new entities have been described in infants and young children, including NEHI and pulmonary interstitial glycogenosis (PIG). A great advance has been the recognition and identification of genetic defects of surfactant function, metabolism, and clearance as causes of ILD, including mutations in the genes producing surfactant protein B, surfactant protein C, member A3 of the ATP binding cassette family of transporters (ABCA3), and the GM-CSF receptor.

This chapter provides an overview of our current state of knowledge of childhood ILD, with particular focus on clinical phenotypes, diagnostic approach, and recognition of entities unique or more prevalent in the pediatric age group.

Epidemiology

ILD is rare in children, and the precise incidence and prevalence are unknown. A combined retrospective and prospective study by Fan et al. performed over a 15-year period identified 99 patients who were evaluated at a large referral center for ILD [1]. The best prevalence data come from a national survey in the UK and Ireland reported by Dinwiddie and co-workers, which estimated a prevalence of 3.6 per million based on the 46 reported cases [2]. During a 3-year period (1995–1998), specialists were asked to report all cases of "idiopathic interstitial pneu-

monitis" in children age 0–16 years, excluding those with immunodeficiency and autoimmune disease. The survey had a remarkably high response rate (93%), though the survey methodology did not include centralized review of radiographic or pathologic material.

Several other working group reports and case series provide some estimates of the frequency of some types of ILD in children. A European task force identified 185 cases of chronic ILD in immunocompetent children age 0–16 years from 1997 to 2002 [3]. Inclusion criteria required symptoms for more than 3 months duration. Data were obtained based on clinical reporting. A North American working group has taken a different approach to case ascertainment, starting with all lung biopsies performed for diffuse lung disease at network referral centers, and including both immunocompetent and immunocompromised children. A first study from 11 referral centers in the USA and Canada over a 5-year period (1999–2004) identified 187 cases in children younger than 2 years of age [4]. A second lung biopsy study of children age 2–18 years identified 199 cases, from among 12 centers over a 4-year time period [5, 6]. All studies identified a slight male predominance (roughly 60%) and definite hereditary component (10–16% familial cases). Further, clustering of cases in infancy was a common feature.

With establishment of consensus case definitions, infrastructure for case ascertainment, and awareness of and access to diagnostic testing, it is anticipated that future studies will likely show higher prevalence/incidence rates.

Pathogenesis

Most forms of ILD share common pathophysiologic features of structural remodeling of the distal airspaces leading to impaired gas exchange. Most research in this field has focused on data from adult lung histopathology and animal models, and similar mechanisms are postulated to apply in children. There are several distinctions which are likely important in considering disease pathogenesis in children. First, when symptom onset occurs early in childhood, there is a greater propensity for disorders to have a heritable basis or be related to developmental abnormalities. Secondly, the injuries and reparative mechanisms occur in an organ that is still developing. If known, pathophysiologic mechanisms are included in the individual disorder subsections detailed later in this chapter.

Approach to Diagnosis

General Approach

Diagnosing ILD requires a high index of suspicion and a careful assessment of the clinical context. The delay between onset of symptoms and ultimate diagnosis ranges from months to years, and many children are treated for asthma before ultimately being diagnosed with ILD [7]. Factors that influence the diagnostic approach and pace include age at presentation, immunocompetence, chronicity, severity of disease, duration of illness, family history, and trend toward improvement. For example, a full-term newborn with respiratory failure will be approached differently from the young child with tachypnea of insidious onset and hypoxemia with feeding or sleep. An age-based general approach to diagnostic testing is summarized in Table 15.1.

As outlined later, some types of ILD may be strongly suggested based on association with systemic disorders and others may be diagnosed on the basis of genetic testing. Chest CT patterns may suggest certain diagnoses, though many forms of ILD in children currently require surgical lung biopsy for definitive diagnosis. Because of the myriad of different types of ILD and the differing associated pathogenesis and prognosis, the diagnosis of ILD alone is rarely sufficient, and instead should be viewed as a starting point for a search for the underlying etiology.

History and Physical Examination

A thorough and systematic clinical history is essential to assess severity, define clinical context, and ascertain clues which may contribute to establishing the diagnosis or alter the diagnostic strategy utilized. Children with ILD often have a constellation of signs and symptoms that largely overlaps with that observed in adults. Common features include tachypnea (75–93% of patients), hypoxemia, and cough [3, 4, 7–9]. Hypoxemia and exercise intolerance may be more evident during feeding in infants. Dyspnea on exertion may be under-reported in children who have gradually accommodated to years to respiratory limitation, or in those who have other comorbidities limiting physical activity such as musculoskeletal disease. Failure to thrive has also been recognized as a frequent clinical feature, particularly in young

Table 15.1 General approach to diagnostic testing for childhood ILD by age

Age of symptom onset	HRCT	PFTs	Bronchoscopy	Genetic Testing	Other considerations	VATS lung biopsy
<2 Years	Yes[a]	Consider infant PFTs[b]	Rule-out structural abnormalities and infection	Yes: *SFTPB, SFTPC, ABCA3, TTFI*	Immunologic assessment Consider evaluation for PCD Consider storage disorders	Consider
2–10 Years	Yes[a]	Yes (for age 5+)	Consider	Yes: *SFTPC, ABCA3, TTFI*	Immunologic assessment	Consider
>10 Years	Yes	Yes	Consider	Consider *SFTPC* and *ABCA3*	Immunologic assessment Evaluate for other systemic diseases including CVD	Consider

HRCT high-resolution computed tomography, *PFT* pulmonary function test, *VATS* video-assisted thoracoscopic surgery, *BPD* bronchopulmonary dysplasia, *ABCA3* ATP-binding cassette A-3 gene, *SFTPB* surfactant protein B gene, *SFTPC* surfactant protein C gene, *PCD* primary ciliary dyskinesia, *CVD* collagen vascular disease
[a]Sedation and controlled ventilation are generally required for children < age 6 years
[b]Infant PFTs are not available at many centers and generally will not obviate the need for other diagnostic testing

children, with reports ranging from 35 to 62% [3, 4, 7]. Because of these common associated clinical findings, the term "childhood ILD syndrome" has recently been adopted to refer to a characteristic clinical phenotype which should prompt further evaluation for ILD [10].

Additional historical features may suggest specific etiologic considerations, such as viral infection precipitating bronchiolitis obliterans, bird or mold exposures causing hypersensitivity pneumonitis, feeding difficulties leading to chronic aspiration, hemoptysis in children with pulmonary hemorrhage syndromes, and musculoskeletal symptoms or rash in connective-tissue associated ILD. An expanded family history should be obtained, as some forms of ILD in children may be associated with widely variable clinical presentation, including neonatal deaths, unexplained childhood respiratory disease, or ILD in adults.

On physical examination, many children with ILD will have crackles on chest auscultation. However, it is important to note that some children with ILD present with wheezing or with normal findings on auscultation [4, 7]. Digital clubbing is present in a minority of cases [7]. Additional physical examination features seen in children with ILD may include chest wall deformity. Pectus excavatum has been reported in children with ABCA3 deficiency [11], and other chest wall deformity may reflect chronic hyperinflation or retraction suggesting chronic lung disease in general. Stigmata of collagen vascular diseases and other systemic disorders should be carefully sought. Physical exam findings such as a right ventricular heave and prominent P2 component may suggest pulmonary hypertension in severe cases.

Initial Clinical Testing

Initial evaluations for a child with symptoms as above should focus on excluding more common causes of such symptoms. Such evaluations will often include an echocardiogram, testing for cystic fibrosis, and investigations for pulmonary infections. General laboratory investigations occasionally point to diagnosis, such as the presence of peripheral eosinophilia, or results of immunologic evaluations or markers of rheumatologic disorders. A step-wise approach is generally indicated, and clinical judgment plays a large role in determining which tests are essential for each individual child. More invasive testing will be required in most, but not all cases [9, 12].

Bronchoscopy and BAL

Bronchoscopy with BAL is a well-established technique utilized in children to assess airway anatomy and obtain samples for microbiologic, cytologic, and biochemical assessment [13]. The technical aspects, normal values, and indications for BAL in children are well outlined in a report by a European Respiratory Society task force [14]. With respect to the evaluation of diffuse lung diseases, BAL is most useful in evaluation of conditions in the differential diagnosis, including infections or airway abnormalities. Because pulmonary infections may complicate many forms of ILD, identification of an infectious etiology may not alleviate the need for further investigations into ILD. Further, there are several categories of diffuse lung diseases which are strongly suggested by BAL findings, including Langerhans cell histiocytosis, pulmonary eosinophilic syndromes, pulmonary hemorrhage syndromes, and alveolar proteinosis. However, histologic, genetic, or molecular testing is still required in most cases to define the specific disease entity. Specifically, findings consistent with alveolar proteinosis on BAL should lead to an investigation of surfactant protein and ABCA3 mutations, GM-CSF antibodies in serum, other abnormalities in GM-CSF signaling, or other rare metabolic disorders such as lysinuric protein intolerance which can result in alveolar proteinosis [15]. Additionally, presence of increased numbers of lipid-laden macrophages (oil-red-O positive) may suggest aspiration, but may also reflect other causes of airway injury or increased endogenous lipid in cases of surfactant dysfunction or storage diseases. When BAL identifies abundant hemosiderin-positive macrophages or acute hemorrhage, lung biopsy may be required to determine whether or not vasculitis or capillaritis is present [4, 16]. In sum, bronchoscopy findings may exclude infections and anatomic abnormalities, but will not be specific or sufficient to establish a diagnosis in most cases [17]; nonetheless, it is routinely performed because of the relative safety, availability, and ease of performance.

Pulmonary Function Testing

Results of pulmonary function tests (PFT) in children with ILD have been widely variable, ranging from restrictive physiology to predominantly obstructive patterns with air-trapping. A relatively recent advance includes the capability to perform infant PFT safely in sedated infants at a large number of pediatric centers [18, 19]. Standard procedures for raised volume rapid thoracic compression (RVRTC) method and normal reference values have been established for spirometric indices and plethysmographic lung volumes [20]. Infant PFT can be performed up until approximately age 3 years for most children, based primarily on the length limitation of the plexiglass box used for plethysmography. Recent publications suggest that these new methods are clinically useful for assessing lung function in infants with cystic fibrosis, airway reactivity, and neonatal lung disease. Case series have suggested utility for infant PFT in diagnosing or monitoring some forms of ILD, and several studies are ongoing.

High-Resolution Computed Tomography

Chest HRCT is essential for most children with ILD and provides a means for determining pattern, extent, and distribution of abnormalities as well as guiding selection of biopsy sites [21]. There are additional considerations for HRCT technique in young children which enable minimizing the radiation risk while optimizing image quality and diagnostic yield [22]. Sedation is generally required in infants and young children to (1) control motion and (2) allow for techniques to control

lung volume thereby facilitating accurate assessment of air-trapping and extent of ground-glass opacities. Poor lung inflation and motion artifact from respiratory motion alone in the tachypneic infant may greatly compromise image quality and even lead to overestimation of parenchymal abnormalities. Therefore, for infants and young children, chest HRCT with inspiratory and expiratory imaging is best performed using sedation and face mask ventilation with a controlled pause for scanning [23], or with endotracheal intubation or laryngeal mask ventilation under general anesthesia.

Terminology for interpretation of pediatric chest CT scans is similar to that utilized in the adult literature. While radiographic patterns of pediatric ILD have been less extensively studied than those in adult ILD, several studies indicate that specific imaging patterns correlate with certain histologic diagnoses. In one study, expert readers were able to accurately predict diagnosis in 61% of cases, and were most likely to correctly diagnose alveolar proteinosis, pulmonary hemosiderosis, and pulmonary lymphangiectasia based on chest HRCT findings [24]. Reports from small numbers of pediatric patients with NEHI, PAP, surfactant mutations, or bronchiolitis obliterans suggest that characteristic HRCT patterns often exist in these entities [11, 24–28].

Genetic Testing

Clinical genetic testing can establish a diagnosis of ILD due to mutations in the genes encoding surfactant protein B, surfactant protein C, or ABCA3, or thyroid transcription factor (TTFI/NKY2.1) [29–31]. Testing is only available in selected Clinical Laboratories Improvement Act (CLIA)-certified diagnostic laboratories (http://www.genetests.org). Testing for *SFTPC* and *ABCA3* mutations should be considered in infants and children with suspected ILD, particularly if they exhibit digital clubbing, diffuse ground-glass opacities, or "honeycomb" changes on HRCT, or if they have a family history of chronic lung disease. Genetic testing for surfactant protein B gene (*SFTPB*) is generally reserved for term or near-term infants with unexplained severe neonatal respiratory distress. This testing allows for a noninvasive diagnosis and generally obviates the need for lung biopsy. However, because of time required for testing, the results of genetic testing may not be timely enough for infants with rapidly progressive disease. Genetic counseling should be made available to family members, particularly in cases of *SFTPC* mutations where asymptomatic family members may be carriers of a dominant gene mutation. TTF1/NKY2.1 testing should be considered for infants and children with ILD and hypothyroidism, hypotonia, or choreoathetosis, though ILD may be the only feature. Testing for mutations in the GM-CSF receptor is currently done on a research basis [25]. Currently, a genetic etiology will not be identified in all cases with clinical and histologic findings to such a disorder of surfactant metabolism and production or a disorder of surfactant clearance. Therefore, genetic testing alone does not definitively exclude disorders of surfactant homeostasis.

Lung Biopsy

Prior studies have demonstrated that a minority of children with ILD will achieve definitive diagnosis without lung biopsy [9, 32]. While lung biopsy is not without risk, clinical experience and several studies suggest that surgical lung biopsy does guide clinical management in children [4, 12]. Transbronchial biopsy can be utilized in children with diffuse lung disease [12], but limitations include the size of the channel and forceps, and the relatively limited tissue sampling achieved. The clinical use of transbronchial biopsy is largely restricted to older pediatric patients undergoing surveillance biopsies after lung transplantation. Therefore, VATS is the preferred method for lung tissue sampling in pediatric patients, having largely replaced open lung biopsy [12, 33, 34]. Advances in the techniques for VATS in young children have led to successful diagnostic sampling with less associated postoperative and long-term morbidity than that associated with open lung biopsy, specifically with respect to surgical time, duration of chest tube placement, and hospital stay [33].

A pediatric lung biopsy protocol has been developed to facilitate the proper processing needed to maximize diagnostic yield in children

[35]. The protocol addresses the importance of decisions regarding biopsy site, the frequent need for biopsy from more than one site, and issues related to biopsy adequacy. Communication between the clinician, surgeon, pathologist, and radiologist before biopsy is essential for determining biopsy sites and prioritizing use of the tissue. Special studies in children which require specific processing include that for electron microscopy, which is of particular importance in diagnosing disorders such as ABCA3 deficiency [11, 29]. It should be acknowledged that despite lung biopsy, a definitive diagnosis is not reached in some patients [4, 12].

While lung biopsy is still considered the gold standard diagnostic method for most forms of childhood ILD, this practice may change over time. Recent advances in the availability of clinical genetic testing and improved recognition of chest HRCT patterns promise to increasingly alter the approach to diagnosis of some specific disorders.

Management

Definitive therapy for most forms of ILD in children is unknown. Most of the available information outlining potential therapeutic strategies is comprised of anecdotal reports or very small case series. If the pulmonary process is secondary to an underlying condition, patients should be treated for the underlying disease. Specific therapeutic considerations will be discussed in the areas on specific disorders where relevant.

Supportive care is the primary management in many patients and is guided by the same principles utilized in managing children with other chronic pulmonary disorders. Extrapolated recommendations include nutritional support, supplemental oxygen, vaccinations, avoidance of environmental tobacco smoke and other irritants, and supervised exercise programs. Management of comorbidities includes evaluation and treatment for gastroesophageal reflux and pulmonary hypertension, and aggressive treatment of secondary infections. Lung transplantation is a consideration for children with severe or progressive disease [36, 37], but must be carefully discussed and undertaken in a center with expertise in children.

Outcome

Overall, pediatric ILD has been associated with high morbidity and mortality. Pulmonary hypertension is consistently a predictor of decreased survival [1, 4]. Several large cohort studies have assessed outcomes for children with a general ILD diagnosis. Fan and Kozinetz reviewed the outcomes of 99 children with ILD over a 15-year period. Survival rates at 24, 48, and 60 months after the appearance of initial symptoms were 83%, 72%, and 64%, respectively [1]. In the European Respiratory Society task force studying immunocompetent children with chronic ILD (>3 month duration), clinical improvement was reported in the vast majority of cases (74%), while stabilized disease occurred in 17%, deterioration in 2%, and mortality of 6% [3]. In the North American Children's Interstitial Lung Disease Network study which included only cases diagnosed by lung biopsy, 30% of children had died and 50% had ongoing pulmonary morbidity [4]. Important differences in the North American study which may explain some of the outcome differences include the case ascertainment from lung biopsies from children under age 2 years, the inclusion of immunocompromised patients, and lack of requirement for chronic symptoms for 3 months, which would otherwise exclude the most severe neonatal cases. Other studies have also suggested that outcomes may be particularly poor for infants and young children.

It is increasingly recognized that the prognosis is variable and depends in large part on the disease etiology.

Approach to Classification and Terminology

Uniform nomenclature and accurate classification are essential to defining the features and natural history of the different forms of pediatric ILD. For forms of ILD occurring in very young children, terminology and disease entities differ greatly from adult ILD (Table 15.2). Indeed it has been increasingly recognized that classification schemes for idiopathic interstitial pneumonias in adults fail to accurately categorize pediatric ILDs. For example, from various reports of children with "IPF" or "cryptogenic fibrosing alveolitis," mortality occurred in only 4 of 99 cases, and these cases failed to demonstrate the histopathologic features of UIP [38]. Furthermore, pediatric cases of desquamative interstitial pneumonia (DIP) have had high mortality and have been subsequently associated with *ABCA3* and *SFTPC* mutations, not tobacco smoke [4, 8]. To address these issues, the Children's Interstitial Lung Disease Research Network has proposed a clinical–histologic classification that emphasizes forms of diffuse lung disease most prevalent or unique to infants and young children [4].

As summarized in Table 15.3, some forms of ILD in children overlap with adult disorders and appropriately share terminology (sarcoidosis, Langerhans cell histiocytosis, follicular bronchiolitis/lymphocytic interstitial pneumonitis). However, the prevalence, clinical features, and outcomes may vary between the pediatric and adult forms. Other forms of pediatric ILD can be best considered in the context of the systemic disease process (i.e., associated with connective tissue disease).

A complete description of all of the entities representing childhood ILD is beyond the scope of this chapter. The following sections will highlight specific disorders which are either among the more common forms seen in children or which have clinical features, diagnostic considerations, or prognosis which may differ from their counterpart forms of adult ILD. Particular emphasis is given to disorders most prevalent or unique to infants and young children, including relatively recently recognized forms of pediatric diffuse lung disease.

Disorders Most Prevalent in Infants and Young Children

Surfactant Protein B Gene Mutations

The disorder is caused by loss of function mutations in the gene encoding surfactant protein B (*SFTPB*) [30, 39]. The most common mutation is 121ins2, but more than 40 mutations have

Table 15.2 Diffuse lung diseases primarily seen in infants and young children

Disorder	Common age of onset	Hereditary basis	Common imaging pattern	Method of diagnosis	Outcome
Alveolar capillary dysplasia with misalignment of the pulmonary veins	Birth	Yes, *FOXF1*; autosomal dominant	Uncertain	Lung biopsy; emergence of genetic testing	Fatal without lung transplant[a]
Lung growth abnormalities (pulmonary hypoplasia, BPD)	Birth	Uncertain; seen in association with chromosomal abnormalities	Uncertain; may include architectural distortion, cystic change	Clinical context, lung biopsy in a typical cases	Variable
Neuroendocrine cell hyperplasia of infancy (NEHI)	Infancy; most first year of life	Suspected; not established	CXR: Hyperinflation, normal, or mild perihilar infiltrates; HRCT: GGO in RML and lingula; air-trapping	Lung biopsy definitive; HRCT and iPFTs may strongly suggest	Gradual improvement (years)
Pulmonary interstitial glycogenosis (PIG)	Neonatal	Unknown	Uncertain	Lung biopsy	Variable
Surfactant protein B gene mutation (*SFTPB*)	Neonatal	Yes, autosomal recessive	CXR: Diffuse hazy infiltrates	Genetic testing definitive; lung biopsy may suggest	Fatal without lung transplant
ABCA3 mutations	Neonatal > childhood	Yes, autosomal recessive	Diffuse ground-glass opacity with thickened intralobular septae	Genetic testing definitive; lung biopsy, particularly EM may suggest	Severe, variable

BPD bronchopulmonary dysplasia, *GGO* ground-glass opacities, *RML* right middle lobe, *EM* electron microscopy, *FOXF1* forkhead box F1 gene, *ABCA3* ATP-binding cassette A-3 gene, *iPFT* infant pulmonary function test
[a]Variable penetrance and phenotype data emerging

Table 15.3 Examples of pediatric diffuse lung diseases which overlap adult disorders

Disorder	Special considerations in children
Surfactant protein C gene mutation (*SFTPC*)	Infancy to older adults
	Highly variable clinical presentation and outcomes
	Variable imaging patterns including reticular-nodular pattern, GGO, thickened intralobular septae, and cystic change
	Variable histologic patterns
	Genetic testing is preferred approach
Hypersensitivity pneumonitis	Rare in infants
	+ Family history in 25%
	Birds most common exposure
Bronchiolitis obliterans	Occurs in children of all ages
	Adenovirus is most common cause in nontransplant population
Sarcoidosis	Pulmonary involvement rare in children
Langerhans cell histiocytosis (LCH)	Peak age in children is 1–3 years
	Multiorgan or single organ disease
	Minority of cases have pulmonary involvement
	Pulmonary involvement rare without other organ involvement
	Not attributable to tobacco smoke
Vascular and lymphatic disorders Lymphangiomatosis Lymphangiectasia	Usually systemic involvement
Follicular bronchiolitis/lymphocytic interstitial pneumonitis	Predominantly associated with immunodeficiency states
Neurocutaneous syndromes	Tuberous sclerosis (LAM in postpubertal females)
	Neurofibromatosis
	Ataxia-telangiectasia
Metabolic and storage disorders	Niemann–Pick disease
	Gaucher's disease
	Pulmonary microlithiasis
Connective tissue disease	Mostly in adolescents; lung disease may precede onset of overt rheumatologic disorder
Pulmonary alveolar proteinosis (PAP)	Autoimmune PAP does occur in school age children
	Other causes include: GMCSF receptor mutations, *SFTPB*, or *ABCA3*, or *TTF1* mutations, lysinuric protein intolerance, or secondary PAP with infection or myelodysplastic disorders
Pulmonary hemorrhage syndromes	Essential to evaluate for capillaritis

GGO ground-glass opacity, *LAM* Lymphangioleiomyomatosis, *GMCSF* Granulocyte macrophage colony stimulating factor, *ABCA3* ATP-binding cassette A-3 gene, *SFTPB* Surfactant protein B gene

been described. The disorder presents with respiratory failure in term infants, at an estimated frequency of one per million live births in the USA [40, 41]. Chest radiographs have diffuse hazy infiltrates similar to neonatal respiratory distress syndrome. Lung biopsies generally show alveolar proteinosis with normal alveolar septae without architectural derangement and a lack of SP-B immunopositivity. Histologic findings in *SFTPB* mutation cases have also been referred to as a DIP pattern based on the presence of "desquamated" alveolar type II cells and accumulation of foamy alveolar macrophages [42]. When SP-B is absent, both in humans and in knockout mice, alveolar type II cells contain inclusions with multiple small vesicles and poorly packed lamellae, but few if any normal-appearing lamellar bodies [41].

The clinical presentation can be similar for cases of *ABCA3* mutations or alveolar capillary dysplasia with misalignment of the pulmonary veins. Furthermore, mutations in the GM-CSF receptor may have similar histologic findings, and SP-B immunostaining may also be absent or weak in lung histology from cases of *ABCA3* mutations [42, 43]. Therefore while lung biopsy may suggest the diagnosis, genetic testing is the most definitive and preferred diagnostic modality.

Mutations in *SFTPB* also cause a block in the processing of pro-SP-C to mature SP-C, and the response to surfactant replacement therapy is transient or unsuccessful [44]. The disorder is almost uniformly fatal without lung transplantation, but very rare cases have been reported with severe chronic lung disease in which partial defects in SP-B production were identified [45, 46].

ABCA3 Gene Mutations

Autosomal recessive mutations in the gene encoding the ATP-binding cassette A-3 (ABCA3) are the primary cause of otherwise unexplained respiratory failure in term infants and are also a cause of ILD in older children [4, 11, 29, 43]. More than 150 mutations have been described to date, resulting in loss of expression, decreased expression, abnormal intracellular trafficking of ABCA3 protein to the lamellar body, abnormal packaging or phospholipids, or defects in ABCA3 functional activity [47–49].

In ABCA3 cases presenting with neonatal respiratory distress syndrome, alveolar proteinosis may be present and pulmonary hypertension may be severe. Chest radiographs may show diffuse hazy infiltrates consistent with RDS in neonates. Chest HRCTs may reveal diffuse ground-glass opacities with thickened intralobular septae (Fig. 15.2a). Lung histology has been classified as consistent with alveolar proteinosis (Fig. 15.2b) or a DIP-like pattern in young children [4, 11, 29]. An adolescent patient was been reported with an UIP histologic pattern, though the chest CT had upper lobe predominant disease [50]. Electron microscopy may reveal small aberrant lamellar bodies with densely packed membranes and eccentric electron-dense inclusion bodies (Fig. 15.2c) [11, 29].

Genetic testing is the primary diagnostic approach. Genetic sequencing results may not be available in time to avoid need for lung biopsy in severe neonatal cases. The diagnosis may be suggested by lung biopsy patterns and electron microscopy, and such findings can be particularly helpful in cases where only one mutation is identified. Not all sequence variants will be pathogenic and consultation may be needed for interpretation of genetic findings. Heterozygosity of ABCA3 has also been found to modify the severity of disease associated with *SFTPC* mutation [51].

Differential diagnostic considerations include mutations in *SFTPB*, *SFTPC*, or the GM-CSF receptor, lysinuric protein intolerance, alveolar capillary dysplasia with misalignment of the pulmonary veins, and PIG.

Substantial mortality has been associated when the neonatal presentation is severe [4, 29]. Genotypes may predict phenotype. Specifically, the missense mutation E292V has been associated with a milder neonatal presentation and survival into the second decade of life in children who were compound heterozygotes for ABCA3 mutations [43]. Currently there are no established pharmacologic therapies, but current preclinical studies are promising and suggest understanding of the molecular biology of different mutations will yield targeted therapeutic approaches. Lung transplantation has been performed for children with severe and progressive disease.

Neuroendocrine Cell Hyperplasia of Infancy

NEHI is a rare disorder previously named "persistent tachypnea of infancy" [52]. Otherwise healthy term or near-term infants present with tachypnea and retractions, generally of insidious onset in the first few months to year of life. Crackles are prominent and hypoxemia is common, while wheezing is rare. Additionally, many patients experience failure to thrive, and upper respiratory infections may lead to exacerbation of symptoms. Chest radiographs are normal or may show hyperinfla-

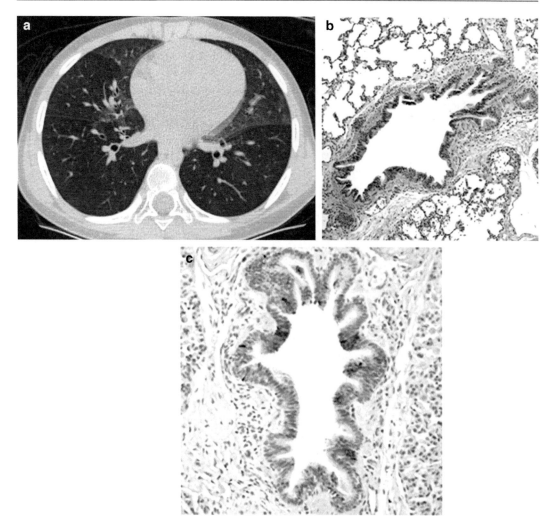

Fig. 15.2 Interstitial lung disease due to ABCA3 gene mutations. (**a**) High-resolution computed tomography scan from a 4-month-old infant with *ABCA3* mutations. The CT scan, which was performed with controlled ventilation under general anesthesia, shows diffuse bilateral ground-glass opacities and thickened interlobular septae. (**b**) Histopathology (hematoxylin and eosin) shows alveolar septal thickening with uniform type II cell hyperplasia and accumulation of granular proteinaceous material within alveolar spaces. (**c**) Electron microscopy demonstrates abnormal lamellar bodies with dense inclusions (image provided by Gail H. Deutsch, MD)

tion or suggest viral disease [52]. High-resolution CT scan findings are distinctive with apparent geographic ground-glass opacity centrally and in the right middle lobe and lingula, with diffuse air-trapping (Fig. 15.2a). No other airway or parenchymal abnormalities are seen. Brody et al. evaluated chest HRCT scans from 23 children with biopsy-proven NEHI and 6 children with other forms of ILD. HRCT specificity for the diagnosis of NEHI was 100% in this study when the CTs were reviewed by two expert radiologists. The sensitivity of HRCT was incomplete, as readers did not suggest NEHI in up to 22% of the cases [28].

Lung histology is near-normal with nonspecific changes including mild airway smooth muscle hyperplasia and mildly increased alveolar macrophages. Increased bronchiolar clear cells are present, which are identified as neuroendocrine cells based on immunopositivity to bombe-sin and serotonin (Fig. 15.2b, c) [52]. The presence of increased numbers of neuroendocrine cells is not sufficient for the diagnosis, as NEC prominence is associated with a variety of other conditions, including bronchopulmonary dyspla-sia (BPD) and airway injury.

The initial diagnostic approach should be to exclude more common causes of the clinical symptoms such as infection, cystic fibrosis, and congenital heart disease. Lung biopsy (via VATS) is currently considered the definitive diagnostic approach. Histologic review should be performed by a pediatric pathologist experienced in this diagnosis, and the histology should be evaluated in the context of the clinical and radiographic findings. Increasingly the diagnosis may be strongly considered based on compatible clinical history, imaging, and infant pulmonary function test data. Studies are ongoing to validate this noninvasive diagnostic approach. Disorders to be considered in the differential diagnosis include acute or chronic infection, lung developmental disorders such as pulmonary hypoplasia, PIG, genetic disorders of surfactant production and metabolism, and airway injury disorders includ-ing bronchiolitis obliterans.

The etiology of NEHI is unknown, but recent data indicate that there are some families with more than one affected individual. There is no known definitive therapy, and therefore manage-ment largely consists of general supportive and preventative care. Most children will require sup-plemental oxygen, and many will require nutri-tional supplementation.

Corticosteroids are not helpful in most cases and therefore establishment of the diagnosis of NEHI helps avoid the complications of corticos-teroids [52]. While long-term outcomes are not well established for this recently recognized dis-order, a diagnosis of NEHI brings a cautious but welcomed good prognosis relative to other forms of childhood ILD. The clinical course is pro-longed but most children demonstrate gradual improvement. The need for supplemental oxygen requirement is variable and may be up to many years. No deaths or need for lung transplantation for NEHI have been reported [4, 52].

Pulmonary Interstitial Glycogenosis

PIG presents with tachypnea and hypoxia, respi-ratory failure, or pulmonary hypertension in pre-term or term infants in the first days to weeks of life [4, 53]. This disorder only occurs in young infants, typically less than at 6 months of age. The severity of the clinical presentation is highly variable. Complicating factors can include prematurity or congenital heart disease.

Case series have reported that chest radio-graphs have diffuse infiltrates or hazy opaci-ties, but no common high-resolution CT scan pattern has been identified [53, 54]. Currently, lung biopsy is the only way to diagnose PIG. Lung histology shows diffuse accumulation of glycogen-laden cells, with diffusely positive immunostaining for Vimentin and PAS-positive immunostaining in the interstitium (Fig. 15.3). Minimal to no inflammation is present. Electron microscopy (EM) shows the interstitium is expanded by primitive interstitial mesenchymal cells with a paucity of organelles and abundant monoparticulate glycogen [53]. PIG may occur as an isolated histologic entity, but is increas-ingly recognized to occur in the setting of other pulmonary conditions, most commonly lung growth abnormalities, including pulmonary hypoplasia and chronic neonatal lung disease due to prematurity [4].

Disorders to be considered in the clinical dif-ferential diagnosis include lung developmental disorders such as alveolar capillary dysplasia with misalignment of the pulmonary veins, pul-monary hypoplasia, pulmonary vascular disease, lymphangiectasia, and genetic disorders of sur-factant production and metabolism. Careful attention is needed to identification of concurrent histologic entities such as lung growth abnormal-ities or vascular abnormalities.

The etiology of PIG is unknown, and there is no known definitive therapy. Most children will require supplemental oxygen and some will require aggressive support including mechanical ventilation and therapies for pulmonary hyper-tension. High-dose pulse corticosteroids have been reported to have benefit in case reports and case series, but no controlled studies have been

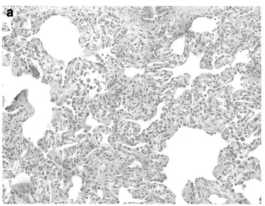
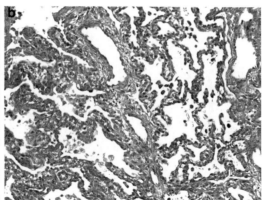

Fig. 15.3 Pulmonary interstitial glycogenosis (PIG). (**a**) H&E of lung histopathology from a 3 week old shows diffuse interstitial widening and cellularity with bland-appearing vacuolated foamy cells containing glycogen, which are weakly PAS positive (**b**). The cells seen in PIG are strongly immunoreactive with vimentin (not shown)

performed [53–55]. Consideration for use of corticosteroids should be assessed in the context of clinical severity and the potential detrimental impact on postnatal alveolarization and neurodevelopment in this patient population. When present, comorbidities such as congenital heart disease or complications of prematurity are often the focus of management.

The natural history is unknown. Reports suggest that the prognosis is favorable in the absence of concurrent disease (i.e., BPD, pulmonary hypertension). Some reports indicate that infants may remain symptomatic for months, but generally improve over time. However, mortality has been associated when other comorbidities are present along with PIG.

Diffuse Lung Diseases Seen in Both Children and Adults: Special Considerations in Pediatrics

Surfactant Protein C Gene Mutations

The clinical presentation of *SFTPC* mutations is highly variable. The relative prevalence of pediatric versus adult cases is not well established, though some pediatric cases present with neonatal respiratory distress syndrome [4, 56]. Other presentations include gradual onset of chronic respiratory symptoms of ILD in young children or presentation with ILD/pulmonary fibrosis in adults [31, 56–61]. Furthermore, some individuals are asymptomatic. Viral infection has been reported to precede symptom onset in some cases [59]. The radiographic appearance may include reticular-nodular pattern, ground-glass opacities, thickened intralobular septae, and peripheral cystic change (Fig. 15.4a) [58, 59].

Histologic findings include hyperplastic type II cells with variable interstitial thickening and fibrosis, granular alveolar proteinosis material and cholesterol clefts, and variable mild lymphocytic inflammation (Fig. 15.4b). The histology has been classified as consistent with patterns of chronic pneumonitis of infancy, NSIP, or a DIP-like pattern in children [4, 31, 42]. UIP and NSIP patterns have been reported in adults [59, 60]. EM generally shows normal lamellar bodies, but disorganized lamellar bodies have been reported in some cases. There are no consistent patterns for immunostaining for the propeptide of SP-C (proSP-C) or mature SP-C, and therefore these immunostains are generally not helpful diagnostically in most *SFTPC* mutation cases [42]. Genetic testing is the preferred and most definitive diagnostic modality. The clinical presentation can be similar for many other causes of diffuse lung disease, and *ABCA3* mutation cases may have considerable clinical and histologic overlap in children [4].

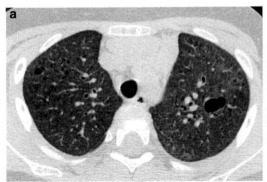 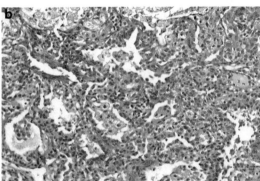

Fig. 15.4 Interstitial lung disease due to *SFTPC* gene mutation. (**a**) High-resolution computed tomography scan from a 2-year-old infant with *SFTPC* mutation. Findings include multiple thin walled cystic lesions and mild diffuse ground-glass opacity. (**b**) Histopathology shows presence of uniform type II cell hyperplasia and prominent intra-alveolar macrophage accumulation and interstitial infiltrate

The pathogenesis of ILD due to *SFTPC* mutations is not simply one of SP-C deficiency. The disorder is due to autosomal dominant or sporadic mutations in *SFTPC* [31, 40, 62], which result in accumulation of the mutant proSP-C peptide leading to cellular toxicity including via ER stress [63, 64]. Abnormal surfactant composition and function may play a role. More than 40 mutations have been described to date [65]. The population frequency is unknown. There are also reports of cases of apparent absence of SP-C despite lack of identified *SFTPC* mutations [66, 67].

The natural history is poorly understood, as the prognosis can be highly variable, even among members of the same family. In children, *SFTPC* mutations may be fatal in the neonatal period or progress to need for lung transplantation. Despite a severe neonatal course, the disorder can show gradual improvement over time including resolution of need for supplemental oxygen [4, 58]. Other children present later with persistent disease requiring supplemental oxygen. Most cases are inherited in an autosomal dominant manner, and relatively or completely asymptomatic family members may also be identified after the presentation of the index case. Genetic counseling should be provided to the family when testing is being considered.

Management consists of supportive care including avoidance of respiratory viral infections. Some case reports suggest response to corticosteroids or other immunomodulatory agents such as hydroxychloroquine [58, 68]. There is compelling scientific rationale for use of RSV immunoprophylaxis (Synagis) in young children with *SFTPC* mutations. Specifically, in in vitro studies, when epithelial cells expressing mutant SP-C are infected with RSV, RSV leads to accumulation of the mutant SP-C proprotein, pronounced activation of the unfolded protein response, and cell death [69].

Aspiration

Gastroesophageal reflux is common in children with ILD, occurring in up to 50% of cases by clinical reports [4]. Infants with tachypnea are particularly prone to feeding incoordination, and it can be quite challenging to determine whether or not aspiration is the primary cause of the lung disease or is a secondary contributor. A multifaceted diagnostic strategy may be needed, including flexible bronchoscopy and BAL, MLB to exclude laryngeal-esophageal cleft, barium study/video swallow study, flexible endoscopic evaluation of swallowing (FEES), and ph/impedance probe. In children with normal airway anatomy and neurocognitive function, aspiration is rarely the primary etiology. Lipoid pneumonia has been reported in children receiving mineral oil for constipation and in older children using lip gloss [70–72]. It is important to remember that increased numbers of lipid-laden macrophages also occur due to abnormalities of surfactant production or clearance, including with surfactant protein or *ABCA3* mutations.

Hypersensitivity Pneumonitis

Hypersensitivity pneumonitis occurs in children of all ages [73], with the youngest reported case in an 8 month old [74]. Bird exposures predominate, but fungal bioaerosols are also a reported cause. The most commonly reported symptoms include cough, weight loss, and fever [73]. Family history of HP has been recognized in 25% of cases [73]. It is essential that the diagnostic approach start with clinical suspicion and a careful exposure history. A multimodal diagnostic strategy is often required incorporating imaging, BAL findings, and sometimes lung biopsy patterns [73]. Serum precipitins fail to distinguish exposure from causality. Lymphocyte proliferation studies are more reliable but not widely available [75]. Treatment approaches have included corticosteroids, but removal from the exposure is essential. Deaths from hypersensitivity pneumonitis have been reported in children as well as in adults, and it is likely that many cases of HP are unrecognized in children.

Pulmonary Hemorrhage Syndromes

Pulmonary hemorrhage may occur in children with already recognized connective tissue disease or in children with no antecedent medical history. Clinical presentation may include hemoptysis or respiratory failure, recurrent pneumonia, lethargy, or chronic cough. Chest imaging shows alveolar infiltrates. Bronchoscopy plays a large role in recognizing pulmonary hemorrhage syndromes. Inflammatory markers and serologies including ANCA, ANA, and anti-GBM antibodies may help suggest an underlying cause. Careful evaluation for renal involvement is warranted. Lung biopsy (via VATS) may be required to determine whether vasculitis or capillaritis are present [4]. In a series of 23 patients who underwent lung biopsy for evaluation of pulmonary hemorrhage, careful histologic review found evidence of capillaritis in eight cases [16]. In this

series, there were no clinical signs to differentiate immune and non-immune-mediated alveolar hemorrhage. High dose corticosteroids were successful in controlling alveolar hemorrhage in these cases. Generally, patients with immune-mediated lung disease require more aggressive pharmacologic intervention including with cytotoxic agents.

Pulmonary Alveolar Proteinosis

Pulmonary alveolar proteinosis occurs in infants and children as well as adults, and variable clinical phenotypes have now been recognized in association with a number of molecular and genetic causes. After recognizing the clinical syndrome of PAP typically by broncho-alveolar lavage and/or chest HRCT, definitive genetic and molecular diagnostics should be pursued to determine the pathogenesis. PAP may be caused by (1) abnormal GM-CSF signaling and a reduction in the ability of alveolar macrophage to catabolize surfactant lipids and proteins (such as with autoantibodies to GM-CSF and GM-CSF receptor mutations), (2) reduction in alveolar macrophage numbers (such as with myelofibrosis causing secondary PAP), or (3) abnormal surfactant production (such as with *SFTPB* mutations).

In adults, PAP is most commonly caused by elevated levels of neutralizing GM-CSF autoantibodies, and thus has been referred to as autoimmune PAP [76]. This autoimmune form of PAP is occasionally seen in adolescents and children. As in adults, secondary PAP can also occur in children in the settings of hematologic malignancies, myelodysplastic syndromes, or certain pulmonary infections.

There are other causes of PAP which to date have only been reported in children. These include GM-CSF receptor β chain deficiency [77], SP-B deficiency [30, 44, 78], or *ABCA3* mutations [4, 11, 29]. Recently, mutations causing GM-CSF receptor α chain dysfunction have been reported in children with insidious onset of chronic respiratory symptoms including exercise intolerance and failure to thrive. These children have high levels of GM-CSF, but impaired or absent GM-CSF signaling and therefore compromised alveolar macrophage function [25, 79]. PAP has also been associated with lysinuric protein intolerance in children [80, 81].

If a genetic or molecular basis for PAP is identified, surgical lung biopsy is usually not needed. However, lung biopsy may be required in cases in which a genetic/molecular basis cannot be identified or when testing cannot be performed in a timely manner given the clinical severity. Lung histology shows simple filling of alveoli with surfactant without significant alveolar wall or interstitial pathology. If alveolar wall or interstitial pathology is present, secondary PAP or disorders of surfactant production and metabolism (such as *ABCA3* or *SFTPC* mutations) should be considered [4, 11].

Whole lung lavage is standard therapy for autoimmune PAP and has also been successfully employed in PAP due to other etiologies. Modified technical approaches are needed but have been accomplished in young children and infants [25, 82]. Experimental therapies for autoimmune PAP include GM-CSF augmentation, plasmapheresis, and anti-B-lymphocyte antibody therapy. Therapy for secondary PAP is usually focused to treating the underlying condition.

While only limited outcome data are available for children with PAP, it should be emphasized that it is increasingly critical to establish the molecular cause of PAP in children in order to inform discussions of prognosis and therapeutic considerations. Some etiologies such as mutations in ABCA3 or SP-B will have a poor prognosis, and lung transplantation may be considered. It has been our experience that children with autoimmune PAP and those with GMCSFRα mutations respond to whole lung lavage [25] (and unpublished observations).

Bronchiolitis Obliterans

Bronchiolitis obliterans has been reported in all pediatric age groups. While common precipitating causes in adults include autoimmune disorders, occupational inhalational injuries, and hypersensitivity pneumonitis, the predominant cause of bronchiolitis obliterans in children is adenovirus infection [83]. Of 109 pediatric cases reported by Colom et al., adenovirus infection was identified in 71% [83]. Of a cohort of 45 infants with adenovirus pneumonia followed prospectively for 5 years after an epidemic outbreak, 47% of the cohort developed bronchiolitis obliterans [84]. Other infectious causes of bronchiolitis obliterans which have been reported in children include influenza, parainfluenza, measles, respiratory syncytial virus, varicella, and mycoplasma [26]. Noninfectious etiologies of bronchiolitis obliterans in children include posttransplant disease, connective tissue disease, toxic fume inhalation, chronic hypersensitivity pneumonitis, aspiration, drug reaction, and Stevens–Johnson syndrome [85, 86].

In children, the diagnosis of bronchiolitis obliterans can be strongly suspected based on clinical features, particularly when fixed obstructive lung disease occurs after a severe infectious or other insult to the lower respiratory tract. A modest bronchodilator response is present in some cases [83]. The severity of clinical findings may wax and wane in some cases, but common features include prolonged tachypnea, hyperinflation, crackles and/or wheezing, and persistent hypoxemia. Characteristic CT imaging patterns include mosaic perfusion, air-trapping, vascular attenuation, and central bronchiectasis, and may obviate the need for lung biopsy in a compatible clinical context [87]. When lung biopsy is performed, histologic features include a spectrum of obliterative bronchiolitis, constrictive bronchiolitis, and cryptogenic organizing pneumonia, with extension of granulation tissue into the alveoli [88]. Because the process can be patchy, lung biopsies may not always be diagnostic or reflect the severity of the disease [85].

There are no controlled therapeutic studies for bronchiolitis obliterans in children. Therapies utilized for bronchiolitis obliterans in children have included bronchodilators, azithromycin, high-dose pulse corticosteroids, IVIG, other immunomodulatory and steroid-sparing agents, and Infliximab in a single case report in a bone marrow transplant recipient [85, 89]. No clinical deterioration or mortality was observed in the report by Castro-Rodriguez [84]. In other case series, mortality and progression to lung transplantation do rarely occur. It has been suggested that bronchiolitis obliterans occurring after Stevens–Johnson syndrome may be associated with a particularly severe course [85].

Follicular Bronchiolitis/Lymphocytic Interstitial Pneumonitis

The histologic patterns of follicular bronchiolitis and lymphocytic interstitial pneumonitis are part of a histologic spectrum most commonly seen in children with immunodeficiency states, and should prompt aggressive evaluation for underlying immune dysfunction if not already recognized [4, 90, 91]. Children may have signs of systemic lymphoproliferative disease or autoimmune disease. LIP has most commonly been associated with HIV infection, but EBV and HHV-6 have also been implicated. Familial cases have also been reported [92, 93]. Other reports indicate a good prognosis and apparent absence of underlying systemic disease [94].

Connective Tissue Disease Associated with ILD

ILD is a relatively rare but well-recognized feature of connective tissue disorders in children. ILD has been reported in particular association with polymyositis/dermatomyositis, systemic sclerosis, mixed connective tissue disease, and Juvenile Inflammatory Arthritis (JIA) [91, 95–97]. A cellular, fibrotic, or mixed NSIP pattern predominates in children, but patterns of lymphoid hyperplasia/follicular bronchiolitis, bronchiolitis obliterans, or alveolar hemorrhage also occur [5, 6, 91]. As in adults, mixed compartment patterns seem to suggest underlying collagen vascular disease. Because pulmonary disease onset may precede overt systemic disease features, these histologic patterns warrant a diligent search for underlying rheumatologic disease. Therapeutic approaches are empirically focused on the systemic disease process, and prognosis is not well established.

References

1. Fan LL, Kozinetz CA. Factors influencing survival in children with chronic interstitial lung disease. Am J Respir Crit Care Med. 1997;156:939–42.
2. Dinwiddie R, Sharief N, Crawford O. Idiopathic interstitial pneumonitis in children: a national survey in the United Kingdom and Ireland. Pediatr Pulmonol. 2002;34:23–9.
3. Clement A. Task force on chronic interstitial lung disease in immunocompetent children. Eur Respir J. 2004;24:686–97.
4. Deutsch GH, Young LR, Deterding RR, et al. Diffuse lung disease in young children: application of a novel classification scheme. Am J Respir Crit Care Med. 2007;176:1120–8.
5. Deterding RR, Young LR, Dishop M, Fan LL, Dell SD, Sweet SC, et al. Diffuse lung disease in older children – report of the child network review. Am J Respir Crit Care Med. 2007;175:A148.
6. Dishop MKAF, Galambos C, White FV, Deterding RR, Young LR, Langston C. Classification of diffuse lung disease in older children and adolescents: a multi-institutional study of the Children's Interstitial Lung Disease Network. Mod Pathol. 2007;20:287–8.
7. Fan LL, Mullen AL, Brugman SM, et al. Clinical spectrum of chronic interstitial lung disease in children. J Pediatr. 1992;121:867–72.
8. Fan LL, Deterding RR, Langston C. Pediatric interstitial lung disease revisited. Pediatr Pulmonol. 2004;38: 369–78.
9. Fan LL, Kozinetz CA, Deterding RR, et al. Evaluation of a diagnostic approach to pediatric interstitial lung disease. Pediatrics. 1998;101:82–5.
10. Deterding R, Fan LL. Surfactant dysfunction mutations in children's interstitial lung disease and beyond. Am J Respir Crit Care Med. 2005;172:940–1.
11. Doan ML, Guillerman RP, Dishop MK, et al. Clinical, radiological and pathological features of ABCA3 mutations in children. Thorax. 2008;63:366–73.
12. Fan LL, Kozinetz CA, Wojtczak HA, et al. Diagnostic value of transbronchial, thoracoscopic, and open lung biopsy in immunocompetent children with chronic interstitial lung disease. J Pediatr. 1997;131:565–9.
13. Wood RE. Pediatric bronchoscopy. Chest Surg Clin N Am. 1996;6:237–51.
14. de Blic J, Midulla F, Barbato A, et al. Bronchoalveolar lavage in children. ERS Task Force on bronchoalveolar lavage in children. European Respiratory Society. Eur Respir J. 2000;15:217–31.
15. de Blic J. Pulmonary alveolar proteinosis in children. Paediatr Respir Rev. 2004;5:316–22.
16. Fullmer JJ, Langston C, Dishop MK, et al. Pulmonary capillaritis in children: a review of eight cases with comparison to other alveolar hemorrhage syndromes. J Pediatr. 2005;146:376–81.
17. Fan LL, Lung MC, Wagener JS. The diagnostic value of bronchoalveolar lavage in immunocompetent

children with chronic diffuse pulmonary infiltrates. Pediatr Pulmonol. 1997;23:8–13.

18. Castile R, Filbrun D, Flucke R, et al. Adult-type pulmonary function tests in infants without respiratory disease. Pediatr Pulmonol. 2000;30:215–27.

19. Feher A, Castile R, Kisling J, et al. Flow limitation in normal infants: a new method for forced expiratory maneuvers from raised lung volumes. J Appl Physiol. 1996;80:2019–25.

20. ATS/ERS statement: raised volume forced expirations in infants: guidelines for current practice. Am J Respir Crit Care Med. 2005; 72:1463–71.

21. Brody AS. New perspectives in imaging interstitial lung disease in children. Pediatr Radiol. 2008;38 Suppl 2:S205–7.

22. Donnelly LF, Emery KH, Brody AS, et al. Minimizing radiation dose for pediatric body applications of single-detector helical CT: strategies at a large Children's Hospital. AJR Am J Roentgenol. 2001;176:303–6.

23. Long FR, Castile RG, Brody AS, et al. Lungs in infants and young children: improved thin-section CT with a noninvasive controlled-ventilation technique–initial experience. Radiology. 1999;212:588–93.

24. Lynch DA, Brasch RC, Hardy KA, et al. Pediatric pulmonary disease: assessment with high-resolution ultrafast CT. Radiology. 1990;176:243–8.

25. Suzuki T, Sakagami T, Rubin BK, et al. Familial pulmonary alveolar proteinosis caused by mutations in CSF2RA. J Exp Med. 2008;205:2703–10.

26. Kim CK, Kim SW, Kim JS, et al. Bronchiolitis obliterans in the 1990s in Korea and the United States. Chest. 2001;120:1101–6.

27. Kim MJ, Lee KY. Bronchiolitis obliterans in children with Stevens-Johnson syndrome: follow-up with high resolution CT. Pediatr Radiol. 1996;26:22–5.

28. Brody A, Guillerman RP, Hay TC, et al. Neuroendocrine cell hyperplasia of infancy: diagnosis with high-resolution CT. AJR Am J Roentgenol. 2010;194(1):238–44.

29. Shulenin S, Nogee LM, Annilo T, et al. ABCA3 gene mutations in newborns with fatal surfactant deficiency. N Engl J Med. 2004;350:1296–303.

30. Nogee LM, de Mello DE, Dehner LP, et al. Brief report: deficiency of pulmonary surfactant protein B in congenital alveolar proteinosis. N Engl J Med. 1993;328:406–10.

31. Nogee LM, Dunbar 3rd AE, Wert SE, et al. A mutation in the surfactant protein C gene associated with familial interstitial lung disease. N Engl J Med. 2001;344:573–9.

32. Barbato A, Panizzolo C, Cracco A, et al. Interstitial lung disease in children: a multicentre survey on diagnostic approach. Eur Respir J. 2000;16:509–13.

33. Rothenberg SS, Wagner JS, Chang JH, et al. The safety and efficacy of thoracoscopic lung biopsy for diagnosis and treatment in infants and children. J Pediatr Surg. 1996;31:100–3. discussion 103–104.

34. Rothenberg SS. Thoracoscopy in infants and children: the state of the art. J Pediatr Surg. 2005;40:303–6.

35. Langston C, Patterson K, Dishop MK, et al. A protocol for the handling of tissue obtained by operative lung biopsy: recommendations of the chILD pathology cooperative group. Pediatr Dev Pathol. 2006;9: 173–80.

36. Hamvas A, Nogee LM, Mallory Jr GB, et al. Lung transplantation for treatment of infants with surfactant protein B deficiency. J Pediatr. 1997;130:231–9.

37. Elizur A, Faro A, Huddleston CB, et al. Lung transplantation in infants and toddlers from 1990 to 2004 at St. Louis Children's Hospital. Am J Transplant. 2009;9:719–26.

38. Fan LL, Langston C. Pediatric interstitial lung disease: children are not small adults. Am J Respir Crit Care Med. 2002;165:1466–7.

39. Nogee LM, Garnier G, Dietz HC, et al. A mutation in the surfactant protein B gene responsible for fatal neonatal respiratory disease in multiple kindreds. J Clin Invest. 1994;93:1860–3.

40. Garmany TH, Wambach JA, Heins HB, et al. Population and disease-based prevalence of the common mutations associated with surfactant deficiency. Pediatr Res. 2008;63:645–9.

41. Cole FS, Hamvas A, Rubinstein P, et al. Population-based estimates of surfactant protein B deficiency. Pediatrics. 2000;105:538–41.

42. Wert SE, Whitsett JA, Nogee LM. Genetic disorders of surfactant dysfunction. Pediatr Dev Pathol. 2009;12:253–74.

43. Bullard JE, Wert SE, Whitsett JA, et al. ABCA3 mutations associated with pediatric interstitial lung disease. Am J Respir Crit Care Med. 2005;172:1026–31.

44. Hamvas A, Cole FS, DeMello DE, et al. Surfactant protein B deficiency: antenatal diagnosis and prospective treatment with surfactant replacement. J Pediatr. 1994;125:356–61.

45. Ballard PL, Nogee LM, Beers MF, et al. Partial deficiency of surfactant protein B in an infant with chronic lung disease. Pediatrics. 1995;96:1046–52.

46. Dunbar 3rd AE, Wert SE, Ikegami M, et al. Prolonged survival in hereditary surfactant protein B (SP-B) deficiency associated with a novel splicing mutation. Pediatr Res. 2000;48:275–82.

47. Cheong N, Madesh M, Gonzales LW, et al. Functional and trafficking defects in ATP binding cassette A3 mutants associated with respiratory distress syndrome. J Biol Chem. 2006;281:9791–800.

48. Matsumura Y, Ban N, Ueda K, et al. Characterization and classification of ATP-binding cassette transporter ABCA3 mutants in fatal surfactant deficiency. J Biol Chem. 2006;281:34503–14.

49. Garmany TH, Moxley MA, White FV, et al. Surfactant composition and function in patients with ABCA3 mutations. Pediatr Res. 2006;59:801–5.

50. Young LR, Nogee LM, Barnett B, et al. Usual interstitial pneumonia in an adolescent with ABCA3 mutations. Chest. 2008;134:192–5.

51. Bullard JE, Nogee LM. Heterozygosity for ABCA3 mutations modifies the severity of lung disease associated with a surfactant protein C gene (SFTPC) mutation. Pediatr Res. 2007;62:176–9.

52. Deterding RR, Pye C, Fan LL, et al. Persistent tachypnea of infancy is associated with neuroendocrine cell hyperplasia. Pediatr Pulmonol. 2005;40:157–65.

53. Canakis AM, Cutz E, Manson D, et al. Pulmonary interstitial glycogenosis: a new variant of neonatal interstitial lung disease. Am J Respir Crit Care Med. 2002;165:1557–65.

54. Onland W, Molenaar JJ, Leguit RJ, et al. Pulmonary interstitial glycogenosis in identical twins. Pediatr Pulmonol. 2005;40:362–6.

55. Deutsch GH, Young LR. Histologic resolution of pulmonary interstitial glycogenosis. Pediatr Dev Pathol. 2009;12(6):475–80.

56. Cameron HS, Somaschini M, Carrera P, et al. A common mutation in the surfactant protein C gene associated with lung disease. J Pediatr. 2005;146:370–5.

57. Guillot L, Epaud R, Thouvenin G, et al. New surfactant protein C gene mutations associated with diffuse lung disease. J Med Genet. 2009;46:490–4.

58. Abou Taam R, Jaubert F, Emond S, et al. Familial interstitial disease with I73T mutation: a mid- and long-term study. Pediatr Pulmonol. 2009;44:167–75.

59. Thomas AQ, Lane K, Phillips 3rd J, et al. Heterozygosity for a surfactant protein C gene mutation associated with usual interstitial pneumonitis and cellular nonspecific interstitial pneumonitis in one kindred. Am J Respir Crit Care Med. 2002;165: 1322–8.

60. Lawson WE, Grant SW, Ambrosini V, et al. Genetic mutations in surfactant protein C are a rare cause of sporadic cases of IPF. Thorax. 2004;59:977–80.

61. Markart P, Ruppert C, Wygrecka M, et al. Surfactant protein C mutations in sporadic forms of idiopathic interstitial pneumonias. Eur Respir J. 2007;29:134–7.

62. McBee AD, Wegner DJ, Carlson CS, et al. Recombination as a mechanism for sporadic mutation in the surfactant protein-C gene. Pediatr Pulmonol. 2008;43:443–50.

63. Wang WJ, Mulugeta S, Russo SJ, et al. Deletion of exon 4 from human surfactant protein C results in aggresome formation and generation of a dominant negative. J Cell Sci. 2003;116:683–92.

64. Mulugeta S, Nguyen V, Russo SJ, et al. A surfactant protein C precursor protein BRICHOS domain mutation causes endoplasmic reticulum stress, proteasome dysfunction, and caspase 3 activation. Am J Respir Cell Mol Biol. 2005;32:521–30.

65. Nogee LM. Genetics of pediatric interstitial lung disease. Curr Opin Pediatr. 2006;18:287–92.

66. Amin RS, Wert SE, Baughman RP, et al. Surfactant protein deficiency in familial interstitial lung disease. J Pediatr. 2001;139:85–92.

67. Tredano M, Griese M, Brasch F, et al. Mutation of SFTPC in infantile pulmonary alveolar proteinosis with or without fibrosing lung disease. Am J Med Genet A. 2004;126A:18–26.

68. Rosen DM, Waltz DA. Hydroxychloroquine and surfactant protein C deficiency. N Engl J Med. 2005;352: 207–8.

69. Bridges JP, Xu Y, Na CL, et al. Adaptation and increased susceptibility to infection associated with constitutive expression of misfolded SP-C. J Cell Biol. 2006;172:395–407.

70. Fan LL, Graham LM. Radiological cases of the month. Lipoid pneumonia from mineral oil aspiration. Arch Pediatr Adolesc Med. 1994;148:205–6.

71. Becton DL, Lowe JE, Falletta JM. Lipoid pneumonia in an adolescent girl secondary to use of lip gloss. J Pediatr. 1984;105:421–3.

72. Zanetti G, Marchiori E, Gasparetto TD, et al. Lipoid pneumonia in children following aspiration of mineral oil used in the treatment of constipation: high-resolution CT findings in 17 patients. Pediatr Radiol. 2007;37:1135–9.

73. Fan LL. Hypersensitivity pneumonitis in children. Curr Opin Pediatr. 2002;14:323–6.

74. Eisenberg JD, Montanero A, Lee RG. Hypersensitivity pneumonitis in an infant. Pediatr Pulmonol. 1992;12: 186–90.

75. Fink JN, Ortega HG, Reynolds HY, et al. Needs and opportunities for research in hypersensitivity pneumonitis. Am J Respir Crit Care Med. 2005;171:792–8.

76. Uchida K, Nakata K, Suzuki T, et al. Granulocyte/macrophage-colony-stimulating factor autoantibodies and myeloid cell immune functions in healthy subjects. Blood. 2009;113:2547–56.

77. Dirksen U, Nishinakamura R, Groneck P, et al. Human pulmonary alveolar proteinosis associated with a defect in GM-CSF/IL-3/IL-5 receptor common beta chain expression. J Clin Invest. 1997;100:2211–7.

78. Nogee LM. Surfactant protein-B deficiency. Chest. 1997;111:129S–35.

79. Martinez-Moczygemba M, Doan ML, Elidemir O, et al. Pulmonary alveolar proteinosis caused by deletion of the GM-CSFRalpha gene in the X chromosome pseudoautosomal region 1. J Exp Med. 2008;205:2711–6.

80. Parto K, Svedstrom E, Majurin ML, et al. Pulmonary manifestations in lysinuric protein intolerance. Chest. 1993;104:1176–82.

81. Santamaria F, Parenti G, Guidi G, et al. Early detection of lung involvement in lysinuric protein intolerance: role of high-resolution computed tomography and radioisotopic methods. Am J Respir Crit Care Med. 1996;153:731–5.

82. McKenzie B, Wood RE, Bailey A. Airway management for unilateral lung lavage in children. Anesthesiology. 1989;70:550–3.

83. Colom AJ, Teper AM, Vollmer WM, et al. Risk factors for the development of bronchiolitis obliterans in children with bronchiolitis. Thorax. 2006;61:503–6.

84. Castro-Rodriguez JA, Daszenies C, Garcia M, et al. Adenovirus pneumonia in infants and factors for developing bronchiolitis obliterans: a 5-year follow-up. Pediatr Pulmonol. 2006;41:947–53.

85. Moonnumakal SP, Fan LL. Bronchiolitis obliterans in children. Curr Opin Pediatr. 2008;20:272–8.

86. Kurland G, Michelson P. Bronchiolitis obliterans in children. Pediatr Pulmonol. 2005;39:193–208.

87. Lynch DA, Hay T, Newell Jr JD, et al. Pediatric diffuse lung disease: diagnosis and classification using

high-resolution CT. AJR Am J Roentgenol. 1999;173: 713–8.

88. Mauad T, Dolhnikoff M. Histology of childhood bronchiolitis obliterans. Pediatr Pulmonol. 2002;33:466–74.

89. Fullmer JJ, Fan LL, Dishop MK, et al. Successful treatment of bronchiolitis obliterans in a bone marrow transplant patient with tumor necrosis factor-alpha blockade. Pediatrics. 2005;116:767–70.

90. Church JA, Isaacs H, Saxon A, et al. Lymphoid interstitial pneumonitis and hypogammaglobulinemia in children. Am Rev Respir Dis. 1981;124:491–6.

91. Langston C, Dishop M. Diffuse lung disease in infancy a proposed classification applied to 259 diagnostic biopsies. Pediatr Dev Pathol. 2009;12(6):421–37.

92. Thomas H, Risma KA, Graham TB, et al. A kindred of children with interstitial lung disease. Chest. 2007;132: 221–30.

93. O'Brodovich HM, Moser MM, Lu L. Familial lymphoid interstitial pneumonia: a long-term follow-up. Pediatrics. 1980;65:523–8.

94. Kinane BT, Mansell AL, Zwerdling RG, et al. Follicular bronchitis in the pediatric population. Chest. 1993;104:1183–6.

95. Kobayashi I, Yamada M, Takahashi Y, et al. Interstitial lung disease associated with juvenile dermatomyositis: clinical features and efficacy of cyclosporin A. Rheumatology (Oxford). 2003;42:371–4.

96. Morinishi Y, Oh-Ishi T, Kabuki T, et al. Juvenile dermatomyositis: clinical characteristics and the relatively high risk of interstitial lung disease. Mod Rheumatol. 2007;17:413–7.

97. Seely JM, Jones LT, Wallace C, et al. Systemic sclerosis: using high-resolution CT to detect lung disease in children. AJR Am J Roentgenol. 1998;170: 691–7.

Rare Interstitial Lung Diseases

16

Tristan J. Huie, Amy L. Olson, Marvin I. Schwarz, and Stephen K. Frankel

Abstract

This chapter details the clinical presentation, pathophysiology, diagnosis, and management of pulmonary alveolar proteinosis and lymphangioleiomyomatosis (LAM). It also highlights other, rarer, interstitial lung diseases (ILDs) including aspiration-related ILD, lipoid pneumonia, amyloidosis, Erdheim–Chester disease, Hermansky–Pudlak syndrome, neurofibromatosis, pulmonary alveolar microlithiasis, bronchioloalveolar cell carcinoma, and lymphangitic carcinomatosis.

Keywords

Pulmonary alveolar proteinosis • Lymphangioleiomyomatosis • Aspiration • Lipoid pneumonia • Amyloidosis • Erdheim–Chester disease • Hermansky–Pudlak syndrome • Neurofibromatosis • Pulmonary alveolar microlithiasis • Bronchioloalveolar carcinoma • Lymphangitic carcinomatosis

T.J. Huie, MD • A. L. Olson, MD, MSPH
Department of Medicine, National Jewish Health,
Denver, CO, USA

M.I. Schwarz, MD
Division of Pulmonary Sciences and Critical
Care Medicine, University of Colorado at Denver,
Aurora, CO, USA

S.K. Frankel, MD (✉)
Health Sciences Center, Division of Pulmonary Sciences
and Critical Care Medicine, University of Colorado at
Denver, Aurora, CO, USA
e-mail: frankels@njhealth.org

R.P. Baughman and R.M. du Bois (eds.), *Diffuse Lung Disease: A Practical Approach*,
DOI 10.1007/978-1-4419-9771-5_16, © Springer Science+Business Media, LLC 2012

Introduction

This chapter reviews those uncommon and rare interstitial lung diseases (ILDs) that have not been discussed elsewhere in this book. As has been highlighted throughout this book, the diagnostic approach to diffuse lung disease relies on a diligent clinical evaluation, chest imaging, and often, histopathology. The history should seek information regarding not only pulmonary manifestations of the disease process, but also occupational and environmental exposures, concomitant extrapulmonary signs and symptoms that may suggest a systemic disorder, and family history. The radiographic pattern, particularly as revealed by high resolution computed tomographic (HRCT) imaging, often suggests a specific and limited differential diagnosis. Still, histopathology is required for definitive diagnosis in many cases. Table 16.1 highlights some key information related to these rarer diseases.

Pulmonary Alveolar Proteinosis

Introduction

Pulmonary alveolar proteinosis (PAP) is a rare, diffuse parenchymal disorder of the lung with a prevalence of 4–10 cases per million [1–3]. PAP is characterized by the accumulation of surfactant phospholipids and proteins in the alveolar spaces and distal airways. While all cases of PAP share a common histopathology, from an etiologic perspective, PAP may occur as (1) an autoimmune-mediated, sporadic disorder secondary to the development of antigranulocyte-macrophage colony-stimulating factor (GM-CSF) autoantibodies that in turn lead to dysregulated macrophage function and dysregulated surfactant homeostasis, (2) as a secondary phenomenon, particularly in response to malignancy, inhalational exposure, or infection, and (3) as a congenital/genetic disorder related to mutation or protein processing of surfactant apoproteins and/or GM-CSF signal transduction. Clinically, patients will generally present with radiographic findings (bilateral alveolar infiltrates) out of proportion to clinical findings that typically include dyspnea, exercise intolerance, cough, and hypoxemia. In addition to the collection of lipoproteinaceous material in the alveolar spaces, PAP is also characterized by impaired macrophage and neutrophil function and susceptibility to infection [4].

Pathogenesis

The identification and reclassification of idiopathic PAP as an autoimmune disorder characterized by the presence of anti-GM-CSF antibodies is a tribute to the power of translational science [5, 6]. PAP was clinically first described as an idiopathic disease by Rosen et al. in 1958 [7]. While advances in the recognition and management of PAP had been made over time, the pathogenesis remained a mystery. In 1994, two groups of researchers created "knock-out" mice that were unable to produce the hematopoietic growth and differentiation cytokine GM-CSF and spontaneously developed a lung condition identical to human PAP [8, 9]. Mice deficient in GM-CSF receptor were then found to have the identical PAP phenotype. Follow-up studies on these mice further revealed that the accumulation of the surfactant-like material in the lung was secondary to impaired macrophage clearance of surfactant proteins and lipids and not related to surfactant synthesis or secretion. Nevertheless, the relationship between the mouse model and the human disease was not readily obvious.

In 1999, Kitamura et al. published a case series of 11 patients with PAP in whom the investigators were able to isolate anti-GM-CSF antibodies from each patient [10]. Other groups have since replicated these findings, identifying blocking anti-GM-CSF antibodies in both the blood and bronchoalveolar lavage (BAL) fluid of patients with primary PAP. What was previously believed to be idiopathic, spontaneous PAP is now known to be an autoimmune disorder related to the development of neutralizing anti-GM-CSF antibodies [11, 12]. The presence of anti-GM-CSF antibodies is not 100% specific for PAP as they can also occasionally be seen in myasthenia

Table 16.1 Highlights of selected rare interstitial lung diseases

Pulmonary alveolar proteinosis	May be primary, secondary (malignancy, infection or inhalation injury), or congenital; most often occurs in male smokers; impaired granulocyte function leads to opportunistic infections	Crazy-paving pattern on CT: septal thickening that outlines secondary pulmonary lobule; reticular abnormalities with bilateral lower lobe alveolar infiltrates	Typical radiographic findings with PAS-staining BAL; anti-GM-CSF antibodies useful	Whole lung lavage; GM-CSF
Lymphangioleiomyomatosis	May present with dyspnea, pneumothorax, or chylothorax; 95% of cases occur in women – most often in premenopausal women; similar pattern in one third of tuberous sclerosis cases; associated with renal tumors	Cystic lung disease with diffusely distributed, thin-walled, uniformly sized cysts; renal angiomyolipomas (renal tumors with fat density tissue on CT)	Typical HRCT findings may be diagnostic; Surgical lung biopsy demonstrates LAM cells staining with HMB-45; Family history of tuberous sclerosis; TSC gene testing for TS	Investigational use of mTOR inhibitors (e.g., sirolimus) for renal tumors; mTOR inhibitors possibly slow progression of lung disease
Langerhans cell histiocytosis	More than 90% of cases occur in smokers; 5–15% of pulmonary LCH have extrapulmonary involvement: especially skin, hypothalamus, bone; may present with pneumothorax; constitutional symptoms present in one third of cases	Thin-walled, irregular cysts and nodules of varying size; upper lobe predominance; lung volumes are usually normal or increased (as opposed to most fibrosing lung diseases)	Typical HRCT findings may be diagnostic; Lung biopsy shows bronchiolocentric stellate lesions of mixed inflammatory cells including CD1a+, S100+ histiocytes (Langerhans' cells); associated fibrosis; pigmented alveolar macrophages in adjacent airspaces (Pseudo-DIP reaction); Birbeck granules (pentalaminar rod-shaped structures) in histiocyte cytoplasm	Smoking cessation; no proven pharmacologic therapy, although corticosteroids often used; other cytotoxic drugs considered if no benefit from steroids and tobacco cessation
Aspiration-related ILD	Less than 50% have reflux symptoms; increased risk in elderly; patients with neurologic disease	Migratory alveolar infiltrates; lower lobe predominant reticular changes, tree-in-bud changes, or centrilobular nodules; airway thickening; associated hiatal hernia or dilated/thickened esophagus	Clinical diagnosis; Biopsy may show foreign body granulomas	Acid-reduction medications; aspiration precautions; fundiplication in resistant cases
Lipoid pneumonia	History of ingestion of mineral oil or use of oily nasal drops; associated with esophageal or neurologic disorders	Lower lobe predominant infiltrates; often alveolar infiltrates with reticular background; infiltrates often have fat density; may have crazy-paving or CT angiogram sign (pulmonary vessels visible against low attenuation consolidation)	BAL shows alveolar macrophages with lipid-laden vacuoles; +Sudan stain or oil red O stain; Biopsy may be required	Avoid offending exposure; steroids may benefit acute cases
Amyloidosis	May present with nodules, airways disease, or diffuse infiltrates; primary amyloid is a systemic disease and is often associated with lymphoproliferative disease; secondary amyloid is associated with chronic inflammatory disease	Depends on type: may be single or multiple nodules; airway thickening; or diffuse infiltrates	Lung biopsy shows eosinophilic material with apple green birefringence under polarized light	Surgical resection for localized disease; limited success with steroids or chemotherapy for diffuse disease

(continued)

Table 16.1 (continued)

Erdheim–Chester disease	Bone pain is most frequent complaint; a systemic disease may affect skin, hypothalamus, posterior pituitary, orbits, heart, and retroperitoneum	Sclerotic bone lesions in long bones may be pathognomonic; lung fibrosis has septal reticulation with ground-glass opacities; pleural and pericardial disease common; "coated aorta" (periaortic fibrosis)	Biopsy shows histiocytic involvement with non-Langerhans cells. Histiocytes stain CD68+ and negative for CD1a	No proven therapy; benefit reported with interferon-α; cyclophosphamide or chemotherapy may provide some benefit
Hermansky–Pudlak syndrome	Classic triad of oculocutaneous albinism, bleeding diathesis, and ceroid deposition in various tissues; associated diseases include pulmonary fibrosis, granulomatous colitis, and renal failure; hereditary disease that most commonly occurs in Puerto Ricans	Nonspecific pattern of reticulation, ground-glass opacities, honeycombing; may also have peribronchovascular fibrosis and bronchiectasis	Lung biopsy demonstrates ceroid deposition, inflammation, and fibrosis Family history helpful	No proven therapy; lung transplant useful in selected cases
Neurofibromatosis	Autosomal dominant disease that most commonly affects CNS and skin (café-au-lait spots and cutaneous neurofibromas)	Nonspecific pattern that often has bullous changes, upper lobe cysts, basilar reticular opacities, and ground-glass opacities	Chest findings in setting of neurofibromatosis	No proven therapy
Pulmonary alveolar microlithiasis	Sporadic or autosomal recessive disease; usually presents between age of 30 and 50; typically very insidious course; one third asymptomatic at diagnosis	Hyperdense or calcified micronodules with lower lobe predominance; "sandstorm appearance"; may also have ground-glass opacities, reticulation and subpleural cysts	Typical chest imaging may be diagnostic	No proven therapy; lung transplant useful in selected cases
Bronchioloalveolar cell carcinoma	Symptoms reflect extent of disease; constitutional symptoms may be present; bronchorrhea (copious sputum production) is a classic symptom; weaker correlation with tobacco than other lung cancers	Diffuse form may show diffuse alveolar nodules or nonresolving pneumonia pattern; CT angiogram sign may be present	Sputum cytology, BAL or transbronchial lung biopsy usually diagnostic Genetic testing for epidermal growth factor receptor (EGFR) mutations may guide therapy	Chemotherapy Tyrosine kinase inhibitors for EGFR mutations
Lymphangitic carcinomatosis	Progressive dyspnea and constitutional symptoms; tumor emboli may result in cor pulmonale	Kerley's B lines; irregularly thickened or beaded septal lines; primary tumor may be observed	Transbronchial or endobronchial biopsy usually diagnostic	Chemotherapy directed at underlying primary cancer

BAL bronchoalveolar lavage, *PAS* periodic acid Schiff stain, *GM-CSF* granulocyte-macrophage colony-stimulating factor, *HRCT* high resolution chest computed tomogram, *mTOR* mammalian target of rapamycin, *DIP* desquamative interstitial pneumonia, *LCH* Langerhans' cell histiocytosis, *CNS* central nervous system gravis, other autoimmune disorders, myeloid leukemias, and even in rare cases in normal, healthy individuals. Conversely, although the sensitivity of the test was initially thought to approach 100%, there are rare cases of primary PAP in which autoantibodies cannot be isolated [1].

Alveolar macrophages from patients with PAP and from GM-CSF deficient mice are phenotypically immature and demonstrate impaired phagocytic function and bacterial killing, impaired cellular adherence, mobility, and chemotaxis, and most importantly, impaired surfactant clearance and catabolism. These deficiencies explain the clinical features of PAP [13]. Restoration of GM-CSF signaling or its down-stream transcription factor, PU.1, restores alveolar macrophage function including both surfactant metabolism and host defense functioning. With our greatly improved understanding of PAP, targeted biologic therapies for PAP have now entered the therapeutic armamentarium. Trials of exogenous GM-CSF to overcome the neutralizing antibodies are described below along with case reports of therapies targeted against antibody production.

The relationship between secondary PAP and anti-GM-CSF antibodies remains a confusing one. In patients in which secondary PAP occurs in the setting of an underlying malignancy, anti-GM-CSF antibodies may or may not be present, and even when present, those antibodies may or may not manifest a neutralizing activity [14, 15]. In those patients in whom the secondary PAP is due to an inhalation exposure, anti-GM-CSF antibodies cannot be demonstrated, but macrophage dysfunction with impaired clearance and catabolism is still hypothesized to be central to the pathogenesis.

Congenital PAP is not associated with anti-GM-CSF antibodies but rather most often results from mutations in surfactant apoprotein B (SP-B), surfactant apoprotein C (SP-C), GM-CSF receptor-α and β-chains, or the ATP-binding cassette transporter A3 (ABCA3) gene [16–22]. The most common of these are SP-B mutations (specifically the 121ins2 frame shift mutation that leads to premature termination and truncation of the SP-B transcript) that lead to SP-B deficiency [23].

Clinical Presentation

More than 90% of PAP is the autoimmune-mediated, sporadic form [1]. Epidemiologically, PAP has a preference for patients who smoke and male gender (2–3 times more common in men), although this may in part be related to increased rates of smoking in men [1, 3]. While it may affect a person at any age, it has a predilection for the 3rd through 6th decades of life [3]. As with other ILDs, patients will complain of insidious, progressive dyspnea on exertion and exercise intolerance, and in point of fact, exertional dyspnea is the single most common presenting complaint of patients with PAP. Cough, chest discomfort, sputum production, hemoptysis, fatigue, malaise, and other constitutional symptoms may also be seen. Patients may also present with incidentally identified abnormal chest imaging but be otherwise asymptomatic. Physical examination, in general, reveals a paucity of findings, and chest auscultation is commonly normal. When abnormalities are present, coarse or bronchial breath sounds, crackles, mild tachypnea, or clubbing may be found [24]. Pulmonary function testing often reveals a reduced diffusing capacity for carbon monoxide. Restrictive physiology may also be seen, but lung volumes and spirometry are commonly within normal limits. Gas exchange assessments may reveal resting or exertional hypoxemia.

Secondary PAP, representing perhaps 7–10% of PAP cases, may occur in a number of clinical settings. These include hematologic malignancies (acute and chronic myelogenous leukemia, acute lymphocytic leukemia, Hodgkin's and non-Hodgkin's lymphomas, myelodysplastic syndrome, and multiple myeloma), inhalation exposures (most notably silica, but also aluminum, cement dust, and titanium), immunodeficiencies (severe common immunodeficiency disorder, IgA deficiency, organ transplantation), lysinuric protein intolerance, and infection, especially HIV, but also potentially including *Pneumocystis jiroveci*, *Nocardia*, cytomegalovirus, and mycobacterial infections. However, it is also important to remember that the macrophage

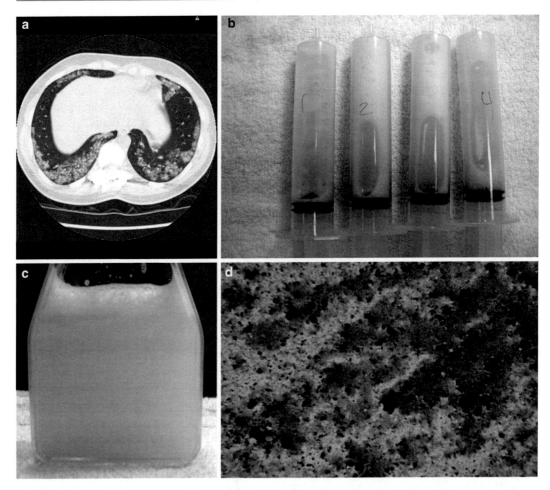

Fig. 16.1 (a) High-resolution computed tomography scan of the chest of a patient with pulmonary alveolar proteinosis (PAP) demonstrating representative, heterogeneous, bilateral ground glass alveolar infiltrates with a "crazy-paving" appearance. (b) Aliquots of bronchoalveolar lavage fluid from a patient with PAP. (c) Pooled aliquots demonstrate the classic "milky" appearance of PAP BALF. (d) Periodic-acid Schiff-positive alveolar lipoproteinaceous, granular material as viewed at ×20 from a patient with PAP. Images courtesy of Dr. Gregory Cosgrove, MD, National Jewish Health, Denver, CO

and neutrophil dysfunction of PAP predispose patients to pulmonary infections, including atypical infections such as *Nocardia*, *Aspergillus* and other fungal pathogens, and mycobacterial infections, such that primary PAP with complicating opportunistic infection must be excluded before settling upon a diagnosis of secondary PAP. Similarly, clinicians must remain vigilant against the possibility of opportunistic infections in their patients with primary PAP.

Congenital PAP presents with neonatal respiratory distress and results from one of a number of genetic abnormalities as outlined earlier. While the histopathology is similar, and the pathogenesis of congenital and autoimmune PAP is related, clinically, congenital PAP remains distinct from primary and secondary PAP.

The "classical" radiologic pattern associated with PAP is the so-called crazy-paving pattern (Fig. 16.1a). The "crazy-paving" appearance takes its name from its visual resemblance to cobblestone masonry. The actual radiologic changes that produce the effect are bilateral, geographic, ground-glass attenuation with an acinar pattern immediately adjacent to inter- and intral-obular septal thickening and/or uninvolved parenchyma creating sharp visual demarcations around the polygonally shaped secondary pulmonary lobules. The crazy-paving pattern is neither sensitive nor specific for PAP. PAP should enter the differential diagnosis of any patient with bilateral, alveolar ground glass or consolidation whether it is symmetric, asymmetric, homogenous, heterogenous, associated with reticular infiltrates or septal thickening or not. Conversely, crazy paving may be seen not only in PAP but also infection, bronchioloalveolar cell carcinoma (BAC), alveolar hemorrhage, acute respiratory distress syndrome, and organizing pneumonia [25]. As mentioned earlier, it is common for the radiographic abnormalities to be much more pronounced than would be anticipated from the clinical symptoms.

Laboratory testing is generally not contributory towards the diagnosis of PAP. Elevated LDH is common but not specific. The presence of anti-GM-CSF antibodies is now the biomarker of choice for PAP and extremely helpful in making a diagnosis of primary PAP when used in conjunction with HRCT imaging and bronchoscopy. While other biomarkers such as KL-6 and SP-A may also be elevated in PAP, these are not generally clinically useful or available in the United States.

Bronchoscopy has traditionally played a key role in the diagnosis of PAP, and PAP is one of the few ILD diagnoses that can be made from BAL [26]. Specifically, patients with suspected PAP should be evaluated via serial instillation and removal of BAL fluid. The lipoproteinaceous material that fills the alveolar spaces confers a "milky" appearance upon the lavagate (Fig. 16.1b, c). The BAL fluid can then be evaluated for the presence of periodic-acid Schiff (PAS) staining positive acellular, granular, amorphous, eosinophilic material characteristic of PAP (Fig. 16.1d). Foamy macrophages filled with diastase-resistant, PAS-positive inclusions can also be identified in the BAL fluid. The combination of a positive lavage and positive anti-GM-CSF antibody is generally sufficient to make a diagnosis of PAP.

In those patients in whom a definite diagnosis of PAP or other diffuse parenchymal lung disease cannot be made, surgical lung biopsy may be required. The histopathology of PAP is characterized by diffuse filling of the airspaces and distal airways with phospholipids and lipoproteinaceous, acellular, granular material that is PAS positive. The alveolar epithelium may be hyperplasic, but the underlying lung architecture is preserved. The presence of an inflammatory infiltrate is uncommon and suggests the presence of a concomitant infection or other secondary process.

Treatment

While a small subset of patients will spontaneously improve or even undergo disease remission (on the order of 8–10%), the majority will develop persistent or progressive disease [3]. Bilateral whole lung lavage (WLL) has served as a mainstay of therapy for PAP, and to date, represents conventional therapy for this disorder [27]. An analysis of the literature by Seymour and Presneill found that patients who have undergone lavage at some point during their illness had a 5-year actuarial survival rate of 94% as compared with 85% for those who did not [3, 28]. WLL is performed in the operating room under general anesthesia with a double lumen endotracheal tube such that the patient is maintained on single lung ventilation while the contralateral lung is lavaged. Specific protocols differ from institution to institution, but the principle of serially instilling and withdrawing (draining to gravity) large volumes of warmed saline until the lavagate "clears" so as to mechanically remove the lipoproteinaceous material from the airspaces is fairly constant. Following WLL, most patients experience an improvement in symptoms and oxygenation. The duration of benefit is variable, but the median time of clinical benefit following WLL is approximately 15 months [3].

Given the recent insights into the pathogenesis of the disorder, and the role of GM-CSF in the pathophysiology of PAP, new targeted biologic therapies have been proposed and have entered into clinical investigation. A number of case series of open label administration of subcutaneous recombinant GM-CSF have been reported in the literature [29]. The largest of these by Venkateshiah et al. described the results of a prospective, open-label trial of subcutaneous GM-CSF in 25 patients with moderately severe PAP [30]. In this group, 21 patients completed the trial, and 12 patients (48% on an intention to treat basis) experienced a beneficial response with improvement in their alveolar-arterial oxygen gradient, room air P_aO_2, DLCO, 6-min walk test distance, and quality of life measures. An earlier study by Seymour et al. of 14 patients similarly found a 35% positive response rate to subcutaneous GM-CSF [31].

More recently, inhaled GM-CSF has been proposed as an alternative method of delivery for patients with PAP [32, 33]. A case series by Wylam et al. of 12 patients who received open-label aerosolized GM-CSF in lieu of WLL or observation alone had a 92% positive response rate [34]. The drug was tolerated well, and patients demonstrated a mean improvement in alveolar-arterial oxygen gradient of 18.4 mmHg and 16.6 percent predicted improvement in DLCO. Other groups of investigators have combined WLL with nebulized GM-CSF theorizing that the aerosolized drug would obtain better lung penetration after WLL [35]. Indeed, this very strategy is the subject of an active, prospective, clinical research trial based in Italy [36]. Still, it is important to remember that GM-CSF therapy remains investigational for the treatment of PAP and should only be offered in centers experienced with its administration. The further question as to whether anti-GM-CSF antibody concentrations can be followed as an adjunct to clinical evaluation to assess a patient's response to therapy also remains an open question [37].

Additional therapies targeted against the production of the blocking autoantibody have been proposed, but to date there is only one case report of open-label, compassionate use of rituximab, a monoclonal antibody directed against the CD20 antigen of antibody-producing B lymphocytes [38]. Nevertheless, given the strong rationale and clinical experience to date with this agent, as of the writing of this chapter, there is an actively enrolling, Phase II, single-center trial prospectively evaluating rituximab for the treatment of

PAP in the United States [39]. Notably, there are also two case reports of plasmapheresis for the treatment of PAP in the literature, one of whom appeared to benefit and another for whom there was a lack of clinical efficacy in spite of a reduction in circulating antibody levels [40, 41].

Lymphangioleiomyomatosis

Introduction

Lymphangioleiomyomatosis (LAM) is a rare multisystem disease that typically occurs in premenopausal women. In the lung, abnormal proliferation of immature-appearing smooth muscle cells (LAM cells) around airways, lymphatic vessels, and blood vessels and within the alveolar interstitium leads to the characteristic pulmonary manifestations, including obstructive lung disease with parenchymal cyst formation and recurrent pneumothorax, chylous pleural effusions, and occlusion of interstitial pulmonary vessels with resultant hemoptysis and hemosiderosis [42]. Extrapulmonary manifestations of disease include benign renal tumors (renal angiomyolipomas) and retroperitoneal or mediastinal lymphangioleiomyomas.

LAM occurs either as a sporadic disease or as a pulmonary manifestation of tuberous sclerosis (TS). TS is an autosomal-dominant neurocutaneous disease classically characterized by seizures, mental retardation, and facial angiofibromas – also called Vogt's triad. Additional features include hamartoma and benign tumor formation in multiple locations. TS results from mutations in one of the TS genes (either the TSC1 or TSC2 gene). In patients with TS, studies have found that approximately one-third of females have TS-associated LAM (cystic lung disease similar to that found in sporadic LAM) [43].

Pathophysiology

Sporadic LAM and TS-associated LAM result from mutations in one of the TS genes. The TSC1 gene encodes the protein hamartin while TSC2 encodes the protein tuberin. Both TSC1 and TSC2 are tumor suppressor genes that regulate intracellular signaling; the loss of either one of these inhibitor proteins results in the constitutive activation of mammalian target of rapamycin (mTOR). This ultimately leads to abnormal cell proliferation, migration, and invasion of these cells – and the clinical manifestations of disease [44]. In sporadic LAM, homozygous mutations in TSC2 have been identified in cells from the lung, lymph nodes, and kidneys of affected patients [45]. TS-associated LAM has been associated with heterozygous germline mutations in TSC1 or TSC2, and lung manifestations may result after the loss of heterozygosity of the normal allele. Thus, as sporadic LAM does not contain germline mutation, it is not transmitted from mother to daughter, whereas TS-associated LAM transmission has been reported [46]. Because LAM is a disease of premenopausal women, estrogen has long been hypothesized to play a role in the disease process. Recent studies suggest that estrogen releases cells from the negative inhibition of downstream mTOR products in those with either of the TS mutations perpetuating this abnormal response of LAM cells [47].

In sporadic LAM, the origin of the LAM cells is unknown. However, these cells have been detected in the blood and lymphatics of patients with LAM. Thus, some hypothesize that LAM represents "the simplest form of human cancers," whereby LAM cells have characteristics of malignancy, including unregulated growth, spread via the blood and/or lymphatics, and invasion of tissue [44, 48].

Gross pathology of the lungs reveals both lung enlargement and cysts ranging from 0.5 to 2.0 cm in diameter. Histopathology characteristically reveals foci of LAM cells, which form nodules, next to areas of cystic change and within the walls of airways, lymphatics, bloods vessels, and the alveolar interstitium (Fig. 16.2). These foci of LAM cells lead to the characteristic manifestations of disease including obstructive lung disease with parenchymal cyst formation and recurrent pneumothorax, chylous pleural effusions, and occlusion of interstitial pulmonary vessels with resultant hemoptysis and hemosiderosis. Foci of LAM cells contain two distinct populations of cells: (1) small spindle-shaped cells located at the center of these nodules, and (2) large epithelioid cells with abundant cytoplasm located at the periphery. Both populations of cells react with antibodies to smooth-muscle specific antigens, but the peripheral cells of the nodules are more likely to be immunoreactive for human melanocyte black 45 (HMB45) antibodies – normally a marker of melanoma cells and immature melanocytes. These LAM cells can also be seen in small cell clusters within the lung parenchyma [49].

Epidemiology

The prevalence of sporadic LAM is estimated between 1 and 5 per 1,000,000 women [50, 51]. Given the prevalence of TS, the predicted prevalence of TS-associated LAM (estimated to be approximately 34% of women with TS) is higher than that of sporadic LAM [43]. However, the National Heart, Lung, and Blood Institute (NHLBI) LAM Registry found that sporadic LAM represented just over 85% of cases. Possible reasons for this discrepancy include that TS-associated LAM clinically manifests as a milder disease and may be unrecognized or that TS-associated LAM is overlooked as other comorbidities (e.g., seizures) receive more attention. In support of the theory that TS-associated LAM may be associated with milder disease, the NHLBI registry found that women with TS-associated LAM had less impaired lung function than those with sporadic disease [52].

Clinical Features

Presenting Features

The mean age of diagnosis ranges between 36 and 43 years. As compared to those diagnosed years ago, those more recently diagnosed tend to be at the older age of this range suggesting the mean age of diagnosis is increasing over time [53]. Although LAM is a systemic disease, pulmonary symptoms typically predominate with

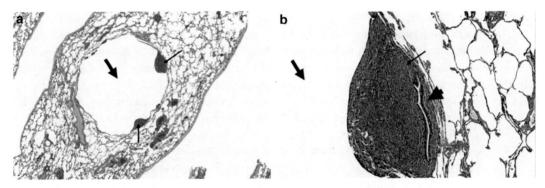

Fig. 16.2 (**a**) Photomicrograph (original magnification, ×2) with hematoxylin and eosin staining of lung tissue from a patient with lymphangioleiomyomatosis (LAM) demonstrates the classic cystic lesion (*thick arrow*) with LAM nodules abutting the cystic space (*thin arrows*). (**b**) Photomicrograph (original magnifi- cation, ×20) with hematoxylin and eosin staining of LAM nodule at higher magnification reveals that the LAM nodule (*thin arrow*) is actually constricting a bronchiole (*arrow head*) thereby possibly leading to the cystic lesion (*thick arrow*) through a ball-valve mechanism

the most common symptoms and manifestations being progressive breathlessness, pneumothorax, fatigue, chest pain, and cough. Dyspnea usually results from progressive cystic involvement of the parenchyma, and tends to be more common in older patients, while pneumothorax, occurring in as many as 76% of patients with disease, tends to be more common in younger patients. Although chylothorax is a classic manifestation of pulmonary disease, studies indicate it occurs in only approximately 20% of patients [53]. Patients with TS-associated LAM tend to be diagnosed at a younger age (36.9 years versus 40.5 years); they are less likely to report dyspnea and more likely to report fatigue [53].

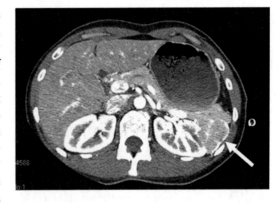

Fig. 16.3 Computed tomography with contrast of the abdomen revealing a left renal angiomyolipoma (*white arrow*) in a lymphangioleiomyomatosis patient

Extrapulmonary Features

In general, renal angiomyolipomas are clinically silent, but flank pain, hematuria, hydronephrosis, renal insufficiency, and rupture resulting in life-threatening retroperitoneal hemorrhage may occur (Fig. 16.3) [54]. These tumors are more common in those with TS-associated LAM (approaching 90%) than in those with sporadic disease (estimated to occur in approximately 35–50% of patients) [53]. Lymphangioleio-myomas, which occur in the retroperitoneum or mediastinum, are present in 20% of patients with sporadic LAM. Symptoms may include abdominal pain, constipation, fecal incontinence, urinary urgency, and peripheral lymphedema.

Pulmonary Physiology

Using data from the NHLBI registry, the most common pulmonary function abnormality is an obstructive pattern occurring in 57.3% of patients followed by a low diffusing capacity occurring in 56.9% of patients. Normal spirometry was noted in 33.9%, whereas a restrictive pattern occurred in 11.4% of patients. Further, several reports have found that in those with obstructive physiology, as many as 25–50% of patients have a significant bronchodilator response [52, 55].

Imaging and Differential Diagnosis

HRCT reveals bilateral thin-walled cysts throughout all lung zones – occasionally with apical

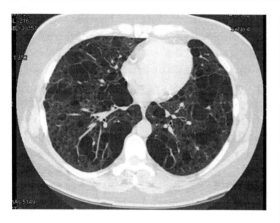

Fig. 16.4 High-resolution computed tomography image of the chest from a 51-year-old female with biopsy proven lymphangioleiomyomatosis demonstrating well-demarcated, large cysts

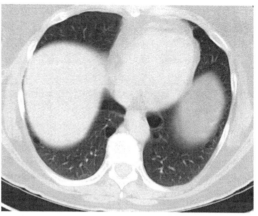

Fig. 16.5 Computed tomography of a 62-year-old woman with genetically proven Birt–Hogg–Dubé demonstrating basilar- and peripheral-predominant cysts

sparing. Less commonly, imaging reveals septal thickening (presumed to be secondary to lymphatic obstruction), ground-glass opacities and/or consolidation (presumed to be secondary to pulmonary hemorrhage), nodular densities, and hilar or mediastinal lymphadenopathy (Fig. 16.4) [50]. The differential diagnosis of cystic lung disease includes Langerhans cell histiocytosis (LCH), cystic emphysema, lymphocytic interstitial pneumonia (LIP)/Sjögrens syndrome, and Birt–Hogg–Dubé (BHD) syndrome. LCH typically spares the costophrenic sulci and is associated with bizarre and irregularly shaped cysts and nodules. Cystic emphysema, unlike LAM, characteristically has vessels in the center of cysts. BHD is an autosomal-dominant genodermatosis characterized by the development of multiple fibrofolliculomas, renal neoplasms, and pulmonary cysts with resultant spontaneous pneumothoraces. BHD results from mutations in the FLCN gene encoding folliculin (another tumor-suppressor protein). While the pulmonary cysts may appear similar to those in LAM, their location tends to be more basilar and peripheral in location (Fig. 16.5).

Diagnosis

The diagnosis of LAM can be made in patients with characteristic thin-walled cystic lesions on HRCT and with either a diagnosis of TS or known

extrapulmonary manifestations of LAM (e.g., renal angiomyolipomas). With isolated lung involvement, however, the gold standard for the diagnosis of LAM remains a surgical lung biopsy demonstrating the characteristic histologic pattern (described above) and HMB-45 antibody positivity. Several reports of transbronchial biopsies with HMB-45 antibody positivity yielding a diagnosis have been published, but the sensitivity of this technique is unknown [56].

Recent efforts have focused on defining possible biomarkers for the diagnosis of LAM and thereby eliminating the need for surgical lung biopsy in those with lung-limited disease. Young et al. found that serum vascular endothelial growth factor – D (VEGF-D) levels were significantly higher in those with LAM than in controls or in other cystic forms of lung disease (i.e., LCH and emphysema) [57]. However, others found that VEGF-D was only a fair marker for diagnosing disease and instead was a better indicator of extent of lymphatic involvement in LAM [58]. Studies regarding additional potential biomarkers are ongoing.

Management

Management of Pulmonary Disease

No therapy has been proven beneficial for the treatment of LAM. Traditional therapies have targeted the antagonism of estrogen based on the observation that the disease generally occurs in premenopausal women and after a case report of significant improvement after progesterone therapy [59]. However, a recent retrospective analysis found that progesterone (either by the IM or oral route) did not slow the decline in FEV_1 in LAM patients, but did accelerate the rate of decline in DLCO compared to untreated patients [60]. Based on these findings, the use of progesterone for the treatment of LAM has been questioned [60]. Because other studies suggest that certain patients may respond to progesterone therapy [61, 62], some experts will treat patients with a documented decline in lung function with a trial of high-dose medroxyprogesterone acetate. Similarly, no convincing data are available regarding the use of other antiestrogen therapies including oophorectomy, gonadotrophin-releasing hormone (GnRH), analogs luteinizing hormone-releasing hormone (LHRH) analogs, and tamoxifen [44].

At this point, supportive care, consideration of enrollment in clinical trials, and referral for lung transplantation when indicated should be employed in management strategies. In patients that exhibit a bronchodilator response, bronchodilator therapy may provide some symptomatic relief [55]. A recent proof-of-principle trial using sirolimus (an mTOR inhibitor) in 20 patients with angiomyolipomas found that tumor volume decreased by nearly 50% after 1 year of therapy. Further, in the 11 of the 20 patients with LAM, significant improvement in FEV_1 and FVC and reduction in residual volume were noted [63]. Thus, clinical trials are underway investigating the effects of mTOR inhibitors (including sirolimus and everolimus). More information regarding these and other clinical trials can be found at http://www.clinicaltrials.gov.

In those with end-stage LAM, lung transplantation may be a therapeutic option. A recent review of transplants for LAM performed from 1987 to 2002 revealed survival rates of 65% at 5 years; these rates were similar to the rates in those who received a transplant for other indications [64]. LAM has been reported to recur after transplantation with the LAM cells originating from the recipient supporting the theory that LAM results from the migration of these abnormal cells to the lungs; however, this complication is rarely reported [65].

Management of Pleural Disease

Pneumothoraces are reported to occur in as many as 76% of LAM patients and may be the presenting manifestation in over half of patients. Because the rate of recurrence is as high as 81% [66], most support an early interventional procedure (either chemical pleurodesis or surgery) after the first pneumothorax. The recurrence rate falls to 27% after chemical pleurodesis and falls to 32% after surgical pleurodesis [67].

Chylothorax is less common occurring in approximately 20% of LAM patients. Conservative treatment includes aspiration or thoracostomy tube drainage with dietary substitution of long- to medium-chain triglycerides; however, patients may ultimately require chemical or surgical pleurodesis to prevent recurrence. Other management strategies (with variable success reported) include thoracic duct ligation, placement of a LeVeen shunt, octreotide, and progesterone therapy [66].

Other Issues

Although the data are limited, reports indicate that some patients with LAM may experience a significant exacerbation of pulmonary symptoms during pregnancy. It is unclear whether pregnancy causes the acute progression of LAM or pregnancy stresses the cardiopulmonary system thereby worsening the symptoms of LAM. In a recent retrospective study of 117 patients with LAM, those who were diagnosed with LAM prior to or during pregnancy had significantly lower pulmonary function when compared to those who were never pregnant supporting the notion that pregnancy adversely affects the natural history of LAM [68]. However, because the data are limited, decisions regarding pregnancy or an unplanned pregnancy should be made after discussion of the risks and on an individual basis.

Given the association of spontaneous pneumothoraces with underlying LAM, air travel represents a special concern for patients. Indeed, pneumothorax with air travel has been reported in individual cases. Nevertheless, air travel is well tolerated by the vast majority of patients with LAM. Still, patients with a history of multiple pneumothoraces may be at higher risk of recurrent pneumothorax during air travel and should be cautioned against air travel.

The risk of angiomyolipoma rupture appears to be related to tumor size (>4 cm) and aneurysm size (>5 mm) [69]. Thus, monitoring of these lesions is warranted and interventions (including embolization and partial nephrectomy) are recommended when tumors exceed 4 cm. Patients with TSC-associated LAM are more likely to have larger tumors and more aneurysms within the tumors. Should atypical renal lesions be detected on imaging, including solid renal masses with little fat, malignancy should be considered as some patients do develop malignant renal angiomyolipomas and renal cell carcinomas.

Prognosis

Using data from case reports and autopsy series, initial estimates of survival were less than 10 years from symptom onset in the majority of LAM patients. However, studies published in the past 10 years indicate a better survival than previously reported. Using a French LAM registry, Urban et al. reported a 10-year survival of 71%, while recent analysis of the UK LAM database found that 10-year survival was 91% from symptom onset [50, 70].

While many patients with LAM appear to have an indolent course of disease, some do have a more rapid deterioration leading to poorer prognosis. Hayashida et al. found that presenting features of LAM affected outcome: the 10-year survival was 89% in those presenting with pneumothorax, whereas the 10-year survival was 60% in those presenting with exertional dyspnea [71]. Further, the histologic severity of lung involvement at surgical lung biopsy also appears to affect survival [72]. The clinical predictors of accelerated disease and the factors that account for these differences in disease course have not been fully elucidated and are under active investigation.

Pulmonary Langerhans Cell Histiocytosis (Eosinophilic Granuloma)

Pulmonary Langerhans cell histiocytosis (PLCH) is a rare ILD that is related to tobacco smoke exposure in ≥90% of cases. As such, it is often found in the differential diagnosis of tobacco-associated ILDs which also includes respiratory bronchiolitis-associated interstitial lung disease (RB-ILD) and desquamative interstitial pneumonia (DIP), and in some cases, PLCH may be found concurrent with COPD, DIP, or RB-ILD. The radiographic appearance of PLCH is one of cysts and nodules, such that PLCH is also often found in the differential diagnosis of cystic lung disease, which in turn may include LAM (discussed earlier), TS, LIP, DIP, sarcoidosis, COPD/emphysema, and pulmonary infections such as *Pneumocystis jiroveci*. However, it should be remembered that PLCH is ultimately a rare ILD that occurs in ≤5% of surgical lung biopsies for ILD and therefore is a diagnostic challenge for the practicing clinician. A full discussion of PLCH is found in Chap. XX, Tobacco-Associated Interstitial Lung Diseases.

Aspiration

Several pulmonary syndromes may develop following the acute aspiration of gastric contents including acute respiratory distress syndrome, worsening asthma, bronchiolitis, infectious pneumonia, and lung abscess. In patients with repeated aspiration events, bronchiolitis, bronchiectasis, organizing pneumonia, or interstitial fibrosis may all occur [73]. Although the injury from an acute aspiration event usually resolves completely, it may lead to persistent interstitial infiltrates [74]. In point of fact, several studies have found a correlation between gastroesophageal reflux and interstitial fibrosis. Additional studies have noted a correlation between gastroesophageal reflux and both IPF and scleroderma lung fibrosis [75, 76]. These studies suggest that repeated aspiration events may contribute to the etiology of these fibrosing lung diseases. The presumed mechanism is that chemical injury due to reflux leads to parenchymal inflammation and then fibrosis [77]. The evidence remains unclear as to the benefit of reflux treatment in affecting disease progression [78].

A more insidious form of fibrosing lung disease has also been reported with recurrent subclinical aspiration of gastric contents [74]. This entity is often associated with hiatal hernia, gastroesophageal reflux, and other esophageal or neurologic problems. Additional risk factors include advanced age, obesity, sleep apnea, and drug and alcohol abuse. Symptoms may include reflux, dyspnea, cough, and bronchospasm. That said, the majority of patients with fibrosing lung disease and manometric or pH probe evidence of esophageal reflux are asymptomatic. Slowly progressive reticulonodular densities appear on the chest radiograph and are located primarily in the lower lung zones. Chest computed tomography (CT) scans often demonstrate migratory alveolar infiltrates, tree-in-bud changes, and centrilobular nodularity. Changes are often most pronounced in the dependent areas of the lungs. Evidence of hiatal hernia or esophageal dysmotility provides further support for aspiration. Histology may show airways inflammation in addition to varying degrees of interstitial inflammation and fibrosis. Foreign body granulomas strongly support the diagnosis, but these are often absent.

Bronchiolar disease is also commonly associated with chronic aspiration. Diffuse aspiration bronchiolitis is typically a disease of the elderly. Symptoms include bronchorrhea, bronchospasm, and dyspnea. More than half of affected patients have dementia or neurologic disease [79, 80].

A diagnosis of aspiration-induced ILD is often difficult to establish. Compatible imaging findings may suggest the diagnosis. Bronchioloalveolar lavage may demonstrate lipid-laden alveolar macrophages [81]. Patients are often poor candidates for lung biopsy. Techniques to prevent aspiration and pharmacologic neutralization of gastric acid are the recommended therapy. Acid suppression alone is often insufficient. Fundoplication may benefit selected patients.

Lipoid Pneumonia

Lipoid pneumonia results from the inhalation or aspiration of an oil-based substance. The most common cause of lipoid pneumonia is aspiration of ingested mineral oil, particularly in patients with esophageal disorders, gastroesophageal reflux, or neurologic disease. Another frequent cause of lipoid pneumonia is the aspiration of

petroleum jelly or an oil-based spray used for nasal lubrication. Lipoid pneumonias from a variety of other oil- or lipid-based products have also been described.

Lipoid pneumonia commonly presents in one of three ways: (1) an incidental finding on the chest radiograph in an asymptomatic patient; (2) an acute or subacute presentation with cough, sputum, fever, and basilar alveolar infiltrates on the chest radiograph; and (3) cough and dyspnea of some duration with reticulonodular bibasilar infiltrates [82]. Community-acquired pneumonia may be superimposed on lipoid pneumonia. Hypercalcemia has been reported in association with lipoid pneumonia, and this may be due to the production of vitamin D by the granulomatous cells similar to that which occurs in sarcoidosis [83].

In the more acute forms, alveolar infiltrates and occasionally consolidation are evident on chest imaging. With repeated aspiration, a granulomatous and fibrotic reaction occurs producing reticulonodular infiltrates and contraction of the involved lobes. The lower lobes, and particularly the right lower lobe, are most affected. Moreover, because this is an ongoing process in most cases, alveolar infiltrates are often superimposed on interstitial infiltrates. A CT scan demonstrating alveolar infiltrates with fat density (low attenuation) is highly suggestive of this diagnosis [84]. The CT angiogram sign, characterized by visible arteries coursing through an area of consolidation, is another description of the low attenuation infiltration. A "crazy-paving pattern" of well-defined areas of ground-glass attenuation with superimposed septal thickening may be seen. Hilar adenopathy, pleural effusions, or cavitation in a known case of lipoid pneumonia should raise suspicion for a complicating infection or malignancy.

Mineral oils and other lipids increase the risk of aspiration [82, 85, 86]. These bland oils do not stimulate a gag reflex or cough, and they inhibit ciliary function. In addition, mineral oil floats to the top of a column of undigested food in the esophagus and is first to be aspirated in patients with esophageal disorders. As alveolar macrophages engulf the aspirated mineral oil, the oil damages the phagocytic cells and is released into the alveolar environment. This results in inflammation, the development of foreign body granulomas with giant cells, and subsequent fibroblastic proliferation and collagen deposition. In more advanced lipoid pneumonia, there is a chronic granulomatous pneumonitis with fibroblastic proliferation, fibrosis, masses of foamy macrophages, and foreign-body giant cells [87]. Various histologic stages of exogenous lipoid pneumonia are present in the same biopsy specimen because the pathophysiologic process spans months to years before coming to clinical attention.

The identification of alveolar macrophages with foamy cytoplasms or abundant free-lipid material in the sputum or BAL confirms the diagnosis [88]. BAL shows alveolar macrophages with abundant lipid-laden cytoplasmic vacuoles that stain positively with Sudan stains or oil red O stains. While alveolar macrophages with vacuolated cytoplasms are also seen with PAP and drug-induced lung disease due to amiodarone, these do not stain positively with the Sudan or oil red O stains. Lung biopsy is sometimes necessary. If a case of unknown ILD proves to be lipoid pneumonia on the biopsy specimen, careful questioning of the patient will reveal the source.

Treatment for lipoid pneumonia focuses on the discontinuation of the offending oil. If discontinued in a timely manner, the prognosis is good. On the other hand, death may occur from an overwhelming aspiration, a superimposed infection, or a comorbid illness. Corticosteroids are effective for the acute pneumonitis and in some chronic cases [89]. Some cases may resolve spontaneously, and success with WLL also has been reported [90].

Amyloidosis

Amyloidosis is characterized by the extracellular accumulation of amyloid fibrils [91]. Pathologically, this appears as amorphous eosinophilic material that stains positively with Congo red dye and reveals a characteristic apple-green birefringence under polarized light (Fig. 16.6). Amyloid material is composed of fibrillary pro-

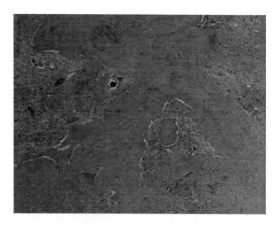

Fig. 16.6 Photomicrograph (original magnification, ×20) from a patient with amyloidosis demonstrating deposition of amorphous eosinophilic material within the airspaces and interstitium (courtesy of Dr. Carlyne Cool, MD, Division of Pathology, National Jewish Health, Denver, CO)

teins arranged in twisted β-pleated sheets. Two amyloid proteins, AA and AL, cause the majority of amyloid-related disease. AA, the major component of secondary amyloidosis, is derived from an acute serum protein of hepatic origin. The AA protein is produced in chronic inflammatory conditions – both autoimmune diseases and chronic infections. The AL protein originates from the variable portion of the immunoglobulin light chain, usually the lambda rather than the kappa light chain. This monoclonal immunoglobulin light chain is produced in patients with systemic primary amyloidosis and amyloidosis associated with multiple myeloma.

Primary amyloidosis is a plasma cell dyscrasia resulting from an abnormal proliferation of plasma cells that produce both a monoclonal gammopathy and excessive light chain deposition in the extracellular matrix of various tissues. In addition to respiratory tract involvement, nephrotic syndrome develops in 33% of patients, cardiomyopathy in 25%, neuropathy in 17%, and gastrointestinal involvement in 8% of cases. Primary amyloidosis can be systemic in nature, or sometimes, can affect a single organ system, such as the respiratory tract. Respiratory tract involvement occurs in 30–90% of cases of primary amyloidosis.

Secondary amyloidosis, with incidental lung involvement, appears with other diffuse lung and systemic diseases such as tuberculosis, lupus erythematosus, alveolar proteinosis, bronchiectasis, Sjögren's syndrome, rheumatoid arthritis, LIP, pulmonary lymphoma, hypersensitivity pneumonitis, cystic fibrosis, and Crohn's disease. Rarely, AA amyloid primarily causes a diffuse ILD.

Tracheobronchial Amyloidosis

Tracheobronchial amyloidosis is a form of primary amyloidosis (AL) that is localized to the respiratory tract and not associated with other systemic involvement [92–96]. This condition usually does not produce symptoms until the fifth or sixth decade. It presents as either an isolated endobronchial or tracheal tumor or as diffuse constricting plaques involving major portions of the tracheobronchial tree. The symptoms relate to the severity, extent, and location of the lesions. Wheezing and hemoptysis often occur, and tracheobronchial amyloid may mimic asthma [97]. A single endobronchial polyp may cause lobar atelectasis or bronchiectasis and obstructive pneumonia. CT demonstrates marked tracheal thickening and narrowing of the main lobar and segmental bronchi. At time of bronchoscopy, submucosal shiny pale plaques are visible, as are regions of localized bronchostenosis. Still, it is often difficult to differentiate between localized endobronchial amyloidosis and endobronchial malignancy on bronchoscopic inspection. Endobronchial resection or lobectomy generally yields an excellent therapeutic result. Laser ablation and external beam radiation also appear to be effective therapeutic modalities.

Nodular Parenchymal Amyloidosis

Nodular parenchymal amyloidosis, similar to the tracheobronchial form, is usually an isolated pulmonary manifestation of primary amyloidosis [93–96]. Approximately 1/3 of cases present as an asymptomatic, single rounded "coin" lesion, or amyloidoma. The other two-third of cases present as the multinodular form of the disease and must be differentiated from malignancy and infection (i.e., miliary tuberculosis). The nodules are slow growing, can cavitate and calcify, but are rarely the cause of significant symptoms or physiologic impairment. The multinodular form has been reported to occur with Sjögren's syndrome, hypergammaglobulinemic purpura, human immunodeficiency virus infection, Crohn's disease, intravenous drug abuse, and asbestos exposure. It has also been associated with isolated low-grade pulmonary lymphomas and Waldenstrom's macroglobulinemia [47]. Histology indicates focal calcification and ossification in addition to the amorphous eosinophilic material. A cellular infiltrate of lymphocytes, histiocytes, and multinucleated giant cells frequently surrounds these lesions. Recurrence of an isolated amyloidoma rarely, if ever, occurs following resection. Multifocal nodular pulmonary amyloidosis, although not a surgically treatable disease, has an excellent prognosis.

Diffuse Alveolar Septal Amyloidosis

Diffuse alveolar septal or interstitial amyloidosis occurs with either primary amyloidosis or multiple myeloma [93–96]. It rarely presents without evidence of systemic involvement. Although diffuse pulmonary involvement frequently occurs with primary amyloidosis, it only contributes to mortality in 5–10% of cases. Once respiratory symptoms develop, survival is usually less than 2 years. Diffuse alveolar septal amyloidosis is often associated with cardiac muscle and pulmonary vascular involvement. Electron microscopic studies demonstrate that the amyloid is deposited within the interstitium, within the walls of small blood vessels, and the alveolar capillary basement membranes.

Progressive dyspnea and cough are the most prominent symptoms and must be differentiated from left ventricular failure due to myocardial amyloid. Recurrent hemoptysis can result from the dissection of involved pulmonary vessels. Severe pulmonary hypertension can appear secondary to diffuse vascular involvement [98]. The chest radiograph shows diffuse reticulonodular infiltrates and occasionally hilar and mediastinal lymph nodes. HRCT scans occasionally demonstrate calcification within the interstitial infiltrates.

Diffuse parenchymal cyst formation has also been seen on HRCT [99]. Pleural effusions result from direct involvement of the pleura or from congestive heart failure. Diagnosis is established on lung biopsy, revealing an eosinophilic, amorphous substance within alveolar walls as well as vessels that exhibit an apple-green birefringence with Congo red stain. Corticosteroids, melphalan, and colchicine have been used with variable results for the treatment of primary systemic amyloidosis. Intensive intravenous melphalan coupled with blood stem cell transplantation eradicates the underlying plasma cell dyscrasia and improves the nephrotic syndrome. The effect of this therapy on the diffuse lung involvement is unknown.

Erdheim–Chester Disease

Erdheim–Chester disease is a non-LCH of unknown etiology that results in xanthomatous and xanthogranulomatous tissue deposition [100]. The most common complaint is bone pain. The pathognomonic finding is symmetric sclerosis of the metaphysis and diaphysis of long bones due to histiocytic infiltration. Extraskeletal involvement affects the skin, hypothalamus, posterior pituitary, orbits, retroperitoneum, and heart. Subglottic stenosis has been reported.

Lung involvement occurs in up to 20% of cases and can cause significant morbidity and mortality [100]. There are diffuse interstitial infiltrates that sometimes demonstrate an upper lobe predominance on the chest radiograph. The CT scan shows thickening of the visceral pleura and interlobular septa with patchy reticular and centrilobular opacities, as well as ground-glass attenuation [101, 102]. Periaortic fibrosis, termed as "coated aorta," is found in at least half of cases. Pericardial effusion and pericardial thickening are common [103].

Lung pathology is characterized by thickening of the visceral pleura, interlobular septa, and bronchovascular bundles with inflammation and fibrosis. The infiltrate consists of foamy histiocytes, lymphocytes, and scattered giant cells in a lymphatic distribution. The histiocytes are invariably CD68-positive, negative for CD1a, and without Birbeck granules on electron microscopy. These findings distinguish Erdheim–Chester from LCH. Variable S-100 staining has been reported [101, 104]. A clonal population of histiocytes has been observed in some patients suggesting this may be a neoplastic disorder [105].

The prognosis is poor with a mortality of 59% over a mean follow-up of 32 months in the largest cohort [100]. There is no effective treatment, although case reports describe some improvement with interferon-α, cyclophosphamide, and chemotherapy regimens.

Hermansky–Pudlak Syndrome

Hermansky–Pudlak syndrome (HPS) is a recessively inherited disease characterized by dysfunctional production or trafficking of organelles that include platelet dense granules, melanosomes, and lysosomes [106–109]. Affected patients may have partial oculocutaneous albinism, a bleeding diathesis due to platelet dysfunction, and complications related to the accumulation of ceroid in the reticuloendothelial system of various tissues. Ceroid deposition may cause pulmonary fibrosis, granulomatous colitis, and renal failure. The bone marrow, heart, spleen, and other tissues may also be involved.

The majority of all HPS cases are from northwestern Puerto Rico and southern Holland. Eight subtypes have been identified. Pulmonary fibrosis is associated with up to 80% of cases with HPS subtypes 1 or 4 [107, 110]. Respiratory symptoms usually appear during the third or fourth decade. Lung involvement is slowly progressive and results in worsening dyspnea and restrictive pulmonary physiology. The chest imaging is nonspecific. A mixed pattern of diffuse, peripheral predominant reticulation, ground-glass opacities and honeycombing often occurs. Peribronchovascular thickening and bronchiectasis may also be seen [110].

The fibrosis appears to be due to the accumulation of ceroid, an insoluble fluorescent lipoprotein, in extracellular spaces and in the lysosomes of alveolar macrophages. Indeed, histology demonstrates patchy fibrosis with macrophages filled with ceroid throughout the interstitium and alveolar spaces. Lymphocytic and histiocytic infiltration in a peri-bronchiolar distribution may result in obliterative bronchiolitis.

There is no effective therapy, although successful lung transplantation has been reported. Lung disease is the most frequent cause of death, followed by complications of inflammatory bowel disease and bleeding complications [109, 111].

Neurofibromatosis

Neurofibromatosis (NF) is an autosomal dominant disease characterized by an abnormal proliferation of neural crest cells [112]. Neurofibromatosis 1, also known as Recklinghausen's disease, may affect any organ system. It occurs in 1 of every 3,500 births, although up to half of cases may be sporadic. The mutation occurs in a tumor suppressor gene on chromosome 17. NF most commonly affects the skin and the central nervous system. Cutaneous findings include multiple café-au-lait spots and cutaneous neurofibromas. Hamartomas of the iris (Lisch nodules) are found in at least 90% of cases. Neurofibromatosis 2, or bilateral acoustic neurofibromatosis, has neither skin nor lung disease.

ILD has been reported to occur in 5–23% of patients with NF [113–116]. Lung disease usually presents between the ages of 35 and 60 years, and dyspnea is the most common symptom. The chest radiograph demonstrates lower zone reticulonodular infiltrates with the eventual appearance of bullous changes in the upper zones [113, 117]. A limited number of HRCT scans have been reported. Findings include bullous changes, upper lung predominant small cysts, basilar reticular opacities, and ground-glass opacities [113]. Physiology typically demonstrates slow progression of a mixed obstructive and restrictive ventilatory defect. Alveolar septal fibrosis is the major histopathologic change, but an alveolitis consisting of mononuclear cell infiltrates is found in earlier disease. Scar carcinoma can complicate the fibrotic lung disease. Severe bullous lung disease with airflow limitation also occurs. It has been postulated that the ILD in neurofibromatosis results from excessive collagen deposition rather than from a postinflammatory scarring process. The association between smoking and diffuse lung disease in neurofibromatosis remains unclear [113].

Pulmonary Alveolar Microlithiasis

Pulmonary alveolar microlithiasis (PAM) is a rare disease in which lamellar concretions composed of calcium and phosphorus form within the alveolar spaces. These microliths are between 0.01 and 3.0 mm in diameter and can fill up to 80% of the air spaces [118–120]. Over time, a fibroproliferative response with elaboration of collagen may develop and result in interstitial fibrosis. Microliths may occasionally be found within alveolar walls or in the bronchial submucosa. Extrapulmonary microliths have been reported in the sympathetic nervous system, the gonads, and the kidneys.

PAM has been linked to a mutation in the SLC34A2 gene, a gene that encodes for a sodium-dependent phosphate transporter that clears phosphate from the alveolar space [121]. Mutations in this gene may result in an accumulation of phosphate that chelates calcium and results in the formation of microliths. The familial form of the disease is autosomal recessive [122].

Most cases present between the ages of 30 and 50 years. There is no sex or racial predisposition. One third of cases are familial. Patients may be asymptomatic when first discovered (usually by chest radiograph) and remain so for 20–30 years. There is a gradual onset of cough and dyspnea. The patient may expectorate microliths. Crackles, clubbing, and cor pulmonale appear with interstitial fibrosis. Lung physiology is often normal or mild at the time of diagnosis. Over time, there is a gradual worsening of a restrictive pattern with reduced gas exchange. There is no evidence of systemic calcium metabolism abnormalities [118, 120].

The chest radiograph shows diffuse bilateral, varying-sized, calcified nodular densities with a lower lung zone predominance. Air bronchograms and air alveolograms are visible.

In long-standing cases, hyperinflation due to bullous emphysema appears in the upper lobes; reticulonodular infiltrates and Kerley's B lines due to interstitial fibrosis also are seen. CT scans demonstrate hyperdense or calcific micronodules predominantly in the lower lung zones. The pattern often has a "sandstorm appearance." Other CT findings include ground-glass opacities, interlobular and intralobular reticulation, pleural calcification, and subpleural cysts that appear as a black line between the pleural surface and the involved lung [123]. The diagnosis is usually established from both the chest radiograph and CT scan appearances.

A major competing diagnostic consideration in patients with PAM is diffuse pulmonary ossification. Pulmonary ossification is the formation of immature bone in the lung. It usually occurs in association with chronic lung injury, especially pulmonary fibrosis. It may also be idiopathic or occur in relation to mitral stenosis or other causes of left ventricular failure. The chest radiograph can be similar to PAM, but the calcified nodules of pulmonary ossification are larger than the microliths found in PAM, and the underlying condition usually points to the correct diagnosis. Metastatic pulmonary calcification, seen primarily in patients on chronic hemodialysis, rarely if ever confounds the differential diagnosis. There is no medical therapy. Lung transplantation offers the best treatment option.

Bronchioloalveolar Cell Carcinoma

BAC accounts for approximately 5% of primary lung tumors. Pure BAC is a subtype of lung adenocarcinoma characterized by growth along intact alveolar septa (this is termed "lepidic growth"). BAC with any evidence of invasion of the alveolar septa defines mixed adenocarcinoma with a BAC component. BAC presents as a solitary nodule, multiple nodules, or lobar consolidation. BAC is divided into mucinous, nonmucinous, and mixed subtypes. Histologic appearance and molecular markers determine this distinction. The distinction between mucinous and nonmucinous BAC has important prognostic and therapeutic

implications [124]. The diffuse forms of BAC tend to be mucinous [125].

Patients with the diffuse form of BAC present with progressive dyspnea, cough, fatigue, weight loss, and fever. Symptoms reflect the extent of disease. Occasionally, sputum production is copious due to excessive secretion of mucus by the malignant cells. Patients with bronchorrhea may produce 30 mL to several liters of sputum per day. Volume depletion and prerenal azotemia may complicate bronchorrhea [126, 127].

Patients with BAC are more likely to be female and younger than other patients with lung cancer. Tobacco use is a risk factor, although the association between tobacco and BAC is weaker than for other lung cancers [128, 129]. BAC has been noted to develop in lung scars, either in a localized scar producing a "scar carcinoma" or arising from diffuse fibrotic lung disease.

The chest radiograph in diffuse BAC demonstrates either a pneumonic consolidation or diffuse alveolar nodules. The radiographic appearance may resemble nonresolving pneumonia or other diffuse alveolar filling disease. The CT angiogram sign may be present as the mucinfilled alveoli highlight the adjacent vessels.

Sputum cytology, BAL, or transbronchial lung biopsy establishes the diagnosis. Surgical lung biopsy is rarely necessary in the diffuse forms of BAC. Therapy is similar to that of other nonsmall cell lung cancers [130]. Tyrosine kinase inhibitors are useful for cancers with activating mutations of the epidermal growth factor receptor. These tend to be the nonmucinous form. Mucinous cancers are treated with standard cytotoxic therapy [131].

Lymphangitic Carcinomatosis

Lymphangitic carcinomatosis is a form of metastatic lung disease that produces an interstitial pattern on the chest radiograph. It originates from adenocarcinomas of the breast, lung, stomach, pancreas, prostate, ovary, and kidney [132]. In one large series, lymphangitic carcinomatosis accounted for 8% of all metastatic malignancies to the lung; the most frequent primary sites were breast and stomach [133].

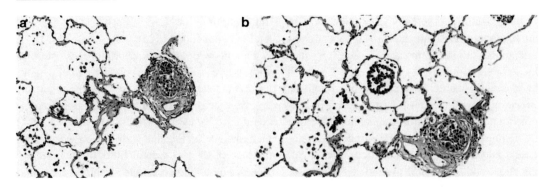

Fig. 16.7 (**a**, **b**) Photomicrographs (original magnification, ×20) from a patient with lymphangitic carcinomatosis (courtesy of Dr. Steve Groshong, MD, Division of Pathology, National Jewish Health, Denver, CO)

Clinically, patients may present with progressive dyspnea, cough, wheezing, or constitutional symptoms. Lymphangitic carcinomatosis progresses rapidly and typically results in cor pulmonale and death within 3–6 months after diagnosis. Tumor emboli, acute cor pulmonale, and severe pulmonary hypertension may also occur [134, 135]. The pulmonary symptoms occasionally precede symptoms referable to the primary tumor site, and thus present as dyspnea with an ILD of unknown etiology. The presence of lymphangitic carcinomatosis in a young adult without an apparent primary site should prompt a search for gastric adenocarcinoma.

The chest radiograph typically demonstrates lower zone Kerley's B lines and reticulonodular infiltrates; extensive involvement of all lung fields occurs over time. The appearance of chest radiographic Kerley's B lines in a patient with ILD with normal left ventricular function should raise the suspicion for lymphangitic carcinomatosis. In addition, pleural effusions and hilar and mediastinal adenopathy may be present. HRCT scans show uneven thickening of bronchovascular bundles, isolated thickening of interstitial lines, and polygonal or septal lines [136, 137]. The physiology demonstrates a restrictive pattern with stiff noncompliant lungs, a reduction in the diffusing capacity for carbon monoxide, and marked gas exchange abnormalities resulting in severe hypoxemia and eventually subacute cor pulmonale.

Histologically, tumor cells fill peribronchial, perivascular, and subpleural lymphatics (Fig. 16.7). In addition, an associated fibrotic reaction in the adjacent alveolar septa accounts for the majority of the parenchymal radiographic findings. The most intriguing histologic feature is an extensive obliterative endarteritis that involves the small muscular pulmonary arteries. Malignant cells are visible within the vessel lumens. This vascular obstruction probably accounts for the development of subacute cor pulmonale [135].

Transbronchial biopsy and bronchial washings are usually diagnostic and obviate the need for a surgical biopsy. Furthermore, endobronchial lymphatic involvement is common, and the diffuse plaque-like infiltrate visible at bronchoscopy is quite accessible to endobronchial biopsy. Therapy is directed at the underlying cancer.

References

1. Inoue Y, Trapnell BC, Tazawa R, et al. Characteristics of a large cohort of patients with autoimmune pulmonary alveolar proteinosis in Japan. Am J Respir Crit Care Med. 2008;177:752–62.
2. Ben-Dov I, Kishinevski Y, Roznman J, et al. Pulmonary alveolar proteinosis in Israel: ethnic clustering. Isr Med Assoc J. 1999;1:75–8.
3. Seymour JF, Presneill JJ. Pulmonary alveolar proteinosis: progress in the first 44 years. Am J Respir Crit Care Med. 2002;166:215–35.
4. Uchida K, Beck DC, Yamamoto T, et al. GM-CSF autoantibodies and neutrophil dysfunction in pulmonary alveolar proteinosis. N Engl J Med. 2007;356: 567–79.
5. Greenhill SR, Kotton DN. Pulmonary alveolar proteinosis: a bench-to-bedside story of granulocyte-macrophage colony-stimulating factor dysfunction. Chest. 2009;136:571–7.

6. Trapnell BC, Whitsett JA, Nakata K. Pulmonary alveolar proteinosis. N Engl J Med. 2003;349:2527–39.
7. Rosen SH, Castleman B, Liebow AA. Pulmonary alveolar proteinosis. N Engl J Med. 1958;258: 1123–42.
8. Dranoff G, Crawford AD, Sadelain M, et al. Involvement of granulocyte-macrophage colony-stimulating factor in pulmonary homeostasis. Science. 1994;264:713–6.
9. Stanley E, Lieschke GJ, Grail D, et al. Granulocyte/macrophage colony-stimulating factor-deficient mice show no major perturbation of hematopoiesis but develop a characteristic pulmonary pathology. Proc Natl Acad Sci USA. 1994;91:5592–6.
10. Kitamura T, Tanaka N, Watanabe J, et al. Idiopathic pulmonary alveolar proteinosis as an autoimmune disease with neutralizing antibody against granulocyte/macrophage colony-stimulating factor. J Exp Med. 1999;190:875–80.
11. Lin FC, Chang GD, Chern MS, Chen YC, Chang SC. Clinical significance of anti-GM-CSF antibodies in idiopathic pulmonary alveolar proteinosis. Thorax. 2006;61:528–34.
12. Bonfield TL, Russell D, Burgess S, Malur A, Kavuru MS, Thomassen MJ. Autoantibodies against granulocyte macrophage colony-stimulating factor are diagnostic for pulmonary alveolar proteinosis. Am J Respir Cell Mol Biol. 2002;27:481–6.
13. Yoshida M, Ikegami M, Reed JA, Chroneos ZC, Whitsett JA. GM-CSF regulates protein and lipid catabolism by alveolar macrophages. Am J Physiol Lung Cell Mol Physiol. 2001;280:L379–86.
14. Sergeeva A, Ono Y, Rios R, Molldrem JJ. High titer autoantibodies to GM-CSF in patients with AML, CML and MDS are associated with active disease. Leukemia. 2008;22:783–90.
15. Huizar I, Kavuru MS. Alveolar proteinosis syndrome: pathogenesis, diagnosis, and management. Curr Opin Pulm Med. 2009;15:491–8.
16. Dirksen U, Hattenhorst U, Schneider P, et al. Defective expression of granulocyte-macrophage colony-stimulating factor/interleukin-3/interleukin-5 receptor common beta chain in children with acute myeloid leukemia associated with respiratory failure. Blood. 1998;92:1097–103.
17. Nogee LM, Dunbar 3rd AE, Wert S, Askin F, Hamvas A, Whitsett JA. Mutations in the surfactant protein C gene associated with interstitial lung disease. Chest. 2002;121:20S–1.
18. Shulenin S, Nogee LM, Annilo T, Wert SE, Whitsett JA, Dean M. ABCA3 gene mutations in newborns with fatal surfactant deficiency. N Engl J Med. 2004;350:1296–303.
19. Nogee LM, Garnier G, Dietz HC, et al. A mutation in the surfactant protein B gene responsible for fatal neonatal respiratory disease in multiple kindreds. J Clin Invest. 1994;93:1860–3.
20. Notarangelo LD, Pessach I. Out of breath: GM-CSFRalpha mutations disrupt surfactant homeostasis. J Exp Med. 2008;205:2693–7.
21. Doan ML, Guillerman RP, Dishop MK, et al. Clinical, radiological and pathological features of ABCA3 mutations in children. Thorax. 2008;63:366–73.
22. Suzuki T, Sakagami T, Rubin BK, et al. Familial pulmonary alveolar proteinosis caused by mutations in CSF2RA. J Exp Med. 2008;205:2703–10.
23. Cole FS, Hamvas A, Rubinstein P, et al. Population-based estimates of surfactant protein B deficiency. Pediatrics. 2000;105:538–41.
24. Goldstein LS, Kavuru MS, Curtis-McCarthy P, Christie HA, Farver C, Stoller JK. Pulmonary alveolar proteinosis: clinical features and outcomes. Chest. 1998;114:1357–62.
25. Rossi SE, Erasmus JJ, Volpacchio M, Franquet T, Castiglioni T, McAdams HP. "Crazy-paving" pattern at thin-section CT of the lungs: radiologic-pathologic overview. Radiographics. 2003;23:1509–19.
26. Milleron BJ, Costabel U, Teschler H, et al. Bronchoalveolar lavage cell data in alveolar proteinosis. Am Rev Respir Dis. 1991;144:1330–2.
27. Shah PL, Hansell D, Lawson PR, Reid KB, Morgan C. Pulmonary alveolar proteinosis: clinical aspects and current concepts on pathogenesis. Thorax. 2000;55:67–77.
28. Presneill JJ, Nakata K, Inoue Y, Seymour JF. Pulmonary alveolar proteinosis. Clin Chest Med. 2004;25:593–613. viii.
29. Kavuru MS, Sullivan EJ, Piccin R, Thomassen MJ, Stoller JK. Exogenous granulocyte-macrophage colony-stimulating factor administration for pulmonary alveolar proteinosis. Am J Respir Crit Care Med. 2000;161:1143–8.
30. Venkateshiah SB, Yan TD, Bonfield TL, et al. An open-label trial of granulocyte macrophage colony stimulating factor therapy for moderate symptomatic pulmonary alveolar proteinosis. Chest. 2006;130: 227–37.
31. Seymour JF, Presneill JJ, Schoch OD, et al. Therapeutic efficacy of granulocyte-macrophage colony-stimulating factor in patients with idiopathic acquired alveolar proteinosis. Am J Respir Crit Care Med. 2001;163: 524–31.
32. Price A, Manson D, Cutz E, Dell S. Pulmonary alveolar proteinosis associated with anti-GM-CSF antibodies in a child: successful treatment with inhaled GM-CSF. Pediatr Pulmonol. 2006;41:367–70.
33. Robinson TE, Trapnell BC, Goris ML, Quittell LM, Cornfield DN. Quantitative analysis of longitudinal response to aerosolized granulocyte-macrophage colony-stimulating factor in two adolescents with autoimmune pulmonary alveolar proteinosis. Chest. 2009;135:842–8.
34. Wylam ME, Ten R, Prakash UB, Nadrous HF, Clawson ML, Anderson PM. Aerosol granulocyte-macrophage colony-stimulating factor for pulmonary alveolar proteinosis. Eur Respir J. 2006;27:585–93.
35. Yamamoto H, Yamaguchi E, Agata H, et al. A combination therapy of whole lung lavage and GM-CSF inhalation in pulmonary alveolar proteinosis. Pediatr Pulmonol. 2008;43:828–30.

36. Luisetti M. Whole lung lavage (WLL)/inhaled granulocyte-macrophage colony-stimulating factor (GM-CSF) in autoimmune pulmonary alveolar proteinosis (PAP). 2009. http://www.clinicaltrials.gov. Last updated 2011.

37. Bonfield TL, Kavuru MS, Thomassen MJ. Anti-GM-CSF titer predicts response to GM-CSF therapy in pulmonary alveolar proteinosis. Clin Immunol. 2002;105:342–50.

38. Borie R, Debray MP, Laine C, Aubier M, Crestani B. Rituximab therapy in autoimmune pulmonary alveolar proteinosis. Eur Respir J. 2009;33:1503–6.

39. Kavuru MS. Prospective trial of rituximab for primary pulmonary alveolar proteinosis (PAP). 2009. http://www.clinicaltrials.gov. Last updated 2011.

40. Luisetti M, Rodi G, Perotti C, et al. Plasmapheresis for treatment of pulmonary alveolar proteinosis. Eur Respir J. 2009;33:1220–2.

41. Kavuru MS, Bonfield TL, Thomassen MJ. Plasmapheresis, GM-CSF, and alveolar proteinosis. Am J Respir Crit Care Med. 2003;167:1036. author reply 1036–1037.

42. Taylor JR, Ryu J, Colby TV, Raffin TA. Lymphangioleiomyomatosis. Clinical course in 32 patients. N Engl J Med. 1990;323:1254–60.

43. Moss J, Avila NA, Barnes PM, et al. Prevalence and clinical characteristics of lymphangioleiomyomatosis (LAM) in patients with tuberous sclerosis complex. Am J Respir Crit Care Med. 2001;164:669–71.

44. McCormack FX. Lymphangioleiomyomatosis: a clinical update. Chest. 2008;133:507–16.

45. Carsillo T, Astrinidis A, Henske EP. Mutations in the tuberous sclerosis complex gene TSC2 are a cause of sporadic pulmonary lymphangioleiomyomatosis. Proc Natl Acad Sci USA. 2000;97:6085–90.

46. Slingerland JM, Grossman RF, Chamberlain D, Tremblay CE. Pulmonary manifestations of tuberous sclerosis in first degree relatives. Thorax. 1989;44:212–4.

47. Okuda M, Okuda Y, Ogura T, et al. Primary lung involvement with amyloid deposition in Waldenstom's macroglobulinemia: observations from over 20 years. Respirology. 2004;9:414–8.

48. Henske EP. Metastasis of benign tumor cells in tuberous sclerosis complex. Genes Chromosomes Cancer. 2003;38:376–81.

49. Krymskaya VP. Smooth muscle-like cells in pulmonary lymphangioleiomyomatosis. Proc Am Thorac Soc. 2008;5:119–26.

50. Urban T, Lazor R, Lacronique J, et al. Pulmonary lymphangioleiomyomatosis. A study of 69 patients. Groupe d'Etudes et de Recherche sur les Maladies "Orphelines" Pulmonaires (GERM"O"P). Medicine (Baltimore). 1999;78:321–37.

51. Chorianopoulos D, Stratakos G. Lymphangioleiomyomatosis and tuberous sclerosis complex. Lung. 2008;186:197–207.

52. Ryu JH, Moss J, Beck GJ, et al. The NHLBI lymphangioleiomyomatosis registry: characteristics of 230 patients at enrollment. Am J Respir Crit Care Med. 2006;173:105–11.

53. Cohen MM, Pollock-BarZiv S, Johnson SR. Emerging clinical picture of lymphangioleiomyomatosis. Thorax. 2005;60:875–9.

54. Maziak DE, Kesten S, Rappaport DC, Maurer J. Extrathoracic angiomyolipomas in lymphangioleiomyomatosis. Eur Respir J. 1996;9:402–5.

55. Taveira-DaSilva AM, Steagall WK, Rabel A, et al. Reversible airflow obstruction in lymphangioleiomyomatosis. Chest. 2009;136:1596–603.

56. Bonetti F, Chiodera PL, Pea M, et al. Transbronchial biopsy in lymphangiomyomatosis of the lung. HMB45 for diagnosis. Am J Surg Pathol. 1993;17:1092–102.

57. Young LR, Inoue Y, McCormack FX. Diagnostic potential of serum VEGF-D for lymphangioleiomyomatosis. N Engl J Med. 2008;358:199–200.

58. Glasgow CG, Avila NA, Lin JP, Stylianou MP, Moss J. Serum vascular endothelial growth factor-D levels in patients with lymphangioleiomyomatosis reflect lymphatic involvement. Chest. 2009;135:1293–300.

59. Sieker HO, McCarty Jr KS. Lymphangiomyomatosis: a respiratory illness with an endocrinologic therapy. Trans Am Clin Climatol Assoc. 1988;99:57–67.

60. Taveira-DaSilva AM, Stylianou MP, Hedin CJ, Hathaway O, Moss J. Decline in lung function in patients with lymphangioleiomyomatosis treated with or without progesterone. Chest. 2004;126:1867–74.

61. Eliasson AH, Phillips YY, Tenholder MF. Treatment of lymphangioleiomyomatosis. A meta-analysis. Chest. 1989;96:1352–5.

62. Schiavina M, Contini P, Fabiani A, et al. Efficacy of hormonal manipulation in lymphangioleiomyomatosis. A 20-year-experience in 36 patients. Sarcoidosis Vasc Diffuse Lung Dis. 2007;24:39–50.

63. Bissler JJ, McCormack FX, Young LR, et al. Sirolimus for angiomyolipoma in tuberous sclerosis complex or lymphangioleiomyomatosis. N Engl J Med. 2008;358:140–51.

64. Kpodonu J, Massad MG, Chaer RA, et al. The US experience with lung transplantation for pulmonary lymphangioleiomyomatosis. J Heart Lung Transplant. 2005;24:1247–53.

65. Bittmann I, Rolf B, Amann G, Lohrs U. Recurrence of lymphangioleiomyomatosis after single lung transplantation: new insights into pathogenesis. Hum Pathol. 2003;34:95–8.

66. Almoosa KF, McCormack FX, Sahn SA. Pleural disease in lymphangioleiomyomatosis. Clin Chest Med. 2006;27:355–68.

67. Almoosa KF, Ryu JH, Mendez J, et al. Management of pneumothorax in lymphangioleiomyomatosis: effects on recurrence and lung transplantation complications. Chest. 2006;129:1274–81.

68. Cohen MM, Freyer AM, Johnson SR, Cohen MM, Freyer AM, Johnson SR. Pregnancy experiences among women with lymphangioleiomyomatosis. Respir Med. 2009;103:766–72.

69. Yamakado K, Tanaka N, Nakagawa T, Kobayashi S, Yanagawa M, Takeda K. Renal angiomyolipoma:

relationships between tumor size, aneurysm formation, and rupture. Radiology. 2002;225:78–82.

70. Johnson SR, Whale CI, Hubbard RB, Lewis SA, Tattersfield AE. Survival and disease progression in UK patients with lymphangioleiomyomatosis. Thorax. 2004;59:800–3.

71. Hayashida M, Seyama K, Inoue Y, Fujimoto K, Kubo K. The epidemiology of lymphangioleiomyomatosis in Japan: a nationwide cross-sectional study of presenting features and prognostic factors. Respirology. 2007;12:523–30.

72. Matsui K, Beasley MB, Nelson WK, et al. Prognostic significance of pulmonary lymphangioleiomyomatosis histologic score. Am J Surg Pathol. 2001;25: 479–84.

73. Morehead RS. Gastro-oesophageal reflux disease and non-asthma lung disease. Eur Respir Rev. 2009;18: 233–43.

74. Pearson JE, Wilson RS. Diffuse pulmonary fibrosis and hiatus hernia. Thorax. 1971;26:300–5.

75. D'Ovidio F, Singer LG, Hadjiliadis D, et al. Prevalence of gastroesophageal reflux in end-stage lung disease candidates for lung transplant. Ann Thorac Surg. 2005;80:1254–60.

76. Raghu G, Freudenberger TD, Yang S, et al. High prevalence of abnormal acid gastro-oesophageal reflux in idiopathic pulmonary fibrosis [see comment]. Eur Respir J. 2006;27:136–42.

77. Knight PR, Davidson BA, Nader ND, et al. Progressive, severe lung injury secondary to the interaction of insults in gastric aspiration. Exp Lung Res. 2004;30:535–57.

78. Raghu G, Yang ST, Spada C, et al. Sole treatment of acid gastroesophageal reflux in idiopathic pulmonary fibrosis: a case series. Chest. 2006;129:794–800.

79. Barnes TW, Vassallo R, Tazelaar HD, Hartman TE, Ryu JH. Diffuse bronchiolar disease due to chronic occult aspiration. Mayo Clin Proc. 2006;81:172–6.

80. Matsuse T, Oka T, Kida K, Fukuchi Y. Importance of diffuse aspiration bronchiolitis caused by chronic occult aspiration in the elderly. Chest. 1996;110: 1289–93.

81. Corwin RW, Irwin RS. The lipid-laden alveolar macrophage as a marker of aspiration in parenchymal lung disease. Am Rev Respir Dis. 1985;132: 576–81.

82. Friedman D, Engelberg H, Merritt W. Oil aspiration (lipoid) pneumonia in adults: A clinical pathological study of 47 cases. Arch Intern Med. 1940;66:11–38.

83. Rolla AR, Granfone A, Balogh K, Khettry U, Davis BL. Granuloma-related hypercalcemia in lipoid pneumonia. Am J Med Sci. 1986;292:313–6.

84. Lee KS, Muller NL, Hale V, Newell Jr JD, Lynch DA, Im JG. Lipoid pneumonia: CT findings. J Comput Assist Tomogr. 1995;19:48–51.

85. Miller A, Bader RA, Bader ME, Teirstein AS, Selikoff IJ. Mineral oil pneumonia. Ann Intern Med. 1962;57:627–34.

86. Hughes RL, Freilich RA, Bytell DE, Craig RM, Moran JM. Clinical conference in pulmonary disease. Aspiration and occult esophageal disorders. Chest. 1981;80:489–95.

87. Weill H, Ferrans VJ, Gay RM, Ziskind MM. Early lipoid pneumonia. Roentgenologic, anatomic, and physiologic characteristics. Am J Med. 1964;36: 370–6.

88. Lauque D, Dongay G, Levade T, Caratero C, Carles P. Bronchoalveolar lavage in liquid paraffin pneumonitis. Chest. 1990;98:1149–55.

89. Chin NK, Hui KP, Sinniah R, Chan TB. Idiopathic lipoid pneumonia in an adult treated with prednisolone. Chest. 1994;105:956–7.

90. Chang HY, Chen CW, Chen CY, et al. Successful treatment of diffuse lipoid pneumonitis with whole lung lavage. Thorax. 1993;48:947–8.

91. Pepys MB. Amyloidosis. Annu Rev Med. 2006;57: 223–41.

92. O'Regan A, Fenlon HM, Beamis Jr JF, Steele MP, Skinner M, Berk JL. Tracheobronchial amyloidosis. The Boston University experience from 1984 to 1999. Medicine (Baltimore). 2000;79:69–79.

93. Hui AN, Koss MN, Hochholzer L, Wehunt WD. Amyloidosis presenting in the lower respiratory tract. Clinicopathologic, radiologic, immunohistochemical, and histochemical studies on 48 cases. Arch Pathol Lab Med. 1986;110:212–8.

94. Cordier JF, Loire R, Brune J. Amyloidosis of the lower respiratory tract. Clinical and pathologic features in a series of 21 patients. Chest. 1986;90:827–31.

95. Smith RR, Hutchins GM, Moore GW, Humphrey RL. Type and distribution of pulmonary parenchymal and vascular amyloid. Correlation with cardiac amyloid. Am J Med. 1979;66:96–104.

96. Utz JP, Swensen SJ, Gertz MA. Pulmonary amyloidosis. The Mayo Clinic experience from 1980 to 1993. Ann Intern Med. 1996;124:407–13.

97. Rajan KG, Reynolds SP, McConnochie K, White JP. Localised amyloid – presenting as bronchial asthma. Eur J Respir Dis. 1987;71:213–5.

98. Sullivan E, Schwarz M. Pulmonary hypertension resulting from primary pulmonary amyloidosis. Semin Respir Crit Care Med. 1994;15:238–42.

99. Graham CM, Stern EJ, Finkbeiner WE, Webb WR. High-resolution CT appearance of diffuse alveolar septal amyloidosis. AJR Am J Roentgenol. 1992; 158:265–7.

100. Veyssier-Belot C, Cacoub P, Caparros-Lefebvre D, et al. Erdheim-Chester disease. Clinical and radiologic characteristics of 59 cases. Medicine (Baltimore). 1996;75:157–69.

101. Egan AJ, Boardman LA, Tazelaar HD, et al. Erdheim-Chester disease: clinical, radiologic, and histopathologic findings in five patients with interstitial lung disease. Am J Surg Pathol. 1999;23:17–26.

102. Wittenberg KH, Swensen SJ, Myers JL. Pulmonary involvement with Erdheim-Chester disease: radiographic and CT findings. AJR Am J Roentgenol. 2000;174:1327–31.

103. Haroche J, Amoura Z, Dion E, et al. Cardiovascular involvement, an overlooked feature of Erdheim-Chester disease: report of 6 new cases and a literature review. Medicine. 2004;83:371–92.

104. Devouassoux G, Lantuejoul S, Chatelain P, Brambilla E, Brambilla C. Erdheim-Chester disease: a primary macrophage cell disorder. Am J Respir Crit Care Med. 1998;157:650–3.

105. Vencio EF, Jenkins RB, Schiller JL, et al. Clonal cytogenetic abnormalities in Erdheim-Chester disease. Am J Surg Pathol. 2007;31:319–21.

106. Hermansky F, Pudlak P. Albinism associated with hemorrhagic diathesis and unusual pigmented reticular cells in the bone marrow: report of two cases with histochemical studies. Blood. 1959;14:162–9.

107. Anderson PD, Huizing M, Claassen DA, et al. Hermansky-Pudlak syndrome type 4 (HPS-4): clinical and molecular characteristics. Hum Genet. 2003; 113:10–7.

108. Gahl WA, Brantly M, Kaiser-Kupfer MI, et al. Genetic defects and clinical characteristics of patients with a form of oculocutaneous albinism (Hermansky-Pudlak syndrome). N Engl J Med. 1998;338:1258–64.

109. Garay SM, Gardella JE, Fazzini EP, Goldring RM. Hermansky-Pudlak syndrome. Pulmonary manifestations of a ceroid storage disorder. Am J Med. 1979;66:737–47.

110. Brantly M, Avila NA, Shotelersuk V, Lucero C, Huizing M, Gahl WA. Pulmonary function and high-resolution CT findings in patients with an inherited form of pulmonary fibrosis, Hermansky-Pudlak syndrome, due to mutations in HPS-1. Chest. 2000;117:129–36.

111. Gahl WA, Brantly M, Troendle J, et al. Effect of pirfenidone on the pulmonary fibrosis of Hermansky-Pudlak syndrome. Mol Genet Metab. 2002;76: 234–42.

112. Mulvihill JJ, Parry DM, Sherman JL, Pikus A, Kaiser-Kupfer MI, Eldridge R. NIH conference. Neurofibromatosis 1 (Recklinghausen disease) and neurofibromatosis 2 (bilateral acoustic neurofibromatosis). An update. Ann Intern Med. 1990;113:39–52.

113. Zamora AC, Collard HR, Wolters PJ, Webb WR, King TE. Neurofibromatosis-associated lung disease: a case series and literature review. Eur Respir J. 2007; 29:210–4.

114. Ryu JH, Parambil JG, McGrann PS, et al. Lack of evidence for an association between neurofibromatosis and pulmonary fibrosis. Chest. 2005;128:2381–6.

115. Massaro D, Katz S. Fibrosing alveolitis: its occurrence, roentgenographic, and pathologic features in von Recklinghausen's neurofibromatosis. Am Rev Respir Dis. 1966;93:934–42.

116. Burkhalter JL, Morano JU, McCay MB. Diffuse interstitial lung disease in neurofibromatosis. South Med J. 1986;79:944–6.

117. Klatte EC, Franken EA, Smith JA. The radiographic spectrum in neurofibromatosis. Semin Roentgenol. 1976;11:17–33.

118. Castellana G, Gentile M, Castellana R, Fiorente P, Lamorgese V. Pulmonary alveolar microlithiasis: clinical features, evolution of the phenotype, and review of the literature. Am J Med Genet. 2002;111:220–4.

119. Castellana G, Lamorgese V, Castellana G, Lamorgese V. Pulmonary alveolar microlithiasis. World cases and review of the literature. Respiration. 2003;70: 549–55.

120. Mariotta S, Ricci A, Papale M, et al. Pulmonary alveolar microlithiasis: report on 576 cases published in the literature [see comment]. Sarcoidosis Vasc Diffuse Lung Dis. 2004;21:173–81.

121. Huqun, Izumi S, Miyazawa H, et al. Mutations in the SLC34A2 gene are associated with pulmonary alveolar microlithiasis. Am J Respir Crit Care Med. 2007;175:263–8.

122. O'Neill RP, Cohn JE, Pellegrino ED. Pulmonary alveolar microlithiasis–a family study. Ann Intern Med. 1967;67:957–67.

123. Deniz O, Ors F, Tozkoparan E, et al. High resolution computed tomographic features of pulmonary alveolar microlithiasis. Eur J Radiol. 2005;55:452–60.

124. Garfield DH, Cadranel J, West HL, Garfield DH, Cadranel J, West HL. Bronchioloalveolar carcinoma: the case for two diseases. Clin Lung Cancer. 2008;9:24–9 [erratum appears in Clin Lung Cancer. 2008;9(2):77].

125. Anonymous. Case records of the Massachusetts General Hospital. Weekly clinicopathological exercises. Case 22-1994. A 57-year-old man with a chronic productive cough, dyspnea, and extensive bilateral air-space disease. N Engl J Med. 1994;330: 1599–606.

126. Dwek JH, Charytan C, Stachura I, Kaganowicz A. Salt-wasting bronchorrhea and its mechanisms. Arch Intern Med. 1977;137:791–4.

127. Homma H, Kira S, Takahashi Y, Imai H. A case of alveolar cell carcinoma accompanied by fluid and electrolyte depletion through production of voluminous amounts of lung liquids. Am Rev Respir Dis. 1975;111:857–62.

128. Falk RT, Pickle LW, Fontham ET, et al. Epidemiology of bronchioloalveolar carcinoma. Cancer Epidemiol Biomarkers Prev. 1992;1:339–44.

129. Morabia A, Wynder EL. Relation of bronchioloalveolar carcinoma to tobacco [see comment]. BMJ. 1992;304:541–3.

130. Regnard JF, Santelmo N, Romdhani N, et al. Bronchioloalveolar lung carcinoma: results of surgical treatment and prognostic factors. Chest. 1998;114:45–50.

131. Yousem SA, Beasley MB, Yousem SA, Beasley MB. Bronchioloalveolar carcinoma: a review of current concepts and evolving issues [see comment]. Arch Pathol Lab Med. 2007;131:1027–32.

132. Goldsmith HS, Bailey HD, Callahan EL, Beattie Jr EJ. Pulmonary lymphangitic metastases from breast carcinoma. Arch Surg. 1967;94:483–8.

133. Harold J. Lymphangitis carcinomatosa of the lungs. Q J Med. 1952;21:353–60.

134. Anonymous. Case records of the Massachusetts General Hospital. Weekly clinicopathological exercises. Case 34-1983. A 32-year-old man with testicular

enlargement and pulmonary intravascular carcinoma. N Engl J Med. 1983;309:477–87.

135. Maza I, Braun E, Plotkin A, Guralnik L, Azzam ZS. Lymphangitis carcinomatosis of unknown origin presenting as severe pulmonary hypertension. Am J Med Sci. 2004;327:255–7.

136. Trapnell DH. Radiological appearances of lymphangitis carcinomatosa of the lung. Thorax. 1964;19: 251–60.

137. Munk PL, Muller NL, Miller RR, Ostrow DN. Pulmonary lymphangitic carcinomatosis: CT and pathologic findings. Radiology. 1988;166:705–9.

Occupational- and Drug-Induced Disorders

17

Michal Pirozynski and John Joseph Borg

Abstract

Occupational, environmental, and medicinal agents remain one of the most common causes for interstitial lung diseases. A major problem with these diseases is recognition, since the number of exposures to new agents increases every year. In some cases, there are characteristics features of the presentation which suggest the diagnosis. For many, the pattern is not specific. In this chapter, these agents and their most common manifestations are presented. The clinician must consider these in evaluating a patient with interstitial lung disease.

Keywords

Drug-induced lung disease • Hypersensitivity pneumonitis • Pneumoconiosis • Silicosis • Alveolar hemorrhage

The views expressed in this article are the personal views of the authors and may not be used or quoted as being made on behalf of, or reflecting the position of any national competent authority or academic institution.

M. Pirozynski, MD, PhD (✉)
Department of Anesthesiology and Critical Care
Medicine CMKP, 231 Czerniakowska Street,
00-416 Warszawa, Poland
e-mail: m.pirozynski@upcpoczta.pl

J.J. Borg, PhD
Post-Licensing Directorate,
Medicines Authority, Rue D'Argens
Gzira GZR 1368 MALTA

Occupational-Induced Lung Disease

Occupational lung diseases constitute an important topic in respiratory disorders. Their diagnosis, treatment, and prevention have major public health implications. Affecting the airways and the lung parenchyma, different pathophysiologic interactions contribute to different disease models, such as pneumoconiosis, occupational asthma, asbestosis, silicosis, berylliosis, irritant inhalant injury, Spanish toxic oil syndrome, occupational bronchitis, paraquat injury, acute silicosis, chronic cadmium exposure, and hard metal disease.

Concern about the respiratory effects of exposure to dust and toxins in the air is far from a modern era preoccupation. Environmental health issues were addressed not only in the Middle Ages, by Ulrich Ellenbog in 1473, but also in Ancient times, as evidenced by descriptions of metalworkers in the ancient Egyptian text Papyrus Sallier [1, 2].

Pneumoconiosis

By the term pneumoconiosis, we understand the accumulation of dust in the lungs and the tissue reaction to its presence. Dust, being an aerosol consisting of solid, inanimate particles, can induce two types of tissue reactions: noncollagenous (when the stromal reaction is minimal, mainly consisting of reticulin fibers) and collagenous (when scarring is permanent). Exposure to many dusts may induce both forms of injury, and transition from one to the other may also take place. The various conditions are compared in Table 17.1.

The deposition of dust articles depends on various factors, such as the size of the particles, their velocity, geometric and aerodynamic properties, interactions between particles and mucociliary clearance mechanisms, individuals' breathing pattern, and airway characteristics (diameter, size, distortion, compression, abnormal movement). Dust accumulation is determined by the nature of the particles, and the particle-tissue biological reaction. Some dusts, such as coal, may accumulate in considerable amounts with minimal tissue response; others, in particular silica and asbestos, have extremely potent properties, contributing to massive tissue response. Tissue responses include nodular fibrosis (the classical example being silicate), diffuse fibrosis (asbestosis), and macule formation with focal emphysema (coal dust macule). Mixed dust exposure leads to irregular and mixed fibrotic patterns. For any given dust exposure, the severity of the parenchyma reaction is related to the cumulative lung dust burden. Unfortunately, in population-based studies the latter can be assessed only indirectly. Exposure can be directly assessed based on job history, environmental measurement data, or personal monitoring [3].

This exposure has clinical implications. For instance, the clinical diagnosis of pneumoconio-sis is greatly strengthened when there has been exposure to dust levels known to produce increased risk of disease. One must bear in mind that rejecting the diagnosis of pneumoconiosis cannot be made solely on the assumption of low exposure dust dose or the duration of its remoteness. The patient may be unusually susceptible, may individually retain more dust or may have an unusual exposure profile. Chest roentgenography remains the cornerstone of surveillance for pneumoconiosis. Computed tomography (CT) and high-resolution computed tomography (HRCT) has revolutionized clinical case evaluation [4, 5]. HRCT allows pulmonary and pleural lesions to be characterized, including their extent, and is considerably more sensitive in detecting disease compared with the conventional chest radiogram [6]. It can also provide a quantitative assessment of emphysema present. Lung function tests are used to assess the degree of impairment caused by pneumoconiosis. This disease may be associated with apparently normal lung function or with predominantly obstructive, restrictive, or mixed patterns of dysfunction. The clinician is faced with two main tasks when evaluating pneumoconiosis: first is to assess the nature of the disease, its site, extent, and whether it has decreased the individual's functional status. Second is the need to determine the possibility of environmental or occupational exposure, its duration, intensity, and character sufficient to account for the patient's condition. Additionally, one must remember that pneumoconiosis may appear and progress after exposure ceases.

Silicosis

Silicosis is a fibrotic lung disease caused by inhalation and lung retention of silicon dioxide or silica, in crystalline form. Silicon dioxide is inhaled as quartz and less commonly as cristobalite and tridymite. Most often exposition to silica is associated with inhalation of silica in the work environment. Three clinicopathologic cases of silicosis have been described: chronic silicosis, accelerated silicosis, and acute silicosis [7]. In chronic silicosis, the exposure period is usually

Table 17.1 Characteristics of the pneumoconioses

Significant positive features	History of exposure
History	
Diagnostic features	*Silicosis*: Cough, chest tightness, wheezes
	Coal workers' pneumoconiosis: Initial lack of symptoms
	Asbestosis: Dyspnea, cough, sputum production
	Berylliosis acute: Cough, chest pain, blood tinged sputum
	Berylliosis chronic: Dyspnea, cough, chest pain, weight loss, fatigue, arthralgias
	Hard metal disease: Cough, dyspnea
Suggests another diagnosis	Chronic bronchitis, emphysema, bronchiectases, lung cancer, pulmonary infections, OLD, circulatory insufficiency
Physical examination	
Diagnostic features	*Silicosis*: Symptom-free individual with abnormal chest radiogram
	Coal workers' pneumoconiosis: Symptom-free individual with abnormal chest radiogram
	Asbestosis: Basal crackles over axillary and basal regions, progressing to whole lungs
	Berylliosis: Lower airway disease
Laboratory tests	
Diagnostic for disease	*Acute silicosis*: Acute airspace disease
	Silicosis: Small rounded opacities initially upper lobe localization, later involving other lung fields, eggshell calcification strongly suggestive of silicosis progressive massive fibrosis, with cavitation in later stages
	Coal workers' pneumoconiosis: Small rounded opacities, initially in upper lung zones, enlargement of hilar lymph nodes, fibrosis seen when opacities exceed diameter of 1 cm
	Asbestosis: Earliest changes – small irregular opacities, seen in lower lung fields, between rib shadows. Progression of disease seen when borders of the heart are obscured; subpleural fibrotic changes; thickening of the intralobar fissures common. Restrictive lung function profile
	Berylliosis: Airspace disease, enlarged hilar lymph nodes
Suggests another diagnosis	*Acute silicosis*: Alveolar proteinosis
	Berylliosis: Sarcoidosis
Pathology	
BAL findings that are useful	*Silicosis*: Presence of silica in BAL; presence of lymphocytes may suggest presence of alveolitis that is likely to progress. Proteinosis suggests acute phase
	Coal workers' pneumoconiosis: Macrophages laden with coal dust
	Asbestosis: "Asbestos bodies" seen after recent exposure or high content of asbestos in lung parenchyma
	Beryllium lung disease: Beryllium lymphocyte proliferate test
	Hard metal disease: BAL lymphocyte transformation on test with cobalt
Bronchoscopy results that are useful	*Silicosis*: Presence of broncholithiasis, intrabronchial polypoid granuloma
Open lung biopsy results that are useful	*Silicosis*: Early injury – hyperplasia, hypertrophy of alveolar II cells. Classic silicotic nodule in hilar nodes. Pulmonary fibrosis, plaque-like lesions involving the visceral pleura. Presence of silica in lung tissue
	Coal workers' pneumoconiosis: Presence of coal macule and focal emphysema. Subpleural dust deposits. Arteries surrounded by coal dust. Enlargement of hilar and mediastinal nodes
	Asbestosis: Macrophage reaction in small airways with alveoli and interstitium. Presence of asbestos in lung parenchyma. Subpleural fibrosis, thickening of pleura
	Beryllium lung disease: Presence of beryllium in lung tissue. Lymphocytic alveolitis. Noncaseating epithelioid granulomas. Interstitial fibrosis in advanced cases
	Hard metal disease: Presence of multinucleated giant cells. Presence of hard metals in lung tissue

over 20 years, with dust containing less than 30% quartz. On chest radiograms, small rounded opacities are seen. Impairment of pulmonary function may occur. Pathological examination reveals the classic silicotic nodule usually involving the hilar nodes. Progression to upper lobe localization is sometimes seen. Less common features include pulmonary fibrosis and plaque-like lesions involving the visceral pleura [8]. With continuing exposure the nodules tend to increase in size, leading in some cases to conglomerate silicosis also termed progressive massive fibrosis [9]. Accelerated silicosis is seen in patients exposed with dusts of higher quartz content for 5–15 years. Pathology reveals numerous nodules of various stages of development. Irregular pulmonary fibrosis may be seen. Clinical features include irregular upper zone fibrosis with a nodular component. A symptomatic course is seen, with functional impairment often progressing to respiratory failure and death. Cavitation and infection with mycobacteria is seen.

Acute silicosis may show all features of pulmonary proteinosis. The exposure period may be measured in months. It is usually seen after exposure to high quartz content dust. On chest radiogram, acute airspace disease is seen. Rapid progression to acute respiratory failure and fulminating mycobacterial infection are common [10].

The lungs of exposed individuals also may demonstrate the features of other diseases associated with occupational dust exposure (chronic bronchitis and emphysema). Extra-thoracic manifestation of silicosis includes lesions in lymph nodes of the neck and abdomen, in the liver, spleen, and bone marrow. Reactions that follow the inhalation of quartz particles are complex. They involve not only all cell components of the air-tissue interspace but also systemic changes. Silica particles of less than 5 μm in diameter reach the lower airways and may enter the alveoli. Silica possesses redox potential and interacts with oxygen, hydrogen, and nitrogen. Low-intensity exposure produces aggregates of fibrosis with relative sparing of the lung architecture, whereas high-intensity exposure causes widespread pulmonary inflammation and collagen deposition. Once silica has been ingested by the macrophages, oxidants, cytokines, and growth factors are produced. Early in the process injury to type I alveolar cells and hyperplasia and hypertrophy of alveolar type II cells occur. The changes in type II cells with progression are thought to lead to fiberogenesis. Other cells that play a role in the development of silicosis are neutrophils, T and B lymphocytes, and mast cells [8].

Clinical Features

The symptoms and signs of chronic silicosis do not differ from signs seen in other chronic focal fibrosis lesions caused by exogenous agents. The main symptom is breathlessness, first noted after exertion and later seen at rest. One must keep in mind that in chronic silicosis and in the absence of other respiratory disease, this symptom may be absent. Often patients present as a symptom-free individuals requiring assessment because of an abnormal chest radiogram [11]. Cough maybe caused by chronic bronchitis, tobacco smoking, with the occupational exposure itself or with presence of airway hyperactivity. Other airway-related symptoms such as chest tightness and wheezing are less common. Chest pains are not a feature nor are systemic symptoms – fever and weight loss. If they do appear, other causes should be looked for – especially cancer or tuberculosis.

Radiographic and Lung Function

Uncomplicated silicosis is characterized by the presence of small round opacities on chest radiograms. Silicotic nodules are usually distributed symmetrically and tend to be initially present in the upper zones, later involving the other lung zones. Occasionally they are calcified. Eggshell calcification is strongly suggestive of silicosis. Enlargement of hilar nodes may precede development of parenchymal lesions. Pleural plaques may occur. Progressive massive fibrosis is characterized by coalescence of small rounded opacities to form larger, more massive lesions. CT and HRCT assessment is superior to chest radiogram in assessing not only the presence and extent of nodulation, but is able to reveal early conglomeration. With time the lesions tend to contract, usually to upper lobes. In this phase, small opacities may disappear, resulting in a picture compatible with tuberculosis. Rapid development of several large lesions suggests rheumatoid silicosis. Changing lesions, especially cavitation, should be regarded as evidence of mycobacterial disease. Acute silicosis is characterized radiologically by diffuse changes that usually display an airspace and interstitial pattern rather than nodularity.

There is no consistent lung function profile associated with silicosis. In chronic silicosis, spirometric test and maximal mid-expiratory flow reflect airflow limitation. Lung volumes (VC, TLC) maybe reduced in advanced disease, but not the functional residual capacity (FRC) and residual volume (RV). Reduction of diffusing capacity is evident in more advanced disease.

Diagnosis and Complications

The diagnosis of silicosis should not be a problem with a history of exposure and characteristic radiological findings. Problems arise when the history of exposure is obscure, remote, or forgotten or when the radiological features are unusual. Detection of silica in bronchoalveolar lavage (BAL) may raise suspicion. Lung biopsy (TBLB, surgical) may be necessary to clarify the diagnosis. Biopsy material should always be processed for presence of dust. Presence of lymphocytes in BAL and an increase in cell number may suggest the presence of alveolitis that is likely to progress [12, 13]. Complications include infection by mycobacteria or fungi, spontaneous pneumothorax, cor pulmonale, broncholithiasis, intrabronchial polypoid granuloma, and lung cancer.

Treatment

Once established, the fibrotic process of silicosis is irreversible. Treatment is directed toward preventing progression and development of complications. Interventions to interrupt the inflammatory process have been tried in the past. There is no evidence that they are of any value. Attracting attention is whole lung lavage to remove the dust, inflammatory cells, and mediator burden. However, there is no proof as yet that this decreases the progression of the disease. Treatment of acute silicosis has been reported in several case reports. This includes the use of BAL, and steroids in cases of alveolar proteinosis [14]. Prognosis depends on the extent of parenchymal response to the silica. Treatment should also be directed toward control of infections, especially tuberculosis.

Coal Workers' Pneumoconiosis

Coal workers' pneumoconiosis is an entity resulting from deposition of coal dust in the lung. Tissue ration to coal dust include coal macule and coal nodule. Coal miners may develop silicotic nodules when a high content of silica is present in the coal seams. Coal mining is also associated with chronic bronchitis, chronic airflow limitation, and emphysema. It proved to be difficult to distinguish the contribution of cigarette smoking from that of occupational exposure. The primary lesion in coal workers' pneumoconiosis is the coal macule. It consists of an aggregation of dust-laden macrophages and fibroblasts accumulated around the respiratory bronchioles filling contiguous alveoli and extending into the interstitium with irregular fibrosis. With time the macule evolves to a nodule which additionally consists of reticulin fibers and irregular fibrosis. In time the respiratory bronchiole weakens and the small airways dilate to create focal emphysema. This form of centriacinar emphysema in combination with a macule forms the characteristic findings of coal workers' pneumoconiosis. Other features include subpleural dust deposits, arteries surrounded by coal dust, enlargement of hilar and mediastinal nodes [15]. Rheumatoid pneumoconiosis is a nodular form of coal workers' pneumoconiosis. One of its variants is termed Caplan's syndrome, a nodular form of coal workers' pneumoconiosis associated with rheumatoid arthritis.

Clinical Features

Simple coal workers' pneumoconiosis is a disease state without symptoms or physical signs. The diagnosis is based on chest radiogram findings in an individual with history of exposition. The symptoms of cough and expectoration are consequences of dust-induced chronic bronchitis [16].

Chest Radiography

Small rounded opacities in the lung parenchyma are characteristic of coal workers' pneumoconiosis. HRCT is helpful in early detection of the disease. Small rounded opacities are observed first in the upper zones and progress to other zones later in the disease. Some enlargement of hilar nodes is possible, eggshell calcification is unusual. Progressive fibrosis is seen when the diameter of the opacities exceed 1 cm [15, 17].

Lung Function

Most of the evidence supports the view that simple coal workers' pneumoconiosis is a condition that does not produce demonstrable effects on pulmonary function [18]. Abnormalities are seen more often in progressive disease.

Diagnosis and Management

The fundamental elements of coal workers' pneumoconiosis are occupational exposure and chest radiogram findings. Complications include mycobacterial infections, Caplan's syndrome, and scleroderma.

Asbestosis: Asbestos-Related Fibrosis of the Lungs and Pleura

Exposure to asbestos fibers tends to be occupational and may occur in mining, milling, transporting, and manufacturing following raw asbestos fiber application. Other forms of exposure are indirect occupational exposure (bystander exposure) seen in those required to work in the vicinity of others who work with asbestos; and domestic exposure occurring primarily as a consequence of fiber-laden work clothes being laundered at home. Environmental and domestic exposure occurs because of living in their neighborhood of asbestos mills or plants that use asbestos and contaminate the environment. Accumulation of asbestos fibers in the lungs is the outcome of exposure, deposition, clearance, and retention. Fiber retention is related to their impaction and accumulation in the airways. Within hours of fiber deposition, they evoke a macrophage reaction in small airways associated with alveoli and interstitium. Fibers (≤ 3 μm) are phagocytosed by activated macrophages, translocated to lymphatic vessels, drained to pleural spaces. Longer fibers are phagocytosed incompletely and become the core of "asbestos bodies." Asbestos bodies may be found in sputum and BAL when lung tissue levels are very high. They are found more frequently when dust exposure is recent. Asbestosis tends to be more common in the lower lobes and in the subpleural area. When disease is advanced, the lungs are quite small; fibrosis outlines the lobar and intralobar septa, with the visceral pleura thickened. Honeycombing may be present in the lower lobes and subpleural areas. Lymph node involvement is rare. The grade of pulmonary fibrosis relates to the asbestos fiber burden carried by the lungs [19].

Clinical Features

Asbestosis is termed the monosymptomatic disease, the most depressing symptom being dyspnea. The initial symptoms start during exertion, and progress to rest dyspnea. Dyspnea precedes other symptoms and therefore may be underrated. Other reported symptoms are cough and sputum production [16]. Basal crackles are heard first over axillary and basal regions, and then generally as the disease progresses.

Radiographic Features

The plain chest radiogram of the chest is the key tool in asbestosis diagnosis. The earliest lesions are termed "small irregular opacities." They are usually seen in the lower regions between the rib shadows. As the disease progresses, the borders of the heart are obscured. HRCT visualizes early fibrotic changes, seen in the subpleural parenchyma. Visceral pleural involvement, thickening of the intralobar fissures, is common. Hilar node enlargement is not a feature of asbestosis [20].

Lung Function

A restrictive lung function profile may be seen in asbestosis.

Diagnosis

Clinical diagnosis depends on establishing the presence, extent, and nature of pulmonary fibrosis and whether there has been exposure of duration to put the individual at risk of developing asbestosis. Most published criteria consider histopathology as the best means of establishing the diagnosis [21]. The individual with asbestos exposure is at risk of developing lung and mesothelioma. Tuberculosis and rheumatoid pneumoconiosis are not frequently seen as complications of pulmonary asbestosis.

Beryllium Lung Disease

Acute beryllium disease is defined as a disease from which the exposed subject recovers within a year. Beryllium enters the body by inhalation and occasionally by the skin. The disease is characterized by acute inflammatory reactions in the upper airways, bronchiolitis, pulmonary edema, and chemically induced pneumonitis. Chronic disease is a multisystem disorder characterized by noncaseating granulomas that occur throughout the body. The lung remains the primary manifestation of this disease. Pathological examination of the lung tissue reveals the presence of a lymphocytic (helper T-cell) alveolitis and noncaseating epithelioid granulomas indistinguishable from those of sarcoidosis [22]. As the disease progresses, interstitial fibrosis develops.

Clinical Features

Acute berylliosis is characterized by the presence of cough, chest pain, blood-tinged sputum, crackles, and the presence of patchy airspace disease on chest radiograms. Chronic disease may develop from acute disease but usually it develops without antecedent events. The clinical features are similar to those of lymphocytes in BAL and an increase in cell number may suggest the presence of alveolitis that is likely to progress [12, 13]. Complications include infection by mycobacteria or fungi, spontaneous pneumothorax, cor pulmonale, broncholithiasis, intrabronchial polypoid granuloma, and lung cancer.

Diagnosis and Treatment

Criteria for diagnosing chronic beryllium diseases is the presence of four out of six features: exposure established on the basis of history; objective evidence of lower airway disease consistent with chronic berylliosis; radiological evidence with diffuse lung disease (DLD); histopathological findings consistent with beryllium disease; and demonstration of the presence of beryllium in biological material (lung, lymph nodes, or urine). Recently, BAL was introduced as a very sensitive diagnostic tool in berylliosis [23]. Most patients present with signs indistinguishable from those of pulmonary sarcoidosis. Evidence of sensitization to beryllium can be obtained by performing BeLPT (beryllium lymphocyte proliferate test) on blood or BAL material [23]. The most important step in treating berylliosis is complete cessation of exposure to beryllium. Steroid therapy has been recommended for chronic berylliosis and long-term steroid therapy has altered favorably the course of the disease.

Hard Metal Disease

Hard metal disease is a disorder related to inhalation of products derived from a sintering process that involves pressurization and heating a mixture of tungsten carbide powder and 10% cobalt to 1,500°C. This work-related disease may present in two forms – acute (rhinitis) and chronic disease (fibrosing alveolitis). The DLD is characterized by the presence of unusual multinucleated giant cells comprising alveolar type II cells and macrophages [24]. Diagnosis is based on exposure history, clinical presentation, pathologic, and mineralogical features on biopsy. Cobalt exposure can be confirmed by patch test, or presence of cobalt in urine or blood. Lymphocyte (blood, BAL) transformation or leukocyte inhibition factor in response to cobalt may be useful [24–26]. Diagnosis and removal of the patient from the harmful environment may reverse the acute phase of the disease and prevent the development of the chronic disease. Steroids and cyclophosphamide have been used with success.

Drug-Induced DLDs

During the past years, drugs used for therapy of various disorders have emerged as a fairly common and significant cause of diffuse interstitial lung disease [27–30]. There are more than 300 drugs known to affect the lungs adversely (Table 17.2). The list is expanding each year. Data are easily accessible through a public domain – Pneumotox® (http://www.medtools.nl/products/pneumotoxframe.html). A considerable amount of information on drug-induced ILD has been gathered and made available regarding the cause of adverse events in the lung and the pattern of lung reaction that can be anticipated with the use of the specific drug [27]. Presently, it is known that not only drugs but also biomolecules can induce ILD (interferons have been linked with development of sarcoidosis and bronchiolitis obliterans; immunoglobulins and antithymocyte globulin may induce pulmonary edema and infiltrates; growth factors can cause acute respiratory distress syndrome (ARDS) and severe ILD; transfusions can cause transfusion-related lung injury syndrome, manifested by rapid development of pulmonary infiltrates or edema) [31, 32]. Up to now drug-induced interstitial lung diseases (DI-DLDs) were regarded as interstitial tissue reactions to drugs, the latter patterns suggest that DI-DLDs may also result from damage to

Table 17.2 Patterns of drug-induced diffuse lung disease (+++, frequent; ++, often; +, rare)

Clinical or radiological feature	Cases	Drugs known to have caused such features
Interstitial lung disease		
Acute hypersensitivity pneumonitis and respiratory failure	+++	Bupropion
		Dasatinib
		Gold salts (aurothiopropanosulfonate)
		Methotrexate
		Nitrofurantoin
	++	Carbamazepine
		Erlotinib
		Fenfluramine/dexfenfluramine
		Nilutamide
	+	Abacavir
		Abciximab
		Celecoxib
		Celiprolol
		Ciprofloxacin
		Clofarabine
		Cotrimoxazole
		Daunorubicin
		Docetaxel
		Doxycycline
		Fludarabine
		Gadopentetate dimeglumine
		Gliclazide
		Haloperidol
		Linezolid
		Lithium
		Losartan
		Mycophenolate
		Peginterferon alfa-2a
		Procarbazin
		Rituximab
		Sunitinib
		Tacrolismus
		Tamoxifen
		Vinblastine
		Voriconazole
Subacute cellular interstitial pneumonitis	+++	Amiodarone
		Bleomycin
		Captopril
		Dasatinib
		Everolimus
		Gefitinib
		Gold salts (aurothiopropanosulfonate)
		Heroin
		Isoniazid
		Methotrexate
		Nitrofurantoin
		Olanzapine
		Phenytoin

(continued)

Table 17.2 (continued)

Clinical or radiological feature	Cases	Drugs known to have caused such features
		Radiation
		Tacrolismus
	++	Carbamazepine
		Carmustine (BCNU)
		Etanercept
		Etoposide
		Fenfluramine/dexfenfluramine
		G(M)-CSF
		Hydrochlorothiazide
		Mitomycin C
		Nilutamide
		Panitumumab
		Pegfilgrastim
		Penicillamine
		Practolol
		Procainamide
		Procarbazine
		Propylthiouracil
		Sulfamides–sulfonamides
		Sulfasalazine
		Sunitinib
	+	Acebutolol
		Acyclovir
		Azathioprine
		Adalimumab
		Ampicillin
		Amrinone
		ACE inhibitors
		Antazoline
		Atenolol
		Azapropazone
		Azathioprine
		BCG therapy
		Bicalutamide
		Chlorambucil
		Cilostazol
		Citalopram
		Clopidogrel
		Cytarabine
		Clozapine
		Cotrimoxazole
		Cromoglycate
		Cyclosporin
		Cyproterone acetate
		Dihydralazine
		Dihydroergocryptine
		Docetaxel
		Doxorubicin
		Dothiepin
		Ergotamine
		Etodolac
		Famotidine

(continued)

Table 17.2 (continued)

Clinical or radiological feature	Cases	Drugs known to have caused such features
		Filgrastim
		Flecainide
		Floxuridine
		Fluorouracil
		Folinic acid
		Fluoxetine
		Gemcitabine
		Glibenclamide
		Hydralazine
		Hydroxycarbamide
		Hydroxyquinoline
		Hydroxyurea
		Ibritumomab
		Ifosfamide
		Imipramine
		Indapamide
		Interferon alfa
		Irbesartan
		Irinotecan
		Itraconazole
		Lamivudine
		Lamotrigine
		Lansoprazole
		Lapatinib
		Leflunomide
		Lenalidomide
		Lenograstim
		Letrozole
		Leuprorelin acetate
		Lopinavir, ritonavir
		Maprotiline
		Mefloquine
		Mercaptopurine
		Metapramine
		Metformine
		Methysergide
		Mitoxantrone
		Measles, mumps and rubella vaccine (live)
		Medroxyprogesterone acetate
		Melphalan
		Meropenem
		Methylprednisolone
		Metoprolol
		Midazolam
		Nadolol
		Natalizumab
		Nomifensine
		Oxprenolol
		Oxyphenbutazone
		Paclitaxel
		Pamidronate disodium
		Paracetamol

(continued)

Table 17.2 (continued)

Clinical or radiological feature	Cases	Drugs known to have caused such features
		Paroxetine
		Penicillins
		Pemetrexed
		Pituitary snuff
		Pranlukast
		Procarbazine
		Pyrimethamine–sulfadoxine
		Quinidine
		Raltitrexed
		Retinoic acid
		Ribavirin
		Rifampicin
		Risperidone
		Sevoflurane
		Simvastin
		Sirolimus
		Sorafenib
		Stavudine
		Tegafur uracil
		Telmisartan
		Teriparatide
		Thalidomide
		Thiotepa
		Tiopronin
		Tocainide
		Topiramate
		Trastuzumab
		Valproate
		Valsartan
		Vindesine
		Vinorelbine
		Zidovudine
		Zoledronic acid
Pulmonary infiltrates and eosinophilia	+++	Amiodarone
		Bleomycin
		Blood transfusions
		Captopril
		Cladribine
		Gold salts (aurothiopropanosulfonate)
		Iodine, radiographic contrast media
		Methotrexate
		Naproxen
		Nitrofurantoin
		Phenytoin
		L-Tryptophan
	++	Acetylsalicylic acid
		Anti-inflammatory drugs
		Carbamazepine
		Fenfluramine/dexfenfluramine
		G(M)-CSF

(continued)

Table 17.2 (continued)

Clinical or radiological feature	Cases	Drugs known to have caused such features
		Hydrochlorothiazide
		Minocycline
		Nilutamide
		Panitumumab
		Penicillamine
		Propylthiouracil
		Sulfamethoxazole, trimethoprim
		Sulfamides–sulfonamides
		Sulfasalazine
	+	Acetaminophen
		Amitriptyline
		Ampicillin
		ACE inhibitors
		Aminoglutethimide
		Azithromycin
		Azacitidine
		Beclomethasone
		Bicalutamide
		Bucillamine
		Camptothecin
		Cefotiam
		Cephalexin
		Cephalosporins
		Cetuximab
		Cladribine
		Chloroquine
		Chlorpromazine
		Chlorpropamide
		Clindamycin
		Clofibrate
		Cotrimoxazole
		Cromoglycate
		Cyproterone acetate
		Dapsone
		Daptomycin
		Darbepoetin alfa
		Dasatinib
		Desipramine
		Diclofenac
		Diflunisal
		Enalapril
		Erythromycin
		Ethambutol
		Febarbamate
		Fenbufen
		Fenoprofen
		Fosinopril
		Furazolidone
		Glafenine
		Ibuprofen
		Imatinib
		Imipramine

(continued)

Table 17.2 (continued)

Clinical or radiological feature	Cases	Drugs known to have caused such features
		Indomethacin
		Interleukin 2
		Isoniazid
		Isotretinoin
		Labetalol
		Levofloxacin
		Lisinopril
		Loxoprofen
		Maprotiline
		Mephenesin
		Mesalamine
		Methylphenidate
		Metronidazole
		Minocycline
		Montelukast
		Moxifloxacin hydrochloride
		Nalfon
		Nalidixic acid
		Naproxen
		Niflumic acid
		Niridazol
		Nomifensine
		Omalizumab
		Omeprazol
		Paclitaxel
		Para-(4)-aminosalicylic acid (PAS)
		Pegfilgrastim
		Penicillins
		Pentamidine
		Perindopril
		Phenylbutazone
		Piroxicam
		Pranoprofen
		Pravastatin
		Procarbazine
		Propranolol
		Pyrimethamine-dapsone
		Pyrimethamine-suifadoxine
		Quetiapine
		Rifampicin
		Roxithromycin
		Serrapeptase
		Sertraline
		Simvastin
		Streptomycin
		Sulindac
		Teicoplanin
		Tenidap
		Tetracycline
		Thalidomide
		Tiaprofenic acid
		Tocilizumab

(continued)

Table 17.2 (continued)

Clinical or radiological feature	Cases	Drugs known to have caused such features
		Tolazamide
		Tolfenamic acid
		Tosufloxacin
		Tramadole
		Trastuzumab
		Trazodone
		Trimipramine
		Troleandomycin
		Vancomycin
		Venlafaxine
		Verapamil
		Warfarin
		Zafirlukast
Organizing pneumonia +/− bronchitis pneumonia (BOOP)	+++	Amiodarone
		Bleomycin
		Gold salts (aurothiopropanosulfonate)
		Nitrofurantoin
		Phenytoin
		Radiation
	++	Carbamazepine
		Cyclophosphamide
		Minocycline
		Nilutamide
		Penicillamine
		Rituximab
	+	Acebutolol
		Amphotericin B
		Atorvastatin
		Barbiturates
		Betaxolol
		Cephalosporins
		Dacarbazine
		Dihydralazine
		Dihydroergocryptine
		Dihydroergotamine
		FK506
		Hydralazine
		Interferon alfa
		Interferon beta
		Mesalamine
		Pravastin
		Simvastin
		Sotalol
		Tacrolismus
		Temozolomide
		Ticlopidine
		Topotecan
Desquamative interstitial pneumonia	+++	Nitrofurantoin
		Temsirolimus
	++	Busulfan
		Docetaxel
		Sulfasalazine

(continued)

Table 17.2 (continued)

Clinical or radiological feature	Cases	Drugs known to have caused such features
	+	Anagrelide
		Interferon alfa
		Lenograstim
		Rituximab
		Ropinirole
		Voriconazole
Lymphocytic pneumonia	+++	Captopril
		Phenytoin
	+	Bortezomib
		Didanosine
		Fludarabine
		Indinavir
		Indometacin
		Lamivudine
		Mercaptopurine
		Nelfinavir
		Nevirapine
		Rabbit human T lymphocyte immunoglobulin
		Ritonavir
		Tenofovir
Pulmonary fibrosis	+++	Amiodarone
		Bleomycin (aurothiopropanosulfonate)
		Methotrexate
		Nitrofurantoin
		Radiation
	++	Bromocryptine
		Busulfan
		Carmustine
		Chlorambucil
		Danazol
		Mitomycin C
		Nitrosoureas
		Penicillamine
		Practolol
		Sulfasalazine
	+	Anti-lymphocyte (thymocyte) globulin
		Bepridil
		Bortezomib
		Bromocriptine
		Cabergoline
		Capecitabine
		Carboplatin
		Chlorozotocin
		Danazol
		Dothiepin
		Ergotamine
		Fluconazole
		5-Fluorouracil
		Flutamide
		Fotemustine
		Hydroxycarbamide

(continued)

Table 17.2 (continued)

Clinical or radiological feature	Cases	Drugs known to have caused such features
		Imatanib
		Indometacin
		Infliximab
		Labetolol
		Lenograstim
		Lomustine (CCNU)
		Medroxyprogesterone
		Melphalan
		Mesalazine
		Methysergide
		Mycophenolate mofetil
		Olanzapine
		Oseltamivir
		Oxaliplatin
		Pegfilgrastim
		Pergolide
		Pioglitazone
		Pindolol
		Procarbazine
		Ropinirole
		Rosuvastatin
		Tamoxifen
		Tocainide
Subclinical cytologic changes in BAL cellular profile	+	Sunitinib
		Clofazamine
Diffuse pulmonary calcification	+	
		Calcium salts
Mineral oil pneumonia with diffuse chronic lung changes	+++	Vitamin D
		Iodine, radiographic contrast media
		Nasal drops (with oil)
	+	Paraffin
Diffuse alveolar damage	+++	Cyclosporin
	++	Amiodarone
	+	Cyclophosphamide
		BCG therapy
		Bevacizumab
		Gemicitabine
		Pranlukast
		Raloxifene
		Telithromycin
		Topotecan
		Verapamil
Pulmonary hemorrhage		
Alveolar hemorrhage	+++	Amiodarone
		Iodine, radiographic contrast media
		Methotrexate
		Nitrofurantoin
		Phenytoin

(continued)

Table 17.2 (continued)

Clinical or radiological feature	Cases	Drugs known to have caused such features
	++	Acetylsalicylic acid
		Arsenic trioxide
		Carbamazepine
		Mitomycin C
		Oral anticoagulants
		Penicillamine
		Propylthiouracil
		Warfarin
	+	Abciximab
		Alcohol
		Alteplase
		Azathioprine
		Capecitabine
		Clopidrogel
		Cyclosporin
		Cytarabine (cytosine arabinoside)
		Dextran
		Dimethylsulfoxide
		Fibrinolytics (including rTPA)
		Fludarabine
		Glibenclamide

(continued)

Table 17.2 (continued)

Clinical or radiological feature	Cases	Drugs known to have caused such features
		Hydralazine
		Moxalactam
		Nitric oxide (NO)
		Quinidine
		Retinoic acid
		Sirolimus
		Streptokinase
		TNFa
		Urokinase
		Valproic acid
Goodpasture-like syndrome	++	Penicyllamine
Pleural involvement		
	+	Alemtuzumab
		Anagrelide
		Arsenic trioxide
		Bromocriptine
		Cabergoline
		Infliximab
		Leflunomide
		Tacrolismus
		Zidovudine

pulmonary vessels during transit of activated blood cells within the pulmonary vasculature. Treatment with natural products also merits attention. Herbs and "dietary supplements" appear capable of inducing serious diseases, including that of the pulmonary parenchyma [33].

The frequency of DI-DLDs is hard to estimate. The reasons for this are multifocal. Use of plain chest radiograms is likely to underestimate subclinical forms of this disease in comparison with HRCT. This has been shown in cases of asymptomatic patients taking amiodarone having opacities detected at HRCT or autopsy [34, 35]. Many drugs are prescribed by nonrespiratory specialists, thus underdiagnosis of respiratory symptoms is possible. In oncological patients where DI-DLD is common, the diagnosis will remain presumptive, because of the severe clinical state of the patient which precludes the use of invasive diagnostic techniques [36, 37]. Estimates of DI-DLD would require notification of drug-induced adverse effects to drug-regulating agencies, which is performed in several countries, but this is needed on a more broadscale basis for accurate epidemiological data [27]. In conclusion, any estimate is rather an underestimate of DI-DLD frequency.

One of the most intriguing questions remains why, out of the whole treated population, only a few develop DI-DLD. For a few of the drugs, a limited dose has been identified [38]. Previously, the pulmonary toxic effects were thought to have been related to the high dose of the used drug. These initial studies were with amiodarone and bleomycin [39–41]. Several reports question this theory, showing that there is no real safe dose for either of these drugs [27]. For most drugs, there is no apparent link between dosage and duration of treatment and pulmonary toxicity; development of pulmonary involvement remains unexpected and idiosyncratic. This unequal risk for developing pulmonary involvement may be due to several factors, including prior respiratory reaction to the drug, occupational factors that potentiate the respiratory effects (exposure to asbestos and use of ergotamine), underlying disease for which the drug was given (ulcerative colitis or rheumatoid arthritis may increase risk of developing respiratory symptoms), interspecies variations in developing adverse reactions to drugs, role of concomitant drugs, and additive effect of therapeutic modalities (administration of several chemotherapeutic agents, use of chemo- and radiotherapy, use of chemotherapy and high concentrations of oxygen) [27, 42]. Mixing of potential pneumotoxic drugs may lead to an unexpected pulmonary toxicity, known as recall pneumonitis. Renal insufficiency may contribute to increased bleomycin pulmonary toxicity. Changing the infusion rate of bleomycin may decrease the likelihood of bleomycin lung toxicity. It is also unclear why only a fraction of patients who develop amiodarone pneumonitis will ultimately develop pulmonary fibrosis. Despite identification of some risk factors, prediction of DI-DLD remains very difficult. Only for a limited number of drugs (i.e., amiodarone, bleomycin, and nitrosoureas), the monitoring of patients who receive these drugs is advisable [43]. Little is known about the mechanism of drug injury to the lungs. Presently four mechanisms are recognized: oxidant injury (as in chronic nitrofurantoin ingestion), direct cytotoxic effects on alveolar capillary endothelial cells (seen in reactions to cytotoxic drugs), deposition of phospholipids within cells (as in amiodarone toxicity), and the immune system-mediated injury (drug-induced lupus erythematosus).

Clinical Patterns of Disease

Patterns of respiratory involvement of the respiratory system following drug toxic reactions may be divided into 11 groups: interstitial lung diseases, pulmonary edema, pulmonary hemorrhage, airways disease, pleural changes, vascular changes, mediastinal changes, major airways involvement, and involvement of muscle and nerve function, systemic symptoms, and others (see Table 17.2).

The clinical and radiological features of DI-DLD vary from subclinical opacities to whole lung involvement with acute respiratory distress consistent with ARDS [44]. In patients with

migratory opacities and infiltrates with or without chest pain suggestive of organizing pneumonia a careful drug history should be taken, as this may relate to drug or radiation exposure [45]. Amongst mild forms of DI-DLD, transient infiltrates have been described following administration of hydrochlorothiazides, nitrofurantoin, anticancer agents, colony-stimulating factors, proteins, and blood products. The histopathological background of these reactions remains unresolved, as no biopsies were taken in the reported cases [27]. In most cases, the reaction to the drug is confined to the lung parenchyma, but it may be part of a generalized and systemic reaction (see Table 17.2). This includes drug-induced systemic lupus erythematosus (SLE) syndrome (seen after administration of beta blockers, nonsteroidal anti-inflammatory drugs, etc.), drug-induced hypersensitivity syndromes with involvement of the brain, digestive system, liver, bone marrow, lymph nodes (after exposure to anticonvulsants), alveolar hemorrhage (penicillamine), drug-induced angiitis ANCA positive (propylthiouracil), and Churg–Strauss syndrome (aspirin, macrolides, leukotriene antagonists) [46–51].

History and Physical Examination

Breathlessness is the most prevailing complaint in patients with DI-DLD. Initially, dyspnea develops only after forced exertion. As the disease progresses, it occurs even at rest. Other prominent complaints include nonproductive cough and fatigue. Cough is most often seen in patients with bronchiolitis obliterans with organizing pneumonia (BOOP), eosinophilic pneumonia, and idiopathic pulmonary fibrosis (IPF). Pleurisy is seen most often in DLD associated with drug-induced lupus-associated syndromes (see Table 17.2). The physical examination may reveal typical findings of DLD. On auscultation bilateral, basilar, and crepitant rales are found in most patients. Only occasionally one hears wheezing, rhonchi, and coarse rales. In some cases, the lung examination may be normal. In advanced cases, patients may exhibit tachypnea and tachycardia. Digital clubbing is seen in many fibrotic lung disorders.

Table 17.3 Patterns of most often seen drug-induced diffuse lung diseases (modified from [27])

Type of DLD	Most common drugs	Course of disease
Nonspecific cellular interstitial pneumonia	Methotrexate, nilutamide	Mild
Granulomatous interstitial pneumonia	Methotrexate, BCG	Mild
Sarcoidosis-like disease	Interferons	Mild
Eosinophylic pneumonia	Antibiotics, nonsteroidal anti-inflammatory, ACE inhibitors	Mild–severe
Organizing pneumonia	Amiodarone, bleomycin, interferons, nitrofurantoin, radiation therapy, statins	Mild–severe
DIP	Nitrofurantoin	Moderate
LIP	Phenytoin	Mild
IPF-like	Amiodarone, gold, methotrexate	Severe
Diffuse alveolar damage	Chemotherapy, gold, methotrexate	Severe
Alveolar filling process with foamy-like macrophages	Amiodarone, mineral oil	Variable
Alveolar hemorrhage	Anticoagulants, fibrinolytic agents, penicyllamine	Variable
Proteinosis-like disease	Busulfan	Variable

The new appearance of this symptom in patients with a known DLD should prompt search for complicating lung malignancy.

Bronchoscopy, Lung Biopsy, and BAL

Bronchoscopy should be performed when tissue abnormalities are distributed in the airways, or there are airspace-filling lesions. Transbronchial lung biopsy is mandatory in all cases suspected of DLD, especially in cases of alveolar-filling disease. Surgical biopsy may not be adequate for establishing a diagnosis. It always should be taken from two distant sites, the choice of which should be based on HRCT findings [52]. BAL can be useful. A predominance of eosinophils in conjunction with a clinical and radiological picture can diagnose eosinophilic pneumonia. BAL can also show subclinical involvement in certain DI-DLD cases [53].

Histopathology

Scant data are available on histological data in DI-DLD [27]. Drugs can induce various histopathological patterns of interstitial lung diseases – nonspecific interstitial pneumonia, granulomatous interstitial pneumonia, eosinophilic pneu-

monia, pseudosarcoidosis, desquamative interstitial pneumonia, lymphocytic interstitial pneumonia, idiopathic interstitial pneumonia, organizing pneumonia, acute interstitial pneumonia, diffuse alveolar damage, proteinosis-like changes, pulmonary hemosiderosis, alveolar hemorrhage, alveolar filling with foamy macrophages, etc. Most usually trigger conventional patterns of ILD nonspecific interstitial pneumonia, eosinophilic pneumonia, or pulmonary fibrosis. Some drugs can elicit less usual patterns of organizing pneumonia or desquamative interstitial pneumonia. Some induce stereotyped changes (nitrofurantoin, minocycline eosinophilic pneumonia, cellular nonspecific interstitial pneumonia), whilst others (amiodarone, bleomycin) can induce a variety of histopathological changes in patients (Table 17.3). Amiodarone toxicity can be described as: nonspecific interstitial pneumonia (cellular or fibrotic), organizing pneumonia, alveolar filling with foamy macrophages, diffuse alveolar fibrosis, usual interstitial pneumonia, and interstitial lung fibrosis. A combination of above-mentioned changes may be seen in the same patient, even in the same biopsy specimen [54]. The reason for such different reactions still remains to be answered. The drug-induced changes of the pulmonary parenchyma are steroid refractory, which may be a clue in distinguishing the etiology of the diffuse changes [55].

Imaging Techniques

The pattern and topographic distribution of changes seen in patients with DI-DLD are highly variable. Nevertheless, in certain cases the imaging features are highly suggestive of certain types of DI-DLD [5, 56, 57]. In mineral oil pneumonia, the "foamy" opacities of lipid density are characteristically seen on HRCT [58]. Amiodarone pneumonitis is characterized by asymmetrical, nonsegmental opacities. The migratory painful opacities seen in BOOP, the "melted candle wax-like" opacities often found in nitrofurantoin lung toxicity, the "photographic negative" of pulmonary edema; and the mosaic pattern of desquamative interstitial pneumonia are further examples of characteristic radiological findings [59–61].

Pulmonary Function Tests

The classic physiologic alterations in DLD include reduced lung volumes (VC, TLC), reduced diffusing capacity (DLco), and a normal or increased ratio of forced expiratory volume in 1 s to forced vital capacity (FEV1/FVC). Static lung compliance is decreased and maximal transpulmonary pressure is increased. A mixed restrictive and obstructive pattern is also seen in BOOP. In advanced DI-DLD, arterial blood gas analysis shows mild hypoxemia.

Most Common DI-DLD

Antimicrobial Agents
Nitrofurantoin
Nitrofurantoin-induced DLD is one of the most commonly reported drug-induced pulmonary diseases. The mechanism of acute and chronic DLD secondary to nitrofurantoin appears to be different. Chronic disease can occur without the acute phase. One of the most common DI-DLDs is nitrofurantoin acute pneumonitis. The Swedish Adverse Drug Reaction Committee reported over 900 cases [62]. The acute stage usually begins 2 h to 10 days after the onset of therapy and is not dose-related. It appears to be much more common in females. Fever is present in most cases; the patients usually experience dyspnea. A reticulonodular or alveolar infiltrate is the most common imaging finding. It is located at the bases of the lungs. Pleural effusion (usually unilateral) has been found in almost one-third of the patients. There is no way to diagnose acute nitrofurantoin pneumonitis other than to suspect that the drug is responsible and to stop its administration. Discontinuation of the drug is the only required treatment. It is not known if steroids accelerate the resolution. No overlap exists between acute and chronic nitrofurantoin pneumonitis, probably because mechanisms of injury are completely different. Chronic reactions occur less frequently. The onset of cough and dyspnea is insidious, beginning months and even years after the chronic use of nitrofurantoin. Radiograms show a diffuse interstitial pattern. The pulmonary functional studies demonstrate a restrictive pattern. Lymphocytosis is seen in BAL. This condition – clinically, radiologically, and histologically – mimics IPF. Data on utility of steroids vary. Most reports have shown that they are usually required before significant resolution occurs [63].

Sulfasalazine
Two separate reactions occur in sulfasalazine-induced toxicity. One is a pulmonary infiltrate and eosinophilia and the other a BOOP. The onset of symptoms (cough, fever, and dyspnea) begins 1–8 months after initiation of therapy. Chest radiograms show a variable pattern of lung infiltrates. Half of the patients demonstrate significant blood eosinophilia. Resolution occurs 1 week to 6 months after discontinuation of therapy; if necessary, steroids may be added.

Miscellaneous Agents
Many reports exist on reactions to various antimicrobial agents (see Table 17.2). The incidence of these is extremely low. Many of these reactions appear to be transient pulmonary infiltrates with eosinophilia. Polymyxin and aminoglycoside antibiotics have been shown to produce respiratory muscle weakness. This occurs especially in patients receiving these agents directly into the pleural or peritoneal space.

Anti-inflammatory Drugs

Aspirin

The most commonly used drugs worldwide are the anti-inflammatory agents. Many of these induce pulmonary toxic effects. Aspirin is the most commonly used drug. It is estimated that 5% of asthmatics are sensitive to aspirin. The aspirin asthma triad consists of asthma, rhinitis, and nasal polyposis. The reactions are not dose-related; they can occur even after indigestion of a small dose. Salicylate-induced noncardiac pulmonary edema can occur when the serum salicylate levels exceed the level of 40 mg/dL. Salicylate toxicity occurs more often in elderly people who are smokers than in young nonsmokers [64].

Gold

Gold salts have been used for treating various disorders, rheumatoid arthritis in particular. Several reports have been published showing diffuse interstitial lung disorders associated with the use of gold that are separate from that of rheumatoid lung [65]. Dyspnea with or without fever begin insidiously several weeks to months after starting intramuscular injections of gold. The chest radiogram shows a diffuse interstitial process. BAL demonstrates a high lymphocyte count [66]. Histologically, fibrosis is seen with interstitial infiltrate of lymphocytes and plasma cells, accompanied by focal hyperplasia of type II pneumocytes. Treatment depends on withdrawal of the drug. A number of patients require addition of steroids for reversal.

Methotrexate

Methotrexate causes granulomatous pneumonitis in 5% of patients on low-dose methotrexate for rheumatoid arthritis or other inflammatory diseases (see Table 17.2). Most patients present with dyspnea, fever, rales, and hypoxemia. Hilar adenopathy is seen in 10–15% of patients, and pleural effusion is present in 10%. When methotrexate is used in low doses, granulomatous pneumonitis is usually

noted after administration of approximately 10 mg/week for an average of 80 weeks. BAL reveals marked lymphocytosis. Most patients respond favorably to discontinuation of methotrexate [67].

Penicillamine

Three pulmonary complications, which do not appear to overlap, exist with the use of penicillamine. They are Goodpasture's syndrome, penicillamine-induced SLE, and bronchiolitis obliterans. Another entity, alveolitis, previously described as another syndrome, should be regarded as a penicillamine-induced SLE. Penicillamine toxicity appears to be one of the most common causes of drug-induced SLE. This condition should always be suspected, especially in the presence of a pleural effusion. A normal concentration of glucose in the effusion fluid eliminates the possibility of rheumatoid effusion. Several case reports of penicillamine-induced Goodpasture's syndrome have been described [68]. If recognized early enough, treatment with hemodialysis, plasmapheresis, and immunosuppression may prevent the fatal outcome.

Leukotriene Antagonists

Several reports have associated the selective leukotriene receptor antagonist zafirlukast with the Churg–Strauss syndrome [47]. Currently, it is not known if the antagonists trigger the reaction or whether they unmask a preexisting eosinophilic disorder as the steroids are withdrawn. In any event, the pulmonary reaction responds to withdrawal of zafirlukast and reinstitution of steroids.

Other Nonsteroidal Anti-inflammatory Drugs

Most of these drugs produce the same side-effects as aspirin. It has been demonstrated that naproxen produces more of these reactions than do other drugs.

Cardiovascular Drugs

Amiodarone

In over 4% of patients receiving amiodarone, a DI-DLD is found [69]. The majority of these cases occur in males. Risk factors include maintenance dose greater than 400 mg/day and previous pulmonary disease. The combination of amiodarone with general anesthesia, pulmonary angiography, and coronary bypass surgery is synergistic of acute lung injury. Two clinical patterns exist. The most common presentation includes the insidious development of dyspnea, cough, fever, and malaise accompanied by weight loss. Pleurisy may be seen in up to 20% of the patients. Diffuse reticulonodular infiltrates are present on radiograms. The other pattern is characterized by an abrupt onset of an acute illness, with localized alveolar infiltrates. The mechanism of amiodarone toxicity is not known. The histological findings generally include foamy alveolar macrophages and pneumocytes containing lamellar inclusions. In over half of the fatalities, macrophages and pneumocytes contain large amount of phospholipids. This presentation may mimic infectious pneumonia or ARDS. Multiple, nodular infiltrates with necrotizing pneumonia and cavitations have been reported. Laboratory studies disclose a mildly elevated leukocyte count, generally no eosinophilia, and increased sedimentation rate with little reactivity to antinuclear antibody. BAL discloses the presence of phospholipid-filled macrophages, and increased counts of leukocytes and lymphocytes [34]. Absence of foamy macrophages eliminates amiodarone toxicity; the presence of foamy macrophages only confirms exposure to amiodarone. Pulmonary function studies show a decrease in total lung capacity as well as hypoxemia. This can also be caused by congestive heart failure. Thus, such findings cannot be diagnostic of amiodarone lung toxicity. Several reports on the use of gallium scans have demonstrated its usefulness in differential diagnosis between congestive heart failure and amiodarone toxicity [70]. Treatment consists of amiodarone withdrawal. In some cases, steroid therapy has been shown to have some benefits. The steroids should be used for a period of 1–6 months or longer.

Beta-Adrenergic Antagonists

These agents are amongst the most commonly prescribed drugs. Propranolol was one of the first beta-adrenergic antagonists introduced. It was quickly recognized that it produced adverse effects in patients with obstructive airway disease. Of the registered drugs, atenolol, metoprolol, and labetalol are the three that can be safely used in patients with obstructive airway disease. Only a few reports have shown beta-blocker-associated pneumonitis.

Protamine

Protamine sulfate is routinely used in reversing the anticoagulant effect of heparin. A number of cases of noncardionegenic edema developing within minutes to hours after administration of protamine have been reported. It was associated with anaphylactic reaction and bronchospasm [71].

Angiotensin-Converting Enzyme Inhibitors

These agents are associated with nonproductive cough and angioneurotic edema [72]. A dry cough occurs in up to 20% of the patients taking angiotensin-converting enzyme (ACE) inhibitors. Treatment involves discontinuation of the drug. Angioneurotic edema is seen less frequently only in 0.1–0.2% of the patients taking ACE inhibitors. Treatment includes the use of epinephrine, antihistamines, and steroid administration. The ACE inhibitor must be discontinued.

Antineoplastic Agents

Drug toxicity may be the cause of over 20% of diffuse pulmonary infiltrates in treated oncology patients. The diagnosis of chemotherapeutic DI-DLD is one of exclusion. Dyspnea occurs within the first few weeks of treatment, followed by cough and intermittent fever. Ten percent of the patients treated with bleomycin may develop drug-induced lung disease. The mortality of this disease is high, approaching 50%. The incidence of DI-DLD increases in the presence of risk factors such as age (>70 years), oxygen therapy, cumulative dose of more than 450 units, concomitant radiation therapy, and multidrug regimens [73].

Busulfan

Busulfan-induced DLD occurs in 2–3% of patients and frequently develops a year after onset of therapy. The onset of dyspnea, cough, and fever is usually more insidious than with other chemotherapeutically induced DI-DLDs. This DLD does not respond to withdrawal of the drug or to administration of steroids [74]. Chest radiograms show an alveolar interstitial process. Alveolar proteinosis has been reported in a few patients receiving busulfan.

Cyclophosphamide

The incidence of this DLD is underestimated. Cyclophosphamide-induced DLD usually begins a few weeks after initiating therapy and has a variable course with steroid-responsive and non-responsive disease [30, 73]. Clinical features include dyspnea, fever, cough, new parenchyma infiltrates, and pleural thickening and gas exchange abnormalities. Early-onset disease occurs within the first months of treatment, and generally responds to withdrawal of the drug. Late-onset disease develops after months to years of cyclophosphamide therapy and is manifested by progressive pulmonary fibrosis and pleural thickening. The late-onset variety has minimal response to withdrawal of cyclophosphamide and institution of steroid therapy.

Nitrosoureas

Nitrosoureas (BCND) and methyl-CCNU DLD have been reported in as many as 50% of patients

undergoing therapy with doses exceeding 1,500 mg/m^2. There have been reports of pulmonary effects occurring with much lower doses [75]. These agents may have a synergistic effect with cyclophosphamide [76]. The clinical course is very similar to that seen in cyclophosphamide- and bleomycin-induced DLD. The outcome is unpredictable and sometimes fatal.

Procarbazine

Procarbazine causes acute DLD with peripheral and pulmonary eosinophilia and pleural effusions [77]. The incidence of this entity is not so frequent.

Bleomycin

Bleomycin-induced lung toxicity is the most common chemotherapeutically induced drug-induced toxicity and the most completely studied one. As many as 20% of the patients treated with bleomycin develop lung toxicity. There is a definite correlation between thoracic radiotherapy and increased incidence of severe bleomycin pulmonary toxicity. Bleomycin-induced DLD may be reversible if only minimal changes have occurred. If significant fibrosis is present, the process may progress despite administration of steroids. In most cases, discontinuation of the drug and introduction of steroid therapy brings about the reversal of the toxic process. A unique complication of bleomycin toxicity and unique to this drug is the presence of nodular changes mimicking metastasis to the lungs [78]. Histologically, most of these lesions consist of bronchiolitis obliterans with organizing pneumonitis.

Mitomycin C

The incidence of mitomycin C-induced lung toxicity ranges from 8 to 32%. The clinical findings are similar to those seen in other toxic syndromes produced by alkylating agents. The response to steroids is very favorable, and more promising than in other cases of lung toxicity [79].

Illicit Drugs

Heroin

Heroin-induced pulmonary edema may be the most common drug-induced pulmonary disease in the world. Several mechanisms of heroin-induced pulmonary edema are currently acknowledged. These include a direct toxic effect on the alveolar capillary membrane leading to increased permeability, a neurogenic response to central nervous system injury, and an allergic reaction [80]. Pulmonary edema may occur during the first intravenous use of the drug. Up to 40% of addicts admitted because of heroin overdose demonstrate acute pulmonary edema with severe hypoxemia and hypercapnia. In chronic heroin abusers, bronchiectases and necrotizing bronchitis have been reported. Treatment consists of assisted ventilation, oxygen, and intravenous naloxone to reverse respiratory depression. Steroids are usually unnecessary.

Methadone and Propoxyphene

Pulmonary toxicity similar to that reported in heroin abusers has been reported with methadone and propoxyphene. Treatment is the same. Propoxyphene, being rapidly absorbed, produced fatal respiratory depression and death within 30 min.

Cocaine

An increasing incidence of pulmonary toxicity to cocaine is being reported worldwide. The pulmonary long-term effects of cocaine use are alveolar damage, alveolar hemorrhage, intraseptal eosinophilic infiltration, lung mass with or without cavitation, and BOOP.

Inhalants

Aspirated oil can produce a variety of pulmonary diseases, ranging from an asymptomatic pulmonary nodule to diffuse disease with respiratory insufficiency [81]. More often, the disease presents in an asymptomatic patient with accidental findings on routine chest radiograms that often mimic a more serious lesion such as lung cancer. Patients rarely consider reporting use of oily nose drops or oily eye lubricants as medication. Three types of oils are used – mineral oils, neutral oils, and animal fats. Mineral oils are the most commonly aspirated oils. Oily drops are taken up by macrophages, released upon disintegration, and taken up again. This inhibits ciliary function of the airways. The cycle is repeated. The oil is not expectorated. Eventually, a granulomatous and fibrotic lesion develops. The diagnosis can be established with the demonstration of oil-laden macrophages in BAL, and of oil in pulmonary tissue. CT is helpful. Treatment includes discontinuation of oil-containing medications.

Transfusion-Related Acute Alveolar Damage

One of the most rarely recognized adverse reactions is acute alveolar damage because of transfusion reaction. This acute reaction is not a hemolytic transfusion reaction or an anaphylactic reaction. The clinical presentation is that of onset of dyspnea, cough, fever, and hypotension within hours after the transfusion. An urticarial rash occurs in approximately half of the patients. Any blood product can produce this reaction. Treatment is supportive, including assisted ventilation and supplemental oxygen. The course of this noncardiac edema is usually limited to only 72 h [31].

Summary

Clinicians must maintain a high index of suspicion that an unexplained pulmonary disease may result from the usage of various medications. Most drug-induced DLDs are reversible if the drug is stopped in time. There is limited knowledge of the mechanisms inducing lung changes, and limited diagnostic tests are available. Seldom is re-challenging the patient with the suspected drug indicated; rather it should be contraindicated.

References

1. Sigerist HE. Civilization and disease. Ithaca: Cornell University Press; 1948.
2. Sigerist HE. The Wesley M. Carpenter Lecture: "Historical background of industrial and occupational diseases". Bull N Y Acad Med. 1936;12(11): 597–609.
3. Bracker A, Storey E. Assessing occupational and environmental exposures that cause lung disease. Clin Chest Med. 2002;23(4):695–705.
4. Henry DA. International Labor Office Classification System in the age of imaging: relevant or redundant. J Thorac Imaging. 2002;17(3):179–88.
5. Cleverley JR, Screaton NJ, Hiorns MP, Flint JD, Muller NL. Drug-induced lung disease: high-resolution CT and histological findings. Clin Radiol. 2002;57(4):292–9.
6. Pipavath SN, Godwin JD, Kanne JP. Occupational lung disease: a radiologic review. Semin Roentgenol. 2010;45(1):43–52.
7. Diseases associated with exposure to silica and nonfibrous silicate minerals. Silicosis and Silicate Disease Committee. Arch Pathol Lab Med. 1988;112(7): 673–720.
8. Mossman BT, Churg A. Mechanisms in the pathogenesis of asbestosis and silicosis. Am J Respir Crit Care Med. 1998;157(5 Pt 1):1666–80.
9. De Vuyst P, Camus P. The past and present of pneumoconioses. Curr Opin Pulm Med. 2000;6(2):151–6.
10. Becklake MR. The mineral dust diseases. Tuber Lung Dis. 1992;73(1):13–20.
11. Becklake MR. When the chest X-ray does not tell the whole story: a tale of miners, selection bias, and the healthy worker effect. Am J Respir Crit Care Med. 2001;164(10 Pt 1):1761–2.
12. Doll NJ, Stankus RP, Barkman HW. Immunopathogenesis of asbestosis, silicosis, and coal workers' pneumoconiosis. Clin Chest Med. 1983;4(1): 3–14.
13. Glaspole IN, Wells AU, du Bois RM. Lung biopsy in diffuse parenchymal lung disease. Monaldi Arch Chest Dis. 2001;56(3):225–32.
14. Wilt JL, Banks DE, Weissman DN, et al. Reduction of lung dust burden in pneumoconiosis by whole-lung lavage. J Occup Environ Med. 1996;38(6):619–24.
15. Pathology standards for coal workers' pneumoconiosis. Report of the Pneumoconiosis Committee of the College of American Pathologists to the National Institute for Occupational Safety and Health. Arch Pathol Lab Med. 1979;103(8):375–432.
16. Jindal SK, Aggarwal AN, Gupta D. Dust-induced interstitial lung disease in the tropics. Curr Opin Pulm Med. 2001;7(5):272–7.
17. Stark P, Jacobson F, Shaffer K. Standard imaging in silicosis and coal worker's pneumoconiosis. Radiol Clin North Am. 1992;30(6):1147–54.
18. Shankar PS. Ventilatory study in simple coal worker's pneumoconiosis. Indian J Med Sci. 1981;35(4):73–6.
19. Ashcroft T. Asbestos bodies. Br Med J. 1968; 2(606):696–7.
20. Akira M, Yamamoto S, Inoue Y, Sakatani M. High-resolution CT of asbestosis and idiopathic pulmonary fibrosis. Am J Roentgenol. 2003;181(1):163–9.
21. Victor LD, Talamonti WJ. Asbestos lung disease. Hosp Pract (Off Ed). 1986;21(4):257–68.
22. Jones-Williams W. On the differential diagnosis of chronic beryllium disease and sarcoidosis. Am Rev Respir Dis. 1990;142(3):739–40.
23. Rossman MD, Kern JA, Elias JA, et al. Proliferative response of bronchoalveolar lymphocytes to beryllium. A test for chronic beryllium disease. Ann Intern Med. 1988;108(5):687–93.
24. Uibu T, Vanhala E, Sajantila A, et al. Asbestos fibers in para-aortic and mesenteric lymph nodes. Am J Ind Med. 2009;52(6):464–70.
25. Fireman E, Greif J, Schwarz Y, et al. Assessment of hazardous dust exposure by BAL and induced sputum. Chest. 1999;115(6):1720–8.
26. Forni A. Bronchoalveolar lavage in the diagnosis of hard metal disease. Sci Total Environ. 1994;150(1–3): 69–76.
27. Camus PH, Foucher P, Bonniaud PH, Ask K. Drug-induced infiltrative lung disease. Eur Respir J Suppl. 2001;32:93s–100.
28. Limper AH, Rosenow III EC. Drug-induced interstitial lung disease. Curr Opin Pulm Med. 1996;2(5):396–404.
29. Rosenow III EC, Myers JL, Swensen SJ, Pisani RJ. Drug-induced pulmonary disease. An update. Chest. 1992;102(1):239–50.
30. Rosenow III EC, Limper AH. Drug-induced pulmonary disease. Semin Respir Infect. 1995;10(2):86–95.
31. Kopko PM, Marshall CS, MacKenzie MR, Holland PV, Popovsky MA. Transfusion-related acute lung injury: report of a clinical look-back investigation. JAMA. 2002;287(15):1968–71.
32. Kopko PM, Holland PV. Transfusion-related acute lung injury. Br J Haematol. 1999;105(2):322–9.
33. Ernst E. Harmless herbs? A review of the recent literature. Am J Med. 1998;104(2):170–8.
34. Bedrossian CW, Warren CJ, Ohar J, Bhan R. Amiodarone pulmonary toxicity: cytopathology, ultrastructure, and immunocytochemistry. Ann Diagn Pathol. 1997;1(1):47–56.
35. Ellis SJ, Cleverley JR, Muller NL. Drug-induced lung disease: high-resolution CT findings. AJR Am J Roentgenol. 2000;175(4):1019–24.
36. Helman Jr DL, Byrd JC, Ales NC, Shorr AF. Fludarabine-related pulmonary toxicity: a distinct clinical entity in chronic lymphoproliferative syndromes. Chest. 2002;122(3):785–90.
37. Wesselius LJ. Pulmonary complications of cancer therapy. Compr Ther. 1999;25(5):272–7.
38. Aronin PA, Mahaley Jr MS, Rudnick SA, et al. Prediction of BCNU pulmonary toxicity in patients with malignant gliomas: an assessment of risk factors. N Engl J Med. 1980;303(4):183–8.
39. Schlaeffer F, Gold B, Hirsch M, Keynan A. A case of interstitial pneumonitis during amiodarone therapy. Isr J Med Sci. 1982;18(7):809–11.

40. Sobol SM, Rakita L. Pneumonitis and pulmonary fibrosis associated with amiodarone treatment: a possible complication of a new antiarrhythmic drug. Circulation. 1982;65(4):819–24.

41. De Lena M, Guzzon A, Monfardini S, Bonadonna G. Clinical, radiologic, and histopathologic studies on pulmonary toxicity induced by treatment with bleomycin (NSC-125066). Cancer Chemother Rep. 1972;56(3):343–56.

42. Salaffi F, Manganelli P, Carotti M, Subiaco S, Lamanna G, Cervini C. Methotrexate-induced pneumonitis in patients with rheumatoid arthritis and psoriatic arthritis: report of five cases and review of the literature. Clin Rheumatol. 1997;16(3):296–304.

43. Cottin V, Tebib J, Massonnet B, Souquet PJ, Bernard JP. Pulmonary function in patients receiving long-term low-dose methotrexate. Chest. 1996;109(4): 933–8.

44. Foucher P, Biour M, Blayac JP, et al. Drugs that may injure the respiratory system. Eur Respir J. 1997;10(2): 265–79.

45. Faller M, Quoix E, Popin E, et al. Migratory pulmonary infiltrates in a patient treated with sotalol. Eur Respir J. 1997;10(9):2159–62.

46. Dhillon SS, Singh D, Doe N, Qadri AM, Ricciardi S, Schwarz MI. Diffuse alveolar hemorrhage and pulmonary capillaritis due to propylthiouracil. Chest. 1999;116(5):1485–8.

47. Green RL, Vayonis AG. Churg-Strauss syndrome after zafirlukast in two patients not receiving systemic steroid treatment. Lancet. 1999;353(9154):725–6.

48. Kastelik JA, Aziz I, Greenstone MA, Thompson R, Morice AH. Pergolide-induced lung disease in patients with Parkinson's disease. Respir Med. 2002;96(7): 548–50.

49. Morita S, Ueda Y, Eguchi K. Anti-thyroid drug-induced ANCA-associated vasculitis: a case report and review of the literature. Endocr J. 2000;47(4): 467–70.

50. Salerno SM, Ormseth EJ, Roth BJ, Meyer CA, Christensen ED, Dillard TA. Sulfasalazine pulmonary toxicity in ulcerative colitis mimicking clinical features of Wegener's granulomatosis. Chest. 1996;110(2):556–9.

51. Skaer TL. Medication-induced systemic lupus erythematosus. Clin Ther. 1992;14(4):496–506.

52. Qureshi RA, Ahmed TA, Grayson AD, Soorae AS, Drakeley MJ, Page RD. Does lung biopsy help patients with interstitial lung disease? Eur J Cardiothorac Surg. 2002;21(4):621–6.

53. Huang MS, Colby TV, Goellner JR, Martin Jr WJ. Utility of bronchoalveolar lavage in the diagnosis of drug-induced pulmonary toxicity. Acta Cytol. 1989;33(4):533–8.

54. Myers JL, Kennedy JI, Plumb VJ. Amiodarone lung: pathologic findings in clinically toxic patients. Hum Pathol. 1987;18(4):349–54.

55. Bone RC, Wolfe J, Sobonya RE, et al. Desquamative interstitial pneumonia following long-term nitrofurantoin therapy. Am J Med. 1976;60(5):697–701.

56. Bergin CJ, Coblentz CL, Chiles C, Bell DY, Castellino RA. Chronic lung diseases: specific diagnosis by using CT. AJR Am J Roentgenol. 1989;152(6):1183–8.

57. Erasmus JJ, McAdams HP, Rossi SE. High-resolution CT of drug-induced lung disease. Radiol Clin North Am. 2002;40(1):61–72.

58. Gondouin A, Manzoni P, Ranfaing E, et al. Exogenous lipid pneumonia: a retrospective multicentre study of 44 cases in France. Eur Respir J. 1996;9(7):1463–9.

59. Gaensler EA, Carrington CB. Peripheral opacities in chronic eosinophilic pneumonia: the photographic negative of pulmonary edema. AJR Am J Roentgenol. 1977;128(1):1–13.

60. Primack SL, Hartman TE, Hansell DM, Muller NL. End-stage lung disease: CT findings in 61 patients. Radiology. 1993;189(3):681–6.

61. Screaton NJ, Hiorns MP, Muller NL. Differential diagnosis in chronic diffuse infiltrative lung disease on high-resolution computed tomography. Semin Roentgenol. 2002;37(1):17–24.

62. Holmberg L, Boman G. Pulmonary reactions to nitrofurantoin. 447 cases reported to the Swedish Adverse Drug Reaction Committee 1966-1976. Eur J Respir Dis. 1981;62(3):180–9.

63. Robinson BW. Nitrofurantoin-induced interstitial pulmonary fibrosis. Presentation and outcome. Med J Aust. 1983;1(2):72–6.

64. Zitnik RJ, Cooper Jr JA. Pulmonary disease due to antirheumatic agents. Clin Chest Med. 1990;11(1): 139–50.

65. Tomioka R, King Jr TE. Gold-induced pulmonary disease: clinical features, outcome, and differentiation from rheumatoid lung disease. Am J Respir Crit Care Med. 1997;155(3):1011–20.

66. Bronchoalveolar T-cell subsets in gold lung. Evidence for a hypersensitivity reaction. Chest. 1985;87(1): 135–6.

67. Zisman DA, McCune WJ, Tino G, Lynch III JP. Drug-induced pneumonitis: the role of methotrexate. Sarcoidosis Vasc Diffuse Lung Dis. 2001;18(3): 243–52.

68. Sternlieb I, Bennett B, Scheinberg IH. D-penicillamine induced Goodpasture's syndrome in Wilson's disease. Ann Intern Med. 1975;82(5):673–6.

69. Martin WJ. Mechanisms of amiodarone pulmonary toxicity. Clin Chest Med. 1990;11(1):131–8.

70. Zhu YY, Botvinick E, Dae M, Golden J, Hattner R, Scheinman M. Gallium lung scintigraphy in amiodarone pulmonary toxicity. Chest. 1988;93(6): 1126–31.

71. Nordstrom L, Fletcher R, Pavek K. Shock of anaphylactoid type induced by protamine: a continuous cardiorespiratory record. Acta Anaesthesiol Scand. 1978;22(3):195–201.

72. Kaufman J, Casanova JE, Riendl P, Schlueter DP. Bronchial hyperreactivity and cough due to angiotensin-converting enzyme inhibitors. Chest. 1989;95(3):544–8.

73. Rossi SE, Erasmus JJ, McAdams HP, Sporn TA, Goodman PC. Pulmonary drug toxicity: radiologic and pathologic manifestations. Radiographics. 2000;20(5):1245–59.

74. Sostman HD, Matthay RA, Putman CE. Cytotoxic drug-induced lung disease. Am J Med. 1977;62(4): 608–15.

75. Smith AC. The pulmonary toxicity of nitrosoureas. Pharmacol Ther. 1989;41(3):443–60.

76. Ewig S, Glasmacher A, Ulrich B, Wilhelm K, Schafer H, Nachtsheim KH. Pulmonary infiltrates in neutropenic patients with acute leukemia during chemotherapy: outcome and prognostic factors. Chest. 1998; 114(2): 444–51.

77. Lauta VM, Valerio G, Greco A, Capece MM. Early-onset diagnosis of lung toxicity caused by cyclophosphamide, melphalan and procarbazine therapy. Tumori. 1987;73(4):351–8.

78. Cohen MB, Austin JH, Smith-Vaniz A, Lutzky J, Grimes MM. Nodular bleomycin toxicity. Am J Clin Pathol. 1989;92(1):101–4.

79. Okuno SH, Frytak S. Mitomycin lung toxicity. Acute and chronic phases. Am J Clin Oncol. 1997;20(3): 282–4.

80. Whitcomb ME. Drug-induced lung disease. Chest. 1973;63(3):418–22.

81. Bandla HP, Davis SH, Hopkins NE. Lipoid pneumonia: a silent complication of mineral oil aspiration. Pediatrics. 1999;103(2):E19.

Bronchiolitis

18

Vincent Cottin and Jean-François Cordier

Abstract

Bronchiolitis is defined as an inflammatory process involving the bronchioles that may be associated with fibrosis of the bronchiolar wall. Bronchiolitis may be classified according to its etiology, onset (acute or chronic), or pathology. Cellular bronchiolitis corresponds to the infiltration of bronchiolar walls by inflammatory cells. Bronchiolitis obliterans is characterized by the narrowing of the caliber of the bronchiole as a consequence of fibrosis, with constrictive bronchiolitis obliterans consisting of concentric fibrosis in the wall of the bronchiole and narrowing of the bronchiolar lumen, and proliferative bronchiolitis obliterans (found in association with organizing pneumonia) characterized by buds of granulation tissue within the lumen of the bronchiole. Bronchiolitis that reduces the caliber of the small airways (constrictive bronchiolitis) typically results in nonreversible airflow obstruction. Characteristic features of bronchiolar disease on high-resolution tomography of the chest consist of a combination of centrilobular nodules, V- or Y-shaped branching linear opacities (tree-in-bud pattern), bronchiolar dilation, and the mosaic attenuation pattern on expiratory images.

The main determined causes of bronchiolitis include infection especially due to respiratory syncytial virus (RSV), acute inhalational injury by toxic gases or fumes, drugs (penicillamine), intake of juice from *Sauropus androgynus*, and occupational exposures (asbestos, nonasbestos mineral dusts, inhaled diacetyl used as butter-flavoring ingredients in

V. Cottin, MD, PhD • J.-F. Cordier, MD (✉)
Department of Respiratory Medicine,
Claude Bernard Lyon I University, Reference
Center for Rare Pulmonary Diseases, Lyon, France

Department of Respiratory Medicine, Louis Pradel
University Hospital, Lyon, France
e-mail: jean-francois.cordier@chu-lyon.fr

R.P. Baughman and R.M. du Bois (eds.), *Diffuse Lung Disease: A Practical Approach*,
DOI 10.1007/978-1-4419-9771-5_18, © Springer Science+Business Media, LLC 2012

microwave-popcorn plants, synthetic polymers in industrial flockers). Bronchiolitis may further occur in well-characterized contexts, especially in rheumatoid arthritis, Sjögren syndrome, following lung transplantation or bone marrow graft, and rarely in paraneoplastic pemphigus. Cryptogenic constrictive bronchiolitis is a rare cause of airflow obstruction predominating in females between 40 and 60 year old. Bronchiolitis may also be observed as an associated pathological finding in a variety of conditions affecting the airways (chronic obstructive pulmonary disease, bronchiectasis, respiratory bronchiolitis) or as a component of diffuse inflammatory lung disease. Management of bronchiolitis depends on the etiological context, pathologic pattern, severity of impairment of pulmonary function, and progression of disease.

Keywords

Bronchiolitis • Organizing pneumonia • Connective tissue disease • Rheumatoid arthritis • Lung transplantation • Graft versus host disease

Bronchiolitis is defined as an inflammatory process involving the bronchioles. Infiltration of the bronchioles by inflammatory cells and fibroblasts may result in fibrosis and/or impairment of their structure and consequently their function. A wide spectrum of diffuse lung diseases includes bronchiolitis as a main or an accessory component. It is thus more important for the clinician to understand the morphological lesions of the bronchioles and their consequences on clinical, imaging, and functional manifestations, rather than to consider bronchiolitis just as a nosologic entity with strict boundaries.

The bronchiole is a small airway without cartilage, less than 1 mm in diameter. The diameter of the bronchiole is approximately the same as that of the accompanying artery. The terminal bronchiole is the bronchiole just proximal to the respiratory bronchioles which have alveoli budging from their walls. The respiratory bronchioles are followed by the alveolar ducts and finally, the alveoli. There are communications between these structures which permit collateral ventilation and prevent distal alveolar collapse when a bronchiole is occluded: between respiratory and terminal bronchioles, between nonrespiratory bronchioles and alveoli (Lambert's canals), and between alveoli (pores of Kohn).

Classification of Bronchiolitis

The etiological classification distinguishes three types of bronchiolitis: bronchiolitis of determined origin, bronchiolitis of undetermined origin but occurring in a well-characterized context (for example, transplantation or connective tissue disease), and solitary bronchiolitis of undetermined origin (cryptogenic or idiopathic). Some other well-individualized entities (e.g., diffuse panbronchiolitis) and disorders with bronchiolitis as a component of another entity (e.g., diffuse bronchiectasis) may be considered separately, although they could be included in the three etiological groups above (Table 18.1). This is the classification for the clinician which will be used in this chapter.

The pathologic classification comprises many entities differing by distinct pathologic lesions affecting the bronchioles [1, 2]. The most characteristic pathologic types of bronchiolitis are cellular bronchiolitis and bronchiolitis obliterans. Cellular bronchiolitis corresponds to the infiltration of the wall of the bronchioles by cells (usually inflammatory cells, occasionally hyperplastic or neoplastic cells). Bronchiolitis obliterans is characterized by the narrowing of the caliber of

Table 18.1 Classification of bronchiolitis

Etiological classification	Individualized entities
Bronchiolitis of determined origin	
• Infectious bronchiolitis	• Smoking-related bronchiolar disorders
• Bronchiolitis by acute inhalation injury	– Respiratory bronchiolitis
• Other known causes of bronchiolitis	– Respiratory bronchiolitis with interstitial lung disease
– Drug-induced bronchiolitis	– Bronchiolitis in COPD
– *Sauropus androgynus* bronchiolitis	• Bronchiectasis as a component of diffuse inflammatory
– Mineral dust airways disease	lung disease of determined origin
– Food flavorer's lung (diacetyl)	– Hypersensitivity pneumonitis
– Flock worker's lung (polypropylene)	– Eosinophilic pneumonia
– Other occupation induced bronchiolitis	• Bronchiectasis and bronchiolitis of determined origin
Bronchiolitis of undetermined origin occurring in a well-characterized context	
• Connective tissue diseases	• Bronchiectasis and bronchiolitis occurring in a
– Rheumatoid arthritis	well-characterized context
– Sjögren's syndrome	• Diffuse panbronchiolitis
– Other connective tissue diseases	• Neuroendocrine cell hyperplasia
• Obliterative bronchiolitis associated with lung	• Malignant bronchiolitis
transplantation or bone marrow graft	• Bronchiolitis as a component of diffuse inflammatory
– Obliterative bronchiolitis after lung transplantation	lung disease
– Obliterative bronchiolitis after bone marrow graft	– Sarcoidosis
• Obliterative bronchiolitis in paraneoplastic pemphigus	– Eosinophilic pneumonia
	• Bronchiolitis in other entities
	– Lymphangioleiomyomatosis
	– Pulmonary Langerhans' cell histiocytosis
	– Sarcoidosis
Cryptogenic (idiopathic) constrictive bronchiolitis	

Table 18.2 Important features of obliterative bronchiolitis

History	
Significant positive features	Progressive dyspnea
Etiology	Acute inhalation injury
	Occupational exposure
	Connective tissue disease
	Transplantation
Physical examination	
Significant positive features	No characteristic physical features (squeaks occasionally)
Suggests another diagnosis	Crackles
Lung function tests and imaging	
Support diagnosis	Decreased FEV1/FVC, FEF 25–75; increased RV/TLC
	Mosaic pattern at HR-CT
Diagnostic for disease	The features above are diagnostic in an appropriate etiologic context
Pathology	
Open lung biopsy (if really needed)	Bronchiolitis obliterans or any type of bronchiolitis reducing the caliber of the bronchiolar lumen

the bronchiole as a consequence of fibrosis (the authors prefer to reserve the terminology of bronchiolitis obliterans for describing pathologic lesions, and to use obliterative bronchiolitis to designate its clinical counterpart and any type of bronchiolitis associated with airflow obstruction) (Table 18.2) [3]. There are two different types of bronchiolitis obliterans. Constrictive bronchiolitis obliterans consists of concentric fibrosis in the wall of the bronchiole; when severe, it may completely occlude the lumen of the bronchiole, leaving just a fibrotic scar. Proliferative bronchiolitis obliterans differs, with buds consisting of connective tissue and mesenchymal cells located within the lumen of the bronchiole, the wall of which is relatively spared by fibrosis; the buds are connected to the bronchiolar wall over a variable part of its circumference. Proliferative bronchiolitis obliterans is the type found in association with organizing pneumonia; however, in this condition bronchiolitis is usually an accessory process and may even be lacking. For this reason, the terminology of idiopathic bronchiolitis obliterans organizing pneumonia has been replaced by cryptogenic organizing pneumonia [4] to emphasize that organizing pneumonia is the main lesion and bronchiolitis obliterans just an accessory component.

If, in some cases, the inflammatory process involving the bronchioles may also concern the alveoli (as seen in bronchiolitis obliterans with organizing pneumonia), in other cases it may involve the large bronchi thus producing a longitudinal airway inflammation from the bronchioles to the large proximal bronchi. Depending on whether inflammation affecting the bronchioles mainly extends to either the alveoli or to the large bronchi, the clinical manifestations will differ markedly. A histopathologic diagnosis of bronchiolitis is not specific of an etiology. In addition, bronchiolitis present on a lung biopsy may represent the predominant condition or may correspond to a secondary phenomenon in another primary pathologic process (e.g., bronchiectasis, hypersensitivity pneumonitis, sarcoidosis, etc.) [1, 2].

In many circumstances of longitudinal airway inflammation, bronchitis associated with bronchiolitis results in damage to the bronchial wall with the development of bronchiectasis. This is especially evident in patients with airway disease of immune origin after lung transplantation or bone marrow graft where the development of bronchiectasis in association with bronchiolitis is rapid, or in patients with impaired defenses of the airways from any origin (e.g., impairment of mucociliary clearance, or hypogammaglobulinemia). It is extremely important for the clinician to identify the bronchial component of airway disease in addition to bronchiolitis since it has major clinical implications, especially for the causal treatment (e.g., immunoglobulin supplemental treatment in severe hypogammaglobulinemia of any cause) and the management of iterative bronchial infections.

Bronchiolitis may be acute or chronic. Acute bronchiolitis usually comprises cellular infiltration of the bronchiolar wall and diffuse damage to the bronchiolar epithelium with desquamation of the injured cells into the bronchiolar lumen. When bronchiolar damage is more severe, necrosis of the bronchiole may occur. When the bronchiolar lesions are mild, adequate repair is the rule, but when damage is more severe, it may result in inappropriate repair with fibrosis reducing the caliber of the bronchiolar lumen (constrictive bronchiolitis) or even in the replacement of the bronchiole by just a fibrous scar.

Constrictive bronchiolitis is more often the consequence of a chronic inflammatory process. It is best illustrated by bronchiolitis obliterans complicating lung transplantation, which is considered as a process of chronic rejection. In parallel, a comparable bronchiolitis may occur as a complication of graft versus host disease (GVHD) in patients after bone marrow allografting. It is clear that in both conditions bronchiolitis obliterans is the consequence of an immune conflict between the host and the transplanted lung or grafted cells.

Chronic bronchiolitis is often associated with bronchiolectasis and mucostasis. Bronchiolectasis is often underestimated and has not been extensively studied for itself. It may accompany emphysema.

Lung Function Tests in Bronchiolitis

Typically, constrictive bronchiolitis, or any other type of bronchiolitis reducing the caliber of the small airways, results in nonreversible airflow obstruction. Airflow obstruction is usually defined by a ratio of forced expiratory volume in 1 s (FEV1) to forced vital capacity (FVC) below 0.7 (FEV1/FVC ratio is nevertheless dependent to some extent on age and height). However, airflow obstruction may be present even in cases where the FEV1/FVC ratio is within normal limits. In such eventuality, the FVC is reduced due to an increase in residual volume (RV) by premature closure of the small airways (air trapping); since the total lung capacity (TLC) is not changed, the RV/TLC ratio increases [3]. It has been proposed that this syndrome be called "small airways obstruction syndrome" [5].

Tests exploring mild airflow obstruction may be useful, but there is much debate about the validity and precise signification of such tests. The forced expiratory flow between 25 and 75% of the FVC (FEF 25–75) is likely a good tool to detect mild airflow obstruction. In particular, it has been demonstrated that FEF 25–75 decline to <70% of the predicted value and of baseline values precedes a 20% reduction in FEV1 by about 4 months [6]. The decline is proportionally greater for FEF 25–75 than for FEV1 and allows an earlier detection of the bronchiolitis obliterans syndrome (BOS) (this is the terminology used to describe airflow obstruction related to bronchiolitis obliterans developing after lung transplantation, whether or not a pathologic confirmation is obtained). This suggests that FEF 25–75 might also be used to detect mild airflow obstruction in other types of bronchiolitis, but this remains to be formally demonstrated.

Imaging Patterns in Bronchiolitis

Although specific differences in imaging pattern between the different types of bronchiolitis exist, the characteristic features identified on thin-section high-resolution computed tomography (HR-CT) and common to various bronchiolitis consist of one or a combination of the following: centrilobular nodules, V- or Y-shaped branching linear opacities representing the tree-in-bud pattern, and later bronchiolar dilation (direct CT signs of small airways disease); and air trapping especially on expiratory HR-CT with alternating geographic areas of decreased and increased attenuation or mosaic pattern (indirect signs of small airways disease) [7–9]. Both inspiratory and expiratory CT images are helpful.

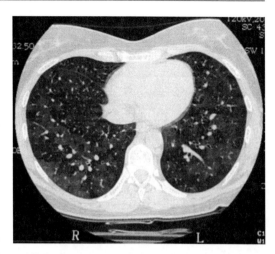

Fig. 18.1 Mosaic attenuation pattern on HR-CT in a patient with obliterative bronchiolitis

The so-called mosaic attenuation pattern results from hypoventilation with air trapping distal to airway obstruction with the consequence of reflex hypoxic vasoconstriction (decreased attenuation, with the lung more lucent than normal) and blood flow redistribution to normal areas (increased attenuation) (Fig. 18.1). Bronchial dilatation is often associated with this pattern. Mosaic attenuation pattern may also be found in infiltrative lung disease, vascular disease, and in a minority of healthy individuals.

Centrilobular nodules may result from bronchiolar wall thickening, bronchiolar dilatation, and bronchiolar impaction; bronchiolar impaction of the bronchioles with mucus or pus may give rise to branching linear structures with more than one branching site (tree-in-bud pattern). Bronchiolectasis is found most commonly in chronic forms of bronchiolitis.

Therapeutic Considerations in Chronic Bronchiolitis

Inhaled bronchodilators are usually poorly effective on the airflow limitation caused by bronchiolar inflammation. Oral corticosteroids and possibly immunosuppressive therapy may contribute to ameliorate airflow obstruction or to limit progression of the disease; however, anti-inflammatory therapy has variable efficacy on the clinical outcome depending on the etiology, stage, and histopathology of the disease. Supplemental nasal oxygen therapy and noninvasive nasal ventilation may be helpful supportive therapy in advanced disease.

Macrolide therapy has dramatically changed the management and the prognosis of diffuse panbronchiolitis, a condition almost unique to the Asian populations, and has shown some efficacy in cystic fibrosis [10]. Following these examples, macrolides have been tested on other chronic airways diseases especially with neutrophilic inflammation, with some beneficial effects documented in posttransplant BOS. The mechanisms of action of macrolides are multifactorial, including antimicrobial properties and modulation of host–pathogen response, inhibition of mucin secretion, and immunomodulation and anti-inflammatory effect through the modulation of cytokine responses and of innate immunity [11].

Bronchiolitis of Determined Origin

Infectious Bronchiolitis

Acute infectious bronchiolitis is rare in adults, but very common in children [12]. In children, it is mainly of viral origin, and especially due to RSV which accounts for ~80% of the cases. It occurs in very young infants (first year of life), usually between 2 and 8 months. Infection is acquired through the upper respiratory tract. Acute bronchiolitis is characterized by a neutrophilic inflammation accompanied by a cascade of inflammatory mediators. Maternal smoking in pregnancy is a predisposing factor. After an incubation of 3–5 days, low grade fever with coryza manifests, and then dry cough with tachypnea. The chest X-ray may show perihilar infiltrates and hyperinflation. Prolonged expiration, ronchi, and wheezes are heard on pulmonary auscultation. Although several therapies including clarithromycin may be promising [13], management is mostly supportive with physiotherapy, fluid supply, and oxygen supplementation to correct hypoxemia. Inhaled bronchodilators may produce short-term improvement, but there is no evidence of benefit for inhaled corticosteroids. Ciliary loss and epithelial abnormalities persist on average for 3–4 months following acute bronchiolitis [14]. RSV bronchiolitis severe enough to cause hospitalization is a risk factor for allergic asthma in early adolescence [15].

Other viruses may cause bronchiolitis, for example, human metapneumovirus, rhinovirus, influenza, parainfluenza viruses (accounting for 15–30% of the cases), adenoviruses, and less commonly viruses of measles, mumps, varicella, influenza, rubeola, and enteroviruses. Some bacteria may occasionally cause bronchiolitis. Obliterative bronchiolitis (with bronchiolitis obliterans) is a rare consequence of viral or bacterial (especially *Mycoplasma pneumoniae*) bronchiolitis. Bronchiolitis is a common feature in infection by nontuberculous mycobacteria, regardless of the specific infective mycobacterial species; thin-section CT findings show bilateral small nodules, cylindric bronchiectasis, and branching centrilobular nodules, corresponding histopathologically to bronchiolectasis and bronchiolar and peribronchiolar inflammation with or without granuloma formation [16]. In invasive aspergillosis of the airways, *Aspergillus* bronchiolitis with peribronchiolar organizing pneumonia and hemorrhage may be observed. Centrilobular nodules, ground-glass opacity, and bronchiectasis corresponding histologically to lymphocytic infiltration along respiratory bronchioles and bronchovascular bundles are frequent in individuals carrying the human T-lymphotropic virus type-1 [17].

Postinfectious constrictive bronchiolitis is very rare in immunocompetent children and may occur especially after acute bronchiolitis due to adenovirus infection, although RSV, measles, and varicella viruses may be involved [18–20]. In recent years, HR-CT of the thorax has enhanced the ability of clinicians to identify bronchiolitis noninvasively in patients with chronic respiratory symptoms after virus infection, and lung biopsy is seldom performed. Bronchoalveolar lavage (BAL) cellular profiles are characterized by an increased percentage of neutrophils (with elevated interleukin-8) [21]. Long-term follow-up may show persistent airflow obstruction [22].

Bronchiolitis by Acute Inhalation Injury

Inhalation of toxic gases or fumes is a well-recognized cause of bronchiolitis. Among toxic gases, nitrogen dioxide (NO_2) is most commonly involved, either directly or by the formation of nitrous or nitric compounds.

The clinical manifestations largely depend on the intensity of inhalation. Symptoms manifest immediately after inhalation by airway irritation, which may be followed by permeability alveolar edema and possible death when inhalation has been massive. However, the immediate evolution is usually favorable, but after a phase of latency of a few (2–4) weeks dyspnea with airflow obstruction may develop. Chest X-ray at the early stage may demonstrate micronodular infiltration corresponding to bronchiolar inflammation with fibrinous or fibro-inflammatory buds within the bronchiolar lumen. Corticosteroid treatment (up to 8 weeks) is useful at the early stage of bronchiolitis, but the persistence of airflow obstruction is common.

Inhalation of toxic gases may occur as occupational hazards for chemical workers, during fires, or in silo filler's disease where the fermentation of grains produces NO_2. Silo filler's disease has been well studied [23]. Mortality may reach 20%, especially by acute respiratory distress syndrome during the initial phase of disease after massive inhalation. When inhalation has been less massive, obliterative bronchiolitis may develop.

Other toxic gases may cause bronchiolitis, including sulfur dioxide, chlorine compounds, and ammonia. Survivors of the Union Carbide gas leak in Bhopal where the inhaled gas was probably methyl isocyanate were found to have airflow obstruction as a consequence of bronchiolitis. Exposure to sulfur mustard (1,5-dichloro-3-thiapentane), a strong vesicant agent used as a weapon, is a cause of late constrictive (obliterative) histologically proved bronchiolitis, with air trapping, mosaic parenchymal attenuation, and bronchiectasis at HR-CT yet mild obstruction or normal lung function [24, 25]. The most common histologic finding is collagen-rich constrictive bronchiolitis, with mild lymphocytic infiltration [24].

Other Known Causes of Bronchiolitis

Drug-Induced Bronchiolitis

Iatrogenic bronchiolitis obliterans is common only in association with organizing pneumonia (with the latter being the main component of the syndrome, thus explaining the lack of airflow obstruction and the characteristic opacities found on imaging). Iatrogenic bronchiolitis obliterans in isolation is usually encountered in the context of disorders which may by themselves be associated with bronchiolitis obliterans in the absence of the drug: one example is that of penicillamine and rheumatoid arthritis (RA) (see below).

Sauropus androgynus Bronchiolitis

An outbreak of bronchiolitis occurred in 1995 in Taiwan in nearly 300 people drinking juice made from the leaves of the plant *Sauropus androgynus* for weight control and containing a high level of the alkaloid papaverine. Airway disease was dose related, developed within 7 months, and was irreversible. Airflow was severe (mean FEV1 at 26% of predicted). At CT scan, bronchiectasis was present in almost all patients as well as mosaic attenuation (notable on expiration or on both inspiration and expiration with FEV1 lower in the latter). The pathologic features consisted of inflammatory and fibrotic lesions of the bronchioles, but also of bronchi less than 3 mm in diameter. Transplantation was necessary in patients who developed end-stage respiratory disease [26, 27]. A smaller outbreak occurred in Japan in 2005 [28].

Mineral Dust Airway Disease

Asbestos and nonasbestos (coal, silica, talc, mica, or iron and aluminum oxides) dust-exposed populations may develop airflow obstruction with pathologic lesions of marked fibrosis (with distortion) and pigmentation of the membranous and respiratory bronchioles (with possible associated centrilobular emphysema) distinct from those induced by smoking. These bronchiolar lesions are largely underestimated and passed off as merely dust macules, but they clearly represent the pathologic basis for significant airflow obstruction of occupational origin resulting from a long-standing inflammatory response to inhaled dust [29].

Other Occupation-Induced Bronchiolitis

Clinical bronchiolitis obliterans has been reported in workers of a small rural microwave-popcorn plant, caused by the inhalation of volatile butter-flavoring ingredients [30]; subsequently, exposure to diacetyl (a diketone that imparts buttery aroma and flavor to foods) was associated with severe fixed obstruction syndrome in many flavoring manufacturing industry workers [31, 32] ("food flavorer's lung") as a result of demonstrated direct toxicity to the airway epithelium in rodents. Many criteria for causal inferences were fulfilled, with about tenfold increased risk of developing severe fixed obstruction in subjects exposed to diacetyl, and exposure–response relation [33]. The latency between the employment and the symptom onset varies between 5 months and 9 years [32], however early identification is difficult, as the diagnosis may be overlooked if not considered by the physicians. Lung function stabilizes within 2 years after exposure cessation. Control of employee exposure and iterative measurement of FEV1 is warranted in workers exposed to respiratory hazards and especially diacetyl. There is no evidence presently to suggest that diacetyl may be hazardous when ingested. Such observations demonstrate that a diagnosis of chronic bronchiolitis of undetermined etiology should hinder investigation of occupational etiology, especially in never-smokers and young smokers with severe obstruction, with likely novel causes present for decades but awaiting recognition [33].

Bronchiolitis obliterans has been reported in some workers exposed to synthetic polymers inhaled as microfibers or "flock," where the offending agent has been identified as polypropylene used for the manufacturing of plastic items; the characteristic histopathological lesion of "flock worker's lung" is a lymphocytic bronchiolitis and peribronchiolitis with lymphoid hyperplasia [34]; HR-CT may show ground-glass opacities, micronodules, and peribronchiolar thickening [35, 36]. Airflow obstruction has also been reported in battery workers exposed to thionyl chloride fumes [37].

Bronchiolitis Occurring in a Well-Characterized Context

Connective Tissue Diseases

Rheumatoid Arthritis

RA is a connective tissue disease with predominant articular signs, but with possible systemic manifestations affecting the bronchopulmonary tract and the pleura. Interstitial lung disease is common in RA whereas bronchiolitis is rather rare; however, both processes are frequently associated. Several types of bronchiolitis may develop in RA, but obliterative bronchiolitis is by far the most characteristic and severe clinically [38–40].

RA is the most common cause of obliterative bronchiolitis in the nontransplant population [41]. Obliterative bronchiolitis usually manifests subacutely over a few weeks in nonsmoking women with RA, sometimes after a flu-like syndrome. The diagnosis of RA precedes the pulmonary symptoms in most cases [40]. There is no cough or bronchorrhea initially. At pulmonary auscultation some crackles may be heard and especially characteristic inspiratory *squeaks*. On lung function tests severe airflow obstruction is present, with a markedly reduced FEV1/FVC ratio and FEV1 often less than 0.8 L. The RV/TLC ratio is increased [40]. Hypoxemia is usually present at rest and especially on exercise. The chest X-ray does not usually show specific abnormalities; however, HR-CT usually shows characteristic mosaic abnormalities, with bronchial dilatation in inspiratory CT scans and air trapping on expiratory CT scans and frequently centrilobular nodules and branching linear structures (Fig. 18.2) [42]. Bronchial wall thickening and bronchiectasis are very frequently found [40]. The course of bronchiolitis is usually severe resulting in chronic respiratory insufficiency despite corticosteroid treatment [40]; cyclophosphamide could prevent or slow airflow deterioration. The development of bronchiectasis is frequent in the evolution.

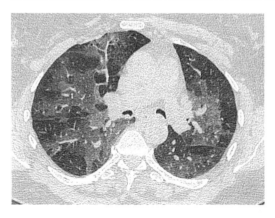

Fig. 18.2 Mosaic attenuation pattern on HR-CT in a patient with rheumatoid arthritis and obliterative bronchiolitis (expiratory views)

The histopathologic lesions underlying this syndrome usually consist of constrictive bronchiolitis with mural inflammation at the early stage, progressing to fibrous concentric constrictive bronchiolitis later. At the early stage, lymphoplasmacytic bronchiolar and peribronchiolar infiltration, when present, may be associated with Sjögren syndrome.

Although obliterative bronchiolitis may develop in RA in the absence of previous penicillamine treatment, this drug is likely to play a role in the occurrence of bronchiolitis, as bronchiolitis is more common in patients treated with penicillamine than in patients not receiving the drug [43]. Bronchiolitis usually occurs after 3–6 months of treatment; the total duration of treatment, total dose received, and daily dose do not seem to play any role in the onset of bronchiolitis. Obliterative bronchiolitis has been only exceptionally reported in patients receiving penicillamine for diseases other than RA.

Other drugs might play a role in the development of obliterative bronchiolitis in RA. Obliterative bronchiolitis has been occasionally reported in patients receiving gold salts or tiopronin but the small number of reported cases does not support a definite causal link.

As penicillamine has been almost abandoned in the treatment of RA, it is worthwhile remarking that the number of cases of obliterative bronchiolitis in RA reported in the literature has markedly decreased. However, whether this reflects

a real change of the incidence of obliterative bronchiolitis (thus indirectly supporting a causal role of penicillamine) or just the lack of publication of such cases is not known.

In addition to severe obliterative bronchiolitis in RA, studies of cohorts of patients with RA have shown an increased incidence of airflow obstruction (as assessed at lung function tests and/or HR-CT) in patients with RA. Furthermore, bronchiectasis is common in RA.

Sjögren Syndrome

Bronchiolar and peribronchiolar lymphocytic infiltration which is common in Sjögren syndrome is likely the cause of the usually mild airflow obstruction and mosaic pattern at expiratory HR-CT encountered in patients with this condition [44]. Interestingly, thin-walled cysts have been reported on HR-CT scan of patients with Sjögren syndrome; these may correspond to dilated airspaces beyond partially obstructed bronchioles (ball-valve mechanism).

Other Connective Tissue Diseases

Obliterative bronchiolitis is far less common in connective tissue diseases other than RA. A few cases of obliterative bronchiolitis have been reported in systemic lupus erythematosus. Follicular bronchiolitis may be commonly found in systemic sclerosis, but constrictive bronchiolitis is exceedingly rare [45]. A case of obliterative bronchiolitis has been reported in a patient with localized scleroderma treated with penicillamine [46].

Obliterative Bronchiolitis Associated with Lung Transplantation or Bone Marrow Graft

Obliterative Bronchiolitis After Lung Transplantation

Lung transplantation is a therapeutic option for patients with end-stage pulmonary diseases. However, obliterative bronchiolitis (and its clinical functional correlate bronchiolitis obliterans), with a prevalence of 35–75% within 5 years of transplantation [47], is the leading cause of death after the first year and the main limiting factor to long-term survival after lung or heart–lung transplantation [47]. The initial stage of bronchiolitis consists of lymphocytic infiltration, with further epithelial cell necrosis and denudation of mucosa (segmental epithelial necrosis). Mesenchymal cells (fibroblasts, myofibroblasts) form intraluminal granulation tissue, resulting in eccentric or concentric fibrotic scars obliterating the bronchioles. Not only the bronchioles, but also the large bronchi are involved in the process of rejection, with lymphocytic bronchitis and finally central bronchiectasis with mucostasis. Histopathological changes associated with allograft obliterative bronchiolitis are described as part of the revised consensus classification for classification and grading of lung allograft rejection (A, acute rejection; B, airway inflammation; C, chronic airway rejection – obliterative bronchiolitis; D, chronic vascular rejection – accelerated graft vascular sclerosis) [48].

The clinical onset of obliterative bronchiolitis is usually insidious with progressively increasing dyspnea and possible cough [49]. However, the onset of BOS may be acute, associated with acute rejection in the first 6 months often triggered by an acute event; it carries a poor prognosis and obliterative bronchiolitis is the main cause of death [50]. The subgroup of patients with BOS developing >3 years after single lung transplantation are less likely to have severe functional impairment on long-term follow-up. In the course of BOS, bronchorrhea develops with bronchiectasis at CT scan and chronic airway colonization by bacteria (including *Pseudomonas* species) and iterative bronchial infections occur. Auscultation findings are poor during the early stage of BOS, with ronchi and crackles or squeaks at a later stage. Infections, acute rejection, and suture complications must be excluded. Lung function tests confirm the presence of obstructive ventilatory defect and reduction in FEV1, the cardinal feature of BOS, and further define the BOS stage (Table 18.3). The diagnosis of BOS is defined by physiologic criteria. Transbronchial or surgical lung biopsies are not necessary to diagnose BOS but may be useful to exclude alternative diagnoses [51]. Imaging by CT scan shows two main

Table 18.3 Diagnostic criteria and classification of bronchiolitis obliterans syndrome (BOS)

BOS 0	FEV1 >90% of baseline[a] *and* FEF 25–75 >75% of baseline
BOS 0-p	FEV1 81–90% of baseline *and/or* FEF 25–75 ≤75% of baseline
BOS 1	FEV1 66–80% of baseline
BOS 2	FEV1 51–65% of baseline
BOS 3	FEV1 50% or less of baseline

BOS bronchiolitis obliterans syndrome, *FEF 25–75* mid-expiratory flow rate, *FEV1* forced expiratory volume in 1 s
[a]The baseline value, to which subsequent measures are referred, is defined as the average of the 2 highest (not necessarily consecutive) measurements obtained at least 3 weeks apart, without the use of inhaled bronchodilators preceding the measurement

abnormalities: bronchiectasis on the inspiratory CT scan, and air trapping with mosaic perfusion on the expiratory CT scan. The combination of these two findings is highly suggestive and they may be an early marker of obliterative bronchiolitis. The progression of obliterative bronchiolitis leads to chronic respiratory insufficiency and eventually death.

Acute cellular rejection is the predominant risk factor for BOS [51, 52], especially in case of multiple and severe episodes, and of late-onset acute rejection, although some patients with BOS have never experienced acute rejection. Additional cofactors for the development of BOS include cytomegalovirus, infections other than cytomegalovirus (including community acquired respiratory viruses, human herpesvirus 6, *Chlamydia pneumoniae*, and *Pseudomonas aeruginosa*), nonspecific injury to the allograft or airways (i.e., primary graft dysfunction, gastroesophageal reflux), HLA mismatching [53], and organizing pneumonia (that may be associated with acute rejection or with infection) [51]. Lymphocytic bronchitis/bronchiolitis may be a precursor of obliterative bronchiolitis and predicts long-term outcome [54].

The pathophysiology of posttransplant obliterative bronchiolitis and BOS is complex, involving allo-immune mechanisms, and allo-immune independent factors such as airway injury from primary graft dysfunction, allograft infections, airway ischemia, and gastroesophageal reflux [51].

Immune-mediated allograft rejection is mainly mediated by T-cells, with demonstrated activation of Th-1, Th-2, Th-17, and T regulatory cells (while Th-1 activation predominates in acute rejection). Autoimmune injury to the allograft airway may also occur.

Because the pathologic diagnosis of bronchiolitis obliterans is difficult to document, the International Society for Heart and Lung Transplantation proposed a clinical definition mainly based on pulmonary function, termed BOS and meaning graft deterioration secondary to persistent airflow obstruction. The diagnostic criteria of BOS [52] take into account an early detection of airflow obstruction by introducing the measurement of FEF 25–75 which is more sensitive than FEV1 (see Table 18.3). Surrogate markers for BOS have been studied, but these are neither sensitive or specific enough to be used reliably in clinical practice: combined lymphocytosis and neutrophilia at BAL without evidence of infection, exhaled NO, exhaled CO, exhaled breath condensate, induced sputum, the slope of the alveolar plateau for helium during a single breath washout, air trapping on expiratory CT scans [55], methacholine challenge, or hyperpolarized 3He magnetic resonance imaging [51]. Surveillance transbronchial biopsies in order to diagnose occult acute rejection (based on the pathologic findings of perivascular and interstitial mononuclear cell infiltrates, or of lymphocytic bronchitis/bronchiolitis) are controversial [56]. Transbronchial biopsies are mostly important to assess potential infection or acute cellular rejection, but their yield in detecting obliterative bronchiolitis is low [57]. The practice of follow-up transbronchial biopsies 3–5 weeks after evidence and treatment of acute cellular rejection is also controversial.

The management of obliterative bronchiolitis is not well established, and there is currently no proven therapy for prevention or treatment of BOS [47]. Because bronchiolitis obliterans is a rejection process, treatment relies on augmentation of immunosuppression or changing immunosuppressive medications, with various approaches of unproven value [51]. Any associated infection requires active treatment. Recent evidence suggests active treatment with augmented immunosuppression of even asymptomatic episodes of minimal (A1) acute cellular rejection [51]. Prevention of cytomegalovirus infection may contribute to reduce the incidence of BOS [51]. Aggressive treatment of gastroesophageal reflux is recommended. Novel strategies of induction immunosuppressive therapy are being evaluated, including with alemtuzumab (a humanized anti-C52 antibody that depletes CD4 lymphocytes). Azithromycin (250 mg daily for 5 days, then thrice weekly), a macrolide displaying immunomodulatory effects, may slow the rate of disease progression and improve survival [58], especially in patients with BAL neutrophilia [10, 47, 59], however placebo-controlled trials are lacking. Aerosolized cyclosporine-A may be beneficial [60]. Infusion of donor bone marrow and extracorporeal photophoresis warrant further experimental studies. The median survival after onset of BOS is 3–4 years [51]. End-stage BOS is the main indication of lung re-transplantation [61].

Obliterative Bronchiolitis After Bone Marrow Graft

Hematopoietic stem cell transplantation from related or unrelated donors after high-dose chemoradiotherapy is an efficient procedure for treating several hematologic, neoplastic, or congenital disorders. However, it may be complicated by infections, veno-occlusive disease of the liver, and acute or chronic GVHD mostly related to an alloreactive immune process. Chronic GVHD presents as an autoimmune disorder, especially with cutaneous features of scleroderma.

Among the manifestations of GVHD, obliterative bronchiolitis is a major complication with a prevalence varying from about 2% (following nonmyeloablative hematopoietic stem cell transplantation) [62] up to about 25% (in patients receiving therapy with busulfan) [63]. It is responsible for an overall survival of only 13% at 5 years [64]. It is quite similar to obliterative bronchiolitis after lung transplantation [65]. It is very rare following autologous hematopoietic stem cell transplantation. The bronchiolar pathologic

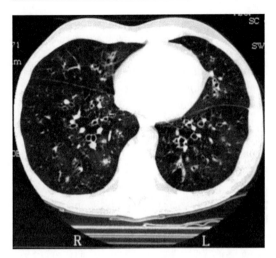

Fig. 18.3 Bronchiectasis and mild mosaic attenuation pattern in a patient with obliterative bronchiolitis and hypogammaglobulinemia after bone marrow graft

Table 18.4 Diagnostic criteria of bronchiolitis obliterans following hematopoietic stem cell transplantation (from ref. [63])

Allogenic stem cell transplantation
Chronic graft versus host disease[a]
Insidious onset of dyspnea, cough, and wheezing after 100 days following transplantation
Normal chest radiograph
HR-CT of the chest (with inspiratory and expiratory views) showing areas of air trapping on expiratory views, hyperinflation or bronchial dilatation, with no parenchymal involvement
Pulmonary function tests showing new onset of airflow obstruction (FEV1/FVC < 0.7 and FEV1 < 75% of predicted), not responsive to bronchodilators
Exclusion of an infectious process by appropriate radiological, serological, and microbiological studies (obtained by sinus aspirate, upper respiratory tract viral screen, sputum culture or BAL)

[a]The risk of bronchiolitis obliterans is highest with progressive chronic graft versus host disease, but it may develop in patients with quiescent or de novo graft versus host disease, or without graft versus host disease

features in bone marrow transplant recipients consist of lymphocytic bronchitis/bronchiolitis (in patients with subacute respiratory manifestations) and cicatricial bronchiolitis obliterans (in patients with chronic manifestations of increasing dyspnea) [66]. Airflow obstruction develops within 1.5 years after the graft, and it is strongly associated with GVHD (with cutaneous and digestive manifestations) [67]. The dermal fibrosis in chronic GVHD may resemble scleroderma, and autoantibodies to nuclear antigens similar to those associated with autoimmune diseases are commonly found. Hypogammaglobulinemia present in about 20% of patients may be a further cause of airway infection and damage. At CT scan mosaic attenuation and bronchiectasis are present in a majority of patients (Fig. 18.3). Risk factors for obliterative bronchiolitis are allogenic hematopoietic stem cell transplantation, GVHD especially progressive chronic GVHD, older age of recipient, airflow obstruction prior to stem cell transplantation, early respiratory viral infection, and, possibly, acute GVHD, busulfan-based conditioning regimen, total body irradiation, methotrexate-based GVHD prophylaxis, CMV infection, older age of donor, decreased level of immunoglobulin G, gastro-esophageal reflux disease, and peripheral blood stem cell transplantation [63]. In contrast to patients with regular respiratory follow-up after lung transplantation,

patients who underwent bone marrow graft are often diagnosed with airflow obstruction once they have developed marked dyspnea (Table 18.4). High dose systemic corticosteroids (prednisone 1–1.5 mg/kg/day, tapered gradually over 6–12 months) and increased immunosuppression may improve or stabilize airflow obstruction [63], but responses are generally marginal. Azithromycin, inhaled bronchodilators, and supportive care may be useful [63, 68]. Whether extracorporeal photodynamic therapy is beneficial requires further evaluation. Once bronchiectasis is present, careful monitoring of airways infection is necessary, with intravenous immunoglobulins if associated hypogammaglobulinemia is present. Lung transplantation is a valuable option at the stage of severe chronic respiratory insufficiency.

Bronchiolitis Obliterans in Paraneoplastic Pemphigus

Paraneoplastic pemphigus is an autoimmune disorder associated with neoplasms (especially lymphomas and Castleman's disease) causing mucosal and skin lesions [69]. It is due to autoantibodies reacting with desmosomal and hemidesmosomal plakin proteins that connect epithelial cells, which may cause acantholytic (loss of cell-to-cell adhesion) changes in the respiratory epithelium and segmental fibrosing bronchiolitis obliterans and airflow obstruction [70]. Respiratory failure occurs in about 30% of patients despite immunosuppressive therapy.

Cryptogenic (Idiopathic) Constrictive Bronchiolitis

This is a rather poorly characterized and heterogeneous entity in nonsmokers with pathologic findings of bronchiolitis (usually constrictive) and often (but not always) airflow obstruction on lung function tests [71, 72]. Published cases are rare, and the real prevalence of this syndrome is not known; 31% of cases of obstructive bronchiolar disease remained cryptogenic in one series [41]. Additional reported cases of presumed cryptogenic constrictive bronchiolitis do not undergo lung biopsy [73], and it is likely that some cases labeled as chronic obstructive pulmonary disease (COPD) in nonsmokers may indeed be bronchiolitis [74], since lung biopsy is not done once a diagnosis of COPD has been clinically accepted.

The majority of patients are female between 40 and 60 years old. Any cause of airflow obstruction has to be carefully excluded (smoking history, inhalation history, viral episode preceding the development of symptoms, connective tissue disease including *formes frustes*, or hypersensitivity pneumonitis). Symptoms usually develop over a few weeks or months, with dyspnea and nonproductive cough. Airflow obstruction is present at lung function tests. Marked neutrophilia (about 50%) is found at BAL differential cell count. The chest X-ray is unremarkable; a mosaic pattern and bronchial dilatation may be found at HR-CT (Fig. 18.4). Improvement with corticosteroids may occur, with BAL neutrophilia returning to normal.

The pathological findings at lung biopsy usually comprise cellular infiltration of the bronchioles with mild submucosal and adventitial fibrosis. Chronic transmural bronchiolitis consists of nonspecific infiltration of the terminal and respiratory bronchioles by lymphocytes, plasma cells, and a few neutrophils. In some

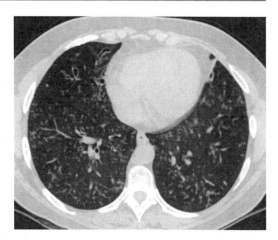

Fig. 18.4 Tree-in-bud pattern, centrilobular nodules, and bronchiectasis in a patient with cryptogenic obliterative bronchiolitis

cases, polypoid buds of granulation tissue within the lumen of the bronchioles (without associated organizing pneumonia) have been reported, with a good response to corticosteroids and possible relapse when the dose of corticosteroids was reduced.

Other Individualized Types of Bronchiolitis

Smoking-Related Bronchiolar Disorders

The role of cigarette smoking in the development of airway disease has been known for a long time, and COPD is presently a major health problem. COPD is usually not included in the category of bronchiolitis, and the involvement of the bronchioles in COPD is often called small airways disease [75]. Nevertheless, COPD is undoubtedly the most common cause of bronchiolitis (or more precisely of longitudinal airway inflammation). Other entities strongly related to cigarette smoking and involving the bronchioles (such as respiratory bronchiolitis and respiratory bronchiolitis-interstitial lung disease) are still included in the group of idiopathic interstitial pneumonias. Surprisingly, it seems that the pathologic analysis of the bronchopulmonary disorders has often considered data obtained by lung biopsy (with examination of the interstitium and the bronchioles as in respiratory bronchiolitis with interstitial lung disease) and that obtained by bronchial biopsy (as in COPD) separately. It is further remarkable that studies of these disorders have often favored either a morphologic or functional analysis. However, the airway disorders related to smoking clearly overlap and should not be considered as entities separated by impenetrable barriers.

Respiratory Bronchiolitis

Respiratory bronchiolitis is the term used to designate a pathologic pattern of bronchiolitis found almost exclusively in smokers, usually asymptomatic. The histopathological lesions consist of accumulation of pigmented macrophages within the respiratory bronchioles and the surrounding airspaces. These findings are encountered in the lungs of current smokers, but also in the lungs of ex-smokers for many years and possibly for decades after stopping smoking, and have been hypothesized to be the precursor of centrilobular emphysema [76]. The yellow-brown pigment present within macrophages is considered to be derived from cigarette smoke. No correlation between the morphologic findings and lung function tests has been established [76, 77]. This is not surprising since all smokers do not develop COPD. Respiratory bronchiolitis is commonly found in patients with primary spontaneous pneumothorax especially relapsing. Other morphologic findings in the small airways of smokers consist of goblet cell metaplasia, smooth muscle hypertrophy, inflammation and fibrosis in the walls of the bronchioles. The findings at HR-CT consist of centrilobular nodules and ground-glass attenuation [78–80].

Respiratory Bronchiolitis with Interstitial Lung Disease

In some patients, respiratory bronchiolitis may be associated with interstitial inflammation and fibrosis, and this entity is thus called respiratory bronchiolitis with interstitial lung disease. Symptoms (dyspnea, cough) are usually mild. On chest X-ray, diffuse fine reticular or reticulonodular opacities may be found. The CT features and the histopathological patterns overlap with those in respiratory bronchiolitis and those in desquamative interstitial pneumonia, the latter being

characterized by the accumulation of macrophages in the alveoli, likely corresponding to a spectrum of pathology in cigarette smokers [78, 79, 81, 82]. Prolonged survival is common, however clinical and physiologic improvement occur in only a minority of patients and is not dramatically affected by smoking cession or immunosuppressive therapy [83].

Bronchiolitis in COPD

COPD is characterized by inflammation of the large and small airways (bronchiolitis) and destruction of lung parenchyma (emphysema). Airflow obstruction (or limitation) results from reduced elastic recoil of the lung (especially due to peribronchiolar parenchymal destruction and loss of alveolar attachment to the bronchioles perimeter) and increased resistance (resulting from increased thickness of the bronchiolar wall by inflammation) [84]. The peripheral airways are the major site of airway resistance in smokers. As COPD develops, the changes of respiratory bronchiolitis progress to changes including airway wall inflammation (macrophages, lymphocytes), fibrosis, smooth muscle hypertrophy, and goblet cell metaplasia with increased mucus production and ensuing mucous plugging of the bronchioles. In parallel, inflammation of the bronchi is characterized by an increase of CD8 lymphocytes and macrophages, together with neutrophils in severe disease; the severity of airflow obstruction is associated with the severity of airway inflammation at bronchial biopsy in smokers, a finding indicating that bronchiolar functional impairment correlates with bronchial inflammation (longitudinal inflammation of the airways).

A consequence of bronchiolar inflammation is emphysema, mainly of the centrilobular type (parenchymal destruction limited to the respiratory bronchioles and the central part of the acinus) [85].

Follicular Bronchiolitis

Follicular bronchiolitis (also called hyperplasia of the bronchus-associated lymphoid tissue) is a non-neoplastic pulmonary lymphoid lesion defined by the presence of abundant peribronchiolar lymphoid follicles with reactive germinal centers that differentiate this condition from lymphocytic bronchiolitis (without follicles). It may compress the airway lumen. Alveolar septal infiltration by lymphocytes, which characterizes lymphoid interstitial pneumonia, is typically not present (but overlap may exist). The bronchiolar epithelium is often infiltrated by lymphocytes. Follicular bronchitis may be associated (especially if there is bronchiectasis). Follicular bronchiolitis is usually a benign condition associated with connective tissue diseases (especially RA and Sjögren syndrome) [86], infections including with human immunodeficiency virus, or immunodeficiencies, and few cases remain idiopathic [87]. The CT findings consist of centrilobular and peribronchial nodules (smaller than 3 mm, sometimes associated with larger nodules, 3–12 mm), and areas of ground-glass opacity.

Primary pulmonary low grade lymphomas, which also usually have a peribronchiolar distribution, may be especially difficult to distinguish from lymphocytic or follicular bronchiolitis. The presence of possible blood or urine monoclonal gammapathy, or demonstration of monotypic lymphocytes or of clonal immunoglobulin gene rearrangements in lung tissue are helpful to distinguish between these conditions (especially in the absence of connective tissue disease), with potential therapeutic consequences.

Bronchiectasis and Bronchiolitis

Bronchiectasis is defined as a permanent dilatation of the bronchi. It is primarily a disease of the airways (bronchi and also the bronchioles) secondary to mural infection and inflammation. Three morphological types of bronchiectasis have been described: cylindrical (uniformly enlarged bronchi), varicose (irregular dilatation of the bronchi with focal constriction), and cystic (with progressive dilatation ending in large cysts). Most localized bronchiectases are due to airway obstruction (e.g., foreign body) or pneumonia. Diffuse bronchiectasis is the consequence of diffuse infection (e.g., pertussis infection) or of

impaired defenses such as impaired mucociliary clearance (ciliary dyskinesia, cystic fibrosis) or humoral immunity deficiency (congenital or acquired hypogammaglobulinemia). As mentioned earlier, bronchiectasis is also a clinically important component associated with bronchiolitis in airway disease of immune origin (RA, lung transplant rejection, bone marrow GVHD).

Bronchorrhea and iterative infections of the dilated bronchi which are almost always colonized by bacteria (especially *Pseudomonas*) are the most common clinical manifestations. However, a majority of patients with diffuse bronchiectasis also have airflow obstruction resulting from bronchiolitis.

Bronchiolitis in bronchiectasis was identified as early as in the first half of the nineteenth century. Interestingly, this was later confirmed by successive technical developments, from bronchography to CT scan, with the finding of absence of peripheral filling resulting in the "leafless tree" or "pruning" pattern at bronchography, and the lack of bronchial tapering and mosaic pattern at CT scan [88]. Pathologic analysis demonstrated that ectasia of the large bronchioles is in continuity with "obliterative bronchitis and bronchiolitis." The heterogeneity of the bronchiolar lesions ranges from ectasia to obliteration, with some bronchioles still normal. Pathologic analysis also demonstrated that the parenchyma beyond the obliterated small bronchi and bronchioles remained aerated, a finding pointing to the role of collateral ventilation. Pathologic studies, and imaging and functional studies, convincingly demonstrated that airflow obstruction in diffuse bronchiectasis results from intrinsic disease of the small and medium airways. Mosaic attenuation, a distinct imaging feature of obliterative bronchiolitis, present in the majority of patients (including in the nonbronchiectatic lobes) is a strong independent determinant of airflow obstruction [89–91]. The severity of airflow obstruction is linked to the extent of mosaic attenuation [91]. Another strong determinant of airflow obstruction is bronchial wall thickness [90] which is moreover the primary determinant of subsequent major functional decline [91].

In cystic fibrosis, patients develop both bronchiectasis and bronchiolar disease. In children, the lesions of the bronchioles mainly consist of inflammation and dilatation. In older patients, chronic inflammation and fibrosis of the bronchioles is evident (with less dilated bronchioles) [92]. CT assessment in children and adults demonstrated, in addition to bronchiectasis, mosaic attenuation suggesting bronchiolar obstruction in about two thirds of the patients, more commonly in patients 17 years and older [93].

Swyer–James (MacLeod) syndrome is characterized by a unilateral small and hyperlucent lung with air trapping and impaired vasculature; it is considered to result from a viral infection in infancy. Bronchiectasis is frequently (but not always) present. Bronchography demonstrated the lack of filling of the peripheral bronchial tree, and CT shows air trapping, which is explained by fibrous obliteration of the small bronchi and bronchioles.

In Kartagener syndrome, the ciliary dyskinesia (immotile cilia syndrome) results in the triad of chronic pansinusitis, bronchiectasis, and situs inversus. Airflow obstruction with diffuse centrilobular nodules on CT scan corresponds to pathologic features of obliterative thickening of the walls of the membranous bronchioles, with infiltration by lymphocytes, plasma cells, and neutrophils (in contrast to the sparing of the respiratory bronchioles) [94].

Whether bronchiectasis precedes the development of bronchiolitis or the reverse is not established. Probably inflammation of the airways is longitudinal, with clinical predominant manifestations of either bronchiectasis or airflow obstruction, with further changes in the course of disease superimposed by bacterial colonization of the airways with iterative infectious exacerbations further damaging both the small and large airways.

Miscellaneous Bronchiolar Disorders

Bronchiolitis as a Component of Diffuse Inflammatory Lung Disease

Bronchiolitis (and bronchitis) is an often underestimated component of hypersensitivity pneumonitis (farmer's lung, pigeon breeder's disease, and other causes). Airflow obstruction is commonly obscured by the restrictive impairment at lung function tests. Interestingly, airflow obstruction and emphysema are more frequent on long-term follow-up of patients with farmer's lung than in farmer controls.

Granulomatous bronchiolitis is found in sarcoidosis and may contribute to the airflow obstruction present in a proportion of patients. Granulomatous bronchiolitis is also found in tuberculosis, in association with Crohn's disease, and in infiltrative lung disease associated with "hot tub lung." Bronchiolitis may be encountered in the eosinophilic pneumonias (eosinophilic bronchiolitis), as well as in allergic bronchopulmonary aspergillosis. Indeed, bronchiolitis as an accessory component of many inflammatory bronchopulmonary processes of any origin is very common. The morphological basis for persistent irreversible airflow obstruction in patients with a long history of asthma is not established.

Malignant Bronchiolitis

Some malignancies may have a predilection for infiltrating the small airways, for example, malignant histiocytosis or primary low grade pulmonary lymphomas.

Diffuse Panbronchiolitis

Diffuse panbronchiolitis is a bronchiolar disease mostly encountered in Japan and other East Asian countries, but very rare in North America and Europe. The disease is closely associated with the HLA Bw54 antigen, itself predominantly found in East Asians, although an HLA-associated major susceptibility gene for diffuse panbronchiolitis remains to be found. As diffuse panbronchiolitis is extremely rare in the Japanese population living outside Japan, the role of an environmental exposure has been hypothesized. The mean age of patients is about 40 years (mostly from 2nd to 5th decade of life), with a male predominance; diffuse panbronchiolitis is not related to smoking. Chronic sinusitis, present in about three quarters of the patients often precedes the bronchopulmonary manifestations, which consist of chronic cough, bronchorrhea, and dyspnea with progressive fixed airflow obstruction. Physical examination reveals crackles, wheezes, or both. Although similarities exist with cystic fibrosis, pancreatic insufficiency, abnormalities of sweat electrolytes, and infertility in males are not present. The CT-scan features are quite characteristic of bronchiolar disease with poorly defined centrilobular nodules up to 3 mm often associated with branched linear opacities and air trapping. Diffuse panbronchiolitis progresses to bronchiectasis and respiratory failure if left untreated. Chronic airway infection, especially with *Hemophilus influenzae* and *P. aeruginosa*, is common. Accumulation of neutrophils in the airways (associated with high secretion of the neutrophil chemoattractant interleukin-8) causes bronchial epithelial cell damage and plays an important role in the pathogenesis of the disease [95]. Neutrophilia is present at BAL.

The diagnosis is established by lung biopsy, demonstrating the prominent involvement of respiratory bronchioles (contrasting with other forms of constrictive bronchiolitis that involve predominantly membranous bronchioles), with interstitial accumulation of foamy macrophages in the wall of respiratory bronchioles and in the surrounding interalveolar septa. Neutrophils are present in the bronchiolar lumen. Lymphoid follicles may be noted in the airways. Narrowing of respiratory bronchioles and ectasia of proximal membranous bronchioles are found in advanced disease [95]. Long-term treatment with low dose macrolides has established efficacy in improving symptoms (reduction in sputum volume), lung function, CT scan changes, and survival rate that has increased to >90% at 10 years [95]. The effect of macrolides is considered to be related to their anti-inflammatory and immunomodulatory effects beyond their antimicrobial properties, including the inhibition of the production of many pro-inflammatory cytokines and down-regulation of neutrophil migration. Guidelines on macrolide therapy recommend erythromycin 400–600 mg/day orally, or alternatively clarithromycin 200 or 400 mg/day orally or roxithromycin 150 or 300 mg/day orally. A series of Caucasian patients has been reported, with similarities with diffuse panbronchiolitis,

although without diffuse pansinusitis and with inconspicuous peribronchiolar alveolar foamy macrophages, possibly representing *formes frustes* of diffuse panbronchiolitis [96]. Overlap between obliterative bronchiolitis (as in RA) and diffuse panbronchiolitis has been mentioned in Japan, but although the clinical features may be similar, the histopathological features are distinct. Recurrence of diffuse panbronchiolitis has been reported after medical therapy and after lung transplantation. One case of diffuse panbronchiolitis associated with microscopic polyangiitis has been reported.

Neuroendocrine Cell Hyperplasia

Idiopathic pulmonary neuroendocrine cell hyperplasia mainly involves the distal bronchi and bronchioles, with hyperplastic neuroendocrine cells and tumorlets (clumps of neuroendocrine cells less than 5 mm) obliterating the bronchioles [97]. This rare disorder occurs mainly in women in their fifth or sixth decade, and is associated with airflow obstruction in a majority of patients. Mosaic attenuation, airway wall thickening, and occasional small nodules are found at CT scan. This disorder may present as obliterative bronchiolitis associated with peripheral carcinoids. Although usually benign, it may result in severe obstructive respiratory insufficiency requiring lung transplantation.

Bronchiolitis in Miscellaneous Entities

Lymphangioleiomyomatosis

Pulmonary lymphangioleiomyomatosis is a rare disorder affecting women, which may be sporadic or part of the tuberous sclerosis complex. It is characterized by a nonneoplastic proliferation of smooth muscle cells involving all parts of the lung, including the bronchioles which are narrowed by muscle cells accumulated in their walls, that may explain air trapping and the development of cystic distal airspaces (ball-valve mechanism) giving a typical pattern on HR-CT scan. Airflow obstruction is present in over one half of the patients.

Pulmonary Langerhans' Cell Histiocytosis (Histiocytosis X)

Pulmonary Langerhans' cell histiocytosis is a disorder strongly correlated with smoking and characterized by granulomas formed by Langerhans' cells, lymphocytes, eosinophils, and macrophages, which are centered around the bronchioles. Therefore, Langerhans' cell histiocytosis may be considered as a bronchiolitis, rather than interstitial lung disease. Inflammatory injury to the bronchioles leads to the formation and to the development of cystic distal airspaces characteristic of the disorder (the HR-CT pattern strongly resembles that in lymphangioleiomyomatosis, with the exception of possible nodules and usual relative sparing of lung bases in Langerhans' cell histiocytosis). Airflow obstruction is common.

Sarcoidosis

In sarcoidosis, granulomas are often located in the bronchial and bronchiolar submucosa and can reduce the bronchiolar lumen [3]. Peribronchiolar fibrosis may contribute to small airways narrowing and airflow obstruction [98].

Other

Various disorders of the small airways have been described by several groups recently, with overlapping histological features, under the terminology of airway-centered interstitial fibrosis, peribronchiolar metaplasia and fibrosis, centrilobular fibrosis, and idiopathic bronchiolocentric interstitial fibrosis. Some cases may be related to underlying connective tissue disease, inhalational injury, or chronic aspiration. Some controversy remains over whether these patterns represent a separate clinicopathological entity [2, 3].

References

1. Visscher DW, Myers JL. Bronchiolitis: the pathologist's perspective. Proc Am Thorac Soc. 2006;3:41–7.
2. Rice A, Nicholson AG. The pathologist's approach to small airways disease. Histopathology. 2009;54:117–33.
3. Cordier JF. Challenges in pulmonary fibrosis. 2: Bronchiolocentric fibrosis. Thorax. 2007;62:638–49.
4. American Thoracic Society/European Respiratory Society International Multidisciplinary Consensus Classification of the Idiopathic Interstitial Pneumonias. Am J Respir Crit Care Med. 2002;165:277–304.
5. Stanescu D. Small airways obstruction syndrome. Chest. 1999;116:231–3.
6. Reynaud-Gaubert M, Thomas P, Badier M, et al. Early detection of airway involvement in obliterative bronchiolitis after lung transplantation. Functional and bronchoalveolar lavage cell findings. Am J Respir Crit Care Med. 2000;161:1924–9.
7. Lynch DA. Imaging of small airways disease and chronic obstructive pulmonary disease. Clin Chest Med. 2008;29:165–79, vii.
8. Kang EY, Woo OH, Shin BK, et al. Bronchiolitis: classification, computed tomographic and histopathologic features, and radiologic approach. J Comput Assist Tomogr. 2009;33:32–41.
9. Pipavath SJ, Lynch DA, Cool C, et al. Radiologic and pathologic features of bronchiolitis. AJR Am J Roentgenol. 2005;185:354–63.
10. Crosbie PA, Woodhead MA. Long-term macrolide therapy in chronic inflammatory airway diseases. Eur Respir J. 2009;33:171–81.
11. Idris SF, Chilvers ER, Haworth C, et al. Azithromycin therapy for neutrophilic airways disease: myth or magic? Thorax. 2009;64:186–9.
12. Bush A, Thomson AH. Acute bronchiolitis. BMJ. 2007;335:1037–41.
13. Tahan F, Ozcan A, Koc N. Clarithromycin in the treatment of RSV bronchiolitis: a double-blind, randomised, placebo-controlled trial. Eur Respir J. 2007;29:91–7.
14. Wong JY, Rutman A, O'Callaghan C. Recovery of the ciliated epithelium following acute bronchiolitis in infancy. Thorax. 2005;60:582–7.
15. Sigurs N, Gustafsson PM, Bjarnason R, et al. Severe respiratory syncytial virus bronchiolitis in infancy and asthma and allergy at age 13. Am J Respir Crit Care Med. 2005;171:137–41.
16. Jeong YJ, Lee KS, Koh WJ, et al. Nontuberculous mycobacterial pulmonary infection in immunocompetent patients: comparison of thin-section CT and histopathologic findings. Radiology. 2004;231: 880–6.
17. Okada F, Ando Y, Yoshitake S, et al. Pulmonary CT findings in 320 carriers of human T-lymphotropic virus type 1. Radiology. 2006;240:559–64.
18. Chang AB, Masel JP, Masters B. Post-infectious bronchiolitis obliterans: clinical, radiological and pulmonary function sequelae. Pediatr Radiol. 1998;28:23–9.
19. Zhang L, Irion K, Kozakewich H, et al. Clinical course of postinfectious bronchiolitis obliterans. Pediatr Pulmonol. 2000;29:341–50.
20. Mauad T, Dolhnikoff M. Histology of childhood bronchiolitis obliterans. Pediatr Pulmonol. 2002;33: 466–74.
21. Koh YY, da Jung E, Koh JY, et al. Bronchoalveolar cellularity and interleukin-8 levels in measles bronchiolitis obliterans. Chest. 2007;131:1454–60.

22. Hardy KA, Schidlow DV, Zaeri N. Obliterative bronchiolitis in children. Chest. 1988;93:460–6.
23. Zwemer Jr FL, Pratt DS, May JJ. Silo filler's disease in New York State. Am Rev Respir Dis. 1992;146:650–3.
24. Ghanei M, Tazelaar HD, Chilosi M, et al. An international collaborative pathologic study of surgical lung biopsies from mustard gas-exposed patients. Respir Med. 2008;102:825–30.
25. Ghanei M, Mokhtari M, Mohammad MM, et al. Bronchiolitis obliterans following exposure to sulfur mustard: chest high resolution computed tomography. Eur J Radiol. 2004;52:164–9.
26. Lai RS, Chiang AA, Wu MT, et al. Outbreak of bronchiolitis obliterans associated with consumption of Sauropus androgynus in Taiwan. Lancet. 1996;348:83–5.
27. Yang CF, Wu MT, Chiang AA, et al. Correlation of high-resolution CT and pulmonary function in bronchiolitis obliterans: a study based on 24 patients associated with consumption of Sauropus androgynus. AJR Am J Roentgenol. 1997;168:1045–50.
28. Oonakahara K, Matsuyama W, Higashimoto I, et al. Outbreak of Bronchiolitis obliterans associated with consumption of Sauropus androgynus in Japan–alert of food-associated pulmonary disorders from Japan. Respiration. 2005;72:221.
29. Wright JL, Cagle P, Churg A, et al. Diseases of the small airways. Am Rev Respir Dis. 1992;146:240–62.
30. Kreiss K, Gomaa A, Kullman G, et al. Clinical bronchiolitis obliterans in workers at a microwave-popcorn plant. N Engl J Med. 2002;347:330–8.
31. Kanwal R, Kullman G, Piacitelli C, et al. Evaluation of flavorings-related lung disease risk at six microwave popcorn plants. J Occup Environ Med. 2006;48:149–57.
32. van Rooy FG, Rooyackers JM, Prokop M, et al. Bronchiolitis obliterans syndrome in chemical workers producing diacetyl for food flavorings. Am J Respir Crit Care Med. 2007;176:498–504.
33. Kreiss K. Occupational bronchiolitis obliterans masquerading as COPD. Am J Respir Crit Care Med. 2007;176:427–9.
34. Eschenbacher WL, Kreiss K, Lougheed MD, et al. Nylon flock-associated interstitial lung disease. Am J Respir Crit Care Med. 1999;159:2003–8.
35. Atis S, Tutluoglu B, Levent E, et al. The respiratory effects of occupational polypropylene flock exposure. Eur Respir J. 2005;25:110–7.
36. Weiland DA, Lynch DA, Jensen SP, et al. Thin-section CT findings in flock worker's lung, a work-related interstitial lung disease. Radiology. 2003;227:222–31.
37. Konichezky S, Schattner A, Ezri T, et al. Thionyl-chloride-induced lung injury and bronchiolitis obliterans. Chest. 1993;104:971–3.
38. Epler GR, Snider GL, Gaensler EA, et al. Bronchiolitis and bronchitis in connective tissue disease. A possible relationship to the use of penicillamine. JAMA. 1979;242:528–32.
39. Geddes DM, Corrin B, Brewerton DA, et al. Progressive airway obliteration in adults and its association with rheumatoid disease. Q J Med. 1977;46:427–44.
40. Devouassoux G, Cottin V, Liote H, et al. Characterisation of severe obliterative bronchiolitis in rheumatoid arthritis. Eur Respir J. 2009;33:1053–61.
41. Parambil JG, Yi ES, Ryu JH. Obstructive bronchiolar disease identified by CT in the non-transplant population: analysis of 29 consecutive cases. Respirology. 2009;14:443–8.
42. Tanaka N, Kim JS, Newell JD, et al. Rheumatoid arthritis-related lung diseases: CT findings. Radiology. 2004;232:81–91.
43. Wolfe F, Schurle DR, Lin JJ, et al. Upper and lower airway disease in penicillamine treated patients with rheumatoid arthritis. J Rheumatol. 1983;10:406–10.
44. Papiris SA, Maniati M, Constantopoulos SH, et al. Lung involvement in primary Sjogren's syndrome is mainly related to the small airway disease. Ann Rheum Dis. 1999;58:61–4.
45. Tzeng DZ, Leslie KO, Shelton D, et al. Unusual dyspnea in a woman with CREST syndrome. Chest. 2008;133:286–90.
46. Boehler A, Vogt P, Speich R, et al. Bronchiolitis obliterans in a patient with localized scleroderma treated with D-penicillamine. Eur Respir J. 1996;9:1317–9.
47. Weigt SS, Wallace WD, Derhovanessian A, et al. Chronic allograft rejection: epidemiology, diagnosis, pathogenesis, and treatment. Semin Respir Crit Care Med. 2010;31:189–207.
48. Stewart S, Fishbein MC, Snell GI, et al. Revision of the 1996 working formulation for the standardization of nomenclature in the diagnosis of lung rejection. J Heart Lung Transplant. 2007;26:1229–42.
49. Knoop C, Estenne M. Acute and chronic rejection after lung transplantation. Semin Respir Crit Care Med. 2006;27:521–33.
50. Jackson CH, Sharples LD, McNeil K, et al. Acute and chronic onset of bronchiolitis obliterans syndrome (BOS): are they different entities? J Heart Lung Transplant. 2002;21:658–66.
51. Belperio JA, Weigt SS, Fishbein MC, et al. Chronic lung allograft rejection: mechanisms and therapy. Proc Am Thorac Soc. 2009;6:108–21.
52. Estenne M, Maurer JR, Boehler A, et al. Bronchiolitis obliterans syndrome 2001: an update of the diagnostic criteria. J Heart Lung Transplant. 2002;21:297–310.
53. Quantz MA, Bennett LE, Meyer DM, et al. Does human leukocyte antigen matching influence the outcome of lung transplantation? An analysis of 3,549 lung transplantations. J Heart Lung Transplant. 2000;19:473–9.
54. Glanville AR, Aboyoun CL, Havryk A, et al. Severity of lymphocytic bronchiolitis predicts long-term outcome after lung transplantation. Am J Respir Crit Care Med. 2008;177:1033–40.
55. Bankier AA, Van Muylem A, Knoop C, et al. Bronchiolitis obliterans syndrome in heart-lung transplant recipients:

diagnosis with expiratory CT. Radiology. 2001;218: 533–9.

56. Glanville AR. The role of bronchoscopic surveillance monitoring in the care of lung transplant recipients. Semin Respir Crit Care Med. 2006;27:480–91.

57. Martinu T, Howell DN, Davis RD, et al. Pathologic correlates of bronchiolitis obliterans syndrome in pulmonary retransplant recipients. Chest. 2006;129:1016–23.

58. Jain R, Hachem RR, Morrell MR, et al. Azithromycin is associated with increased survival in lung transplant recipients with bronchiolitis obliterans syndrome. J Heart Lung Transplant. 2010;29:531–7.

59. Vanaudenaerde BM, Meyts I, Vos R, et al. A dichotomy in bronchiolitis obliterans syndrome after lung transplantation revealed by azithromycin therapy. Eur Respir J. 2008;32:832–43.

60. Iacono AT, Johnson BA, Grgurich WF, et al. A randomized trial of inhaled cyclosporine in lung-transplant recipients. N Engl J Med. 2006;354:141–50.

61. Brugiere O, Thabut G, Castier Y, et al. Lung retransplantation for bronchiolitis obliterans syndrome: long-term follow-up in a series of 15 recipients. Chest. 2003;123:1832–7.

62. Yoshihara S, Tateishi U, Ando T, et al. Lower incidence of Bronchiolitis obliterans in allogeneic hematopoietic stem cell transplantation with reduced-intensity conditioning compared with myeloablative conditioning. Bone Marrow Transplant. 2005;35: 1195–200.

63. Soubani AO, Uberti JP. Bronchiolitis obliterans following haematopoietic stem cell transplantation. Eur Respir J. 2007;29:1007–19.

64. Williams KM, Chien JW, Gladwin MT, et al. Bronchiolitis obliterans after allogeneic hematopoietic stem cell transplantation. JAMA. 2009;302:306–14.

65. Philit F, Wiesendanger T, Archimbaud E, et al. Post-transplant obstructive lung disease ("bronchiolitis obliterans"): a clinical comparative study of bone marrow and lung transplant patients. Eur Respir J. 1995;8:551–8.

66. Yousem SA. The histological spectrum of pulmonary graft-versus-host disease in bone marrow transplant recipients. Hum Pathol. 1995;26:668–75.

67. Clark JG, Crawford SW, Madtes DK, et al. Obstructive lung disease after allogeneic marrow transplantation. Clinical presentation and course. Ann Intern Med. 1989;111:368–76.

68. Khalid M, Al Saghir A, Saleemi S, et al. Azithromycin in bronchiolitis obliterans complicating bone marrow transplantation: a preliminary study. Eur Respir J. 2005;25:490–3.

69. Nikolskaia OV, Nousari CH, Anhalt GJ. Paraneoplastic pemphigus in association with Castleman's disease. Br J Dermatol. 2003;149:1143–51.

70. Maldonado F, Pittelkow MR, Ryu JH. Constrictive bronchiolitis associated with paraneoplastic autoimmune multi-organ syndrome. Respirology. 2009;14: 129–33.

71. Kraft M, Mortenson RL, Colby TV, et al. Cryptogenic constrictive bronchiolitis. A clinicopathologic study. Am Rev Respir Dis. 1993;148:1093–101.

72. Dorinsky PM, Davis WB, Lucas JG, et al. Adult bronchiolitis. Evaluation by bronchoalveolar lavage and response to prednisone therapy. Chest. 1985;88:58–63.

73. Turton CW, Williams G, Green M. Cryptogenic obliterative bronchiolitis in adults. Thorax. 1981;36:805–10.

74. Salvi SS, Barnes PJ. Chronic obstructive pulmonary disease in non-smokers. Lancet. 2009;374:733–43.

75. Hogg JC. State of the art. Bronchiolitis in chronic obstructive pulmonary disease. Proc Am Thorac Soc. 2006;3:489–93.

76. Niewoehner DE, Kleinerman J, Rice DB. Pathologic changes in the peripheral airways of young cigarette smoker's. N Engl J Med. 1974;291:755–8.

77. Fraig M, Shreesha U, Savici D, et al. Respiratory bronchiolitis: a clinicopathologic study in current smokers, ex-smokers, and never-smokers. Am J Surg Pathol. 2002;26:647–53.

78. Galvin JR, Franks TJ. Smoking-related lung disease. J Thorac Imaging. 2009;24:274–84.

79. Wells AU, Nicholson AG, Hansell DM. Challenges in pulmonary fibrosis. 4: smoking-induced diffuse interstitial lung diseases. Thorax. 2007;62:904–10.

80. Heyneman LE, Ward S, Lynch DA, et al. Respiratory bronchiolitis, respiratory bronchiolitis-associated interstitial lung disease, and desquamative interstitial pneumonia: different entities or part of the spectrum of the same disease process? AJR Am J Roentgenol. 1999;173:1617–22.

81. Craig PJ, Wells AU, Doffman S, et al. Desquamative interstitial pneumonia, respiratory bronchiolitis and their relationship to smoking. Histopathology. 2004; 45:275–82.

82. Ryu JH, Myers JL, Capizzi SA, et al. Desquamative interstitial pneumonia and respiratory bronchiolitis-associated interstitial lung disease. Chest. 2005;127: 178–84.

83. Portnoy J, Veraldi KL, Schwarz MI, et al. Respiratory bronchiolitis-interstitial lung disease: long-term outcome. Chest. 2007;131:664–71.

84. Barnes PJ. Small airways in COPD. N Engl J Med. 2004;350:2635–7.

85. Leopold JG, Gough J. The centrilobular form of hypertrophic emphysema and its relation to chronic bronchitis. Thorax. 1957;12:219–35.

86. Aerni MR, Vassallo R, Myers JL, et al. Follicular bronchiolitis in surgical lung biopsies: clinical implications in 12 patients. Respir Med. 2008;102: 307–12.

87. Romero S, Barroso E, Gil J, et al. Follicular bronchiolitis: clinical and pathologic findings in six patients. Lung. 2003;181:309–19.

88. Kang EY, Miller RR, Muller NL. Bronchiectasis: comparison of preoperative thin-section CT and pathologic findings in resected specimens. Radiology. 1995;195:649–54.

89. Hansell DM, Wells AU, Rubens MB, et al. Bronchiectasis: functional significance of areas of decreased attenuation at expiratory CT. Radiology. 1994;193:369–74.

90. Roberts HR, Wells AU, Milne DG, et al. Airflow obstruction in bronchiectasis: correlation between

computed tomography features and pulmonary function tests. Thorax. 2000;55:198–204.

91. Sheehan RE, Wells AU, Copley SJ, et al. A comparison of serial computed tomography and functional change in bronchiectasis. Eur Respir J. 2002;20:581–7.

92. Sobonya RE, Taussig LM. Quantitative aspects of lung pathology in cystic fibrosis. Am Rev Respir Dis. 1986;134:290–5.

93. Helbich TH, Heinz-Peer G, Eichler I, et al. Cystic fibrosis: CT assessment of lung involvement in children and adults. Radiology. 1999;213:537–44.

94. Homma S, Kawabata M, Kishi K, et al. Bronchiolitis in Kartagener's syndrome. Eur Respir J. 1999;14:1332–9.

95. Poletti V, Casoni G, Chilosi M, et al. Diffuse panbronchiolitis. Eur Respir J. 2006;28:862–71.

96. Poletti V, Chilosi M, Trisolini R, et al. Idiopathic bronchiolitis mimicking diffuse panbronchiolitis. Sarcoidosis Vasc Diffuse Lung Dis. 2003;20:62–8.

97. Davies SJ, Gosney JR, Hansell DM, et al. Diffuse idiopathic pulmonary neuroendocrine cell hyperplasia: an under-recognised spectrum of disease. Thorax. 2007;62:248–52.

98. Naccache JM, Lavole A, Nunes H, et al. High-resolution computed tomographic imaging of airways in sarcoidosis patients with airflow obstruction. J Comput Assist Tomogr. 2008;32:905–12.

Pulmonary Vasculitis

19

Ulrich Specks and Karina A. Keogh

Abstract

Pulmonary vasculitis is usually but one manifestation of a systemic auto-immune disease. Primary vasculitis syndromes commonly affecting the respiratory tract are Wegener's granulomatosis (WG), microscopic poly-angiitis (MPA), and the Churg–Strauss syndrome. They are small-vessel vasculitides characterized by the presence of antineutrophil cytoplasmic autoantibodies (ANCA). This chapter provides an overview for a diagnostic approach to these patients that enables disease severity-adapted therapy. The respiratory manifestations of other vasculitides including Takayasu's arteritis, Behcet's disease, and Goodpasture's disease are also discussed.

Keywords

Pulmonary vasculitis • Wegener's granulomatosis • Microscopic poly-angiitis • Churg–Strauss syndrome • Antineutrophil cytoplasmic autoantibodies

The vasculitides are a group of systemic disorders characterized by inflammation and necrosis of blood vessel walls. This chapter focuses on those that predominantly affect the respiratory system. A logical approach toward the differential diagnosis and management of the patient with pulmonary vasculitis is provided with emphasis on disease manifestations and appropriate use of diagnostic tools including serology. Because of the systemic nature of these illnesses, the comments made in this chapter frequently go beyond the mere respiratory manifestations and pulmonary subspecialty concerns.

Different vasculitic conditions have a predilection for vessels of different size [1]. Pulmonary involvement is generally a feature of those vasculitides which primarily affect small vessels – arterioles, capillaries, and venules. The three most common forms of pulmonary vasculitis are Wegener's granulomatosis, microscopic poly-angiitis, and Churg–Strauss syndrome. The majority of patients with these three syndromes have autoantibodies directed against neutrophil cytoplasmic granule components called antineutrophil

U. Specks, MD (✉) • K.A. Keogh, MB, BCh
Division of Pulmonary and Critical Care Medicine,
Mayo Clinic, Rochester, MN, USA
e-mail: specks.ulrich@mayo.edu

R.P. Baughman and R.M. du Bois (eds.), *Diffuse Lung Disease: A Practical Approach*,
DOI 10.1007/978-1-4419-9771-5_19, © Springer Science+Business Media, LLC 2012

cytoplasmic antibodies (ANCA). For reasons that include the shared clinico-pathologic features, the strong association with ANCA, and the similar response to immunosuppressive agents, Wegener's granulomatosis and microscopic polyangiitis, and to a lesser extent, Churg–Strauss syndrome, are usually referred to as "the ANCA-associated vasculitides" [1].

The term "Goodpasture's syndrome" has been used with variable implications. Originally, it designated patients presenting with alveolar hemorrhage and glomerulonephritis, a combination that has also been referred to as "pulmonary-renal syndrome." These terms have not been used consistently, and it is now well recognized that the majority of cases presenting as "pulmonary-renal syndrome" are ANCA-associated. Autoantibodies directed against basement membrane components of the kidney glomeruli (anti-GBM) can also cause glomerulonephritis and alveolar hemorrhage. When this syndrome occurs in the presence of anti-GBM, it is now referred to as "anti-GBM disease" or "Goodpasture's disease" [2]. Because of these clinical similarities anti-GBM disease will also be discussed in this chapter, even though it is not a vasculitic disorder per se.

The connective tissue disorders including systemic lupus erythematosus and rheumatoid arthritis may be complicated by vasculitis affecting the lung. These are addressed in a separate chapter.

The primary vasculitides are rare. Hence, epidemiologic data are limited. The estimated incidence of small-vessel vasculitis is 20 cases per million population per year [3]. The average age of onset is past the fifth decade, but these diseases may occur at any age. The incidence of different types of ANCA-associated vasculitis seems to vary between different ethnic groups and latitude [3].

Prior to modern immunosuppressive therapy, these disorders were almost universally fatal. Today, their prognosis has improved significantly. However, the chronic relapsing nature of these diseases and the resulting need for long-term therapy continue to impart significant morbidity.

The etiologies of the various pulmonary vasculitides remain unclear. However, they are immune-mediated and respond to immunosuppressive therapy. Wegener's granulomatosis,

microscopic polyangiitis, and Churg–Strauss syndrome are all associated with ANCA. The target antigens for these autoantibodies are neutrophil granule proteins. ANCA are classified into two groups, cytoplasmic (C-ANCA) or perinuclear ANCA (P-ANCA), based on the location of immunofluorescent staining in ethanol-fixed neutrophils [4]. The granular cytoplasmic staining pattern of C-ANCA is generally caused by antibodies against proteinase 3 (PR3). The perinuclear staining pattern of P-ANCA may be caused by antibodies reacting with a variety of different neutrophil granule constituents that have been dislodged from the granule and rearranged around the nucleus as an artifact of ethanol fixation. Only P-ANCA reacting with myeloperoxidase (MPO) are of diagnostic utility. The C-ANCA/PR3-ANCA combination and the P-ANCA/MPO-ANCA combination are highly specific for Wegener's granulomatosis, microscopic polyangiitis, and the Churg–Strauss syndrome. ANCA that do not match this immunofluorescence pattern and antigen specificity combination are caused by antibodies reacting with other neutrophil proteins. They may occur in the context of connective tissue diseases including rheumatoid arthritis or systemic lupus erythematosus, inflammatory bowel disease, various infections or cocaine-induced midline destructive lesions [4, 5]. Such ANCA are nonspecific.

Most patients with ANCA-associated vasculitis present with symptoms caused by multi-organ involvement. Frequently, they appear ill and have constitutional symptoms such as malaise, fever, night sweats, weight loss, and acute renal dysfunction or neurological symptoms. The acute and potentially life-threatening presentation as diffuse alveolar hemorrhage syndrome is not unusual. Patients with pulmonary vasculitis require prompt diagnosis and intervention with immunosuppressive therapies. The individual disorders are characterized by the clinical pattern of disease manifestations, pathology, and serology. Table 19.1 compares these features for the three most common pulmonary vasculitides. These disorders are discussed below, in the order of their frequency and likelihood to present with respiratory symptoms.

Table 19.1 Clinical features

	Feature	Frequency WG	MPA	CSS
History: significant positive features				
Pulmonary	Hemoptysis	++	+	
	Stridor	+		
	Asthma			+++
General	Fever, weight loss, malaise, arthralgias	++	++	++
ENT	Sinus pain, discharge, epistaxis, hearing loss	+++	+	+++
Neurological	Weakness, numbness, tingling, headache.	++	++	+++
Opthalmologic	Painful eye, red eye, blindness	++		
Gastrointestinal	Pain, bleeding, small bowel obstruction		+	+
Physical examination: significant positive features				
Pulmonary	Pleural effusion	+		
Skin	Palpable purpura, ulceration, pyoderma gangrenosum, urticaria	++	++	++
ENT	Nasal erosions and crusting, septal destruction, serous otitis	+++		
Neurological	Mononeuritis multiplex, sensory peripheral neuropathy, paresis or paralysis, cranial nerve palsy	++	++	+++
Opthalmologic	Conjunctivitis, episcleritis, uveitis, retro-orbital mass/ proptosis, corneal ulceration, retinal vasculitis	++		
Gastrointestinal	Acute abdomen – bowel perforation, pancreatitis		+	+
Joints	Symmetric polyarthritis, oligo or monoarthritis, rarely erosive	++	++	++
Diagnostic features	Saddle nose deformity	☐		
	Strawberry gingival hyperplasia	☐		
Suggests other diagnosis	Ear cartilage destruction – *relapsing polychondritis*			
	Septal destruction in the absence of systemic manifestations – *digital trauma/cocaine induced*			
Pathology	C-ANCA/PR3	75–90%	10–50%	0–10%
	P-ANCA/MPO	Up to 20%	Up to 80%	60–80%
	Necrotizing granulomatous inflammation			
	Necrotizing vasculitis of the small arteries and veins			
	Necrotizing glomerulonephritis			
BAL findings that are useful	Sequentially bloody aliquots hemosiderin-laden macrophages	☐	☐	
	Microbiology to rule out infection			
	Eosinophils			☐
Bronchoscopy results that are useful	Tracheobronchial ulceration	☐		
	Cobblestoning	☐		
	Pseudotumor	☐		
	Bronchomalacia	☐		
Open lung biopsy results that are useful	Necrotizing granulomas, neutrophilic microabscesses, geographic necrosis, giant cells	☐		
	Vasculitis, capillaritis	☐	☐	☐
	Eosinophilic inflammation			☐

Wegener's Granulomatosis

Clinical Presentation

Wegener's granulomatosis is the most common form of vasculitis to involve the lung. It has a prevalence of up to 63 per million, and an annual incidence of 10 per million [6]. Symptoms and clinical disease manifestations are the result of necrotizing granulomatous inflammation and small-vessel vasculitis occurring at variable degrees of combination [7–9]. Granulomatous inflammation may affect any organ. Involvement of the upper respiratory tract occurs in almost all patients and usually causes the first symptoms [10, 11]. These include chronic rhinitis with or without epistaxis, nasal crusting, chronic sinusitis, and serous otitis media. Destruction of the nasal cartilage may lead to septal perforation or saddle nose deformity. Oropharyngeal ulcerations or salivary gland involvement may also occur. Inflammation and vasculitis involving the interdental papillae results in gingival hyperplasia with clefting and petechiae. This manifestation is rare but almost pathognomonic of Wegener's granulomatosis (Fig. 19.1).

Necrotizing granulomatous inflammation of the lung parenchyma may present radiographically as nodules or masses (Fig. 19.2). They cavitate when the necrotic center gets access to

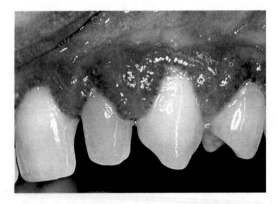

Fig. 19.1 "Mulberry" or "strawberry" gums, a rare but pathognomonic feature of Wegener's granulomatosis, are due to vasculitis involving the interdental papillae, which results in gingival hyperplasia with clefting and petechiae. Such findings may occur at disease onset or with a flare of the disease

an airway. These lesions are frequently asymptomatic. Occasionally, they are associated with cough and mild hemoptysis. Necrotizing granulomatous inflammation of the tracheobronchial tree may cause ulcerative lesions, so-called "cobble-stoning" or inflammatory pseudotumors of the airways detectable by bronchoscopy [12, 13]. Symptoms caused by these lesions include dyspnea, cough and stridor, which should not be mistaken for asthma. There is a predilection of the inflammation for the immediate subglottic area, and subglottic inflammation affects younger patients preferentially [14]. Persistent inflammation and subsequent scarring may lead to bronchomalacia or stenosis with airway obstruction. Necrotizing ulcerative airway inflammation with similar functional outcome may also be encountered in relapsing polychondritis [15].

Alveolar hemorrhage occurs in approximately 15% of patients and indicates the presence of capillaritis [16]. It is usually associated with other signs of severe systemic disease including renal involvement but may precede them. Alveolar hemorrhage in Wegener's granulomatosis has a mortality in the order of 50%. Therefore, prompt implementation of aggressive immunosuppressive therapy is essential. Hemoptysis is a prominent symptom of alveolar hemorrhage. However, up to a third of patients with alveolar hemorrhage have no hemoptysis. In these cases, a reduced hemoglobin level in association with roentgenographic evidence of diffuse alveolar infiltrates may be the only indication of alveolar hemorrhage (Fig. 19.3). In severe cases dyspnea secondary to gas exchange abnormalities is common, and represents an emergency which may require management in the intensive care unit, with oxygen supplementation, mechanical ventilation and possibly blood transfusion.

The differential diagnosis of significant hemoptysis includes bleeding from an endobronchial source, an underlying bleeding diathesis, cardiac disease, other form of vasculitis, anti-GBM disease, connective tissue disease, or exposure to inhalational toxins, therapeutic or illicit drugs. If the patient is already on immunosuppressive medication, exclusion of an infectious etiology such as pneumocytis carinii pneumonia is imperative. Toxicity from methotrexate, and more rarely

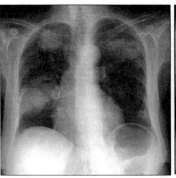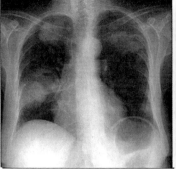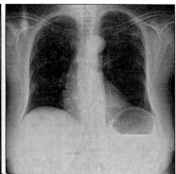

Fig. 19.2 Wegener's granulomatosis with granulomatous involvement of the pulmonary parenchyma may present radiographically with nodules or masses. Characteristically these lesions cavitate, become progressively more thin-walled, before they collapse on themselves and disappear or leave a fibrotic scar. Shown are serial chest roentgenograms of an 85-year-old woman who presented with a cough and constitutional symptoms. The diagnosis was established by transbronchial lung biopsy and a positive C-ANCA/PR3-ANCA test. She was treated with prednisone and cyclophosphamide with good clinical and radiographic response. At 3 and 5 months, the nodules were seen to be getting progressively smaller. On the last film, air-fluid levels had developed. In the absence of systemic signs of either disease activity or infection, no changes were made to her treatment regimen

cyclophophamide, may also be the cause of pulmonary infiltrates (see Alveolar Hemorrhage Algorithm, Fig. 19.4). The frequency of subclinical alveolar hemorrhage may be largely underestimated as one report stated that half of the patients with ANCA-associated vasculitis had more than 5% iron-laden alveolar macrophages on bronchoalveolar lavage [17].

Renal involvement, occurring in up to 80% of patients, is another manifestation of capillaritis, which requires urgent immunosuppressive therapy, in order to preserve renal function [7, 9]. The creatinine level at initiation of treatment predicts the ultimate renal outcome [18].

Neurological involvement is rare as an initial manifestation, but ultimately may affect up to 40% of patients with Wegener's granulomatosis [19, 20]. It is usually a result of vasculitis affecting the vasa nervorum. Mononeuritis multiplex and symmetric peripheral neuropathies are common. Cranial nerve function may be impaired due to compression by necrotizing granulomatous lesions. Inflammation of the pachymeninges may be the cause of severe headache. Cerebrovascular events and seizures are other potential manifestations of CNS vasculitis in the setting of Wegener's granulomatosis.

Ophthalmologic involvement may be due to granulomatous inflammation (orbital pseudotumors and lacrimal duct stenosis) or vasculitis (episcleritis, scleritis, uveitis, retinal vasculitis, or optic neuropathy) [21].

The skin is most frequently affected by leukocytoclastic vasculitis presenting clinically as palpable purpura. Up to 50% of patients develop some skin lesions over the course of their disease [22]. Pyoderma gangrenosum-like ulcerations, bullae, and granulomatous lesions may also be seen [22].

The classic diagnostic triad for Wegener's granulomatosis consists of necrotizing vasculitis, necrotizing granulomatous inflammation of the upper and lower respiratory tracts, and necrotizing glomerulonephritis [23]. However, limited forms of disease with less prominent vasculitic features have been recognized since the 1960s [24–26]. These cases are characterized by predominantly necrotizing granulomatous pathology, a more protracted clinical evolution and less imminent risk to organ function or life of the patient [27]. The limited disease state may persist for a variable time period, however, if left untreated, the majority of patients will progress to generalized vasculitis, with kidney involvement. Up to 30% of these patients do not have ANCA,

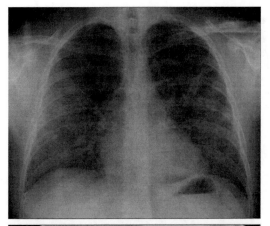

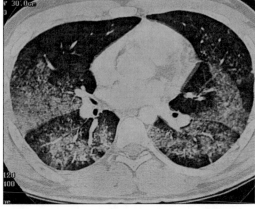

Fig. 19.3 Alveolar hemorrhage may be indicated by diffuse or patchy alveolar infiltrates on radiographic studies. This patient had Wegener's granulomatosis confirmed by open lung biopsy. He was initially treated with prednisone and cyclophosphamide which was subsequently changed to methotrexate. After 2 years of treatment the medications were stopped and several months later he presented with hemoptysis, dyspnea, fever, and a falling hemoglobin level. Both his chest roentgenogram and the thoracic computed tomogram show a patchy alveolar filling process consistent with alveolar hemorrhage. The presence of alveolar hemorrhage was further documented by bronchoalveolar lavage. He quickly responded to the reintroduction of immunosuppression

but the presence of C-ANCA is indicative of a higher likelihood of progression [28, 29].

Investigations

The goals of diagnostic evaluations are: (1) to accurately diagnose the disease and estimate the severity; (2) monitor the response to therapy and detect any relapse of disease; (3) detect both disease sequelae and adverse events secondary to therapy.

Blood Counts and Serology

Routine testing includes a complete blood count. The hemoglobin and hematocrit may be low in the setting of alveolar hemorrhage, or as a result of chronic illness or renal insufficiency. The white blood cell count and platelet count may be elevated as an acute phase reaction. Prominent eosinophilia would be suggestive of Churg–Strauss syndrome. Erythrocyte sedimentation rate and C-reactive protein levels should be measured as markers of inflammation. In patients with limited disease these may be normal, whereas in the setting of active vasculitis they are usually markedly elevated. Serum chemistry, urine analysis, and urine microscopy should be performed to assess renal function and to search for signs of glomerulonephritis. If there is any suggestion of renal involvement, renal function should be quantified formally by determination of creatinine or iothalamate clearance.

Serologic testing for specific autoantibodies is crucial in the differential diagnosis of patients suspected to suffer from a systemic vasculitic illness. Eighty to 95% of patients with Wegener's granulomatosis are positive for C-ANCA. Depending on the clinical presentation, additional serologic testing should be performed. The finding of other autoantibodies may suggest alternative diagnoses, such as antiglomerular basement membrane antibodies indicative of Goodpasture's disease, or antinuclear antibodies and anti-double-stranded DNA, elevated creatine kinase levels, and antiphospholipid antibodies, all of which may be suggestive of specific connective tissue diseases.

Radiographic Studies

Radiographic studies primarily consist of chest roentgenogram and/or computed tomography. Pulmonary parenchymal granulomatous involvement may present radiographically as nodules or masses. Characteristically these lesions cavitate, then become progressively more thin walled as

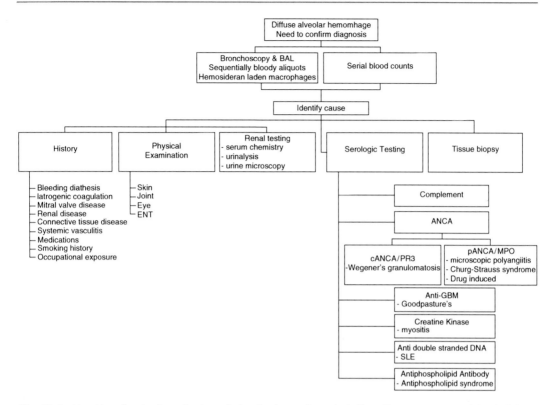

Fig. 19.4 Algorithm for the investigation of alveolar hemorrhage including diagnoses suggested by individual findings

they heal (see Fig. 19.2). Ultimately, they collapse on themselves and either disappear or leave a fibrotic scar. On rare occasions, they can persist and get superinfected with nosocomial organisms or *Aspergillus fumigatus*. The granulomatous lesions are frequently asymptomatic, occasionally they are associated with cough and mild hemoptysis. The differential diagnosis includes malignancy, including lymphomatoid granulomatosis (which however does not cavitate), infection, e.g., fungal or nocardia, and other idiopathic pulmonary processes such as necrotizing sarcoid granulomatosis.

Localized or diffuse infiltrates may also be seen. Localized infiltrates may be postobstructive in nature. Diffuse alveolar infiltrates are usually caused by alveolar hemorrhage, even in the absence of hemoptysis. Other less common pulmonary manifestations include pleural effusions, pleural inflammatory pseudotumors, and hilar adenopathy [30]. The effusions are generally small and insignificant. Similarly, mediastinal adenopathy, which may be seen in approximately 10% of patients, is usually small and clinically insignificant.

High-resolution computed tomography is more sensitive than standard chest roentgenography. It may be helpful in the assessment of bronchial and peri-bronchial involvement, and for the demonstration of residual scarring [31]. Three-dimensional reconstructive CT-imaging may be useful to assess bronchial involvement, and particularly the poststenotic airway caliber beyond the reach of bronchoscopy [13, 32].

Computed tomography is indispensable in the evaluation of patients' ear, nose and throat symptomatology and eye involvement. Sinus disease and orbital inflammatory pseudotumors are best visualized by this imaging modality. Magnetic resonance imaging is another useful diagnostic modality to assess inflammatory abnormalities of the sinuses and orbits [33].

Magnetic resonance imaging should be performed in patients with Wegener's granulomatosis who complain of headaches and/or cranial nerve function abnormalities, to identify granulomatous lesions of the base of the skull, pituitary gland involvement, meningeal involvement, or cerebral vasculitis.

Pulmonary Function Testing

Pulmonary function testing should be an integral part of the initial evaluation of patients suspected of Wegener's granulomatosis. Dyspnea is one of the most frequent complaints of patients with Wegener's granulomatosis. Therefore, it is useful to have baseline pulmonary function data early in the course of the disease, when they are frequently normal. As the pulmonary parenchymal pathology and airway manifestations of Wegener's granulomatosis are highly variable, pulmonary function testing may reveal a wide spectrum of flow and lung volume abnormalities. The diffusing capacity is often low. It may be elevated in the acute setting of alveolar hemorrhage. However, its determination is rarely practical in this clinical setting, and by the time the patient with acute alveolar hemorrhage is stable enough to undergo formal pulmonary function testing the diffusion capacity is usually reduced. A low diffusion capacity that cannot be easily explained by parenchymal abnormalities should raise the suspicion of thromboembolic events which are very common in the acute setting of active Wegener's granulomatosis.

The flow–volume loop is particularly useful in the evaluation of patients with stridor or wheezing, as these clinical symptoms should raise the suspicion of subglottic, tracheal or endobronchial stenosis [13]. Characteristic examples of flow–volume loop abnormalities indicative of fixed airway obstructions caused by Wegener's granulomatosis are shown in Fig. 19.5. The shape of the flow–volume curve is representative of the functional, rather than the anatomic degree of obstruction. It has been demonstrated that with tracheal lesions the flow–volume loop may be relatively well preserved until the lumen is less than 8 mm in diameter (an 80% reduction in area). Therefore, visual inspection via bronchoscopy or laryngoscopy is warranted if airway involvement is suspected, even if the flow–volume loop appears well preserved.

Bronchoscopy

Flexible fiberoptic bronchoscopy with or without bronchoalveolar lavage may be utilized in Wegener's granulomatosis to establish the initial diagnosis, assess disease activity, document alveolar hemorrhage, and rule out an infectious etiology. Characteristic findings include ulcerating tracheo-bronchitis, cobble-stoning of the mucosa, and inflammatory pseudotumors [12, 13]. These lesions may cause stenosis acutely or chronically due to scar tissue formation. All patients with symptoms or findings on pulmonary function testing suggestive of airway involvement should undergo bronchoscopy. These lesions may also be clinically occult. In one study one-third of patients who underwent bronchoscopy for radiographic abnormalities, and denied airway symptoms, were found to have endobronchial lesions [12, 13]. Biopsies obtained at bronchoscopy are diagnostic of Wegener's granulomatosis only approximately 20% of the time. However the pathologic findings when taken in conjunction with the clinical and serologic findings may establish the diagnosis, and thus obviate the need for an open lung biopsy in about half of patients. Bronchoscopic manifestations of alveolar hemorrhage include bronchoalveolar lavage fluid aliquots that are sequentially bloodier and contain hemosiderin laden macrophages. Microbiological stains and cultures are needed to exclude an infectious etiology. Bronchoalveolar lavage must be preformed cautiously as it may cause deterioration in an already tenuous patient.

Biopsy

Biopsy evidence remains the gold standard in making the diagnosis of Wegener's granulomatosis. Because of the side effects of long-term immunosuppressant therapy, the diagnosis should be established as firmly as possible – ideally with a biopsy, though in certain settings a classic presentation in conjunction with the appropriate serological markers may be sufficient. Biopsies should be obtained in the least invasive manner (e.g., from nose or skin).

Fig. 19.5 Pulmonary function flow–volume loops may be helpful in the diagnosis of upper airway obstruction in patients with Wegener's granulomatosis. (**a**) Fixed airway obstruction with a plateau seen on both the inspiratory and expiratory loops, in a patient with subglottic stenosis, (**b**) intra-thoracic bilateral proximal airway obstruction. The shape of the inspiratory curve is preserved, however the expiratory curve after an initial downward slope reaches an early plateau. The same findings would be expected in a patient with an intrathoracic tracheal lesion

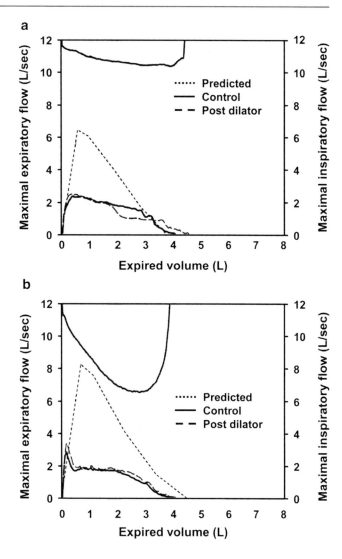

Renal biopsy with direct immunofluorescence should be performed if there is laboratory evidence for renal insufficiency (elevated creatinine) or glomerulonephritis (active urinary sediment). The classic renal lesion on light microscopy is focal segmental necrotizing glomerulonephritis. This may also be seen in other conditions including microscopic polyangiitis, Goodpasture's disease, and systemic lupus erythematosus. These different disorders can at least in part be distinguished on the basis of direct immunofluorescence. This shows few or no immune deposits (pauci-immune) in Wegener's granulomatosis or microscopic polyangiitis. Linear deposition of immunoglobulins is characteristic of Goodpasture's disease, and clumpy granular deposits of immune complexes are seen in systemic lupus erythematosus. Granulomatous inflammation is rarely seen on kidney biopsy in Wegener's granulomatosis. Renal biopsy is not only of diagnostic but also of prognostic value [18]. The role of transbronchial biopsy, as discussed previously, is limited, with pathology often nondiagnostic. Open lung biopsy has the highest diagnostic yield but should be considered only in the absence of more accessible biopsy sites.

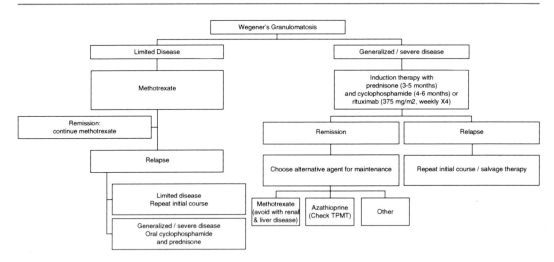

Fig. 19.6 Algorithm for the treatment of Wegener's granulomatosis, stratified by disease severity and the different phases of treatment

Clinical Management

When left untreated, Wegener's granulomatosis is a universally fatal disease [34]. However, with introduction of cyclophosphamide-based immunosuppressive therapy the median survival is 22 years [9]. Treatment needs to be individualized for extent and severity of disease, taking into account whether the disease is limited or generalized. There are separate protocols for induction therapy to achieve remission, and to maintain remission.

Limited disease is disease characterized predominantly by necrotizing granulomatous pathology, and no affected organ is at risk for irreversible damage [27]. In contrast, generalized or severe disease includes all patients with vasculitic symptoms including alveolar hemorrhage, glomerulonephritis, or nervous system involvement [27]. In addition, cardiac involvement, scleritis, sensorineural hearing loss, and leukocytoclastic vasculitis of the skin should be categorized as severe or generalized disease because they represent clinical manifestations of systemic small-vessel vasculitis with the potential for life- or organ function-threatening outcome [27]. Rarely localized necrotizing granulomatous lesions may be in life-threatening locations, and in these cases are treated in the same aggressive manner as generalized disease.

The principles of a stage-adapted individualized treatment approach are summarized in the Wegener's granulomatosis treatment algorithm (Fig. 19.6).

Remission Induction

For the last four decades, the standard regimen for remission induction in severe or generalized disease has consisted of oral cyclophosphamide (2 mg/kg/day, adjusted for renal function) and prednisone (1 mg/kg/day, not to exceed 80 mg/day). Once disease activity is controlled, the prednisone dose is tapered with the goal of complete discontinuation after about 3 months. Cyclophosphamide is continued for up to 6 months. At that stage, provided that the patient has achieved remission, the cyclophosphamide should be changed to a less toxic immunosuppressive agent for remission maintenance [35–37]. This standard regimen induces complete remission in 70–93% of patients [9, 35–37]. However, there is a greater than 50% relapse rate over 5 years. The treatment itself may cause significant morbidity and mortality [7, 9, 36]. Up to 46% experience serious infectious complications, other complications include hemorrhagic cystitis (up to 50%), bladder cancer (up to 11%), and myelodysplasia (up to 8%). Other significant management problems are osteoporosis, diabetes control, and cyclophosphamide-induced infertility.

In an attempt to the limit toxicity associated with oral cyclophosphamide use, intermittent high-dose (pulse) intravenous cyclophosphamide in conjunction with oral prednisone has also been used. A recent randomized controlled trial compared oral daily cyclophosphamide application to a pulse regimen [38]. There was no difference in efficacy for remission induction, mortality, toxicity, or relapse rate between the regimens. Only the observed frequency of leucopenia was lower in the pulse than in the oral cyclophosphamide treatment arm. However, the infection rate was not different between the two regimens. It should be noted that the frequency of pulses given in this trial was higher than the monthly application, customarily used in the United States [38]. Because the cumulative cyclophosphamide dose is lower when pulsed cyclophosphamide is given, this approach is most appropriately utilized in select groups such as young women who want to maximize their chances of future fertility.

The introduction of rituximab for treatment of Wegener's granulomatosis and microscopic polyangiitis represents a paradigm shift for remission induction therapy of these diseases [39–41]. A recently completed randomized controlled trial that compared rituximab head to head to daily oral cyclophosphamide for remission induction of severe ANCA-associated vasculitis showed that rituximab is not inferior to cyclophosphamide [42]. For patients who had entered the trial with a severe disease flare rituximab proved superior to cyclophosphamide [42]. For the first time there is now a proven alternative to cyclophosphamide for patients with Wegener's granulomatosis and microscopic polyangiitis. This is of particular interest for young patients who want to preserve their fertility, and for patients who suffer a severe disease flare rituximab represents the preferable treatment alternative.

Induction Therapy for Limited Disease

In limited disease methotrexate (at a target dose of 25 mg once a week) is used in conjunction with prednisone (1 mg/kg/day, not to exceed 80 mg/day), rather than cyclophosphamide. It is less toxic and appears to have similar efficacy, with regards to inducing remission in these patients [36, 43, 44]. Patients receiving methotrexate also need to receive folic acid 1 mg/day to minimize toxicity. In order to prevent *Pneumocystis jerovecii* pneumonia, prophylaxis with trimethoprim/sulfamethoxazole or alternate agents is imperative.

Remission Maintenance

Methotrexate was the first drug demonstrated to be an efficacious alternative to cyclophosphamide for remission maintenance, without comparable side effects [45]. However, methotrexate is contraindicated in patients with significant renal dysfunction. Liver function and white cell count need to be monitored while on this drug. The methotrexate dose used for remission maintenance is the same as used for remission induction. *Azothioprine* appears to be as effective as methotrexate for remission maintenance [35, 37]. It may be the preferred agent as it can be used in patients with diminished renal function, and hepatotoxicity is less frequent and reversible. Prior to its administration patients should be tested for thiopurine-methyltransferase deficiency, to identify patients who are at high risk for profound and prolonged pancytopenia. Azathioprine should not be used in patients deficient in this enzyme that is required for normal metabolization of the drug. Azathioprine is usually given at a dose of 2 mg/kg/day. Both white cell counts and liver function tests need to be monitored on at least a monthly basis. *Mycophenolate mofetil* is a second-line agent for remission maintenance, used when the above two agents are contraindicated. It is dosed at 1,500–2,000 mg/day orally. Initial reports suggest that it can be used successfully to maintain remission after standard induction therapy. The drug is generally well tolerated [46].

Trimethoprim/sulfamethoxazole There is some evidence that this drug may have a beneficial effect on disease activity. After initial observations, it has become apparent that patients with mild upper respiratory tract disease who lack ANCA may be treated with this drug at a dose of 800/240 mg twice a day under careful observation [47]. This agent also seems to be beneficial by reducing the rate of disease relapse [48].

It remains unclear whether this agent exerts its effect by suppressing upper respiratory tract infections that may trigger relapses or whether the drug has immune modulatory properties.

The optimal duration for remission maintenance is not well defined. Generally, the remission induction phase is of 6 months duration followed by 12 months of remission maintenance therapy. Patients who have suffered repeated relapses subsequently require more prolonged remission maintenance therapy.

Beyond Standard Therapy

Patients with vasculitic disease who do not respond to current immunosuppressive therapy represent a considerable clinical challenge. The addition of intravenous immunoglobulin therapy to standard therapy has been advocated as one potential option for these patients [49, 50]. The rationale for this approach is the presence of anti-ANCA idiotype antibodies in pooled gamma globulin preparations [51]. However, the outcome of this treatment modality is unpredictable, possibly because of batch-to-batch variability and differences between preparations from different manufacturers.

Plasma exchange has also been used in the most seriously ill patients. It may of particular benefit in patients who present with rapidly progressive renal disease or severe alveolar hemorrhage [52, 53]. The rationale for this somewhat invasive approach is to remove circulating pathogenic ANCA or other relevant inflammatory mediators quickly.

A number of biologic agents have been or are also under investigation, including the tumor necrosis factor alpha antagonists etanercept and infliximab, B-cell-targeted therapy with the anti-CD20 monoclonal antibody, rituximab, and most recently, the anti-CTLA 4 agent, abatacept. Etanercept has no effect on disease activity, but when given to patients who have been exposed to cyclophosphamide increases the risk for solid malignancy significantly [36, 54]. Infliximab may have some efficacy when added to failing standard remission induction therapy. However, this approach seems to be associated with an excessive risk of severe infections [55–57]. For these reasons, antitumor necrosis factor therapy is not advocated for Wegener's granulomatosis. Therapeutic agents targeting T-cell function either directly or indirectly remain under investigation and are currently not recommended for standard practice. In contrast, the anti-CD20 monoclonal antibody, rituximab, which specifically targets B cells, is now firmly established as the agent of choice for patients with refractory or chronically relapsing disease [41, 58, 59].

Management of Disease Sequelae

Even after the inflammation has resolved, scaring from the disease may result in damage which requires further treatment. Examples of damage causing significant morbidity include saddle nose deformity, tracheobronchial stenosis, and end-stage renal disease [60]. Nasal deformities may be safely reconstructed once the patient is in stable remission [61]. Similarly, nasolacrimal duct patency may be restored surgically.

Subglottic stenosis represents another challenging management problem. Inflammation in this region may occur even when disease is quiescent elsewhere. Symptoms such as stridor and dyspnea usually do not become manifest until scarring has occurred. In the past, trachoeostomy has frequently been required. However, with the use of intra-tracheal dilatation and the intralesional injection of long-acting glucocorticoids, tracheostomy may be prevented [62].

Stenosis and obstruction may also occur more distally in the bronchial tree. Airway patency may be improved by selective placement of silastic airway stents, which may be deployed in the trachea and mainstem bronchi [12, 13]. Careful balloon dilatation may also alleviate airway obstruction at a more segmental level. These are specialized procedures, which should only be performed by experienced otolarynologists and interventional bronchoscopists working in interdisciplinary teams caring for Wegener's granulomatosis.

Monitoring Therapy

Many of the immunosuppressive agents used for the treatment of Wegener's granulomatosis and other pulmonary vasculitides are associated with significant toxicities. These can be avoided or

Table 19.2 Monitoring for morbidity due to therapeutic agents

Medication	Potential morbidity	Monitoring/management
Corticosteroids	Opportunistic infection	PCP prophylaxis with trimethoprim/sulphamethoxazole for daily doses >20 mg
	Osteoporosis	Baseline bone density scan, repeated every 1–2 years
		Calcium + vitamin D supplementation +/– bisphosphonates
	Diabetes mellitus	Fasting glucose levels
Cyclophosphamide	Opportunistic infection	PCP prophylaxis with trimethoprim/sulphamethoxazole
	Myelosuppression	Weekly CBC. Hold drug for WBC < 4
	Bladder toxicity	Drug administered in morning. 3–4 L fluid consumption/day
		Regular urinalysis. Cystoscopy for hematuria or yearly if on agent for >1 year
Methotrexate	Opportunistic infection	PCP prophylaxis with trimethoprim/sulphamethoxazole
	Myelosuppression	CBC every 2 weeks. Folic acid 1 mg po qd
	Hepatotoxicity	Monthly LFT's
Azothioprine	Allergic reaction	TPMT blood test prior to drug administration
	Opportunistic infection	PCP prophylaxis with trimethoprim/sulphamethoxazole
	Myelosuppression	Initially CBC every 2nd week, then monthly
	Hepatotoxicity	Monthly LFTs

minimized through specific preventive measures, careful laboratory monitoring, and appropriate dose adjustments (Table 19.2).

Microscopic Polyangiitis

Clinical Presentation and Diagnosis

Microscopic polyangiitis is a nongranulomatous form of necrotizing vasculitis, which shares many of the features with Wegener's granulomatosis [1, 63]. It has an annual incidence of 8.4 cases per million population [6]. Pulmonary capillaritis, resulting in alveolar hemorrhage, occurs in 10–30%. As in Wegener's granulomatosis, necrotizing glomerulonephritis is very common, occurring in almost 80%, and may deteriorate rapidly. Ocular, ear, nose, and throat involvement are much less common. However approximately 30% of patients with microscopic polyangiitis have gastrointestinal involvement, as opposed to Wegener's granulomatosis in which gastrointestinal tract involvement is very rare [63, 64]. As with Wegener's granulomatosis essentially any organ may be involved.

Microscopic polyangiitis is associated with P-ANCA, reacting with MPO in 40–80% of cases [63]. Less frequently, C-ANCA with reactivity to PR3 is seen. Occasionally, some patients with microscopic polyangiitis later develop granulomatous inflammation and are reclassified as having Wegener's granulomatosis; this usually occurs in patients who are positive for C-ANCA. Microscopic polyangiitis may occasionally be associated with pulmonary fibrosis, which may have the radiographic appearance of acute interstitial pneumonia or idiopathic pulmonary fibrosis. There are also reports of an association between microscopic polyangiitis and severe obstructive airways disease and bronchiectasis. Visceral angiography is generally not helpful even in the presence of abdominal symptoms as the vessels involved are too small to be visualized [64]. As in Wegener's granulomatosis, biopsy specimens should be obtained from the most accessible site. Renal biopsy shows pauci-immune focal segmental necrotizing glomerulonephritis, with extracapillary proliferation forming crescents. Unless granulomas are present in the biopsy specimen (which would identify it as being Wegener's granulomatosis), the two conditions are indistinguishable, and the same treatment principles apply [35, 42, 53].

Treatment and Prognosis

A 5-year survival of 74% is reported [63]. As in patients with Wegener's granulomatosis, the most significant negative prognostic factor appears to be alveolar hemorrhage [65]. Patients who are C-ANCA positive also seem to have a greater mortality than those with P-ANCA [66]. The treatment regimen is the same as that for generalized Wegener's granulomatosis (see Wegener's granulomatosis treatment algorithm) [35, 42, 53]. This regimen induces remission in 70–93%, however 25–30% of patients will relapse within 18–24 months. Most of these appear to respond to retreatment [67]. Patients with microscopic polyangiitis, mild renal disease, P-ANCA/MPO-ANCA and no life-threatening disease manifestation may respond well to mycophenolate mofetil and may not require cyclophosphamide or rituximab for remission induction [68, 69].

Classic Polyarteritis Nodosa

While microscopic polyangiitis was initially felt to be part of the polyarteritis nodosa spectrum it is now known to be a distinct entity. Classic polyarteritis nodosa is now recognized to be a very rare form of vasculitis [70]. In contrast to microscopic polyangiitis, it does not affect capillaries and therefore does not cause either glomerulonephritis or alveolar hemorrhage [1]. On the rare occasion that classic polyarteritis nodosa does affect the lung, it is usually in the form of bronchial or bronchiolar artery vasculitis [71]. Only 10–20% with polyarteritis nodosa have ANCA, and it is unclear if these patients have classic polyarteritis nodosa or an overlap syndrome [72, 73]. Classic polyarteritis nodosa is far less likely to relapse than microscopic polyangiitis, and therefore can generally be treated with a shorter 1 year course of immunosuppression. Classic polyarteritis nodosa has also been associated with viral infections, specifically hepatitis B and C, and therefore may respond to antiviral therapy [72].

Churg–Strauss Syndrome

Clinical Presentation and Diagnosis

Churg–Strauss syndrome is the third type of vasculitis which commonly affects the lung. It remains however a rare diagnosis with an estimated annual incidence of 3.1 per million [6]. It is primarily distinguished from Wegener's granulomatosis and microscopic polyangiitis by a high prevalence of asthma and peripheral blood and tissue eosinophilia. Churg–Strauss syndrome has also been described as having three distinct phases [74]: The first is a prodromal allergic/asthmatic phase. This phase may last for a number of years and consists of allergic rhinitis, nasal polyposis and/or asthma. Second is an eosinophilic phase where both peripheral and tissue eosinophilia may be seen. This phase may also last a number of years and the manifestations may remit and recur over this time period. The differential diagnosis for patients in this phase of the disease includes Loeffler's eosinophilic pneumonia and chronic eosinophilic pneumonia. The third vasculitic phase consists of systemic vasculitis and may be life-threatening. The three phases are not seen in all patients and do not necessarily occur in this order, in fact they may all be seen concurrently. However, in general, asthma predates vasculitic symptoms by a mean of 7 years (range 0–61) [75]. Formes frustes of Churg–Strauss syndrome have also been described where eosinophilic vasculitis and/or eosinophilic granulomas are seen in an isolated organ without evidence of systemic disease [76].

Lung involvement occurs in 38% of patients [75, 77]. Transient alveolar-type infiltrates are most common, but occasionally nodular lesions may be seen. In contrast to Wegener's granulomatosis and microscopic polyangiitis, alveolar hemorrhage is exceedingly rare [75, 77–79]. Renal involvement in Churg–Strauss syndrome is less prominent than in Wegener's granulomatosis and microscopic polyangiitis and does not generally lead to renal failure [75, 77, 80]. In contrast, peripheral nerve involvement, typically in the form of mononeuritis multiplex, is more frequent [75, 77–79]. Skin, heart, central nervous system, and abdominal viscera may also be involved [75, 77–79].

The classic histopathologic picture consists of necrotizing vasculitis, eosinophilic tissue infiltration, and extravascular granulomas [1, 74, 81]. However, not all features are found in every case, and they are not pathognomonic of the condition. Particularly, the finding of a "Churg–Strauss granuloma" on skin biopsy should not be confused with the diagnosis of Churg–Strauss syndrome. While this type of necrotizing extravascular granuloma may be seen in Churg–Strauss syndrome, other systemic autoimmune diseases occur including Wegener's granulomatosis and rheumatoid arthritis [82].

ANCA are present in 50–80% of patients with Churg–Strauss syndrome [75, 77–79]. Typically, these are P-ANCA reacting with MPO. When ANCA is present, it appears to correlate with disease activity [75]. Some studies have suggested that the presence of ANCA portends a more vasculitic disease phenotype but this was not confirmed by all [75, 78, 79]. Recently, as leukotriene receptor antagonists are being used more frequently in the treatment of asthma, there has been speculation that they are playing a causative role in the development of Churg–Strauss syndrome, and that they may be contributing to an increased incidence of this disease. Alternatively, these agents may unmask previously unrecognized Churg–Strauss syndrome by facilitating a taper of the corticosteroid dose given for asthma control [83]. The onset of Churg–Strauss syndrome has also been reported in association with other drugs, which allow a reduction in corticosteroid use. According to a National Institutes of Health workshop 88% of patients developed CSS in conjunction with a steroid taper, with no single compound or class of anti-asthmatic agent associated with Churg–Strauss syndrome [84].

Prognosis and Treatment

Most deaths in Churg–Strauss syndrome are secondary to cardiac involvement rather than pulmonary or renal disease [77]. In contrast to Wegener's granulomatosis or microscopic polyangiitis, the overall mortality of Churg–Strauss syndrome is lower and not significantly different from the normal population [75]. Corticosteroids are the mainstay of therapy. In cases of cardiac or neurologic involvement, cyclophosphamide should be considered early as in the treatment of Wegener's granulomatosis and microscopic polyangiitis. However, no significant improvement in outcomes has been documented by the addition of cyclophosphamide. In refractory cases, a number of drugs have been used experimentally including hydroxyurea, alpha-interferon, and rituximab [85–87].

Isolated Pauci-Immune Pulmonary Capillaritis

There have been several reports of an isolated pauci-immune pulmonary capillaritis causing diffuse alveolar hemorrhage in patients with variable P-ANCA positivity. In a series of eight ANCA negative patients with pulmonary capillaritis on biopsy, no evidence for a systemic disease could be detected after a mean follow up of 43 months [88]. Therapeutically these patients should be approached in the same way as microscopic polyangiitis and Wegener's granulomatosis, e.g., remission induction with prednisone and cyclophosphamide, followed by remission maintenance with azathioprine.

Giant Cell Arteritis

This is the most common form of systemic vasculitis in Caucasians. However, it generally does not cause significant pulmonary symptoms. The inflammation involves the medium and large blood vessels. It predominantly affects the elderly, and is more common in women. It is often associated with polymyalgia rheumatica. It may present subacutely with malaise, fatigue, weight loss and fever, in conjunction with a very high sedimentation rate. Alternatively it may present acutely with abrupt painless visual loss (15% of patients), due to vasculitic involvement of the ophthalmic or posterior ciliary artery. Other common symptoms are headache, tenderness over the temporal arteries and jaw claudication. The aortic arch and its branches are involved in 10–15% of cases. This may cause cough and aortic arch syndrome. Pulmonary artery involvement has also been reported [89]. One epidemiological study documented the presence of pulmonary symptoms in up to 25% of patients [90]. Rarely, an unexplained cough in an elderly patient may be the first manifestation of giant cell arteritis [91]. Isolated cases of giant cell arteritis with pulmonary nodules, pleural effusion, lymphocytic alveolitis, and follicular bronchiolitis have also been described [92–95]. However, in clinical practice, pulmonologists seldom have to manage respiratory complications of giant cell arteritis. Chest roentgenography and pulmonary function testing are generally unremarkable. Diagnostic findings on biopsy of the temporal arteries are the presence of giant cells and lymphocytes, intimal proliferation, and destruction of the elastic membranes. Bilateral biopsies should be sought as skip lesions are common. Very occasionally, Wegener's granulomatosis can present with vasculitis involving the temporal arteries [96, 97]. The histological findings can be very similar. The main distinguishing features indicating Wegener's granulomatosis are the presence of small-vessel involvement in other organs (e.g., alveolar hemorrhage secondary to pulmonary capillaritis and glomerulonephritis) and positive ANCA serology. Giant cell arteritis responds well to prednisone therapy, and seldom requires the use of additional immunosuppressive agents [98].

Takayasu's Arteritis

Takayasu's arteritis is another large-vessel vasculitis [99, 100]. It affects vessels with abundant elastic tissue. The disease is most commonly seen in young women. It predominantly affects the aorta and its major branches. The peripheral lobular branches of the pulmonary vasculature also have an elastic component, and may be involved in up to 50% of patients. Pulmonary involvement is usually clinically occult, however mild to moderate pulmonary hypertension occurs in up to 70% [101]. Fistula formation between pulmonary artery branches and bronchial arteries has also been reported, as has nonspecific inflammatory interstitial lung disease. Initial symptoms in patients with Takayasu's arteritis often consist of malaise and arthralgias. Later, patients may develop symptoms of cerebral ischemia including headaches, dizziness, and visual disturbances. If the coronary ostia are involved, angina may develop. Limb claudication and intra-abdominal

ischemia may also occur. On examination, most patients have an asymmetrical reduction in peripheral pulses, with blood pressure differences of >10 mmHg. Bruits may be heard over the large vessels, and aortic root dilatation with aortic insufficiency may cause a cardiac murmur. The electrocardiogram may show signs of ischemia, and a dilated aortic arch may be detectable on chest roentgenography. Computed tomography of the chest may demonstrate areas of low attenuation (felt to represent regional hypoperfusion), subpleural reticulolinear changes, and pleural thickening [102]. The diagnosis is made based on classic or magnetic resonance angiography demonstrating aneurysms with smooth tapered narrowings and occluded vessels [103]. Biopsy is generally not performed because of the size of vessel involved. These patients are followed with computed tomography and magnetic resonance angiography. The mainstay of therapy is immunosuppression with glucocorticoids, which has led to 15-year survival rates of over 80%. However, relapses are common. Methotrexate as well as infliximab may be used in refractory or relapsing cases [104, 105]. Surgical bypass or vascular dilatation procedures may be considered for severe disease in individual cases but their benefit is only temporary [106–108].

Behçet's Disease

Behçet's disease is characterized by recurrent apthous oral ulcerations, and two or more of the following: genital ulcers, uveitis, skin involvement with cutaneous nodules or pustules or meningoencephalitis. Pulmonary symptomatology includes cough, hemoptysis, dyspnea, chest pains, and fever [109, 110]. This form of vasculitis can affect vessels of all sizes. Involvement of veins frequently leads to secondary thrombosis. Involvement of the pulmonary arteries may cause aneurysms and arterial-bronchial fistulae, which may clinically present as massive hemoptysis. For the diagnosis of pulmonary artery aneurysms, angiography has largely been replaced by noninvasive computed tomography and magnetic resonance angiography [111–113].

The prognosis in the setting of pulmonary involvement is poor, due to the high mortality from pulmonary hemorrhage [110]. All patients require immunosuppressive therapy with prednisone [114]. Azothioprine and cyclophosphamide have been used effectively and have resulted in the resolution of pulmonary aneurysms [112]. Anticoagulation must be avoided in the setting of documented pulmonary arteritis, but 80 mg of aspirin a day may be considered to prevent secondary thrombosis [114]. Embolization therapy may prevent and treat hemorrhage from pulmonary aneurysms.

Goodpasture's Disease

In the past, the term Goodpasture's syndrome has been used synonymously with pulmonary-renal syndrome. Now only the specific entity of glomerulonephritis and pulmonary hemorrhage secondary to anti-GBM should be referred to as Goodpasture's disease. The term anti-GBM disease is also used to describe patients with disease secondary to serum antibodies against basement membrane, with or without pulmonary involvement. Anti-GBM disease is not classified as a form of primary systemic vasculitis as it is not a systemic disease, as generally only the kidney and lung are affected. Furthermore, inflammation and destruction of the blood vessel walls is not a prominent histopathologic feature. Anti-GBM disease is very rare with an estimated annual incidence of 0.5–3 cases per million population. It has been described in many racial groups but primarily affects Caucasians. It occurs most commonly in young males 10–40 years of age. There is a second peak in the sixth decade, where the sex distribution is relatively equal, but this group of patients suffers less frequently from alveolar hemorrhage.

Goodpasture's disease is caused by anti-GBM antibodies with a specificity for the NC1 domain of the alpha-3 chain of type IV collagen [115]. The expression of the alpha-3 collagen chain is most abundant in the basement membranes of the lungs and kidneys, and specific epitopes to which the antibodies bind appear to be particularly accessible in these organs [116]. In patients with anti-GBM, inhalational lung injury by a variety of agents, and particularly by smoking seems to enhance the pathogenic effect of anti-GBM by facilitating access of the antibodies to their target antigen. This explains the significantly higher frequency of alveolar hemorrhage in active smokers compared to nonsmokers [117]. Other examples of predisposing insults include upper respiratory tract infections or exposure to volatile hydrocarbons. Genetic factors also influence the development of Goodpasture's disease. Patients with HLA type DRw15 and DR4 are at increased risk, whereas those with DR1 are at lesser risk [118].

Pulmonary involvement rarely occurs in the absence of renal disease [119]. The pulmonary symptoms are those of diffuse alveolar hemorrhage. These patients generally develop relatively acute renal failure with a nephritic sediment on urinalysis. Systemic symptoms such as malaise, fevers, and arthralgias are less prominent than in the systemic vasculitides. The most significant predictor of outcome is the degree of renal insufficiency at the time of treatment initiation [119].

Diagnosis

The diagnosis is established by immunologic testing for anti-GBM antibodies. The indirect immunofluorescence test, in which the patient's serum is incubated with normal renal tissue, has largely been replaced by antigen-specific solid phase assays (ELISA). ELISA assays for anti-GBM may have variable sensitivity and specificity [120]. A renal biopsy specimen demonstrating linear deposition of IgG along the basement membranes is diagnostic. Similar linear IgG deposits along the basement membranes are seen by direct immunofluorescence of affected lung tissue. A frozen specimen of lung tissue should therefore be saved if patients with isolated alveolar hemorrhage undergo open lung biopsy and serology is inconclusive. Standard light microscopy is nonspecific in anti-GBM disease. Most frequently it shows alveolar hemorrhage with little destruction of the alveolar architecture (bland alveolar hemorrhage). Occasionally, capillaritis or diffuse alveolar damage with hemorrhage may be detected.

Approximately 30% of patients with anti-GBM antibodies are also ANCA-positive [121]. Most commonly the ANCA are of the P-ANCA variety without specificity for MPO. This is a nonspecific finding, and these patients have Goodpasture's disease. However, if patients have a coexistent PR3-/C-ANCA or an MPO-/P-ANCA, their illness usually behaves like an ANCA-associated vasculitis [122, 123].

Treatment

Treatment of anti-GBM disease is aimed at suppression of inflammation and elimination of the pathogenic autoantibodies [2]. High-dose corticosteroids should be given as soon as possible, followed by plasma-exchange to remove anti-GBM and other inflammatory mediators as quickly as possible. The efficacy of plasma-exchange has been documented only in small, uncontrolled series. Nevertheless, it has become standard therapy. Initially, patients receive either daily or alternate day 4-l exchanges for 2–3 weeks. Longer course of plasma-exchange are only given to those patients, who continue to have hemoptysis or elevated anti-GBM titers. In order to suppress continued antibody production and prevent their recurrence after plasma-exchange, cyclophosphamide is usually added. The immunosuppressive regimen given for Goodpasture's disease resembles that for ANCA-associated vasculitis. In contrast to Wegener's granulomatosis or microscopic polyangiitis, Goodpasture's disease has a low tendency to relapse.

References

1. Jennette JC, Falk RJ, Andrassy K, et al. Nomenclature of systemic vasculitides: the proposal of an international consensus conference. Arthritis Rheum. 1994;37:187–92.
2. Levy JB, Turner AN, Rees AJ, Pusey CD. Long-term outcome of anti-glomerular basement membrane antibody disease treated with plasma exchange and immunosuppression. Ann Intern Med. 2001;134: 1033–42.
3. Watts RA, Scott DG. Epidemiology of the vasculitides. Semin Respir Crit Care Med. 2004;25:455–64.
4. Hoffman GS, Specks U. Anti-neutrophil cytoplasmic antibodies. Arthritis Rheum. 1998;41:1521–37.
5. Wiesner O, Russell KA, Lee AS, et al. Antineutrophil cytoplasmic antibodies reacting with human neutrophil elastase as a diagnostic marker for cocaine-induced midline destructive lesions but not autoimmune vasculitis. Arthritis Rheum. 2004;50: 2954–65.
6. Watts RA, Lane SE, Bentham G, Scott DG. Epidemiology of systemic vasculitis: a ten-year study in the United Kingdom. Arthritis Rheum. 2000;43: 414–9.
7. Hoffman GS, Kerr GS, Leavitt RY, et al. Wegener granulomatosis: an analysis of 158 patients. Ann Intern Med. 1992;116:488–98.
8. Colby TV, Specks U. Wegener's granulomatosis in the 1990s – a pulmonary pathologist's perspective. Monogr Pathol. 1993;36:195–218.
9. Reinhold-Keller E, Beuge N, Latza U, et al. An interdisciplinary approach to the care of patients with Wegener's granulomatosis: long-term outcome in 155 patients. Arthritis Rheum. 2000;43:1021–32.
10. Rasmussen N. Management of the ear, nose, and throat manifestations of Wegener granulomatosis: an otorhinolaryngologist's perspective. Curr Opin Rheumatol. 2001;13:3–11.
11. Cannady SB, Batra PS, Koening C, et al. Sinonasal Wegener granulomatosis: a single-institution experience with 120 cases. Laryngoscope. 2009;119:757–61.
12. Daum DE, Specks U, Colby TV, et al. Tracheobronchial involvement in Wegener's granulomatosis. Am J Respir Crit Care Med. 1995;151:522–6.
13. Polychronopoulos VS, Prakash UB, Golbin JM, Edell ES, Specks U. Airway involvement in Wegener's granulomatosis. Rheum Dis Clin North Am. 2007;33:755–75.
14. Langford CA, Sneller MC, Hallahan CW, et al. Clinical features and therapeutic management of subglottic stenosis in patients with Wegener's granulomatosis. Arthritis Rheum. 1996;39:1754–60.
15. Ernst A, Rafeq S, Boiselle P, et al. Relapsing polychondritis and airway involvement. Chest. 2009;135: 1024–30.
16. Lee AS, Specks U. Pulmonary capillaritis. Semin Respir Crit Care Med. 2004;25:547–55.
17. Schnabel A, Reuter M, Csernok E, Richter C, Gross WL. Subclinical alveolar bleeding in pulmonary vasculitides: correlation with indices of disease activity. Eur Respir J. 1999;14:118–24.
18. de Lind van Wijngaarden RA, Hauer HA, Wolterbeek R, et al. Clinical and histologic determinants of renal outcome in ANCA-associated vasculitis: a prospective analysis of 100 patients with severe renal involvement. J Am Soc Nephrol. 2006;17:2264–74.
19. Nishino H, Rubino FA, DeRemee RA, Swanson JW, Parisi JE. Neurologic involvement in Wegener's granulomatosis: an analysis of 324 consecutive patients at the Mayo Clinic. Ann Neurol. 1993;33:4–9.

20. de Groot K, Schmidt DK, Arlt AC, Gross WL, Reinhold-Keller E. Standardized neurologic evaluations of 128 patients with Wegener granulomatosis. Arch Neurol. 2001;58:1215–21.

21. Harper SL, Letko E, Samson CM, et al. Wegener's granulomatosis: the relationship between ocular and systemic disease. J Rheumatol. 2001;28:1025–32.

22. Daoud MS, Gibson LE, DeRemee RA, el-Azhary RA, Su WPD. Cutaneous Wegener's granulomatosis: clinical, histopathologic, and immunopathologic features of thirty patients. J Am Acad Dermatol. 1994;31:605–12.

23. Godman GC, Churg J. Wegener's granulomatosis. Pathology and review of the literature. AMA Arch Path. 1954;58:533–53.

24. Carrington CB, Liebow AA. Limited forms of angiitis and granulomatosis of Wegener's type. Am J Med. 1966;41:497–527.

25. DeRemee RA, McDonald TJ, Harrison EG, Coles DT. Wegener's granulomatosis. Anatomic correlates, a proposed classification. Mayo Clin Proc. 1975;51: 777–81.

26. Fienberg R. The protracted superficial phenomenon in pathergic (Wegener's) granulomatosis. Hum Pathol. 1980;12:458–67.

27. Stone JH. Limited versus severe Wegener's granulomatosis: baseline data on patients in the Wegener's granulomatosis etanercept trial. Arthritis Rheum. 2003;48:2299–309.

28. Nölle B, Specks U, Lüdemann J, Rohrbach MS, DeRemee RA, Gross WL. Anticytoplasmic autoantibodies: their immunodiagnostic value. Ann Int Med. 1989;111:28–40.

29. Finkielman JD, Lee AS, Hummel AM, et al. ANCA are detectable in nearly all patients with active severe Wegener's granulomatosis. Am J Med. 2007;120:643. e9–14.

30. Travis WD. Common and uncommon manifestations of Wegener's granulomatosis. Cardiovasc Pathol. 1994;3:217–25.

31. Maskell GF, Lockwood CM, Flower CDR. Computed tomography of the lung in Wegener's granulomatosis. Clin Radiol. 1993;48:377–80.

32. Summers RM, Aggarwal NR, Sneller MC, et al. CT virtual bronchoscopy of the central airways in patients with Wegener's granulomatosis. Chest. 2002;121:242–50.

33. Muhle C, Reinhold-Keller E, Richter C, et al. MRI of the nasal cavity, the paranasal sinuses and orbits in Wegener's granulomatosis. Eur Radiol. 1997;7:566–70.

34. Walton EW. Giant-cell granuloma of the respiratory tract (Wegener's granulomatosis). Br Med J. 1958;2: 265–70.

35. Jayne D, Rasmussen N, Andrassy K, et al. A randomized trial of maintenance therapy for vasculitis associated with antineutrophil cytoplasmic autoantibodies. N Engl J Med. 2003;349:36–44.

36. The WGET Research Group. Etanercept plus standard therapy for Wegener's granulomatosis. N Engl J Med. 2005;352:351–61.

37. Pagnoux C, Mahr A, Hamidou MA, et al. Azathioprine or methotrexate maintenance for ANCA-associated vasculitis. N Engl J Med. 2008;359:2790–803.

38. de Groot K, Harper L, Jayne DR, et al. Pulse versus daily oral cyclophosphamide for induction of remission in antineutrophil cytoplasmic antibody-associated vasculitis: a randomized trial. Ann Intern Med. 2009;150:670–80.

39. Specks U, Fervenza FC, McDonald TJ, Hogan MC. Response of Wegener's granulomatosis to anti-CD20 chimeric monoclonal antibody therapy. Arthritis Rheum. 2001;44:2836–40.

40. Keogh KA, Wylam ME, Stone JH, Specks U. Induction of remission by B lymphocyte depletion in eleven patients with refractory antineutrophil cytoplasmic antibody-associated vasculitis. Arthritis Rheum. 2005;52:262–8.

41. Keogh KA, Ytterberg SR, Fervenza FC, Carlson KA, Schroeder DR, Specks U. Rituximab for refractory Wegener's granulomatosis: report of a prospective, open-label pilot trial. Am J Respir Crit Care Med. 2006;173:180–7.

42. Stone JH, Merkel PA, Spiera R, et al. Rituximab versus cyclophosphamide for ANCA-associated vasculitis. N Eng J Med. 2010;363(3):221–32.

43. De Groot K, Rasmussen N, Bacon PA, et al. Randomized trial of cyclophosphamide versus methotrexate for induction of remission in early systemic antineutrophil cytoplasmic antibody-associated vasculitis. Arthritis Rheum. 2005;52:2461–9.

44. Villa-Forte A, Clark TM, Gomes M, et al. Substitution of methotrexate for cyclophosphamide in Wegener granulomatosis: a 12-year single-practice experience. Medicine (Baltimore). 2007;86:269–77.

45. Langford CA, Talar-Williams C, Barron KS, Sneller MC. A staged approach to the treatment of Wegener's granulomatosis: induction of remission with glucocorticoids and daily cyclophosphamide switching to methotrexate for remission maintenance. Arthritis Rheum. 1999;42:2666–73.

46. Koukoulaki M, Jayne DR. Mycophenolate mofetil in anti-neutrophil cytoplasm antibodies-associated systemic vasculitis. Nephron Clin Pract. 2006;102: c100–7.

47. DeRemee RA, McDonald TJ, Weiland LH. Wegener's granulomatosis: observations on treatment with antimicrobial agents. Mayo Clin Proc. 1985;60:27–32.

48. Stegeman CA, Cohen Tervaert JW, de Jong PE, Kallenberg CG. Trimethoprim-sulfamethoxazole (cotrimoxazole) for the prevention of relapses of Wegener's granulomatosis. N Engl J Med. 1996;335: 16–20.

49. Jayne DR, Chapel H, Adu D, et al. Intravenous immunoglobulin for ANCA-associated systemic vasculitis with persistent disease activity. Q J Med. 2000;93: 433–9.

50. Martinez V, Cohen P, Pagnoux C, et al. Intravenous immunoglobulins for relapses of systemic vasculitides associated with antineutrophil cytoplasmic autoantibodies: results of a multicenter, prospective,

open-label study of twenty-two patients. Arthritis Rheum. 2008;58:308–17.

51. Rossi F, Jayne DR, Lockwood CM, Kazatchkine MD. Anti-idiotypes against anti-neutrophil cytoplasmic antigen autoantibodies in normal human polyspecific IgG for therapeutic use and in the remission sera of patients with systemic vasculitis. Clin Exp Immunol. 1991;83:298–303.

52. Klemmer PJ, Chalermskulrat W, Reif MS, Hogan SL, Henke DC, Falk RJ. Plasmapheresis therapy for diffuse alveolar hemorrhage in patients with small-vessel vasculitis. Am J Kidney Dis. 2003;42:1149–53.

53. Jayne DR, Gaskin G, Rasmussen N, et al. Randomized trial of plasma exchange or high-dosage methylprednisolone as adjunctive therapy for severe renal vasculitis. J Am Soc Nephrol. 2007;18:2180–8.

54. Stone JH, Holbrook JT, Marriott MA, et al. Solid malignancies among patients in the Wegener's Granulomatosis Etanercept Trial. Arthritis Rheum. 2006;54:1608–18.

55. Lamprecht P, Voswinkel J, Lilienthal T, et al. Effectiveness of TNF-alpha blockade with infliximab in refractory Wegener's granulomatosis. Rheumatology (Oxford). 2002;41:1303–7.

56. Bartolucci P, Ramanoelina J, Cohen P, et al. Efficacy of the anti-TNF-alpha antibody infliximab against refractory systemic vasculitides: an open pilot study on 10 patients. Rheumatology (Oxford). 2002;41:1126–32.

57. Booth A, Harper L, Hammad T, et al. Prospective study of TNFalpha blockade with infliximab in antineutrophil cytoplasmic antibody-associated systemic vasculitis. J Am Soc Nephrol. 2004;15:717–21.

58. Golbin JM, Keogh KA, Fervenza FC, Ytterberg SR, Specks U. Update on Rituximab use in patients with chronically relapsing Wegener's Granulomatosis. Clin Exp Rheumatol. 2007;25:S-111.

59. Jones RB, Ferraro AJ, Chaudhry AN, et al. A multicenter survey of rituximab therapy for refractory antineutrophil cytoplasmic antibody-associated vasculitis. Arthritis Rheum. 2009;60:2156–68.

60. Hernandez-Rodriguez J, Hoffman GS, Koening CL. Surgical interventions and local therapy for Wegener's granulomatosis. Curr Opin Rheumatol. 2010;22: 29–36.

61. Congdon D, Sherris DA, Specks U, McDonald T. Long-term follow-up of repair of external nasal deformities in patients with Wegener's granulomatosis. Laryngoscope. 2002;112:731–7.

62. Hoffman GS, Thomas-Golbanov CK, Chan J, Akst LM, Eliachar I. Treatment of subglottic stenosis, due to Wegener's granulomatosis, with intralesional corticosteroids and dilation. J Rheumatol. 2003;30: 1017–21.

63. Guillevin L, Durand-Gasselin B, Cevallos R, et al. Microscopic polyangiitis: clinical and laboratory findings in eighty-five patients. Arthritis Rheum. 1999;42: 421–30.

64. Pagnoux C, Mahr A, Cohen P, Guillevin L. Presentation and outcome of gastrointestinal involvement in

systemic necrotizing vasculitides: analysis of 62 patients with polyarteritis nodosa, microscopic polyangiitis, Wegener granulomatosis, Churg-Strauss syndrome, or rheumatoid arthritis-associated vasculitis. Medicine (Baltimore). 2005;84:115–28.

65. Lauque D, Cadranel J, Lazor R, et al. Microscopic polyangiitis with alveolar hemorrhage. A study of 29 cases and review of the literature. Medicine (Baltimore). 2000;79:222–33.

66. Hogan SL, Nachman PH, Wilkman AS, Jennette JC, Falk RJ. Prognostic markers in patients with antineutrophil cytoplasmic autoantibody-associated microscopic polyangiitis and glomerulonephritis. J Am Soc Nephrol. 1996;7:23–32.

67. Nachman PH, Hogan SL, Jennette JC, Falk RJ. Treatment response and relapse in antineutrophil cytoplasmic autoantibody-associated microscopic polyangiitis and glomerulonephritis. J Am Soc Nephrol. 1996;7:33–9.

68. Hu W, Liu C, Xie H, Chen H, Liu Z, Li L. Mycophenolate mofetil versus cyclophosphamide for inducing remission of ANCA vasculitis with moderate renal involvement. Nephrol Dial Transplant. 2008;23:1307–12.

69. Silva F, Specks U, Kalra S, et al. Mycophenolate mofetil for induction and maintenance of remission in microscopic polyangiitis with mild to moderate renal involvement – a prospective, open-label pilot trial. Clin J Am Soc Nephrol. 2010;5(3):445–53.

70. Watts RA, Jolliffe VA, Carruthers DM, Lockwood M, Scott DGI. Effect of classification on the incidence of polyarteritis nodosa and microscopic polyangiitis. Arthritis Rheum. 1996;39:1208–12.

71. Nick J, Tuder R, May R, Fisher J. Polyarteritis nodosa with pulmonary vasculitis. Am J Respir Crit Care Med. 1996;153:450–3.

72. Guillevin L, Lhote F. Distinguishing polyarteritis nodosa from microscopic polyangiitis and implications for treatment. Curr Opin Rheumatol. 1995;7: 20–4.

73. Guillevin L, Lhote F, Amouroux J, Gherardi R, Callard P, Casassus P. Antineutrophil cytoplasmic antibodies, abnormal angiograms and pathological findings in polyarteritis nodosa and Churg-Strauss syndrome: indications for the classification of vasculitides of the polyarteritis Nodosa Group. Br J Rheumatol. 1996;35:958–64.

74. Lanham JG, Elkon KB, Pusey CD, Hughes GR. Systemic vasculitis with asthma and eosinophilia: a clinical approach to the Churg-Strauss syndrome. Medicine. 1984;63:65–81.

75. Keogh KA, Specks U. Churg-Strauss syndrome. clinical presentation, antineutrophil cytoplasmic antibodies, and leukotriene receptor antagonists. Am J Med. 2003;115:284–90.

76. Churg A, Brallas M, Cronin SR, Churg J. Formes frustes of Churg-Strauss syndrome. Chest. 1995;108: 320–3.

77. Guillevin L, Cohen P, Gayraud M, Lhote F, Jarrousse B, Casassus P. Churg-Strauss syndrome. Clinical

study and long-term follow-up of 96 patients. Medicine. 1999;78:26–37.

78. Sinico RA, Di Toma L, Maggiore U, et al. Prevalence and clinical significance of antineutrophil cytoplasmic antibodies in Churg-Strauss syndrome. Arthritis Rheum. 2005;52:2926–35.

79. Sable-Fourtassou R, Cohen P, Mahr A, et al. Antineutrophil cytoplasmic antibodies and the Churg-Strauss syndrome. Ann Intern Med. 2005;143: 632–8.

80. Sinico RA, Di Toma L, Maggiore U, et al. Renal involvement in Churg-Strauss syndrome. Am J Kidney Dis. 2006;47:770–9.

81. Churg JC, Strauss L. Allergic granulomatosis, allergic angiitis and periarteritis nodosa. Am J Pathol. 1951;27:277–301.

82. Finan MC, Winkelmann RK. The cutaneous extravascular necrotizing granuloma (Churg-Strauss granuloma) and systemic disease: a review of 27 cases. Medicine (Baltimore). 1983;62:142–58.

83. Hauser T, Mahr A, Metzler C, et al. The leucotriene receptor antagonist montelukast and the risk of Churg-Strauss syndrome: a case-crossover study. Thorax. 2008;63:677–82.

84. Weller PF, Plaut M, Taggart V, Trontell A. The relationship of asthma therapy and Churg-Strauss syndrome: NIH workshop summary report. J Allergy Clin Immunol. 2001;108:175–83.

85. Tatsis E, Schnabel A, Gross WL. Interferon-a treatment of four patients with the Churg-Strauss syndrome. Ann Intern Med. 1998;129:370–4.

86. Koukoulaki M, Smith KG, Jayne DR. Rituximab in Churg-Strauss syndrome. Ann Rheum Dis. 2006;65:557–9.

87. Pepper RJ, Fabre MA, Pavesio C, et al. Rituximab is effective in the treatment of refractory Churg-Strauss syndrome and is associated with diminished T-cell interleukin-5 production. Rheumatology (Oxford). 2008;47:1104–5.

88. Jennings CA, King Jr TE, Tuder R, Cherniack RM, Schwarz MI. Diffuse alveolar hemorrhage with underlying isolated, pauciimmune pulmonary capillaritis. Am J Respir Crit Care Med. 1997;155: 1101–9.

89. Glover MU, Muniz J, Bessone L, Carta M, Casellas J, Maniscalco BS. Pulmonary artery obstruction due to giant cell arteritis. Chest. 1987;91:924–5.

90. Machado EB, Michet CJ, Ballard DJ, et al. Trends in incidence and clinical presentation of temporal arteritis in Olmsted County, Minnesota, 1950-1985. Arthritis Rheum. 1988;31:745–9.

91. Larson TS, Hall S, Hepper NGG, Hunder GG. Respiratory tract symptoms as a clue to giant cell arteritis. Ann Intern Med. 1984;101:594–7.

92. Bradley JD, Pinals RS, Blumenfeld HB, Poston WM. Giant cell arteritis with pulmonary nodules. Am J Med. 1984;77:135–40.

93. Zenone T, Souquet PJ, Bohas C, Vital Durand D, Bernard JP. Unusual manifestations of giant cell arteritis: pulmonary nodules, cough, conjunctivitis

and otitis with deafness. Eur Respir J. 1994;7: 2252–4.

94. Blockmans D, Knockaert D, Bobbaers H. Giant cell arteritis can be associated with T4-lymphocytic alveolitis. Clin Rheumatol. 1999;18:330–3.

95. Roddy E, Summers G, Chaudry Z, Bateman R. Follicular bronchiolitis, an unusual cause of haemoptysis in giant cell arteritis. Clin Rheumatol. 2006;25:433–5.

96. Small P, Brisson M-L. Wegener's granulomatosis presenting as termporal arteritis. Arthritis Rheum. 1991;34:220–3.

97. Nishino H, DeRemee RA, Rubino FA, Parisi JE. Wegener's granulomatosis associated with vasculitis of the temporal artery: report of five cases. Mayo Clin Proc. 1993;68:115–21.

98. Mazlumzadeh M, Hunder GG, Easley KA, et al. Treatment of giant cell arteritis using induction therapy with high-dose glucocorticoids: a double-blind, placebo-controlled, randomized prospective clinical trial. Arthritis Rheum. 2006;54:3310–8.

99. Seo P, Stone JH. Large-vessel vasculitis. Arthritis Rheum. 2004;51:128–39.

100. Maksimowicz-McKinnon K, Clark TM, Hoffman GS. Takayasu arteritis and giant cell arteritis: a spectrum within the same disease? Medicine (Baltimore). 2009;88:221–6.

101. Lupi E, Sanchez G, Horwitz S, Gutierrez E. Pulmonary artery involvement in Takayasu's arteritis. Chest. 1975;67:69–74.

102. Takahashi K, Honda M, Furuse M, Yanagisawa M, Saitoh K. CT findings of pulmonary parenchyma in Takayasu arteritis. J Comput Assist Tomogr. 1996;20:742–8.

103. Yamada I, Nakagawa T, Himeno Y, Kobayashi Y, Numano F, Shibuya H. Takayasu arteritis: diagnosis with breath-hold contrast-enhanced three- dimensional MR angiography. J Magn Reson Imaging. 2000;11:481–7.

104. Hoffman GS, Leavitt RY, Kerr GS, Rottem M, Sneller MC, Fauci AS. Treatment of glucocorticoid-resistant or relapsing Takayasu arteritis with methotrexate. Arthritis Rheum. 1994;37:578–82.

105. Hoffman GS, Merkel PA, Brasington RD, Lenschow DJ, Liang P. Anti-tumor necrosis factor therapy in patients with difficult to treat Takayasu arteritis. Arthritis Rheum. 2004;50:2296–304.

106. Miyata T, Ohara N, Shigematsu H, et al. Endovascular stent graft repair of aortopulmonary fistula. J Vasc Surg. 1999;29:557–60.

107. Liang P, Tan-Ong M, Hoffman GS. Takayasu's arteritis: vascular interventions and outcomes. J Rheumatol. 2004;31:102–6.

108. Maksimowicz-McKinnon K, Clark TM, Hoffman GS. Limitations of therapy and a guarded prognosis in an American cohort of Takayasu arteritis patients. Arthritis Rheum. 2007;56:1000–9.

109. Efthimiou J, Johnston C, Spiro SG, Turner-Warwick M. Pulmonary disease in Behçet's syndrome. Q J Med. 1986;58:259–80.

110. Raz I, Okon E, Chajek-Shaul T. Pulmonary manifestations in Behçet's syndrome. Chest. 1989;95: 585–9.
111. Winer-Muram HT, Gavant ML. Pulmonary CT findings in Behçet's disease. J Comput Assist Tomogr. 1989;13:346–7.
112. Tunaci M, Ozkorkmaz B, Tunaci A, Gul A, Engin G, Acunas B. CT findings of pulmonary artery aneurysms during treatment for Behcet's disease. AJR Am J Roentgenol. 1999;172:729–33.
113. Berkmen T. MR angiography of aneurysms in Behcet disease: a report of four cases. J Comput Assist Tomogr. 1998;22:202–6.
114. Uzun O, Akpolat T, Erkan L. Pulmonary vasculitis in Behcet disease: a cumulative analysis. Chest. 2005;127:2243–53.
115. Kalluri R, Wilson CB, Weber M, et al. Identification of the alpha 3 chain of type IV collagen as the common autoantigen in antibasement membrane disease and Goodpasture syndrome. J Am Soc Nephrol. 1995;6:1178–85.
116. Weber M, Pullig O, Kohler H. Distribution of Goodpasture antigens within various human basement membranes. Nephrol Dial Transplant. 1990;5:87–93.
117. Donaghy M, Rees AJ. Cigarette smoking and lung haemorrhage in glomerulonephritis caused by autoantibodies to glomerular basement membrane. Lancet. 1983;2:1390–3.
118. Dunckley H, Chapman JR, Burke J, et al. HLA-DR and -DQ genotyping in anti-GBM disease. Dis Markers. 1991;9:249–56.
119. Herody M, Bobrie G, Gouarin C, Grunfeld JP, Noel LH. Anti-GBM disease: predictive value of clinical, histological and serological data. Clin Nephrol. 1993;40:249–55.
120. Litwin CM, Mouritsen CL, Wilfahrt PA, Schroder MC, Hill HR. Anti-glomerular basement membrane disease: role of enzyme-linked immunosorbent assays in diagnosis. Biochem Mol Med. 1996;59: 52–6.
121. Short AK, Esnault VLM, Lockwood CM. Anti-neutrophil cytoplasm antibodies and anti-glomerular basement membrane antibodies: two coexisting distinct autoreactivities detectable in patients with rapidly progressive glomerulonephritis. Am J Kidney Dis. 1995;26:439–45.
122. Weber MFA, Andrassy K, Pullig O, Koderisch J, Netzer K. Antineutrophil-cytoplasmic antibodies and antiglomerular basement membrane antibodies in Goodpasture's syndrome and in Wegener's granulomatosis. J Am Soc Nephrol. 1992;2:1227–34.
123. Bosch X, Mirapeix E, Font J, et al. Prognostic implication of anti-neutrophil cytoplasmic autoantibodies with myeloperoxidase specificity in anti-glomerular basement membrane disease. Clin Nephrol. 1991;36:107–13.

Index

R.P. Baughman and R.M. du Bois (eds.), *Diffuse Lung Disease: A Practical Approach*,   387
DOI 10.1007/978-1-4419-9771-5, © Springer Science+Business Media, LLC 2012

Printed by Publishers' Graphics LLC
MO20120716